# Applied Therapeutic Drug Monitoring

*Volume II: Review and Case Studies*

# Applied Therapeutic Drug Monitoring

*Volume II: Review and Case Studies*

*Editors*
Thomas P. Moyer
Roger L. Boeckx

*Editorial Board*
Christopher Frings
Virginia Marcum
Kent E. Opheim
Paul J. Orsulak
Charles E. Pippenger
Steven J. Soldin
Jim C. Standefer

The American Association for Clinical Chemistry
1725 K Street, N.W.
Washington, DC 20006

*Related books from the American Association for Clinical Chemistry:*

**The Drug Monitoring Data Pocket Guide,** Roger Boeckx, Ed.

**Effects of Drugs on Clinical Laboratory Tests,** Donald Young, L.C. Pestaner, and Val Gibberman, Eds. (*Clin. Chem.* Vol. 21, #5)

**The Therapeutic Drug Monitoring Program Syllabus**
Proceedings from the Four Travelng TDM Programs

**The Future of Therapeutic Drug Monitoring,** Reprinted from *Clinical Chemistry News*

**Zeroing in on TDM,** Reprinted from Clinical Chemistry News

**Therapeutic Drug Monitoring Comprehensive Reference Source, Volume 1**

**Applied Therapeutic Drug Monitoring, Volume 1: Fundamentals**

Library of Congress Catalog Card No. 82-72107
ISBN 0-915274-23-X

Printed in the United States of America.

# Preface

This second volume presents a continuation of the organized publication of educational material collected by the Therapeutic Drug Monitoring Laboratory Improvement Program, sponsored by the American Assocation for Clinical Chemistry. The purpose of this volume is, like the first, to provide an organized compendium on therapeutic drug monitoring. It is not complete because this field continues to grow. New developments occur weekly.

The Laboratory Improvement Program is a continuously evolving effort. Since publication of Volume I, George F. Johnson, Ph.D., R. Thomas Chamberlain, Ph. D., J.D., and Vijay Aggarwal, Ph.D., have joined the Task Force, replacing us. This turnover keeps the program active, innovative and timely. Mrs. Diane Breunsbach left the program as Director to raise her new family and was replaced by Mr. Don Kaveny. The efforts of both of these individuals have been essential in keeping the program on schedule.

We again wish to acknowledge those laboratorians, researchers, and clinicians throughout North America and Europe who have donated their time to review manuscripts for scientific content. Without their review, this program would have floundered years ago.

**Thomas P. Moyer**
**Roger L. Boeckx**

# Contents of Volume II

# List of Contributors

J. Eric Ahlskog, Ph.D., M.D.
Instructor in Neurology
Mayo Medical School
Mayo Clinic
Rochester, MN

John P. Anhalt, Ph.D., M.D.
Associate Professor of Laboratory Medicine and
Microbiology
Mayo Medical School
Mayo Clinic
Rochester, MN

Paul S. Appelbaum, M.D.
Associate Professor of Psychiatry and Law
Western Psychiatric Institute and Clinic
Pittsburgh, PA

Leonas G. Bekeris, M.D.
Assistant Clinical Professor of Pathology
Loyola University Medical Center
MacNeil Memorial Hospital
Berwyn, IL

Edward W. Bermes, Jr., Ph.D.
Professor of Pathology and Biochemistry
Loyola University Medical Center
Maywood, IL

Roger L. Boeckx, Ph.D.
Associate Professor of Child Health and Development
George Washington University
Children's Hospital National Medical Center
Washington, DC

Larry D. Bowers, Ph.D.
Associate Professor of Laboratory Medicine
University of Minnesota
Minneapolis, MN

John F. Bresnahan, M.D.
Assistant Professor of Medicine
Mayo Medical School
Mayo Clinic
Rochester, MN

Larry A. Broussard, Ph.D.
Assistant Director, Clinical Chemistry and Toxicology
Medical Laboratory Associates
Birmingham, AL

Margan J. Chang, M.D.
Associate Professor of Child Health and Development
George Washington University
Children's Hospital National Medical Center
Washington, DC

Robert J. Cipolle, Pharm.D.
Associate Professor of Pharmacy Practice
Unversity of Minnesota
Minneapolis, MN

Christine Collier, M.S.
Graduate Student in Biochemistry
University of Toronto
Sick Children's Hospital
Toronto, Ontario, Canada

Paul Didisheim, M.D.
Professor of Laboratory Medicine
Mayo Medical School
Mayo Clinic
Rochester, MN

W. Edwin Dodson, M.D.
Associate Professor of Pediatrics and Neurology
Washington University School of Medicine
St. Louis Children's Hospital
St. Louis, MO

Alexander Duncan, M.D.
Senior Resident in Internal Medicine
Mayo Clinic
Rochester, MN

Jacob Federman, M.D.
Consultant in Cardiology
Alfred Hospital
Melbourne, Australia

Juan-Ramon de la Fuente, M.D.
Associate Professor of Psychiatry
National Autonomous University of Mexico
Mexican Institute of Psychiatry
Mexico City, Mexico

Andrew L. Finn, Pharm.D.
Associate Director, Clinical Research
Glaxo, Inc.
Research Triangle Park, NC

Christopher S. Frings, Ph.D.
Director, Clinical Chemistry and Toxicology
Medical Laboratory Associates
Birmingham, AL

Edwin Grab, B.A.
Senior Chemist
Harvard Medical School
Massachusetts Mental Health Center
Boston, MA

Robert V. Groover, M.D.
Associate Professor of Pediatric Neurology
Mayo Medical School
Mayo Clinic
Rochester, MN

Dan Haidukewych, Ph.D.
Director, Clinical Chemistry and Pharmacology Laboratory
Epilepsy Center of Michigan
Detroit, MI

J. Gilbert Hill, M.D., Ph.D.
    Associate Professor of Clinical Biochemistry
    University of Toronto
    Hospital for Sick Children
    Toronto, Ontario, Canada

Gordon Ireland, Pharm.D.
    Associate Professor of Clinical Pharmacy
    St. Louis College of Pharmacy
    The Jewish Hospital of St. Louis
    St. Louis, MO

William H. Jeffery, Pharm.D.
    Associate Professor of Pharmacy
    University of New Mexico
    Albuquerque, NM

H. William Kelly, Pharm.D.
    Associate Professor of Pharmacy
    University of New Mexico
    Albuquerque, NM

Henn Kutt, M.D.
    Associate Professor of Neurology and Pharmacology
    Cornell University Medical College
    New York, NY

Sten Lofgren, M.D.
    Associate Professor of Psychiatry
    Harvard Medical School
    McLean Hospital
    Boston, MA

Alexander G. Logan, M.D., F.R.C.P.(C)
    Associate Professor of Medicine
    University of Toronto
    Mount Sinai Hospital
    Toronto, Ontario, Canada

Sandra Lipchus, M.S.
    Associate in Psychiatry
    Harvard Medical School
    Massachusetts Mental Health Center
    Boston, MA

Carl Ludvigson, M.D., Ph.D.
    Assistant Professor of Pathology and Laboratory Medicine
    University of Nebraska Medical Center
    Omaha, NE

Mhairi G. MacDonald, M.B.Ch.B., F.R.C.P.(E)., F.A.A.P.,
    D.C.H.
    Associate Professor Child Health and Development
    George Washington University
    Children's Hospital National Medical Center
    Washington, DC

Janis J. MacKichan, Pharm.D.
    Assistant Professor of Pharmacy
    Ohio State University
    Columbus, OH

Stuart M. MacLeod, M.D., Ph.D.
    Professor of Clinical Pharmacology
    University of Toronto
    Sick Children's Hospital
    Toronto, Ontario, Canada

Thomas P. Moyer, Ph.D.
    Associate Professor of Laboratory Medicine
    Mayo Medical School
    Mayo Clinic
    Rochester, MN

Paul M. Orsulak, Ph.D.
    Associate Professor of Psychiatry
    Southwestern Medical School
    Veterans Administration Medical Center
    Dallas, TX

Michael A. Pesce, Ph.D.
    Associate Professor of Clinical Pathology
    Columbia University, College of Physicians and Surgeons
    The Presbyterian Hospital
    New York, NY

C.E. Pippenger, Ph.D.
    Head, Section of Applied Pharmacology
    Department of Biochemistry
    Cleveland Clinic Foundation
    Cleveland, OH

Philip R. Reid, M.D.
    Associate Professor of Medicine
    Sinai Hospital of Baltimore
    Baltimore, MD

Mario L. Rocci, Jr., Ph.D.
    Research Assistant Professor of Medicine
    Jefferson Medical College
    Philadelphia, PA

Dan M. Roden, M.D.
    Assistant Professor of Medicine and Pharmacology
    Vanderbilt University
    Nashville, TN

Deborah H. Schaible, Pharm.D.
    Assistant Professor of Pharmacy
    University of Pennsylvania School of Medicine
    Children's Hospital of Philadelphia
    Philadelphia, PA

Alan F. Schatzberg, M.D.
    Associate Professor of Psychiatry
    Harvard Medical School
    McLean Hospital
    Boston, MA

Joseph J. Schildkraut, M.D.
    Professor of Psychiatry
    Harvard Medical School
    New England Deaconess Hospital
    Boston, MA

Dorothy Schottelius, Ph.D.
Assistant Professor of Neurology
University of Iowa
Iowa City, IA

F. Estelle R. Simons, M.D., F.R.C.P.(C)
Associate Professor of Allergy and Clinical Immunology
University of Manitoba
Children's Hospital
Winnipeg, Manitoba, Canada

Steven J. Soldin, Ph.D.
Associate Professor of Clinical Biochemistry and Pharmacology
University of Toronto
Hospital for Sick Children
Toronto, Ontario, Canada

Jim Standefer, Ph.D.
Associate Professor of Pathology
University of New Mexico School of Medicine
Albuquerque, NM

Daniel T. Teitelbaum, M.D.
Associate Professor of Preventive Medicine
University of Colorado Health Sciences Center
Denver Clinical Medical Center, P.A.
Denver, CO

James M. Thornbery, M.D.
Assistant Clinical Professor of Pathology
University of Wisconsin Medical School
Madison General Hospital
Madison, WI

Hilde M. Vandenberghe, Ph.D.
Postdoctoral Fellow in Biochemistry
University of Toronto
Toronto General Hospital
Toronto, Ontario, Canada

Russell G. Vasile, M.D.
Assistant Professor of Psychiatry
Harvard Medical School
New England Deaconess Hospital
Boston, MA

Ronald E. Vlietstra, M.D.
Associate Professor of Medicine
Mayo Medical School
Mayo Clinic
Rochester, MN

Mark R. Wick, M.D.
Instructor in Laboratory Medicine and Pathology
University of Minnesota
Minneapolis, MN

Anthony J. Windebank, M.D.
Assistant Professor of Neurology
Mayo Medical School
Mayo Clinic
Rochester, MN

Raymond L. Woosley, M.D., Ph.D.
Associate Professor of Medicine and Pharmacology
Vanderbilt University
Nashville, TN

Darwin Zaske, Pharm.D., F.C.P.
Associate Professor of Pharmacy
University of Minnesota
St. Paul-Ramsey Medical Center
St. Paul, MN

# I. Antiepileptic Drugs

# 1

# Seizure Disorders and Epilepsy

W. Edwin Dodson, M.D.

A seizure is an abrupt alteration of brain function due to excessive neural activity in gray matter. The ictus, or sudden attack, can affect mental function and movement. A seizure which causes violent involuntary muscular contraction is a convulsion; a seizure may be convulsive or nonconvulsive. Nonconvulsive seizures, also called absence seizures, are characterized by staring or subtle movements. Although seizures indicate excitatory brain dysfunction, they are nonspecific symptoms which have many causes. A diagnosis of epilepsy is made when seizures recur over time and are not caused by transient metabolic or toxic disorders.

Seizures are relatively common; at least 4% of the population are expected to have seizures sometime during their lives (1). The estimated prevalence of epilepsy is 1%. New cases of epilepsy occur in the population at a rate of approximately 0.4/1000 annually. Among new cases of epilepsy, 77% occur in people less than 20 years old. In the United States approximately 2.3 million citizens have epilepsy and 92 652 will develop epilepsy in 1982.

## Pathogenesis of Seizure Disorders

The normal cerebral cortex in all higher animals has the intrinsic capacity to manifest seizure discharges (2). In experimental animals, normal cerebral cortex develops recurrent paroxysmal discharges when it is surgically isolated from surrounding neural tissue. During a seizure, brain neuronal activity is both qualitatively and quantitatively different from normal. Individual neurons undergo a marked depolarization that is abnormal in both extent and duration.

Different mechanisms appear important in experimental models of absence seizures on the one hand and focal or tonic clonic seizures on the other. In the case of focal and generalized tonic clonic seizures, the seizure activity begins in a localized area of cere-

*Dr. W. Edwin Dodson is affiliated with the Edward Mallinckrodt Department of Pediatrics and the Department of Neurology and Neurological Surgery (Neurology) and the Division of Clinical Neuropharmacology, Washington University School of Medicine, St. Louis, and The Division of Pediatric Neurology, St. Louis Children's Hospital. Correspondence to Dr. Dodson should be addressed to St. Louis Children's Hospital, 500 S. Kingshighway, P.O. Box 14871, St. Louis, MO 63178.*

bral cortex. The seizure discharge may remain localized or it may spread to involve other areas of brain. If the seizure activity becomes generalized to the entire cortex, it is thought to spread first down to nuclei located in the thalamus and then project back upwards to cortex via the diffusely projecting thalamocortical pathways. Although it was previously thought that generalized seizures began deep in the thalamus or upper brainstem, experimental evidence has not indicated a deep thalamic origin. Thus, it appears that in focal and generalized tonic clonic seizures, the discharge begins in the cortex and secondarily spreads via diffuse brain pathways even when the focal cortical origin is not clinically apparent.

Focal cortical activity can also spread superficially over the cortex to involve contiguous areas. As the seizure discharge spreads to involve larger areas of the cortex, the areas of the body which are involved are progressively enlarged. Consciousness is usually preserved until the discharge involves both cerebral hemispheres simultaneously.

In absence seizures, there appears to be a widespread cortical susceptibility to hypersynchronization by thalamic input. Diffuse synchronous discharges in abnormal cortex can be triggered by what is normally nonepileptogenic stimulation of thalamic nuclei. The spike-and-wave pattern in the surface EEG is associated with alternating discharges of excitatory and inhibitory neurons.

The seizure discharge in brain is associated with marked increases in brain electrical and metabolic activity (2). Approximately 50 years ago Hans Berger discovered that abnormal electrical brain rhythms are associated with seizures. The excessive electrical activity of the brain during a seizure can be measured at the scalp with the electroencephalograph. Between the brain and the scalp, electrical potentials are attenuated 58-fold by intervening tissue. Surface potentials must be amplified 1 000 000 times to produce the electroencephalogram (EEG). When a convulsive discharge is localized, it has been estimated that at least 6 cm$^2$ of cortical surface must be involved to produce a spike of electrical activity on the EEG. When seizure discharges occur only on the inferior surface of the brain, they are undetectable in routine EEG tracings.

At the time of the seizure, the metabolic rate in brain tissue also increases markedly. Within an area of focal seizure discharge, the cerebral metabolic rates for glucose and oxygen increase and blood flow increases. These phenomena permit the specific area of brain involved to be visualized. Radiolabeled substrates can be administered and the area of excessive metabolism can be visualized by autoradiography in experimental animals or by positron emission transaxial tomography (PET) scans in patients. Between seizures, in the interictal period, the seizure focus may have a reduced rate of glucose metabolism.

The alterations of behavior and mental function that occur during seizures depend on the location of the seizure discharge in the brain. The discharge may be restricted to a small area of cortex or generalized over both cerebral hemispheres. When the epileptic discharges are localized, patients may have focal movements of parts of the body or perceive sensations or psychic experiences. If the discharge involves the limbic system, patients may have a variety of emotional and cognitive experiences.

Seizures which originate in the temporal lobe are the second most frequent seizure type, following generalized tonic clonic seizures. Partial complex (psychomotor) seizures arising in the temporal lobe are the principal seizure type in an estimated 20 to 44% of patients with epilepsy (1). The temporal lobe has widespread effects on mental and motor functioning. Temporal lobe structures, specifically the amygdala and hippocampus, are important components of a network of structures called the limbic system. The limbic system participates in brain functions of emotion, awareness, and memory. Within the temporal lobe, the amygdala is prone to developing seizure discharges. When the amygdala is stimulated over a period of weeks with subconvulsive electrical shocks, the response to the stimulus becomes progressively abnormal, a procedure called *kindling* (2). Ultimately, the stimulus, which previously had no effect, elicits a generalized convulsion.

## Seizure Types

The international classification of seizure types is the most widely used classification system (Table 1) (3). It was developed by a panel of epileptologists, who reviewed videotapes and EEG patterns of patients actually having seizures. The first distinction of the classification system is between localized and generalized seizures. Seizures that begin focally in restricted area of brain and have limited effects are called *partial seizures*. The manifestations of partial seizures may be discrete or simple, or complex when the seizures involve bilateral brain structures and produce unconsciousness.

In partial seizures, the symptoms are referable to the normal function of the involved brain tissue. If the seizure process involves a region of brain which causes

**Table 1. International Classification of Seizure Types**

I.  **Partial seizures**
    A.  Simple partial (consciousness not impaired)
        1. With motor signs
        2. With somatosensory or special-sensory symptoms
        3. With autonomic signs
        4. With psychic symptoms
    B.  Complex partial (consciousness impaired)
    C.  Partial seizures, secondarily generalized

II.  Generalized seizures
    A.  Absence
    B.  Myoclonic
    C.  Clonic
    D.  Tonic
    E.  Tonic clonic
    F.  Atonic

III.  Unclassified epileptic seizures (e.g., neonatal)

IV.  Addendum

movement, a focal twitching occurs. Partial motor seizures most commonly originate in body areas which have the largest cortical topographic representation, such as the face, the thumb, or the great toe. Seizures can also begin in brain areas which are involved primarily with perceiving tactile sensation. In these circumstances, the patients experience tingling or buzzing in the body part represented by that area of brain. When the seizure causes an elementary movement or sensation, the seizure is said to be a partial seizure with simple symptoms (*simple partial seizure*).

Simple partial seizures produce motor signs, sensory symptoms, autonomic manifestations, and psychic symptoms. Autonomic manifestations include flushing, piloerection, pallor, localized or diffuse sweating. Somatosensory or special sensory symptoms can involve any sensory modality. Special sensory symptoms include hallucinated odors, tastes, visual patterns, or sounds. The sensations are most often vague or amorphous but occasionally are intricate and detailed. The psychic symptoms which occur as a manifestation of partial simple seizures are particularly intriguing. Abnormalities of speech are dysphasic symptoms. Dysmnesic psychic symptoms refer to exaggerated feelings of recognition or familiarity about the environment. A feeling of heightened familiarity is termed *deja vu* (already seen) whereas the feeling of unfamiliarity is termed *jamais vu* (never seen). Seizures can cause a variety of illusions or misperceptions of the environment. The most common are macropsia and micropsia in which objects are perceived as inappropriately large or small, respectively. Psychic symptoms may involve the cognitive processes such as memory; the most common example is forced thinking. During episodes of forced thinking, the patient recalls a specific event or sequence of events. The recollection is stereotyped from one seizure to the next. Structured or unstructured hallucinations can occur during seizures, although the latter are more common. The most common psychic symptoms caused by partial seizures are affective. Any mood or feeling which is normally experienced can occur; fear is most common. Ecstatic or pleasurable seizures such as those experienced by Dostoevsky are rare (4). "...suddenly amid the sadness, spiritual darkness and depression, his brain seemed to catch fire at brief moments, and with an extraordinary momentum his vital forces were strained to the utmost all at once ... all his agitation, all his doubts and worries, seemed composed in a twinkling, culminating in a great calm, full of serene and harmonious joy . . ."

Localized seizure discharges that impair consciousness are termed *complex partial seizures*. Complex partial seizures most often are associated with abnormal discharges in the temporal lobe and often are associated with other manifestations of partial seizures. As noted previously, if the seizure discharge spreads diffusely throughout the cortex, the *partial seizure* evolves into a *secondarily generalized* tonic clonic seizure.

*Generalized seizures* are characterized by the loss of consciousness, most often with abnormal convulsive movements on both sides of the body. The most common type of convulsion is the *tonic clonic* generalized (*grand mal*) *seizure*, the sole seizure type in approximately 50% of patients with epilepsy (1). Tonic clonic seizures, either alone or in combination with other types of seizures, occur in an estimated 85% of patients who have epilepsy. Tonic clonic convulsions are the most dramatic and easily recognized type of seizure. They either occur following secondarily generalization of a partial seizure or appear *de novo* without warning.

An *aura* is a stereotyped sensory or psychic experience which precedes a generalized seizure. Auras in fact are partial seizures. Auras sometimes warn the patient that a generalized seizure is about to occur.

Tonic clonic seizures evolve in a characteristic sequence beginning with the abrupt loss of consciousness and an inarticulate cry. This utterance is created when the patient's diaphragm contracts spasmodically forcing air through the tonically opposed vocal cords. The initial movement culminates in a tonic contraction of body musculature usually lasting 10-20 s. During the period of sustained muscular contraction there is initially a predominance of the flexor muscles followed by the predominance of the extensor muscles causing the patient to first bend then extend. Following the initial tonic contraction, rhythm clonic jerking ensues lasting 3-5 times longer than the tonic phase,

ordinarily less than 1 min. The tonic jerking gradually abates into a state of severely reduced muscle tone. During this phase the relaxation of the sphincters may lead to incontinence of urine and feces. The phase of muscular relaxation blends imperceptibly into a period of postictal unresponsiveness from which the patient gradually recovers normal mental functioning, **usually in a fragmentary, erratic pattern. In the postictal period, as the patient is awakening, he may be confused and is usually sleepy. Patients who have** seizures are consistently amnestic for the time while they were unconscious. However, if the generalized tonic clonic seizure is preceded by a partial seizure, the **patient sometimes recalls the sensory or psychic experience which occurred during the prior partial seizure.**

Generalized *absence seizures* are characterized by a brief period of staring with loss of contact with the environment (3). After absence seizures the recovery of normal consciousness and function is prompt, seemingly immediate. In contrast to generalized tonic clonic seizures, postictal relaxation and sleepiness do not occur. In the most restricted forms, absence seizures are characterized only by interruption of normal behavior with staring. A staring episode due to an absence seizure is often clinically indistinguishable from staring episodes caused by partial complex seizures, but seizure types can be differentiated with the EEG pattern. In an absence seizure, the EEG characteristically indicates the sudden onset of a diffuse bilateral 3/s spike-and-wave pattern. Staring spells caused by partial complex seizures are associated with focal electrical discharge over the temporal lobe. The distinction between absence seizures and partial complex seizures is clinically important because different treatments are required.

**Patients with absence seizures often have subtle myoclonic movements involving the eyelids, fingers, arms or shoulders, brief alterations of postural tone, autonomic symptoms or automatisms. Automatisms** are stereotyped repetitive complex movements which occur during a seizure, presumably when patterned movements represented in lower brain structures are released from cortical inhibition. Automatisms consist of movements such as chewing, swallowing or fumbling with the clothes. They occur in partial complex seizures, in absence seizures, or sometimes during the recovery period after a generalized tonic clonic seizure.

*Clonic seizures, tonic seizures*, and certain atonic seizures may be regarded as fragments of an abortive generalized tonic clonic seizure. These seizure types are most often seen when patients are treated with antiepileptic drugs which apparently interrupt the orderly convulsive sequence.

*Myoclonic seizures* are characterized by the diffuse synchronous body jerks and are usually unassociated with the postictal depression. *Atonic seizures* are characterized by a sudden loss of postural tone causing a sudden fall or drop attack if the patient is standing. A mild, brief atonic seizure may cause only a head nod. Atonic and myoclonic seizures usually occur in patients who also have other types of seizures.

Certain types of seizures are not classified by the international classification. Specifically, *neonatal seizures* are not included. The most common seizures in newborn infants are subtle (5). Examples of subtle seizures include tonic eye deviation with eye jerking, repetitive fluttering of the eye lids, rowing, swimming or pedaling movements. Infrequently, apnea, the cessation of respiration, is an isolated manifestation of a neonatal seizure. The second most common seizure type in newborn infants is generalized tonic seizures. These are followed in frequency by multifocal clonic seizures and focal clonic seizures. The least common type of neonatal seizure, myoclonic, is characterized by single or multiple flexor jerks of the arms or legs.

## Causes of Seizures and Epilepsy

Diseases which affect the brain may cause transient or permanent alterations of brain structure and functioning. The most common transient disorders which cause seizures are metabolic or toxic. Although these transient disorders do not necessarily lead to structural brain damage, brain damage causing later epilepsy can result if the extent and duration of the metabolic derangements are excessive (6). Thus, transient metabolic abnormalities that cause acute seizures variably produce permanent brain damage leading to later epilepsy. A classification of seizure disorders is shown in Table 2.

Among the many causes of *nonepileptic seizure disorders*, fever is most common (7). In febrile seizures, the transient metabolic abnormality that causes the seizure is fever. Febrile seizures occur in children between the ages of six months and six years. Genetic studies suggest that the propensity to this disorder is inherited. In various studies, from 7.6 to 50% of patients have a positive family history. Although febrile seizures occur in 3.5% of children, only 2% of these children develop epilepsy by age seven. After febrile seizures, the chance of later epilepsy is increased when certain risk factors are present. These include a family history of epilepsy, abnormal development or neurological examination, and a febrile seizure that was focal, prolonged more than 20 min, or recurred within a 24-h period.

Other causes of nonepileptic seizures will be discussed only briefly here. Certain metabolic abnormalities such as hypoxia, ischemia and hypoglycemia

---

**Table 2.   Classification of Seizure Disorders**

I.   Nonepileptic (nonrecurrent) seizure disorders

Seizures are prominent or major symptoms of transient brain dysfunction. Later epilepsy may or may not occur.

A.   Neonatal seizures

B.   Febrile seizures

C.   Metabolic disorders
Cerebral ischemia
Hypoxia
Hypoglycemia
Divalent cation deficiency ($Ca^{2+}$, $Mg^{2+}$)
Hyponatremia/hypernatremia
Uremia
Fever

D.   Toxic disorders
Drug abstinence syndromes
Drug intoxications
Other chemicals

E.   Nutritional deficiency states

F.   CNS infections

G.   CNS neoplasia

H.   Trauma

I.   Cerebrovascular disease

II.   Epileptic (recurrent) seizure disorders — epileptic syndromes

Seizures, convulsive or nonconvulsive, recur due to a long-lasting abnormality of brain physiology or structure. An epileptic syndrome may have multiple causes.

A.   Infantile spasms (West syndrome)

B.   Multiple types of seizures with encephalopathy (Lennox-Gastaut syndrome)

C.   Benign Rolandic epilepsy

D.   Petit mal epilepsy

E.   Myoclonic epilepsy

F.   Epilepsy symptomatic of identified brain disease. The epilepsy is characterized by seizure type and cause, for example, posttraumatic epilepsy with generalized tonic clonic seizures.

G.   Epilepsy due to unidentified brain disease (idiopathic, cryptogenic).
The epilepsy is characterized by typical seizure type, e.g., epilepsy with generalized tonic clonic (grand mal).

H.   Reflex epilepsy
The epilepsy is characterized by the stimulus which produces seizures.

III.   Status epilepticus

---

are more likely to cause brain damage than others because of their vital role in brain metabolism. Drugs are the most common toxic cause of seizures, usually when doses are excessive. The most common offenders are penicillin, theophylline, tricyclic antidepressants, local anesthetics, phenothiazines, and meperidine. Seizures are common during withdrawal from addiction to barbiturates or alcohol but rare during withdrawal from narcotics.

The term *epileptic seizure disorder* or epilepsy implies that the brain abnormality which causes recurrent seizures is long lasting, though not necessarily permanent. Whereas the international classification categorizes seizure types, it does not classify the epilepsies; the nomenclature of the epilepsies has never been standardized. The most prevalent diagnostic labels are descriptive. Among patients with seizures, certain groups of patients have clinical features and natural histories that are sufficiently unique to merit syndromic labels. Examples include petit mal epilepsy and infantile spasms. The most useful diagnostic terminology includes the patient's seizure type and etiology, but abbreviated terms abound. For example pyschomotor epilepsy is better labeled as epilepsy with complex partial seizures due to unknown cause.

Infantile spasms are an example of an epileptic syndrome that occurs uniquely in childhood (8). Although patients can have several types of seizures, the major seizure type is flexor or extensor spasms. When a cause is identified it is often associated with widespread brain dysfunction. The causes of infantile spasms are identified in approximately 60% of patients and include, in order of decreasing frequency, perinatal asphyxia, tuberous sclerosis, brain malformation, hypoglycemia, hydrocephalus, intraventricular hemorrhage, and certain genetic disorders. Any disease which causes widespread brain damage can cause infantile spasms. As these patients grow older, the infantile spasms abate, but are replaced by other seizure types in at least half of the patients.

In a majority of patients with epilepsy, the cause cannot be identified. Using clinical means, chemical laboratory tests, and the EEG, the cause of seizures can be determined in approximately 25% of older children and adults (1). The leading causes of epilepsy are birth injuries, cerebrovascular disease, and head trauma. Among 516 patients in Olmstead County, MN, who developed epilepsy between 1935 and 1967, the cause was identified in 23.3%. In this particular series, birth asphyxia was less prominent than in other series; trauma accounted for 5.2%, vascular disease 5.2%, brain tumor 1%, congenital or genetic disorders 3.9%, infections 2.9% and birth asphyxia 1.4%. Overall, the cause of epilepsy is more easily identified among the very young and old patients.

Since the advent of computerized transaxial tomography (CT brain scanning), approximately one-third of epileptic patients have been found to have brain lesions (9,10). Conversely, even with CT scanning no cause for the epilepsy is found in two-thirds of the patients. Among patients with generalized absence epilepsy (petit mal) the incidence of CT abnormalities is very low. Partial motor seizures have the highest probability of being associated with abnormal CT scans, followed by partial complex seizures. The type

of abnormality which is found varies with age. Among children with generalized seizures 32% have abnormal CT scan findings, most commonly brain atrophy (9).

Among children with partial epilepsy, 43% have CT scan abnormalities whereas with generalized epilepsy only 20% have abnormal CT scans (9). Among older patients, atrophic lesions and brain tumors are increasingly common. In one study, brain tumors were found in 37.5% of patients with partial seizures and CT scans were abnormal in nearly 2/3 of adult epileptic patients with partial seizures (11). Even among older patients with generalized seizures, only 8.5% had brain tumors.

Brain tumors are a relatively infrequent cause of epilepsy. A brain tumor is more likely to be found when the epilepsy begins in adulthood, particularly after the age of 40 (12). Approximately 30% of brain tumors cause seizures although certain types of tumors may cause seizures in more than 50% of cases. The tumors which are most likely to produce seizures grow slowly, gradually encroaching on the cerebral cortex. Brain tumors account for approximately 1-2% of epilepsy in children and in young adults. The incidence of brain tumors causing the onset of epilepsy peaks in the fifth decade. When epilepsy begins after the age of 50, the leading causes are cerebrovascular disease 69%, brain tumors 15.4%, trauma 5.1%, with only 9% of the new cases being undiagnosed.

Epilepsy results from the interaction of multiple factors, one of which is a genetic predisposition. Studies on the inheritance of epilepsy are conflicting (13). This is not surprising, because epilepsy is a symptom of brain dysfunction and not a specific disorder. Certain diseases which often cause seizures such as tuberous sclerosis are clearly genetic. In tuberous sclerosis, the inheritance pattern is autosomal dominant and approximately 50% of the patient's offspring will be affected. Metabolic disorders which are associated with seizures such as maple syrup urine disease or phenylketonuria have an autosomal recessive inheritance. When the asymptomatic parents carry the trait, one-fourth of their children manifest the disease. The 3/s generalized spike wave abnormality on the EEG is thought to be inherited as autosomal dominant with an age-dependent expression in the affected offspring. Thirty-five percent of offspring at risk demonstrate the EEG abnormality and 8% have epilepsy. Genetic studies of epilepsy generally indicate that a propensity to develop certain types of seizures can be inherited but other factors are important.

Among patients who undergo surgery to treat intractible seizures the most common causes of seizures are perinatal brain injury (43.3%), followed by infection (26.7%), trauma (16.7%), and brain tumor (5%) (1). In 3-5% of surgical specimens the cause of the seizure cannot be demonstrated pathologically. The most common brain lesion found in these patients is mesial temporal sclerosis. The cause of this lesion is not fully understood, but it may in part be related to previous asphyxia or prolonged seizure activity, plus a special vulnerability of hippocampal brain tissue to metabolic injury.

In *status epilepticus*, seizures are either long lasting or so frequently recurrent as to result in a continuously abnormal mental state (6,14). Among various studies the duration of seizures necessary to be defined as status has varied, but 30 min is sufficient, because serious changes in brain metabolism begin to occur after 20 min and progress if the seizure is not stopped. Although any seizure type can occur in status epilepticus, generalized tonic clonic seizures are most common and the most dangerous for the patient.

Status epilepticus with generalized tonic clonic seizures is a medical emergency which requires aggressive, intensive treatment to interrupt the seizures and support the patient's vital functions. Because the chance of permanent brain injury increases as status is prolonged, it should be stopped within 20 min whenever possible. Because the occurrence of status epilepticus often indicates acute brain disease, the cause should be sought aggressively and treated specifically.

## Diagnosis and Management of Epilepsies

In the evaluation of patients with seizures, it is important first to document that the abnormal behavior is indeed due to seizures and to obtain a careful description of the ictal experience and behavior. The description of the seizure is used to classify the seizure type and may indicate where the seizure originated in the brain. The physician must first differentiate those patients who have seizures due to transient disorders affecting the brain from those who have recurrent seizures (epilepsy) due to long-lasting alterations of brain physiology or structure (15,16).

The initial evaluation includes a careful history and both physical and neurological examinations. Laboratory tests are utilized to rule out infectious, toxic, or metabolic causes of seizures which should be treated specifically when they are present.

The EEG is helpful in characterizing the seizure type and looking for a focal origin of the seizure (2). It is particularly valuable if it is obtained fortuitously during a seizure. But this is rare. Usually, the EEG is obtained in the interictal period between seizures. Under these conditions the EEG provides only circumstantial evidence about the origin of the behavior in question. In difficult cases, prolonged EEG recordings or videotapings with EEG may be necessary to determine the nature of a specific recurrent behavior

or experience. The finding of an abnormal EEG does not prove that epilepsy is present, nor does the finding of a normal EEG rule out the epilepsy. Among patients with confirmed epilepsy, initial interictal EEG's are normal in 20%, but with repeated interictal recordings the chance of detecting an abnormality increases. Among patients with epilepsy due to focal brain discharges on the inferior brain surface, an EEG abnormality may not be detected at the scalp. If the focus responsible for the seizures is quiescent when the EEG is obtained, it will not be detected.

CT scanning is indicated for those patients who have partial seizures, focal EEG abnormalities, or epilepsy which begins after the age of 20 years. Although middle-aged patients developing epilepsy have the highest probability of brain tumor, brain tumors are found in less than half of this group (12). Overall the most common CT scan abnormalities are atrophic lesions with focal or diffuse loss of brain substance (10).

Antiepileptic drugs (AEDs) are utilized to prevent seizures in patients with epilepsy (17). AEDs are symptomatic therapy which do not treat the underlying cause of seizures. Most of the AEDs are anticonvulsant, that is, they prevent or interrupt seizures. The first chemical to be used as an anticonvulsant was bromide which was introduced by Locock in 1857 (16). In 1912, phenobarbital was introduced and in 1937 diphenylhydantoin, later called phenytoin, became available. AEDs are given continuously to prevent the recurrence of seizures.

The selection of the appropriate AED is based upon a careful characterization of the patient's most frequent seizure type (17). From a practical point of view, AEDs can be grouped by whether they are effective in treating absence seizures, generalized tonic clonic seizures plus partial seizures, or both of the previous categories (Table 3). AEDs that are effective only against absence seizures are ethosuximide and trimethadione. Anticonvulsants that are effective only against generalized tonic clonic seizures and partial seizures include carbamazepine and phenytoin. Anticonvulsant drugs that are effective against both categories of seizures include valproic acid and certain benzodiazepines. In practice, the physician first determines the patient's seizure type and frequency, considers factors such as potential drug toxicity and unique patient variables such as associated systemic disease and allergic history, and then selects an appropriate AED.

The manner in which the AED is initially administered depends on the urgency of the clinical situation. Status epilepticus is a medical emergency and AEDs must be administered intravenously in high doses to rapidly stop the seizures (14). Usually, seizures are

**Table 3. The principal AEDs and their clinical spectrum**

| Drug | Year Introduced | Absence (petit mal) | Partial and generalized tonic clonic |
|---|---|---|---|
| Phenobarbital | 1912 | ± | + |
| Phenytoin | 1938 | 0 | + |
| Trimethadione | 1946 | + | 0 |
| Primidone | 1954 | 0[a] | + |
| Methsuximide | 1957 | 0 | + |
| Ethosuximide | 1960 | + | 0 |
| Carbamazepine | 1974 | 0 | + |
| Clonazepam | 1975 | + | ± |
| Valproic acid | 1978 | + | + |

Primidone is metabolized to phenobarbital.

relatively mild and infrequent, making it preferable to initiate treatment slowly, and avoid early inebriating and sedative side effects to which patients become tolerant as the AED level gradually increases (15). In this situation, patients begin taking the medication at a low or average dose and the drug level gradually is increased until a steady state is obtained (17). At steady state, the rate of drug intake is equal to the rate of drug elimination and drug levels are relatively constant. To avoid neurological side effects, the physician strives to treat the patient with as little medication as possible. Thus, the dose of AED is gradually increased until either the seizures are stopped or until the patient experiences toxicity.

The effective use of AEDs depends on knowing a patient's seizure type, the selection of an appropriate AED, and the careful follow-up of the patient to evaluate AED efficacy and toxicity (16). A knowledge of pharmacokinetics of the AED being given helps the physician use it optimally. The most important pharmacokinetic parameter is the half-life. The half-life of a drug is the amount of time required for one half of the drug to be eliminated from the body. Inter-patient variability in the half-life of AEDs is a major determinant of the different dosage requirements among patients. The half-life is clinically important for several reasons. First, the half-life is directly related to the steady-state concentration, which occurs after chronic dosing. Second, doses should be given at intervals equal to or less than the half-life to avoid excessive fluctuations in drug levels. Third, approximately five half-lives are required for a patient to achieve a steady state after a constant dose is given chronically. Thus, when a physician initiates drug therapy, it is best to wait, whenever possible, until the drug has had time to reach steady state before the patient is reevaluated. Because AEDs have side effects which are additive, it is best to obtain the maximal benefit from an initial AED before adding others. If the initial AED is ineffective, it should be discontinued while a second is tried. The smallest number of AEDs that is sufficient to do the job is preferable. When it is necessary to administer more than one AED, drug concentration measurements are particularly valuable in helping to maximize the effectiveness of each of the AEDs.

AEDs act in the brain to prevent either the spread of seizure activity from the focus or to suppress the abnormal discharges which occur in the focus. When AEDs are given in high doses, the principal toxicities are neurological or neuropsychiatric (16,17).

The measurement of AED levels is a valuable clinical adjunct. AED measurements allow a physician to individualize drug doses to produce an appropriate therapeutic concentration for each patient. AED levels should be drawn whenever the physician needs to know them. If a patient has symptoms which might be due to drug toxicity, levels obtained when the symptoms are present are most valuable. If the patient continues to have seizures despite presumably adequate doses, levels are best measured when the AED level is expected to be at its lowest point, usually just prior to taking a dose. Noncompliance in taking AEDs is a prevalent problem. AED levels provide an objective means of assessing compliance and can indicate those patients who need additional encouragement to take their medications regularly.

How effective are AEDs? Although early studies suggested that drug therapy was effective in controlling seizures in most patients, more careful analysis indicate that only 30 to 50% of patients enjoy complete prevention of their seizures for a prolonged period of time (1). Certain types of seizures are more easily controlled than others. For example, more than 50% of patients with absence seizures can be controlled with either ethosuximide or valproic acid. When patients are not controlled by one medication alone, an estimated 90 to 95% of patients with absence seizures can be controlled by the combination of these medications. Generalized tonic clonic seizures are the second most easily controlled by AEDs. Patients with multiple seizure types, usually including atonic and myoclonic seizures, appear to have an epileptic process which is very intense and often difficult to control. Although patients with these types of epilepsy syndromes may expect relatively good control of generalized tonic clonic seizures, complete prophylaxis of myoclonic or atonic seizures is more difficult; probably less than half of patients with this epilepsy syndrome enjoy complete seizure control with current AEDs. Among these types of patients the ketogenic diet is helpful (*18*).

Recurrent partial seizures are the most common form of refractory epilepsy among older children and adults. Patients who have partial seizures which originate in well localized areas of the brain, areas which are not involved in critical brain functions, may be candidates for surgical treatment of epilepsy (*18*). The criteria for selecting patients for surgical therapy of epilepsy include the failure of AEDs to control the seizures, the occurrence of seizures with a well localized origin, and a persistent seizure frequency which prevents the patient's carrying out age-appropriate activities of living. For those patients with severe epilepsies which are not adequately controlled by medications, thoughtful evaluation and skillful surgery may allow half of surgical candidates to resume a normal level of functioning.

## References

1.  U.S. Commission for the Control of Epilepsy and Its Consequences, *Plan for Nationwide Action on Epilepsy,* Vol. 1, DHEW Publications No. (NIH) 78-276, 1978.
2.  Goldensohn, E., The epilepsies. In *Scientific Approaches to Clinical Neurology,* Eli S. Goldensohn and Stanley H. Appel, Eds., Lea & Febiger, Philadephia, 1977, pp 654-692.
3.  Commission on Classification and Terminology of the International League Against Epilepsy, Proposal for revised clinical and electroencephalographic classification of epileptic seizures. *Epilepsia* **22**, 489-501 (1981).
4.  Cirignotta, F., Todesco, C.V, and Lugaresi, E., Temporal lobe epilepsy with ecstatic seizures (so-called Dostoevsky epilepsy). *Epilepsia* **21**, 705-710 (1980).
5.  Volpe, Joseph J., *Neurology of the Newborn,* W. B. Saunders Co., Philadelphia, 1981, pp 111-137.
6.  Delgato-Escueta, A.V., Wasterbain, C., Treiman, D.M., and Porter, R.J., Current concepts in neurology: Management of status epilepticus. *N. Engl. J. Med.* **306**, 1337-1340 (1982).
7.  Nelson, Karin, B., and Ellenberg, Jonas H., *Fibrile Seizures,* Raven Press, New York, 1981, pp 1-17.
8.  Kurokawa, T., Goya, N., Fukuyama, Y., Suzuki, M., Seki, T., and Ohtahara, S., West syndrome and Lennox syndrome: A survey of natural history. *Pediatrics* **65**, 81-88 (1980).
9.  Bachman, D.S., Hodges, F.J., and Freeman J.M., Computerized axial tomography in chronic seizure disorders of childhood. *Pediatrics* **58**, 828-832 (1976).
10.  Gastaut, H., and Gastaut, J.L., Computerized transverse axial tomography in epilepsy. *Epilepsia* **17**, 325-336 (1976).
11.  Scollo-Lavizzari, G., Eichhorn, K., and Wuthrich, R., Computerized transverse axial tomography (CTAT) in the diagnosis of epilepsy. *Eur. Neurol.* **15**, 5-8 (1977).
12.  Merlis, J.K., Epilepsy of late onset. In *The Epilepsies, Handbook of Clinical Neurology,* P.J. Vinken and G.W. Bruyn, Eds., North Holland Publishing Co., New York, 1974, pp 264-270.
13.  Newmark, M.E., and Penry, J.K. *Genetics of Epilepsy,* Raven Press, New York, 1980.
14.  Dodson, W.E., Prensky, A.L., DeVivo, D.C., Goldring, S., and Dodge, P.R., Management of seizure disorders: Selected aspects. Part 1. *J. Pediatr.* **89**, 522-540 (1976).
15.  Dodson, W.E., Pharmacology and therapeutics of epilepsy in childhood. *Clin. Neuropharm* **4**, 1-29, (1979).
16.  Wilder, B.J., and Bruni J., *Seizure Disorders. A Pharmacological Approach to Treatment,* Raven Press, New York, 1981.
17.  Woodbury, D.M., Penry, J.K, Pippenger, C.E., *Antiepileptic Drugs,* Second edition, Raven Press, New York, 1982.
18.  Dodson, W.E., Prensky, A.L., DeVivo, D.C., Goldring, S., and Dodge, P.R., Management of seizure disorders: Selected aspects. Part 2. *J. Pediatr.* **89**, 695-703 (1976).

# 2

# Therapeutic Drug Monitoring of Phenytoin

**Andrew L. Finn, Pharm.D.**

Phenytoin (Dilantin®) was introduced as an anti-convulsant by Merritt and Putnam in 1938. Since then, it has become the most frequently prescribed drug for the management of seizure disorders. Phenytoin has assumed this position because of its demonstrated efficacy in a group of commonly encountered seizure disorders and relative freedom from serious side effects. This situation has evolved despite phenytoin's unusual pharmacokinetic properties and relatively poor correlation between administered dose and seizure control.

More than twenty years after phenytoin's introduction, a relationship was demonstrated between serum phenytoin concentrations and seizure control (1). In the early seventies, phenytoin's unusual pharmacokinetic properties became apparent as did information that maximal efficacy was obtained at serum concentrations of 10 to 20 mg/L (39-79 mmol/L) (2). These factors coupled with technologic improvements have led to the widespread availability and utilization of therapeutic drug monitoring. Serum concentration determinations have enabled the physician to compensate for the unusual pharmacokinetic properties of phenytoin and therefore increase the likelihood of obtaining optimal seizure control while avoiding unnecessary toxicity.

Extended availability of therapeutic drug monitoring technology has enabled the medical practitioner to take full advantage of the defined therapeutic range. Recent studies indicate that optimum utilization of phenytoin alone avoids the need and risk of multiple anticonvulsant therapy.

## Clinical Pharmacology
## Clinical Indications

Currently, phenytoin is the drug of choice for generalized major motor and focal seizures with or without secondary generalization. Though not the preferred drug, it can also be used to treat elementary partial (focal) or complex partial (psychomotor, temporal lobe) seizures. Phenytoin is considered to be ineffective for petit mal seizures. It has been used to treat status epilepticus and in some institutions is the

*Dr. Finn is Clinical Assistant Professor of Family Medicine, Duke University Medical Center, Durham, NC.*

preferred treatment for this disorder. Clinical studies have defined phenytoin's therapeutic range as 10 to 20 mg/L (39-79 mmol/L).

The therapeutic range should be thought of as a continuum, with the probability of seizure control increasing as the serum concentration increases from the lower portion of the therapeutic range to the upper portion. Thus, a 50% reduction in seizure activity is likely to occur when serum concentrations are greater than 10 mg/L (39 mmol/L), and an 86% reduction will occur with concentrations greater than 15 mg/L (59 mmol/L) (3). It has been estimated that 90% of new epileptic patients with generalized seizures can be satisfactorily controlled on phenytoin alone, without the unnecessary risk and expense of additional medications (4). Further evidence suggests that approximately half of this group would be started on a second medication in addition to phenytoin if the serum concentrations were not evaluated. The failure of the medical community to realize the importance of the therapeutic range is depicted in a 1977 publication describing a population of previously treated epileptics. In this study, patients were receiving an average of three anticonvulsants and 69 out of 100 patients did not have a single therapeutic serum concentration (5).

## Mechanism of Anticonvulsant Action

Despite extensive investigation, the basic mechanism through which phenytoin exerts its antiepileptic activity is unknown. In animal studies, phenytoin diminishes the duration of afterdischarge and limits the spread of seizure activity, possibly by reducing post-tetanic potentiation. These electrophysiological actions are more prominent than any elevation of the seizure threshold, which is principally an occurrence of the cerebral cortex and hippocampus.

At the biochemical level, studies of the effect of phenytoin on sodium potassium ATPase have been conflicting. Some portion of phenytoin's anticonvulsant activity may be mediated through an increase in active potassium influx and sodium extrusion by normal cells. Alternatively, phenytoin has been demonstrated to inhibit calcium uptake into brain synaptosomes leading some investigators to conclude that its anticonvulsant activity is a result of a reduction in central synaptic transmission. Another theory which has some support is that phenytoin's anticonvulsant activity is mediated by an increase in benzodiazepine receptor binding sites in brain membranes, which may enhance endogenous control of abnormal neuronal excitability.

The principal difficulty in evaluating these observations is that the brain mechanism responsible for seizure activity is unknown. Thus, complete understanding of phenytoin's anticonvulsant activity depends upon elucidation of the basic mechanisms responsible for epileptic activity.

## Adverse Reactions

As stated earlier, one of the reasons for phenytoin's acceptance as an anticonvulsant is that intolerable side effects are uncommon and only rarely necessitate its discontinuation. A number of side effects, however, do occur, and these range from predictable dose-related toxicities to unpredictable hypersensitivity reactions. Serum concentration determinations can be extremely valuable in avoiding those toxicities that are dose-related and in evaluating those that occur despite precautionary measures.

Commonly encountered dose-related toxicities begin to develop at serum concentrations in excess of 20 mg/L (79 mmol/L). The symptoms usually progress as follows: nystagmus, blurred vision, ataxia, dysarthria, drowsiness and coma. This progression, however, does not hold for every patient. It has been noted that only a small portion of patients with serum concentrations less than 30 mg/L (99 mmol/L) will exhibit any toxic side effects. However, approximately half the patients with serum concentrations above 30 mg/L (99 mol/L) will have side effects. The frequency and severity of side effects increases with the serum concentration. It is worth noting that in some cases the total serum concentration is not the most sensitive index of dose-related toxicity. Variations in the protein binding of a patient may produce substantial alterations in the free phenytoin concentration. This free fraction may be elevated and produce toxicity in patients where the total serum concentration is within the accepted therapeutic range.

Another group of adverse reactions associated with phenytoin has a more insidious onset, does not appear to be dose-related, and occurs in enough patients to speculate that these may be additional pharmacologic effects. Phenytoin has been associated with a folic acid deficiency and megaloblastic anemia. Prospective evaluation of this association demonstrated a reduction in serum and red blood cell folic acid levels, but there was no evidence of anemia or alterations of other hematologic parameters. Thus, the anemia may result from some other complicating factor, such as

diet. Rickets, osteomalacia, and an increased number of fractures have been attributed to phenytoin's effects on calcium and vitamin D homeostasis. Phenytoin appears to stimulate the catabolism of 25-hydroxy vitamin D and its active metabolites to inactive products. Some institutions are now recommending prophylactic use of vitamin D, particularly in children and possibly for some adults.

A benign morbilliform skin rash frequently occurs one to fourteen days after initiation of therapy. It is generally self-limited despite the continuation of therapy. Rarely does it progress to the more severe toxic epidermal necrolysis, exfoliative dermatitis, or Stevens-Johnson syndrome. A pseudolymphoma syndrome has been described in which there is a generalized, histologically benign lymphadenopathy in association with the skin rash. Some cases are reported to progress to a malignant lymphoma picture. Hepatitis has been associated with the pseudo-lymphoma syndrome, but has also been noted as an isolated entity.

There is two- to threefold increase in the frequency of congenital malformation in infants born to mothers who have been taking phenytoin. Craniofacial anomalies, particularly cleft lip and/or palate have been most widely reported, although mental deficiency, growth deficiency, and digital hypoplasia have been observed as part of a "fetal hydantoin syndrome." It is currently recommended that a pregnant epileptic controlled on phenytoin be maintained on this medication. Multiple medications should be avoided.

## Pharmacokinetics

*Systematic Availability.* The efficacy and toxicity of phenytoin are influenced by the product selected and route of administration. Phenytoin chewable tablets, capsules and suspension are available for oral administration. Because phenytoin is insoluble in aqueous mediums, the actual dosage administered may vary when the liquid suspension is used. If not properly mixed, the phenytoin concentration may be lower at the top of the bottle than at the bottom, resulting in significant fluctuations in phenytoin serum concentrations and seizure control. Another significant concern is the different absorption characteristics and bioinequivalence of generic brands of phenytoin. The generic brands tend to have faster absorption characteristics and significantly different bioavailability than the market standard Dilantin® (6).

Approximately 90% of orally administered phenytoin reaches the systemic circulation with absorption ocurring in the small intestine. Peak serum concentrations will be noted 3-9 after an oral dose of the market standard Dilantin®, and 1½-3 h after generic preparations. Because of its insolubility, complete absorption may require 48 h with Dilantin® (7). Multiple daily doses are necessary with the generic brands, but a single daily dose is adequate in most adult patients treated with Dilantin® (8).

When rapid anticonvulsant activity is necessary, phenytoin may be administered by the intravenous route. Whether administered by direct intravenous injection or as an infusion, the administration rate should not exceed 25-50 mg/min because of the risk of cardiac arrhythmia and respiratory depression. The diluent, propylene glycol, in the intravenous preparation may be responsible for these side effects.

Intramuscular injection of phenytoin results in slow and erratic absorption of the medication because it precipitates at intramuscular pH. Fifty percent or more of the dosage may remain at the injection site 24 h after administration, Because of the delay in absorption, serum concentrations should be very low, but may increase to toxicity after multiple injections and unexpected release from muscle sites.

*Volume of Distribution.* Phenytoin's apparent volume of distribution ranges from 0.7 L/kg in adults and children to 1.2 L/kg in infants and neonates. Because of its lipid solubility, only 5% of the drug is contained within the intravascular space. In adults, 88-92% of intravascular phenytoin is bound to albumin. The free fraction (8-12%), is assumed to be the pharmacologically active portion and may correlate best with seizure control and toxicity. After intravenous administration, phenytoin rapidly diffuses into brain tissue where its binding characteristics and concentrations are similar to those in serum. Diffusion into the cerebrospinal fluid occurs at a slightly slower rate, but eventually concentrations in this fluid approximate the free plasma concentrations.

Presently, investigators are concerned with factors that may affect phenytoin's binding characteristics. Reductions in serum albumin and changes in the binding characteristics of the albumin molecule may increase the free phenytoin fraction. Phenytoin may also be displaced from its albumin binding sites by increases in serum bilirubin in neonates and patients with liver disease. A binding inhibitor has been postulated to accumulate in free phenytoin concentration. Addition of various acidic drugs such as valproic acid, sulfonylureas, and salicylates to a patient receiving phenytoin will result in an increase in the free phenytoin fraction. This may not be reflected in the total serum concentration, which may remain within normal limits. In these situations, the free phenytoin concentration may be a more accurate

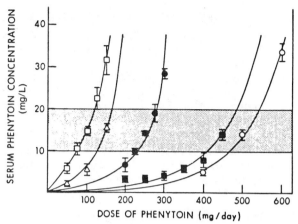

**Fig. 1. Relationship between serum concentration and daily dose in five epileptic patients. (Adapted from A. Richens and A. Dunlop: Serum phenytoin levels in the management of epilepsy. Lancet 2:247, 1975.)**

indicator of clinical efficacy and toxicity than the total serum concentration.

*Metabolism.* The principal route of phenytoin elimination is through liver metabolism to 5-(*p*-hydroxyphenyl)-5-phenylhydantoin (HPPH), an inactive metabolite. This metabolite is conjugated with glucuronic acid and then eliminated in the urine. A small portion, approximately 5%, of phenytoin is excreted unchanged in the urine. There appears to be a limited hepatic capacity to metabolize phenytoin which accounts for its unusual elimination characteristics. Saturation of this process generally occurs within the therapeutic range and results in a disproportionate increase in the serum concentration when the daily dosage exceeds the metabolic capacity (See figure 1). Conversely, as the dosage is increased in the patient, a point is reached at which the serum concentration begins to rise much faster than the proportionate increase in dose. Clinically, phenytoin doses that produce a therapeutic serum concentration are very close to those which yield toxicity. For these reasons, it is extremely difficult to identify a therapeutic dosage and avoid toxicity without the benefit of serum concentration monitoring. The clinical implication is that small increments in dosage must be used as the serum concentration approaches the therapeutic range to avoid dose-related side effects. Saturation is generally seen at dosages of 4 mg/kg per day in adults and 6 mg/kg per day in children.

Because of phenytoin's limited capacity for hepatic metabolism, it cannot be described by first order kinetics, and thus the term half-life is inaccurate. its use here is not an attempt to perpetuate this inaccuracy, but reflects a realization that the term is broadly understood while other nomenclature, such as clearance, are not as widely used. In most adults, the half-life of phenytoin is approximately 20 h when serum concentrations are in the lower portion of the therapeutic range. As the serum concentration is increased, the half-life will also increase, and adult values have been reported to range from 10 to 95 h. Longer periods of time are required to attain a steady state as the serum concentration increases.

## Clinical Use of Phenytoin

Optimal anticonvulsant efficacy can only be attained from phenytoin when its use is individualized according to population groups, disease states and concurrent medications. Therapeutic drug monitoring will enable the clinician to evaluate the effect of these parameters on phenytoin kinetics and to insure that a therapeutic level has been attained. A number of studies have documented the relationship between serum concentration and anticonvulsant efficacy of phenytoin. The 10-20 mg/L (39-79 mmol/L) therapeutic range is intended as a guideline for the management of epileptic patients. In a small percentage of patients, seizure control may be obtained with serum levels below 10 mg/L (39 mmol/L). Another small percentage of patients will benefit from serum concentrations slightly higher than the therapeutic range, while other patients exhibit an increase in seizure frequency at these concentrations.

### Adults

Individual differences in absorption, metabolism, compliance, disease states and concomitant medications combine to produce considerable variation in the responsiveness of the adult patient to phenytoin therapy. The importance of therapeutic drug monitoring in attaining maximal efficacy and avoiding dose-related toxicity cannot be overstated. The half-life of phenytoin in adults generally ranges from 20 to 40 h necessitating a period of 4-8 days to attain a steady-state following initiation of maintenance therapy. As dosages and serum concentrations are progressively increased to achieve maximal efficacy, longer half-lives will be observed, and 2-4 weeks may be necessary to attain a new steady-state.

In the average adult, phenytoin therapy is started at a dose of 5 mg/kg/day by the oral route. The serum phenytoin concentration should be checked in one week to establish that a therapeutic value has been attained. Dosages are then increased until either seizure control or the upper limit of the therapeutic range is reached. There is generally no advantage to divided daily doses in adults taking Dilantin®, and a single dose in the morning or evening is preferred. Serum phenytoin concentrations should be checked approximately once each year even in compliant patients with good seizure control who have had therapeutic serum concentrations in the past.

In the management of status epilepticus, phenytoin is administered intravenously in order to rapidly attain a therapeutic serum concentration. The recommended loading dose is 15 mg/kg of body weight administered by direct intravenous injection. It should be administered at a rate not exceeding 25-50 mg/minute while monitoring the patient's cardiac and respiratory functions. Therapeutic serum concentrations can be achieved within 30 min using this dosage schedule. If seizures persist, a serum concentration should be measured approximately 30 min after the loading dose is completed, and additional medication administered accordingly. If the seizure is broken, a serum concentration measured within 4 h will

## Pharmacokinetic Summary Table

| | Daily Maintenance Dose (mg/kg) | Volume of Distribution (L/kg) | Half-life (h) | Recmnd. Plasma Concs. (mg/L) |
|---|---|---|---|---|
| Pre-term neonate | 5.9 | 1.2 | 75 ± 64.5 | 6-14 |
| Term neonate (<2 week old) | 5.9 | 0.8 | 21 ± 11.6 | 6-14 |
| Infants (>2 week old) | 8 (2-4 doses) | 0.8 | 7.6 ± 3.5 | 6-14 (<3 mo. of age) 10-20 (>3 mo. of age) |
| Adults | 5 | 0.7 | 20-40 | 10-20 |
| Pregnancy | Increased | Increased (?) | Decreased | 10-20 |

establish a reference point for determining the adequacy of maintenance therapy and the maximum delay that can occur before maintenance therapy is initiated. Generally, maintenance therapy should be initiated within 12 h of the loading dose.

## Pediatrics

The variability in dosage requirements seen in the adult population is magnified substantially in children. Age-related changes in volume of distribution and elimination rates necessitate a stricter approach to phenytoin titration in the pediatric population. The pre-term neonate has an average volume of distribution of 1.2 L, which is unaffected by gestational age. The term neonate has a volume of distribution of 0.8 L, which remains constant through 96 weeks of age. A marked reduction in phenytoin binding will be noted during the first three months of life due to either competition with bilirubin for albumin binding sites or alteration in the binding characteristics of the albumin molecule itself. This increase in the free fraction should result in antiepileptic activity at lower total serum concentrations in this population, and the suggested range is 6-14 mg/L (23-56 mmol/L).

The hepatic immaturity in the pre-term infant is reflected in a markedly prolonged phenytoin half-life. In utero exposure to phenytoin results in increased metabolic rates presumably as a consequence of hepatic enzyme induction. In the term infant, less than 2 weeks of age, the half-life is approximately 20 h. However, the metabolic capacity increases during this period such that past the age of 2 weeks, the half-life and small body size necessitates multiple daily doses to sustain a therapeutic level. When immediate anticonvulsant activity is necessary in the pre-term neonate, loading doses on the order of 15-20 mg/kg are required because of the large volume of distribution. Phenytoin should not be administered orally in neonates as the absorption is very poor, and intravenous administration must be used to maintain adequate levels.

In the preschool child, serial serum levels may be necessary to establish the total daily dosage and schedule of administration. Some children have subtherapeutic concentrations despite doses of 5-10 mg/kg/day and may require 15 mg/kg/day to sustain therapeutic concentrations. Because of the rapid elimination rate, adequate average serum concentrations may be associated with toxic peaks or subtherapeutic troughs. This problem may be circumvented by multiple daily doses and sufficient serum drug determinations to characterize the daily fluctuations in the serum concentration. The change

from childhood metabolic rates is a gradual process occurring throughout adolescence, that is best compensated for by periodic phenytoin serum concentration monitoring.

## Liver and Renal Disease

Few pharmacokinetic studies on phenytoin in patients with liver and renal disease have been done. Those that are available indicate that the problems are similar. The presence of hypoalbuminemia in either liver or renal disease results in an increased fraction of free phenytoin. Metabolic waste products such as bilirubin and urea can also displace phenytoin from its albumin binding sites. This issue may be of particular importance in the patient with renal failure where there is an accumulation of phenytoin's metabolite HPPH glucuronide or a binding inhibitor. With the expected increase in the free fraction, therapeutic phenytoin activity should be expected at total serum concentrations below the normally cited range. A direct measurement of the free fraction would be the best index of anticonvulsant activity.

Phenytoin metabolism may be impaired in patients with chronic liver disease, while its degradation is increased in patients with acute hepatitis and mononucleosis. Hepatic metabolism may also be increased in patients with renal disease, resulting in a reduced phenytoin half-life. Many physicians administer supplemental dosages of phenytoin to patients after dialysis. Recent data indicate that serum phenytoin concentrations are unaltered by dialysis and supplemental doses are therefore unnecessary.

## Drug Interactions

The majority of drug interactions with phenytoin alter the pharmacokinetic handling of one or both drugs. The clinical significance of each interaction depends on variables that are not within the scope of this paper. Intelligent use of serum phenytoin concentrations will help assess the effect of various drugs on phenytoin metabolism.

Barbiturates in high concentrations, chloramphenicol, disulfiram, isoniazid, and dicumarol have all been demonstrated to impair the hepatic metabolism of phenytoin. As a result the addition of one of these agents to a patient maintained on phenytoin may produce an increase in the serum concentration. Patients whose seizure activity has been uncontrolled in the past may suddenly become controlled, while those who had serum concentrations in the upper therapeutic range may develop symptoms of phenytoin toxicity. Patients who have been receiving one of these five drugs and then have phenytoin added to it should require lower doses of phenytoin for adequate seizure control. Upon discontinuation of one of these drugs, the serum phenytoin level may decline with resultant loss of seizure control.

Alcohol, barbiturates in low concentrations, and carbamazepine may increase the hepatic metabolism of phenytoin. Thus the addition of one of these agents to a patient on phenytoin will likely produce a decline in the serum concentration. Discontinuation of one of these medications in a patient receiving chronic phenytoin therapy may result in an increase in the phenytoin serum concentration and potential toxicity. The addition of phenytoin to a patient routinely ingesting one of these substances will likely necessitate higher than expected dosages for adequate serum concentrations and anticonvulsant activity.

Salicylates, valproic acid, phenylbutazone, and sulfonylureas may displace phenytoin from its albumin binding sites. As a result the total serum phenytoin concentration may decline as more drug is available for hepatic metabolism. However, the free phenytoin concentration remains unchanged and dosage adjustments are probably unnecessary.

Phenytoin itself is a potent stimulator of hepatic microsomal enzyme systems. It can in turn increase the elimination rate of other drugs that are eliminated through hepatic metabolism. Importantly, reduced pharmacologic activity should be expected when corticosteroids and oral anticoagulants are combined with phenytoin therapy.

## Summary

The development of technology for measuring serum phenytoin concentrations has expanded the role of therapeutic drug monitoring in the management of epileptic patients. Therapeutic drug monitoring helps the clinician obtain maximal efficacy, avoid dose-related toxicity, and avoid the unnecessary risk and cost of polypharmacy.

The following principles should be considered when interpreting serum concentration data: (1) Optimal anticonvulsant activity occurs with serum phenytoin concentrations between 10 and 20 mg/L (39-79 mmol/L); (2) When serum concentrations are below 10 mg/L (39 mmol/L); phenytoin is less effective, while dose-related side effects occur with serum concentrations above 20 mg/L (79 mmol/L); (3) These ranges apply to the population in general and must be interpreted in light of the clinical status of the patient

undergoing treatment; (4) In initiating phenytoin therapy with maintenance level dosages, steady state is attained after approximately 3-5 days; (5) As the serum concentration increases to the upper portion of the therapeutic range, the half-life also increases and a period of 2-4 weeks may be required to attain steady state following a dosage change; (6) For neonates and patients with hepatic or renal disease, free serum concentrations of phenytoin may be a better index of pharmacologic activity than total serum concentrations.

## References

1. Buchthal, F., Svensmark, O., and Schiller, P.J., Clinical and electroencephalographic correlations with serum levels of diphenylhydantoin. *Archives of Neurology* **2**, 624-630 (1960).
2. Richens, A., and Dunlop, A., Serum phenytoin levels in the management of epilepsy. *Lancet* **2**, 247-248 (1975).
3. Lund, L., Anti-convulsant effect of diphenylhydantoin relative to plasma levels; a prospective 3-year study in ambulant patients with generalized epileptic seizures. *Archives of Neurology* **31**, 289-294 (1974).
4. Reynolds, E.H., Chadwick, D., and Galbraith, A.W., One drug (phenytoin) in the treatment of epilepsy. *Lancet* **1**, 923-926 (1976).
5. Meinaridei, H., van Heycopten Ham, M.W., Meijer, J.W.A., and Bonger, E., Long term control of seizures in epilepsy. *The 8th International Symposium*, J.K. Penry, Ed., Raven Press, New York, N.Y., 1977, pp 17-26.
6. Melikian, A.P., Straughn, A.B., Slywka, G.W.A., Whyatt, P.L., and Meyer, M.C., Bioavailability of 11 phenytoin products. *J. Pharmacokinet & Biopharm.* **5**, 133-146 (1977).
7. Jusko, W.J., Koup, J.R., and Alvan, G., Non-linear assessment of phenytoin bioavailability. *J. Pharmacokinet. & Biopharm.* **4**, 326-327 (1976).
8. Anonymous, FDA Drug Bulletin, August-September, 1978.

## Recommended Reading:

Olanow, C.W., and Finn, A.L., Phenytoin: Pharmacokinetics and clinical therapeutics. *Neurosurgery* **8**, 112-117 (1981).

# 3

# Phenytoin: Adult and Pediatric Case Histories

J.G. Hill, Ph.D., M.D.

## Case History (Adult)

This case illustrates the most common single problem in long-term phenytoin therapy—noncompliance—and indicates how monitoring phenytoin in plasma may be of value in dealing with the problem.

## Case Presentation

T.G., a 27-year-old unemployed white man, was brought to the hospital emergency department by ambulance in a semi-conscious state. His wife, who accompanied him and who had called the ambulance, reported that he had been under treatment for epilepsy since childhood, but had been seizure-free for almost two years. For the past month the patient had been severely depressed because of his inability to find work, and had been irregular in his sleeping and eating habits. In addition, he had sometimes neglected to take his prescribed phenytoin, and on the morning in question he had had a typical grand mal seizure.

He was of average height and weight, apparently in a post-ictal state. His vital signs were normal, as were the results of the rest of the physical examination.

Immediate management consisted only of observation and monitoring of vital signs. After about 4 h he awoke from his deep sleep and, except for mild confusion with respect to time and place, appeared to be perfectly normal.

Additional history obtained at that time revealed that the patient had for the past three weeks taken less than one-quarter of his prescribed daily dose of 400 mg of phenytoin. He justified this action to himself on the basis of his long freedom from seizures, which led him to believe he no longer needed the medication. Moreover, he related his inability to find work to his continuing dependence on phenytoin, and he hoped that stopping the drug would in some way help him to find a job.

A plasma phenytoin assay showed a concentration of 3.5 mg/L. The patient was then given a single oral loading dose of phenytoin of 700 mg, and urged to

*Dr. Hill is the Head of the Service Division, Department of Biochemistry at the Hospital for Sick Children, Toronto, Ontario*

resume his regular daily maintenance dose of 200 mg twice daily.

Seen one week later in clinic, he reported that he felt well and had not had another seizure. The plasma phenytoin concentration was now 14.7 mg/L, so he was advised to carry on with his established drug regimen. In addition, arrangements were made for a return to the clinic in six months for repeat of the plasma phenytoin measurement, and reassessment.

## Discussion

As with any other disease that requires long-term medication, patient compliance is a major factor in the success or failure of drug therapy in epilepsy. In the case of phenytoin, it has been estimated that 30-40% of plasma values of < 10 mg/L are the result of the patient failing to take (or receive) his prescribed medication. This may be done inadvertently, through misunderstanding or carelessness, or deliberately, in an attempt to deny the need, or for various other reasons. In any case, the situation is further complicated by the unpredictability of seizures, so that there may be long non-compliance before the consequences become apparent.

In a patient with a history of non-compliance, it has been shown that regular clinic visits, with measurement of plasma phenytoin at each visit, serve as an effective stimulus to improve compliance. In addition, such visits provide a valuable opportunity to help the patient understand his condition, as well as objective data on which to base logical decisions about modifying drug dosage.

## Measurement of Plasma Phenytoin

Plasma phenytoin may be measured by spectrophotometry, gas-liquid chromatography, "high-performance" liquid chromatography, enzyme-multiplied immunoassay, or radioimmunoassay. Each of these techniques can provide reliable results; thus the choice of a particular method will be influenced by volume of work, equipment and technical expertise available, requirements for micro-scale sample handling, and the like. Irrespective of the method selected, however, care and attention to detail are required if the benefits of drug monitoring are to be made available to patients.

## PHENYTOIN PROFILE

**Trade name:**       Dilantin, Epanutin
**Chemical name:**   5,5-diphenylhydantoin

**Chemical Structure:**

| | |
|---|---|
| **Molecular Weight:** | 252.3 |
| **Melting point, °C:** | 295-298 |
| **Solubility in water, mg/L:** | 14 |
| **pK$_a$:** | 8.3 |
| **Partition coefficient:** | 28.8 (chloroform/water at pH 3.4) |
| **Dose absorption—** | |
| time to peak plasma conc., h: | 4-8 |
| percentage dose absorbed: | 90 |
| **Percentage protein bound:** | 87-93 |
| **Tissue distribution (V$_d$, L/kg):** | 0.5-0.8 |
| **CSF/plasma:** | 0.1 |
| **Brain/plasma:** | 1.2-1.6 |

| Urinary excretion, % daily dose - | | Active | Detectable in Blood |
|---|---|---|---|
| **as unchanged drug:** | 1-5 | yes | yes |
| **as 5-(4-Hydroxyphenyl) -5-phenylhydantoin (HPPH):** | 60-80 | no | yes |
| **as 5-(3,4-Dihydroxyphenyl) -5-phenylhydantoin:** | — | no | no |
| **as 5-(3-O-Methyl -4-hydroxyphenyl)-5- phenylhydantoin:** | — | no | no |

| | Adults | Children |
|---|---|---|
| **Recommended dose, mg/kg:** | 5 | 5-8 |
| **Half-life, h:** | 22 | 18-22 |
| **Time to steady state, d:** | 5-7 | 5-7 |
| **Effective levels, µg/mL:** | 10-20 | 5-20 |
| **Toxic levels, µg/mL:** | >25 | >25 |
| **Steady-state level expected from 1 mg/kg/d, µg/mL:** | 2-3 | 1-2 |

## Bibliography

Pippenger, C.E., Penry, J.K. and Kutt, H. (Eds). *Antiepileptic Drugs: Quantitative Analysis and Interpretation.* Raven Press, New York, NY, 1978.

Hvidberg, E.F., and Dam, M., Clinical pharmacokinetics of anticonvulsants. *Clin. Pharmacokinet.* 1 161-168 (1976).

Richens, A., Clinical pharmacokinetics of phenytoin. *Clin. Pharmacokinet.* 4 153-169 (1979).

Mucklow, J.C. and Dollery, C.T. Compliance with anticonvulsant therapy in a hospital clinic and in the community. *Br. J. Clin. Pharmacol.* 6 75-79 (1978).

## Case History (Pediatric)

This case illustrates the importance of monitoring the concentration of phenytoin in plasma at appropriate intervals, especially when dosages are being altered in an attempt to control the underlying disease without toxic side effects, and when the patient is at a stage of rapid growth and development.

## Case Presentation

H.S., a 10-year-old white girl, was brought to a neurology clinic because of a one-month history of lack of interest in school, lethargy, and a tendency to stumble.

The patient, who lived 240 kilometers from the clinic, had been admitted to the hospital nine months previously because of the sudden onset of seizures. After appropriate investigation, grand mal epilepsy had been diagnosed, and she was started on therapy with phenobarbital. However, this drug led to disabling drowsiness, without controlling the seizures, so that it was discontinued after one month and replaced with phenytoin.

The initial dose of phenytoin was 60 mg twice daily (this total daily dose of 120 mg was equivalent to 4 mg/kg body weight), but in the face of continuing seizures, and a plasma phenytoin concentration of 8.1 mg/L, the dose was increased to 100 mg twice daily (6.7 mg/kg per day). Ten days later, the plasma phenytoin concentration was 13.4 mg/L.

The patient appeared to do very well on this regimen, so was discharged home from the hospital, to be followed by her family physician. However, occasional seizures still occurred, and the patient's family, aware of the beneficial effect of the previous increase in amount of medication, added a second 100-mg capsule to the morning dose of phenytoin (bringing the total daily dose to 300 mg, equivalent to 10 mg/kg).

About a week later, the family realized that the frequency of the patient's seizures had actually increased, and that she was having some difficulty in walking about the house.

The remainder of the history and functional inquiry were noncontributory.

At the time of this examination the girl was seen to be well developed, well nourished, but lethargic, and in no acute distress. Her weight was 30 kg, her height 136 cm. Her vital signs were within normal limits, as were results of the rest of the physical examination, except for the presence of moderate ataxia. There were no physical signs of the onset of puberty.

The concentration of phenytoin in her plasma was found to be 41 mg/L.

## Discussion

In a patient being treated with phenytoin the development of ataxia and, less frequently, the recurrence of seizures are characteristic of phenytoin toxicity. In this case, the diagnosis was confirmed by the finding that the plasma phenytoin concentration was 41 mg/L (usual therapeutic range in children, 5-20 mg/L). How did this situation develop?

In seeking the explanation, one must consider two possible mechanisms: (a) the decreased ability to metabolize a given amount of the drug, that frequently occurs just before the onset of puberty, and (b) saturation of the phenytoin metabolizing pathway. In the present case, it is not possible to attribute the problem exclusively to one or other of these mechanisms and, in fact, it is likely that both are implicated:

(a) It has long been recognized that many drugs are metabolized faster during infancy and childhood than in later life; this shift from the childhood pattern to the adult pattern of drug metabolism usually occurs at or just before puberty. The mechanism of the change is still being actively investigated, but it appears probable that it reflects the result of a competition between drug and sex steroids for the limited capacity of the hepatic microsomal enzyme systems. In the present case, the patient was at an age that suggests that she may have been about to enter puberty, and consequently was decreasing her capacity to metabolize phenytoin.

(b) In adjusting the dosage of phenytoin in an individual patient, it is essential to realize that a change in the dosage and the resulting change in its concentration in plasma are not always linearly related. Thus, at relatively low plasma phenytoin concentrations the rate of metabolism of the drug is proportional to drug concentration (first-order kinetics), but at some point within the therapeutic range (10-20 mg/L) the metabolizing system may become saturated and the rate of metabolism will be unable to increase, regardless of drug concentration (zero-order kinetics). Under these conditions, a relatively small dose increase may lead to a very large change in its circulating concentration. In this patient, whose plasma phenytoin concentration was 13.4 mg/L while she was receiving 200 mg of phenytoin per day, the increase to 300 mg would be more than enough to account for the subsequent toxicity.

## Follow-up

The patient's phenytoin was reduced to 200 mg/day, and within two weeks signs of toxicity had disappeared and the concentration in plasma was 15.2 mg/L. Strict instructions were given to the patient and her family to adhere to the prescribed dosage regimen, and arrangements were made to follow the course of the patient closely in the clinic.

## Bibliography

Wilson, J.T., Special Problems for Drugs Use In Children *Southern Med. J.* 69 779-785 (1976).

Rane, A., and Wilson, J.T., Clinical Pharmacokinetics in Infants and Children. *Clin. Pharmacokinet.* 1 2-24 (1976)

Morselli, P. (Ed.) *Drug Disposition During Development: An Overview.* Spectrum Publications, Inc., New York, NY, 1977.

# 4

# Phenytoin and Isoniazid Coadministration: Two Case Histories

## Henn Kutt, M.D.

These case histories illustrate a clinical problem that occurs in about 15% (12,15,17) of patients who are given isoniazid together with phenytoin in the usual clinical doses. The problem is based on drug-drug interaction in genetically determined susceptible individuals (2). It is easily detected by monitoring phenytoin concentrations in the blood. It is solved by adjusting phenytoin dosage (12). If unrecognized, it may clinically simulate more serious conditions such as a brain tumor.

### Case 1

A 23-year-old white man, weighing 64 kg, started to have generalized tonic-clonic seizures at the age of 17 years. For the past two years, his antiepileptic medication had consisted of 300 mg phenytoin daily. This regimen had reduced the seizure frequency to about one per year and caused no side effects other than modest gum hypertrophy. On regular visits to a seizure clinic, periodic monitoring of circulating phenytoin revealed values between 8 and 13 mg/L.

Three months before admission, the patient started to feel continuously tired, have night sweats, and developed a chronic cough associated with slightly blood-tinged sputum. A roentgenogram of the chest was interpreted as indicating pulmonary tuberculosis and the patient was hospitalized on the chest service.

Sputum examination revealed tuberculosis bacilli and the patient was started on 300 mg of isoniazid with 600 mg rifampin daily; the 300 mg phenytoin daily was continued. About two weeks after the onset of antitubercular chemotherapy, the patient started to complain of episodes of double vision and at the end of the third week he became unsteady. The patient stated that he felt "like being drunk without the benefit of whiskey." Examination revealed marked horizontal nystagmus on lateral gaze, broad-based staggering gait with inability to walk tandem, and some dysmetria in finger-to-nose testing. There was no papilledema. Because of cerebellar signs and symptoms, the provisional clinical diagnoses included cerebellar tuberculoma and

phenytoin intoxication. Further neurological work-up regarding cerebellar mass lesion was contemplated; and the concentration of phenytoin in blood was measured along with liver-function tests and hematological profile. The latter were within normal limits but the phenytoin concentration was 37 mg/L. Thereupon, phenotyping with respect to isoniazid inactivation was carried out. This revealed that the patient was a very slow isoniazid acetylator.

Phenytoin was withheld for two days, then resumed at a dosage of 100 mg daily. The blurred vision and unsteadiness slowly improved and disappeared two weeks later. By that time, the circulating phenytoin had declined to 6 mg/L, whereupon the dosage was increased, first to 125 mg and then to 150 mg daily. This raised and maintained the phenytoin concentration at about 14 mg/L for the duration of antitubercular chemotherapy period. When the latter was completed 14 months later and isoniazid was discontinued, the phenytoin dose had to be increased again to 300 mg daily, to maintain the concentration near 10 mg/L.

### Case 2

A 62-year-old oriental man had pulmonary tuberculosis and had been treated for the past six months with 300 mg of isoniazid and 600 mg rifampin daily. He then had two tonic-clonic seizures in three days, following which antiepileptic therapy was started with 300 mg of phenytoin daily.

Four weeks later, the patient started to complain about blurred vision and difficulties with reading his newspaper. By the sixth week he became unsteady on his feet and frequently bumped into objects while walking. Examination then revealed mild lethargy, nystagmus on lateral gaze and broad-based gait with inability to stand in tamdem position. Finger-to-nose and heel-to-shin tests were performed with overshooting and inaccuracy, but the rest of the results of neurological examination were normal.

Laboratory studies at that time revealed normal liver functions except for a mild increase in aspartate- and alanine aminotransferase activities, but the circulatory phenytoin concentration was 44 mg/L. The clinical suspicion of phenytoin intoxication was thus confirmed.

Phenytoin was withheld for three days and then begun with 100 mg daily. Phenytoin in the blood de-

*Dr. Kutt is in the Depts. of Neurology and Pharmacology, Cornell University Medical College, New York, NY.*

clined, the signs and symptoms of intoxication diminished, and by the 12th day the neurological status returned to normal. The phenytoin dose was later readjusted to 200 mg daily, which maintained a concentration in the low teens for the rest of the therapy period. No seizures occurred.

## Comment

Phenytoin therapy is usually started with a dose of 300 mg daily (4-6 mg/kg) in adults and 5-8 mg/kg in children. The dose is then later adjusted to meet the individual patient's need, which is best accomplished under the guidance of monitoring phenytoin concentration in the blood (6,7,10,13,14). Renal elimination of phenytoin is preceded by hepatic microsomal action in which aromatic hydroxylation followed by conjugation is the major pathway (9). If the biotransformation of phenytoin is inhibited, the parent compound accumulates in the organism, with ensuing intoxication.

The development of signs and symptoms of phenytoin intoxication in individuals receiving the usual clinical doses of both phenytoin and isoniazid was first reported from the Monson State School for Epileptics in 1962 (17). The epileptic residents of that institution had been given isoniazid as tuberculosis prophylaxis. About 11% of individuals receiving the combined medication became unsteady. At that time, this was thought to be due to an increased sensitivity to phenytoin, perhaps within the brain cell. Since then, other clinical studies in which phenytoin was monitored in the blood revealed that an accumulation of phenytoin was provoked by isoniazid and that this was the mechanism of phenytoin intoxication (2,12,15). The extent to which isoniazid caused phenytoin accumulation, however, varied in different individuals from nearly no change to a three-to four-fold increase in the phenytoin in the blood from the previous maintenance concentration. The reason for such variation of response between different individuals was found to be related to the individual's phenotype for isoniazid inactivation: the slow isoniazid acetylators accumulated more phenytoin than the fast acetylators and phenytoin concentrations were greatest in the slowest isoniazid acetylators (2,12).

Isoniazid is inactivated in the organism by acetylation, catalyzed by enzymes present in the soluble fraction of the liver cells. The general population appears to be divided into genetically determined two phenotype groups: "fast" and "slow" acetylators (8,18); most recent studies even indicate the presence of a third, the "intermediate", group (3). The determination of isoniazid acetylator phenotype is usually carried out by giving a test-dose of isoniazid (5-10 mg/kg) and taking a blood sample at a set interval (4-6 hour); or by taking serial blood samples and calculating the apparent half-life of isoniazid (8). Sulfamethazine, which also under-

goes acetylation, may be used instead of isoniazid to determine the acetylator phenotype (3,18). A test-dose, usually 20 mg/kg of sulfamethazine, is given and blood and urine samples collected. Sulfamethazine concentration is then determined by using Bratton and Marshall diazotizing system (1); or fluorometrically after combining sulfamethazine with fluorescamine (4). Those individuals with a high concentration of the test-drug at the set interval or with a long half-life are termed "slow acetylators", those with a low concentration of test-drug or a short half-life are the "fast acetylators". Slow acetylators usually have relatively high isoniazid concentrations for several hours after dosing and they are generally the ones who develop complications of isoniazid therapy, such as systemic lupus erythematosus (SLE) or pyridoxine deficiency syndromes including peripheral neuropathy (5). The fast acetylators, on the other hand, are subject to liver damage (16).

In vitro studies have shown that isoniazid is a potent inhibitor of phenytoin biotransformation (11). A concentration of 0.1 mmol of isoniazid per liter caused a 50% noncompetitive inhibition of phenytoin hydroxylation by rat liver microsomal preparations; a 0.01 mmol/L concentration inhibited it by 15%. The exact mechanism of this inhibition is not clear, because phenytoin hydroxylation is a function of microsomal enzymes whereas isoniazid acetylation occurs in the soluble fraction. It may be postulated that utilization of common cofactors is involved; interference with glucuronidation may occur; or it could be an effect analogous to that of general enzyme inhibitors such as disulfiram.

Rifampin does not affect phenytoin kinetics but may act as an inducer of metabolism of some other drugs (19).

It appears then that the individuals who are very slow isoniazid acetylators are candidates for significant phenytoin accumulation during combined therapy and cannot tolerate the usual clinical doses of phenytoin. They usually constitute 10-20% of all patients on such regimen. It is therefore advisable to ascertain the isoniazid acetylator phenotype of a patient before starting the combined therapy. As such phenotyping is not routinely available, the alternative commonly used approach is to monitor phenytoin in the blood at least weekly after beginning the co-administration of these drugs. If by the sixth week there is no increase, or only a modest one, in phenytoin concentration, there is little reason for further concern, because the patient apparently is a fast or intermediate acetylator of isoniazid. In contrast, continuous increase during the initial weeks of combined therapy indicates very slow isoniazid acetylation and the need to decrease the phenytoin dosage. The new dosage is then titrated, based on phenytoin blood levels until the concentration is stabilized in the desired range.

## References

1. Bratton, A.C. and Marshall, E.K., A new coupling component for sulfanilamide determination. *J. Biol. Chem* **128**, 537-550 (1939).
2. Brennan, R.W., Dehejia, H., Kutt, H. et al., Diphenylhydantoin intoxication attendant to slow inactivation of isoniazid. *Neurology* **20**, 687-693 (1970).
3. Chapron, D.J., Kramer, P.A. and Mercik, S.A., Kinetic discrimination of three sulfamethazine acetylation phenotypes. *Clin. Pharmacol. Ther.* **27**, 104-113 (1980).
4. de Silva, J.A.F. and Strojny, N., Spectrofluorometric determination of pharmaceuticals containing aromatic or aliphatic primary amino groups as their fluorescamine (fluram) derivatives. *Anal. Chem.* **47**, 714-718 (1975).
5. Drayer, D.E. and Reidenberg, M.M., Clinical consequences of polymorphic acetylation of basic drugs. *Clin. Pharmacol. Ther.* **22**, 251-258 (1977).
6. Eadie, M.J., Plasma level monitoring of anticonvulsants. *Clin. Pharmacol.* **1**, 52-66 (1976).
7. Eadie, M.J. and Tyrer, J.H., *Anticonvulsant Therapy*. Churchill Livingstone, Edinburgh, London and New York, pp 63-82 (1980).
8. Evans, D.A.P., Storey, P.B., Wittstadt, R.B., and Manley, K.A., The determination of the isoniazid inacticator phenotype *Am. Rev. Respir. Dis.* **82**, 853-856 (1960).
9. Glazko, A.J., Antiepileptic drugs: biotransformation, metabolism and serum half-life, *Epilepsia* (Amst.) **16**, 367-391 (1975).
10. Hvidberg, E.F. and Dam, M., Clinical pharmacokinetics of anticonvulsants. *Clin. Pharmacokin.* **1**, 161-188 (1976).
11. Kutt, H., Verebely, K., and McDowell, F., Inhibition of diphenylhydantoin metabolism in rats and in rat liver microsomes by antitubercular drugs. *Neurology* **18**, 706-710 (1968).
12. Kutt, H., Brennan, R., Dehejia, H., and Verebely, K., Diphenylhydantoin intoxication: A complication of isoniazid therapy. *Am. Rev. Respir. Dis.* **101**, 729-732 (1970).
13. Kutt, H. and Penry, J.K., Usefulness of blood levels of antiepileptic drugs. *Arch. Neurol.* **31**, 283-288 (1974).
14. Lund, L., Anticonvulsant effect of diphenylhydantoin relative to plasma levels. *Arch. Neurol.* **31**, 289-294 (1974).
15. Miller, R.R., Porter, J., and Greenblatt, D.J., Clinical importance of the interaction of phenytoin and isoniazid. *Chest* **75**, 356-358 (1979).
16. Mitchell, J.R., Thorgeirsson, U.P., Black, M., Timbrell, J.A., et al. Increased incidence of isoniazid hepatitis in rapid acetylators: Possible relation to hydrazine metabolites. *Clin. Pharmacol. Ther.* **18**, 70-79 (1975).
17. Murray, F.J., Outbreak of unexpected reactions among epileptics taking isoniazid. *Am. Rev. Respir. Dis.* **86**, 729-732 (1962).
18. Olsen, W., Micele, J. and Weber, W., Dose-dependent changes in sulfamethazine kinetics in rapid and slow isoniazid acetylators. *Clin. Pharmacol. Ther.* **23**, 204-211 (1978).
19. Twum-Barima, Y. and Carruthers, S.G., Evaluation of rifampin-quinidine interaction. *Clin. Pharmacol. Ther.* **27**, 290 (1980).

# 5

# Phenytoin: Methods for Analysis

**Dan Haidukewych, Ph.D.**

Phenytoin (5,5-diphenylhydantoin) was introduced in 1938 as a major drug in the treatment of seizures. Currently, it is the most widely used anticonvulsant for treating all varieties of epilepsy except petit mal and myoclonic seizures.

In the past, dosage was regulated on the basis of giving the drug until signs of toxicity appeared, then decreasing the dose enough to avoid toxicity and, it was hoped, adequately control seizures. In the absence of methods for determination of drugs in biological fluids and of an appreciation of therapeutically effective concentrations this approach necessarily generated multiple drug use, remnants of which are more persistent than is desirable.

Along with the development of new and more potent agents has come understanding of the relation between seizure control and concentration of anticonvulsants in plasma. This relation was demonstrated for phenytoin in 1960 (*1*). The development of methods for determining phenytoin (as well as other common anticonvulsants) in plasma parallels the development of new analytical techniques.

## Methods of Historical Interest

### Spectrophotometric Procedures

The first major breakthrough in methodology came in 1956, with simultaneous reports of spectrophotometric and colorimetric methods. With both methods the problem of interference by phenobarbital was clearly recognized, and subsequent efforts were directed at eliminating it. The colorimetric method involves initial extraction of the drug from acidified plasma with chloroform. The extract is then subjected to a three-plate countercurrent extraction. The clean extract is then subjected to quantitative aromatic nitration of phenytoin, reduction of the nitro group with stannous chloride to the amine, and diazotization and coupling with Bratton-Marshall reagent to form a highly colored azo dye. This procedure is highly specific (*2*) but time consuming. Nevertheless, its use in the decade after its development added considerably to our knowledge

*Dr. Haidukewych is the Clinical Chemistry and Pharmacology Laboratory Director at the Epilepsy Center of Michigan, Detroit, MI 48201.*

concerning the relation between phenytoin dosage and concentration in plasma.

### Thin-Layer Chromatography

After initial attempts to use thin-layer chromatography (TLC) to (at best) semiquantitatively estimate phenytoin, perhaps the most exacting TLC studies to give a fair degree of accuracy were reported in 1971 (*3*). Phenytoin was extracted from plasma, concentrated by evaporation, and subjected to TLC on silica gel plates. After the phenytoin spot was scraped off, the colorimetric procedure was applied directly to the scrapings.

### Benzophenone-Extraction Procedure

A novel approach to phenytoin assays was introduced in 1965: benzophenone, formed from phenytoin by heating with alkali and bromine, was separated by steam distillation, then extracted from the distillate with an organic solvent and its ultraviolet absorbance measured. The advantage of this procedure is that neither phenobarbital nor most other drugs interfere, and blanks prepared with normal plasma are low. However, the orginal procedure required such large volumes of blood that many modifications were made before the technique was suitable for clinical application (*4*).

For a fascinating panorama of these early developments for phenytoin assays the reader is directed to an excellent monograph (*5*).

## Major Current Methods

### Gas-Liquid Chromatography (GLC)

The laborious wet-chemistry techniques generated unprecedented activity to develop analytical procedures that would be both accurate and precise, sensitive, technically easy, rapid, and inexpensive. The application of GLC to anticonvulsant drug analysis provides an example of this effort. In the last 10 years, more than 100 papers have described methods for the gas-chromatographic determination of antiepileptic drugs. A recent comprehensive systematic review (*6*) lists exhaustive information on the following: anticonvulsant determined, internal standard, amount of sample, extraction procedure, preparation of derivative, sample injection, detection, column support and temperature, and stationary phase.

An integrated method with use of six internal standards for GLC determination of seven antiepileptic agents in 1 mL of plasma has recently been published (7).

Simultaneous determination of the "panel of drugs" by GLC predominates currently, so few papers in the last 10 years give procedures that are specific for phenytoin (8). Therapy with phenytoin alone is uncommon. Therefore, the GLC procedure for phenytoin is most useful when simultaneous determination of its metabolite, 5-(4-hydroxyphenyl)-5-phenylhydantoin (HPPH) is needed (9). In cases of unsuspected noncompliance or for occasional patients who are either fast or slow phenytoin metabolizers, determination of HPPH can be most helpful and can avoid frustration of both physicians and laboratory personnel.

The disadvantages of GLC methods are: (a) difficulty in maintaining reproducible extraction; (b) the need for highly trained and dedicated analysts; (c) the need for extensive specimen extraction and clean-up procedures leads to attempted short cuts that negate the value of results; (d) derivatization is usually required for better volatility, sensitivity, and reduction of peak tailing; (e) only thermally stable and volatile analytes can be used; and (f) urgently needed results cannot be provided in emergencies.

## "High-Performance" Liquid Chromatography (HPLC)

One of the most significant advances in clinical laboratory practices in recent years has been the application of HPLC to therapeutic drug monitoring (10). It obviates most of the disadvantages listed above.

Most prominent advantages of HPLC are: sensitivity down to 10-20 ng/L is often achievable, an impossibility with GLC when flame-ionization detectors are used, and HPLC methods (including extraction steps) are readily automated, reducing analyst error and time. The thermally mild conditions used in HPLC make the method ideal for metabolite determination.

Some disadvantages of HPLC are: (a) the analyte in question must absorb light, fluoresce, or be electroactive, because most commonly, spectrophotometric, fluorometric, and amperometric detectors are used; and (b) administrators hesitate to spend over $30,000 for an automated HPLC system when fully amortized GLC equipment (usually more than one) meets the immediate needs.

Short column life used to be a major disadvantage of HPLC. A recent development, which has significantly reduced column costs and increased column life, is the advent of radial compression columns (11).

There is no doubt that HPLC will retain a prominent place in routine as well as research laboratories.

## Homogenous Enzyme Immunoassay (EMIT®)

The introduction of the EMIT technique into clinical laboratories has been hailed as the most significant breakthrough in therapeutic drug monitoring. This is especially true for small laboratories.

The technique is based on competitive protein binding with an enzyme as label and an antibody as the binding protein. When the enzyme-labeled drug becomes bound to an antibody to the drug, the activity of the enzyme is decreased. Drug in the patient's specimen competes with the enzyme-labeled drug for the antibody and thereby decreases the antibody-induced inactivation of the enzyme. Thus the enzyme activity correlates directly with the concentrations of the drug.

The most significant advantages are the simplicity of the procedure, its speed, and its adaptability to routine laboratory operations. Emergency results can be provided without undue effort.

The EMIT technique has been automated with the KA-150 Kinetic Analyzer, the CentrifiChem centrifugal analyzer, the ABA-100 bichromatic analyzer, the Gilford 3500, the DuPoint Automatic Clinical Analyzer, the Chemetrics Analyzer, the Multistat III, and the Aminco Rotochem II. The technique will continue to be adapted to use with other clinical analyzers, and reagent cost and analyst time will be reduced considerably.

The major disadvantages of EMIT are the high reagent cost and its inapplicability to simultaneous analysis for a series of drugs.

With the EMIT technique caution should be exercised when one approaches low level of reagent in the bottle. The "Bottom of the Bottle Effect" produces values that are at least 30% higher than GLC (12). To correct for this unexplained phenomenon, when a level of approximately 1 mL is reached, the left-overs should be added to another set of appropriate reagents with *identical* lot number. After mixing the contents, the control and at least one earlier specimen should be checked before further analysis is attempted.

A potentially serious disadvantage has surfaced on a recent report (13) showing that for uremic patients, EMIT plasma phenytoin values significantly exceed values by GLC or HPLC.

The vendor of EMIT reagents tested the extent of HPPH and HPPH-glucuronide cross-reactivity and reported (*14*) that three factors influence the apparent increase in phenytoin observed in uremic sera: (*a*) interpatient variability in phenytoin disposition; (*b*) lot-to-lot variation of the EMIT reagent response to HPPH and HPPH-glucuronide; and (*c*) the concentration of phenytoin and its metabolites in a particular sample.

Knowledge that the patient is uremic would be grounds not to use the EMIT technique. On the other hand, determination of plasma phenytoin for uremic patients is of no value; rather, free phenytoin should be determined.

A cursory look at data generated by AACC-TDM Program shows that 90% of the reporting laboratories use EMIT, GLC, or HPLC to measure phenytoin.

## Other Current Methods

### Radioimmunoassay (RIA)

Phenytoin, as well as other anticonvulsants, can be determined by RIA (*15*). Although very sensitive, this technique has the same disadvantages as EMIT that simultaneous assay of drugs in patients who are on multiple drug regimens is not possible. A liquid-scintillation counter is required. Specialized RIA laboratories provide excellent service, but the cost per analysis is high and RIA has not been popular.

### Gas Chromatography-Mass Spectrometry (GC/MS)

The most accurate and sensitive means of phenytoin determination is GC/MS (*16*). Nevertheless, because of the expense of the equipment, this technique has made no significant impact on routine therapeutic drug monitoring.

### Fluorescent Immunoassay (FIA)

FIA methods have recently been reviewed (*17, 18*) and methods specific for phenytoin reported (*19-21*). The impact of this latest addition to the clinical laboratory's choice of methods remains to be established.

The choice of any one of the current methods depends on expertise of laboratory personnel, existing equipment, and workload. The recent development of practical methods for determining the pharmacologically active portion (i.e., the free drug) in plasma suggests that in the decade ahead those methods that are most accurate and precise in the 10- to 100-fold more sensitive range will predominate. Currently, the most common methods applicable to free drug determination are RIA, HPLC, and GLC with nitrogen-phosphorus detector (*22*).

## References

1. Buchthal, F., Svensmark, O., and Schillar, P.J., Clinical and electroencephalographic correlation with serum levels of diphenylhydantoin. *Arch. Neurol.* **2**, 624-630 (1960).
2. Kristensen, M., Molholm Hansen, J., Hansen, O.E., and Lund, V., Sources of error in the determination of phenytoin (Dilantin®) by Svensmark and Kristensen's method. *Acta. Neurol. Scand.* **43**, 447-450 (1967).
3. Simon, G.E., Jatlow, P.I., Seligson, H.T., and Seligson, D., Measurement of 5, 5-diphenylhydantoin in blood using thin layer chromatography. *Am. J. Clin. Pathol.* **55**, 145-151 (1971).
4. Morselli, P.L., An improved technique for routine determination of diphenylhydantoin in plasma and tissues. *Clin. Chim. Acta* **28**, 37-40 (1970).
5. Glazko, A.J., Diphenylhydantoin-chemistry and methods for determination. In *Antiepileptic Drugs*, D.M. Woodbury et al., Eds., Raven Press, New York, N.Y., 1972, pp 103-112.
6. Rambeck, B., and Meijer, J.W.A., Gas chromatographic methods for determination of antiepileptic drugs: A systematic review. *Ther. Drug. Monitor.* **2**, 385-396 (1980).
7. Patton, J.R., Hershey, A.E., Bius, D.L., and Dudley, K.H., Integrated method for the gas chromatographic determination of antiepileptic drugs in human plasma. *Ther. Drug. Monitor.* **2**, 397-409 (1980).
8. Gordos, J., Schaublin, J., and Spring, P., Microdetermination of plasma diphenylhydantoin by gas-liquid chromatography. *J. Chromatogr.* **143**, 171-181 (1977) and references therein.
9. Estas, A., and Dumont, P.A., Simultaneous determination of 5, 5-diphenylhydantoin and 5-(*p*-hydroxyphenyl)-5-phenylhydantoin in serum, urine and tissues by gas-liquid chromatography, after flash heater methylation. *J. Chromatogr.* **82**, 307-314 (1973).
10. Kabra, P.M., MacDonald, D.M., and Marton, L.J., A simultaneous high-performance liquid chromatographic analysis of anticonvulsants and their metabolites. *J. Anal. Toxicol.* **2**, 127-133 (1978).
11. Soldin, S.J., High performance liquid chromatographic analysis of anticonvulsant drugs using radial compression columns. *Clin. Biochem.* **13**, 99-101 (1980).

12. Nandedkar, A.K.N., Kutt, H., and Fairclough, Jr., G.F., Correlation of the "EMIT" with a gas-liquid chromatographic method for determination of antiepileptic drugs in plasma. *Clin. Toxicology* **12**, 483-494 (1978).

13. Nandedkar, A.K.N., Williamson, R., Kutt, H., and Fairclough, Jr., G.F., A comparison of plasma phenytoin level determinations by EMIT and gas-liquid chromatography in patients with renal insufficiency. *Ther. Drug Monitor.* **2**, 427-430 (1980).

14. Aldwin, L., and Kabakoff, D.S., Metabolite interference in homogenous enzyme immunoassay of phenytoin. *Clin. Chem.* **27**, 770-771 (1981).

15. Cook, C.E., Christensen, H.D., et al., Radio-immunoassay of anticonvulsants: Phenytoin, phenobarbital, and primidone. In *Quantitative Analytic Studies in Epilepsy*, P. Kellaway and I.S. Petersen, Eds., Raven Press, New York, N.Y., 1976.

16. Horning, M.G., et al., Anticonvulsant drug monitoring by GC-MS-COM techniques. *J. Chromatogr. Sci.* **12**, 630-631 (1974).

17. Soini, E., and Hemmila, I., Fluoroimmunoassay: Present status and key problems. *Clin. Chem.* **25**, 351-353 (1979).

18. O'Donnell, C.M., and Suffin, S.C., Fluoresence immunoassays. *Anal. Chem.* **51**, 33A-40A (1979).

19. Wong, R.C., et al., Substrate-labeled fluorescent immunoassay for phenytoin in human serum. *Clin. Chem.* **25**, 686-691 (1979).

20. Wong, R.C., et al., A comparison of serum phenytoin determination by the substrate-labeled fluorescent immunoassay with gas chromatography, liquid chromatography, radioimmunoassay and "EMIT", *Clin. Chim. Acta* **100**, 65-69 (1980).

21. McGregor, A.R., et al., Polarisation fluoro-immunoassay of phenytoin. *Clin. Chim. Acta* **83**, 161-166 (1978).

22. Joern, W.A., Gas-chromatographic assay of free phenytoin in ultrafiltrates of plasma: Test of a new filtration apparatus and specimen stability. *Clin. Chem.* **27**, 417-421 (1981).

# 6

# Clinical Pharmacology of Phenobarbital and Primidone: A Review

**Dorothy D. Schottelius, Ph.D.**

## Introduction

The antiepileptic drugs provide us with an excellent example of the importance that therapeutic drug monitoring and the application of pharmacological principles can have on the treatment of a patient. From approximately 1912 to 1970 the utilization of these drugs in the treatment of the epileptic patient was based completely on trial and error, with only clinical signs for guides—continuing seizures or toxic manifestations—at recommended doses. This means of adjustment of therapeutic regimens often resulted in addition of another drug, failure to control seizures, or control seizures only with adverse side-effects. The availability of assay procedures has made possible a more rational approach to the treatment of the epilepsies and has stimulated many investigations into the pharmacology of the antiepileptic drugs. Application of information concerning the clinical pharmacology of the drugs will enhance the usefulness and benefits of drug monitoring in the case of the epileptic patient.

The clinical pharmacology of two antiepileptic drugs, phenobarbital and primidone, will be considered in one review because of their closely related chemical structures (Figure 1). Phenobarbital is a derivative of barbituric acid and primidone may be viewed as a congener in which a carbonyl oxygen is replaced by two hydrogen ions.

Phenobarbital, the first effective organic anti-epileptic agent, was marketed in 1912 and was the major drug for the treatment of epilepsy until the late 1930s. The drug continues to have widespread use because of its relative safety, its relative inexpensiveness and its well documented effectiveness against many types of seizures.

Primidone, a deoxybarbiturate, was synthesized in 1949 and was marketed in 1954. It is effective for the treatment of all types of seizures with the exception of absence.

Further references concerning the chemical synthesis of both of these compounds may be found in the bibliographies contained in Vida and Gerry (1) and Rall and Schleifer (2).

The following topics will be discussed for pheno-

barbital and primidone: absorption, distribution, biotransformation, excretion, relation of plasma drug concentrations to clinical control, toxicity, and drug interactions.

## Phenobarbital

### Absorption

Primary sites of absorption after the oral administration of phenobarbital are the stomach and small intestine. Because this drug is a weak acid, $pK_a$ 7.3, it is mostly unionized in the acidic gastric secretions and capable of passing through lipid membranes. The amount that may be absorbed through the gastric mucosa is highly variable and depends on the degree of gastric acidity, the rate of gastric emptying, and the solubility of the drug in water. In the small intestine the pH rises considerably and absorption might be expected to slow with the increase in the ionized fraction. Apparently, maximum absorption occurs in the small intestine between pH 6.5 and 7.5 and it has been speculated that protein binding in the mucosal membrane of the small intestine is the critical factor rather than the degree of ionization. Indirect evidence supports the assumption that phenobarbital is nearly completely absorbed in the adult in doses ranging from 0.5 to 3.2 mg/kg. Calculations of plasma concentrations of phenobarbital have agreed very well with the actual values found.

Although textbooks often state that the rate of absorption is rapid, only a few quantitative studies have been performed. The rate of absorption is determined by several factors: $pK_a$, pH of the medium, solubility, gastric emptying, rapidity of transit through the gastrointestinal tract, interaction with the mucosal membrane, presence of drugs that may affect circulation and motility of the gastrointestinal tract, and even

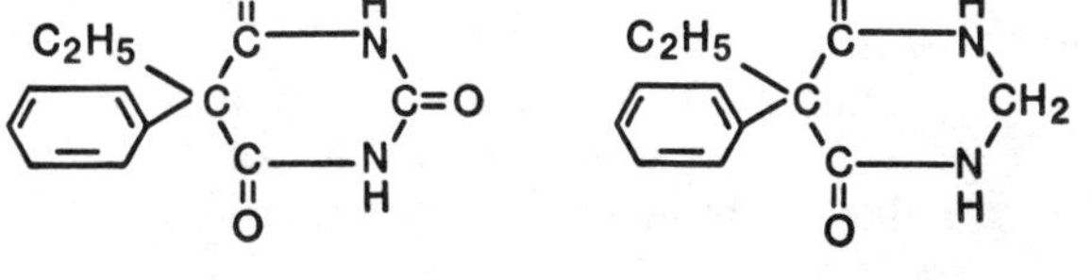

*Dr. Schottelius is an Assistant Professor of Neurology at the University of Iowa, Iowa City, IA 52242.*

**PHENOBARBITAL**          **PRIMIDONE**

**Fig. 1. Chemical formulas of phenobarbital and primidone.**

the size of the dose. When 750 mg of phenobarbital was administered to young adults maximum plasma concentrations occurred within 9 to 12 h; however, two other studies utilizing a much smaller dose (200 and 30 mg) revealed peak plasma concentrations 3.5-4 hours after dose. Infants and children have the same rapid absorption, with peak concentrations generally attained 2-4 hours after oral dose.

Intramuscular doses of phenobarbital may be preferable in acute treatment since peak concentrations are attained somewhat more rapidly (approximately 2 hours after injection).

Complete references to these absorption studies, as well as studies of distribution and excretion, may be obtained by consulting reviews listed in references 3, 4 and 5.

## Distribution

Phenobarbital is present in high concentrations in the more vascular organs of the body shortly after absorption. Because the drug has a significant unionized, lipid-soluble fraction at the pH of plasma, it is capable of rapidly diffusing from blood into other tissues. The plasma concentration and thus the tissue distribution of phenobarbital are particularly sensitive to blood pH changes; with lower pH the plasma concentration is decreased (increased unionized, diffusible phenobarbital); conversely, the phenobarbital concentration increased with increasing pH. Metabolic and respiratory alkalosis and acidosis can thus cause important shifts in the tissue concentrations of this drug.

Despite the rapid distribution of this drug into other tissues, it is presumed from animal experiments that phenobarbital enters the human brain slowly; consequently when this drug is used to treat status epilepticus, immediate efficacy cannot be expected.

Protein binding occurs in both plasma and tissue proteins, and brain tissue concentrations more closely reflect the concentration in cerebrospinal fluid than total plasma concentrations. Approximately 45-50% of phenobarbital is bound to plasma proteins, chiefly albumin.

The actual volume of distribution ($V_d$) is somewhat variable, averaging 0.7 L/kg; the range was 0.36 to 0.73 in normal adults after oral or intramuscular doses.

Phenobarbital can cross the placental barrier and enter the fetus. Distribution in the fetus appears to be similar to that in the adult. Phenobarbital also crosses the blood-milk barrier.

## Biotransformation

As with other drugs containing a phenyl ring, phenobarbital is hydroxylated in the *para* position to form *p*-hydroxyphenobarbital. The liver is apparently the sole organ concerned with the metabolism of this drug. This compound, and its glucuronide conjugate, appears to be the most common metabolite in man. There has been no isolation of a sulfate ester in human urine. The data on excretion of unchanged phenobarbital, *p*-hydroxyphenobarbital and the glucuronide clearly indicate that the fate of the drug has not been fully accounted for by these three compounds. In various studies the sum has been reported to be 42%, 25% and 50% of the dose. Recent reports indicate the presence of a diol structure and *N*-hydroxyphenobarbital (now presumed to be phenobarbital *N*-β-D glucopyranoside) in human urine. Other metabolites have also been suggested, but the amount and significance remain to be clarified; clearly the complete fate of phenobarbital remains to be elucidated in man. It has been shown that *p*-hydroxyphenobarbital has no pharmacological activity and the same is probably also true for the other metabolites.

Interestingly, phenobarbital, generally recognized as a powerful enzyme inducer of the cytochrome P-450 system, has little effect on its own metabolism. The serum half-life is apparently shorter after a single dose than after repeated doses (95 versus 150 hours) and there is no alteration in the elimination rate after repeated doses.

## Excretion

The half-life of phenobarbital is the longest of any of the commonly used antiepileptic drugs, ranging from 53 to 140 h in adults. The half-life in infants and children is somewhat shorter. Neonates, however, exhibit a somewhat prolonged half-life. Between 10 and 30% of the drug is excreted unchanged. The clearance of the drug is increases markedly with urinary flow. Clearance can be increased from 2-3 mL/min to 4.3 to 7.5 mL/min with diuresis. The pH of the urine will also alter the clearance and a change in urinary pH from 6.1 to 8.0 increases clearance to 9.8 mL/min. It can be readily concluded from this information and the prior discussion of tissue levels that increasing the plasma pH by infusing or ingesting sodium bicarbonate would increase the removal of phenobarbital from the tissues and increase the excretion of the drug from the body; this procedure is valuable in cases of intoxication.

The renal clearances of the metabolites have not been measured but various physical factors would suggest that they are not reabsorbed from the kidney.

## Concentration in Plasma and Clinical Control

The frequently quoted therapeutic concentration for phenobarbital is between 10 and 40 mg/L (10-40 μg/mL; conversion factor 4.306 from μg to μmol). It should be remembered that therapeutic concentration is a statistical concept and some patients will be seizure-free with levels below 10 mg/L and therefore will not need a higher dose of phenobarbital. Various studies show a significant increase in therapeutic efficiency when the plasma level has been above 10 mg/L but only a slight increase in efficacy when the levels are increased above 40 mg/L.

The dose necessary to achieve a steady state concentration is somewhat more predictable with phenobarbital than with other antiepileptic drugs and in adults each mg/kg/day gives a plasma level of approximately 10 mg/L (steady state is achieved in 16-21 days). For children doses need to be approximately double the dose for adults to achieve the same steady state plasma concentration. The transition to adult values of plasma clearance may be abrupt as children reach puberty and there may be problems in maintaining a stable plasma concentration at that time.

The upper limit of the therapeutic range is somewhat difficult to determine. The adverse effects are difficult to evaluate as some individuals remain ambulatory and do not complain even with levels of 80 mg/L. Recent investigations have shown impairment of cognitive and adaptive abilities, even though the individuals had no complaint of sedation. Short and long term memory may also be affected in a dose-dependent manner. Future research must be done to allow treatment with this drug to be guided not only by relating plasma concentrations to seizure control but also to subtle but definite subclinical toxicities. See reference 6 for additional references.

## Toxicity

As mentioned in the previous section, adverse changes may occur with chronic use even with doses that produce plasma concentrations within the therapeutic range. High plasma concentrations cause neurological signs including nystagmus, dysarthria, incoordination, and ataxia. Upon initiation of therapy patients will complain of sedation during the first few days. Paradoxically, in children and the very elderly, phenobarbital may produce insomnia and hyperkinetic activity, but these findings may not be dose-related phenomena. Frank overdose with high drug concentrations produces the usual symptoms, progressing to stupor and coma. The severity of the symptoms and central nervous system depression is much greater in the drug-naive patient, in whom a concentration of 80 mg/L is potentially lethal. Sufficiently high concentrations may lead to depression of cardio-respiratory function and death.

Phenobarbital as a sole drug is particularly benign in its likelihood of producing serious hematological changes. However, megaloblastic anemia, folate deficiency and decrease in production of vitamin K-dependent clotting factors have occurred.

Phenobarbital is a potent inducer of hepatic microsomal enzymes which can lead to enhanced metabolism of other drugs. The drug is hepatotoxic only in unusually susceptible individuals. Hereditary acute porphyria can be exacerbated if phenobarbital is used.

Hypersensitivity reactions can cause various types of skin reactions, usually maculopapular, morbilliform or scarlatiniform rashes that fade rapidly when the drug is stopped. More serious reactions may include eosinophilia and fever. There have been reports of fatalities from sensitivity to phenobarbital.

Abrupt discontinuation of phenobarbital may lead to withdrawal symptoms, especially after chronic use of high doses. Even though the drug has a long half-life, it should be tapered rather than abruptly withdrawn.

## Drug Interactions

Since many patients are treated with a combination of antiepileptic drugs, the interaction of phenobarbital with these agents is clinically important. The addition of phenobarbital to a regimen of phenytoin may cause the phenytoin concentration to increase, decrease or remain unaltered in an individual patient. We have noted that when patients are withdrawn from phenobarbital (especially if the plasma concentrations are quite high) their phenytoin concentrations also decrease and both drugs may reach subtherapeutic levels at the same time, resulting in seizure exacerbation; therefore it is advisable to closely monitor plasma concentrations (Schottelius and Fincham, unpublished). The addition of valproic acid to a regimen of phenobarbital has resulted in rapid marked increases in plasma concentrations of phenobarbital and clinical intoxication.

The influence of phenobarbital on the metabolism of other drugs has usually been to decrease their plasma concentration and their activity. This can cause bleeding problems with anticoagulant drugs if the phenobarbital is stopped without altering the anticoagulant dose. With other drug combinations phenobarbital can increase the level of metabolites to a toxic concentration with resulting symptoms.

Additional discussions of phenobarbital interactions may be found in *Antiepileptic Drugs*, 2nd Edition (see references).

## Summary

Phenobarbital, the oldest antiepileptic drug still in use in clinical practice, is an effective and relatively safe compound in the treatment of seizures. It has a long half-life (90-150 h), the therapeutic range is relatively broad (10-40 mg/L). The drug is well absorbed when given by oral and intramuscular routes. Plasma protein binding (~50%) does not play a significant role in the distribution of this drug, and it is widely distributed in the body. The dose:plasma ratio of this drug is predictable with each 1 mg/kg dose resulting in approximately a 10 mg/L drug concentration in adults. Two-fold higher doses are required in children. The drug is excreted unchanged as *p*-hydroxyphenobarbital **and a glucuronide conjugate of that** metabolite; the relative proportions of these products are partly pH dependent.

## Primidone
### Absorption

Several chemical factors may influence the rate and **extent of absorption, including its relative molecular mass (218.25), its neutral properties, and its** solubility in water (600 mg/L at 37° C). The latter appears to be the only factor that might alter a predictable rapid rate of absorption. Gastric and intestinal absorption have been studied in a variety of laboratory animals; in all instances the compound was rapidly absorbed after oral administration, peak concentrations occurring from 0.5 to 1 h after dose. The rate and extent of **absorption in humans have not been completely investi**gated. Peak plasma concentrations have been determined after various single and multiple doses. Low single doses (500 mg) peak in 2.5 h, whereas higher doses (750 mg) prolonged the peak time (4.2 h). Multiple doses on chronic administration were found to prolong time to peak plasma concentrations as much as 5.5-fold. A low single dose of 125 mg was approximately 60% absorbed in 30 min with a plasma concentration of 3.6 mg/L at that time.

From these indirect studies it would appear that primidone is rapidly and completely absorbed from the gastrointestinal tract and that initial therapy may result in high plasma concentrations very rapidly. Therefore this drug must be started at low doses and gradually increased to the effective dose to avoid side-effects. Tablet disintegration and solubility are apparently the dominant features of the rate and extent of absorption of primidone.

### Distribution

Distribution studies in man are also incomplete. From animal investigations utilizing intravenous administration there appears to be a rapid distribution into tissues. Peak brain concentrations have been found in 1 to 2 hours following a single oral dose to animals; the brain to plasma ratios were approximately 0.56. Data from human brains indicate an average brain to plasma ratio of 0.87 after multiple doses. Primidone has also been found in muscle, skin, and bone, but the distribution correlates poorly with concentration in plasma. The cerebrospinal fluid to plasma ratio has been reported from 0.53 to 1.13. We have shown that this ratio varies markedly and is dependent on the dose-sample interval (*7,10*).

Transplacental passage of primidone has been demonstrated in humans and this compound also has been found in breast milk.

The volume of distribution in humans has been given as 1 L/kg but more recent evidence would indicate the value is 0.6 L/kg (*7*).

The drug appears to be variably bound to plasma proteins with approximately 20-25% binding.

### Biotransformation

The primary metabolic pathways in the biotransformation of primidone with the formation of two metabolites, phenylethylmalonamide (PEMA) and phenobarbital, are illustrated in Figure 2. Both of the metabolites possess anticonvulsant activity, which has made the interpretation of pharmacological and clinical studies of primidone more complex.

PEMA was the first substance to be identified as a possible metabolic product of primidone when crystals of this substance were found in rat urine. Phenobarbital and *p*-hydroxyphenobarbital were isolated and identified in dog urine and human urine and phenobarbital in plasma of both following the administration of primidone. The finding that primidone was metabolized to PEMA and phenobarbital stimulated several studies into the relative importance of these pathways in man. These studies show that the presence of other **drugs, either prior to or concomitant with the presence of primidone, has a marked influence on the** relative amounts of the metabolites. In patients who had no prior anticonvulsant therapy, primidone is largely not metabolized to either phenobarbital or PEMA. In one retrospective study with primidone as a sole drug, little relationship was found between plasma primidone and phenobarbital concentrations when phenobarbital levels were less than 15 mg/L. In these individuals the plasma phenobarbital/primidone ratio was 0.87 which indicates little conversion to this metabolite. When plasma phenobarbital concentrations were in excess of 15 mg/L, the phenobarbital primidone was 2.25 and there was a more linear relationship between concentrations of phenobarbital and primidone. All of the subjects studied were in steady state and plasma samples were obtained 2-4 h after dose.

**The principal site of biotransformation appears to be the liver, but the enzyme systems involved are unknown. The proportions of the three compounds are highly variable and apparently differ in patients** who have been on chronic doses of primidone as a sole drug. The influence of other drugs on this metabolic pathway will be further discussed under the section on drug interactions.

### Excretion

Various factors must be considered in evaluating data concerning the half-life of primidone and its

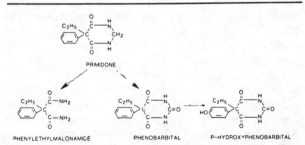

**Fig. 2. Biotransformation of primidone.**

active metabolites, PEMA and phenobarbital. Among these factors are dose, presence of other drugs, age of the patient, and individual variability. In patients given a single dose of 500 or 750 mg the mean half-life was 8.0 h (range 3.3 - 19.0 h); there was some tendency for half-life to increase with chronic medication. The half-lives of both PEMA and primidone were found to be shorter in patients who were taking other anti-epileptic drugs in addition to primidone. Few studies have been done in children but the half-life is apparently similar or slightly shorter, with 6-8 h usually cited. The relative half-lives seem to be consistently primidone < PEMA < phenobarbital when all three compounds are present.

Regardless of the proportions in which the compounds are present, primidone and its metabolites are primarily excreted throught the renal pathway. When no other antiepileptic drugs are present approximately 85% is excreted as unchanged primidone, 9% as PEMA, and 3% as phenobarbital. With concomitant administration of other antiepileptic drugs 51% is excreted as unchanged primidone, 36% as PEMA and 5% as phenobarbital. Detailed references for absorption, distribution, excretion and biotransformation of primidone are given in references 7 and 8.

## Relation of Concentration in Plasma to Clinical Control

Correlation of the plasma concentration of primidone with the clinical control of seizures is complicated by the concern as to whether primidone itself is an effective anticonvulsant or whether its effect is due to phenobarbital, one of its metabolites. Primidone has been shown to effectively control chemical and electrical seizures in animals when little or no PEMA or phenobarbital was found in either plasma or brain. Prospective and controlled human trials utilizing primidone have not been performed, so the therapeutic range has been established from a variety of data obtained in retrospective studies. Dr. Fincham and I have followed a rather large group of patients (80) who have been treated with primidone as a sole agent. These patients were experiencing tonic-clonic and/or partial seizures with either simple or complex symptomatology. These patients have been followed for a period of years and all drug concentrations were determined when the same dose had been maintained for at least a month. The blood samples were obtained 2-4 h after dose because of the relatively short half-life of primidone. Poor correlation was found between the dose of primidone and either the primidone or phenobarbital concentration in plasma. Good to excellent seizure control was obtained when primidone concentrations were between 6 and 15 mg/L, when phenobarbital levels were less than 15 mg/L. In patients where phenobarbital levels were above 15 mg/L control was excellent to good with the same concentration of primidone. Plasma phenobarbital/primidone ratios in all 80 patients averaged 1.45±0.1 (S.E.) indicating a relatively low conversion to phenobarbital. Other studies, which are referred to in reference 9, have also indicated a definite antiepileptic effect of primidone itself.

On the basis of data presented in the literature a therapeutic range for primidone is probably between 6 and 15 mg/L and dose adjustments of primidone must be made utilizing the plasma concentrations of both primidone and phenobarbital. Effective seizure control can be obtained when only the primidone is within the therapeutic range. Adding additional phenobarbital to increase the concentration in plasma of that compound is not advised (10).

## Toxicity

A special kind of toxicity frequently appears with the first dose of primidone and may appear as early as 30 minutes after ingestion. This toxic state includes feelings of drowsiness, gastrointestinal distress and, rarely, hallucinations and feelings of drunkenness. These difficulties can be minimized by starting with 125 mg or less of primidone taken at night and by giving appropriate forewarnings to the adult patient.

**Table 1.** Properties of Phenobarbital and Primidone

|  | PHENOBARBITAL | PRIMIDONE |
|---|---|---|
| Relative molecular mass | 232.23 | 218.25 |
| Melting point | 176°C | 182°C |
| Conversion factor (g/L to mol/L) | 4.306 | 4.581 |
| pK$_a$ | 7.3 | -- |
| Solubility in H$_2$O | salt freely soluble | 600 mg/L at 37°C |
| Partition coefficient (chloroform/water) | 4.2 | 0.7 |
| Protein binding, % bound | 45-50 | 20-30 |
| Absorption |  |  |
| Time to peak, h | 6-18 | 2-4 |
| % absorbed | 80 | 90-100 |
| Tissue distribution |  |  |
| V$_d$, L/kg. | 0.7 | 0.6 |
| Brain/plasma | 0.9-1.0 | 0.87 |
| CSF/plasma | 0.5 | 0.62-1.0 |
| Primary excretion products | Phenobarbital, | primidone, PEMA, phenobarbital |

**Table 2.** Clinical Pharmacology

|  | Phenobarbital | | Primidone | |
|---|---|---|---|---|
|  | Adults | Children | Adults | Children |
| Half-life, h | 50-120 | 40-70 | 6-8 | 5-8 |
| Time to reach steady state, days | 14-21 | 10-18 | 2-3 | 2-3 |
| Effective concentrations, mg/L | 15-40[a] | 15-40[a] | 6-15 | 6-15 |
| Toxic concentration, mg/L | >50 | >50 | >18 | >18 |
| Steady state level expected from 1 mg/kg/day (mg/L) | 10 | 5 | 0.5-1.0 | 0.5-1.0 |

[a] The author suggests an upper value of 30 based on recent studies.

Other side-effects may occur with high plasma concentrations of primidone, including ataxia, sedation and nystagmus. These symptoms appear without abnormally high phenobarbital concentrations.

Hematological and dermatological reactions are rare but have been reported. Personality and behavior changes have been mentioned with primidone therapy. Impotence has been reported.

### Drug Interactions

The most relevant drug interaction of primidone appears to be the alteration in biotransformation of this drug by the addition or presence of phenytoin in the same therapeutic regimen. This combination results in significantly higher plasma concentrations **of phenobarbital, and phenobarbital to primidone** ratios may be as high as 12 or 18:1 (average is 4.0:1). Several instances of phenobarbital intoxication have occurred when phenytoin has been added to a regimen containing primidone. Obviously a combination of phenytoin, primidone and phenobarbital is very likely to lead to such a toxicity problem. Again, the individual variability in the biotransformation necessitates monitoring of plasma concentrations when adjusting therapeutic regimens.

Carbamazepine and primidone are also frequently used together and carbamazepine may increase the metabolism of primidone. Lower carbamazepine concentrations than expected may occur.

Valproic acid may also influence the metabolism of primidone, and plasma concentrations should be closely monitored if these two drugs are used in combination.

References to various drug interactions with primidone are listed in reference *10*.

### Summary

Primidone, a deoxybarbituric acid, is a drug useful in the treatment of tonic-clonic and partial seizures. It has a short half-life (6-8 h) and its therapeutic range is 6-15 mg/L. It is metabolized to two metabolites, phenylethylmalonamide and phenobarbital, both of which have anticonvulsant activity. The proportion of these three compounds is highly variable and influenced by the presence of other antiepileptic medications. Primidone is rapidly absorbed and distributed following oral administration. Unpleasant side-effects may occur early in therapy so initiation of the drug must be with small doses. From the available clinical evidence primidone is an effective anticonvulsant and it is important to measure both the primidone and phenobarbital concentrations in plasma to obtain the best therapeutic results with this drug.

Several important parameters of phenobarbital and primidone are summarized in Table 1 and their clinical pharmacology in Table 2.

The information in this review will help you in answering questions the physician may have regarding appropriate sampling intervals and times for appropriate dosage adjustments.

### References

1. Vida, J.A., and Gerry, E.H., Cyclic ureides. In *Anticonvulsants*, J.A. Vida. Academic Press, New York, NY 1977, pp 151-212.
2. Rall, T.W., Schleifer, L.S., Drugs Effective in the Therapy of the Epilepsies. In *The Pharmacological Basis of Therapeutics*, 6th ed. A.G. Gilman, L.S. Goodman, and A. Gilman, Eds., Macmillan Publishing Co., Inc., New York, NY, 1980, pp 448-474.
3. Maynert, E.W., Phenobarbital: Absorption, Distribution and Excretion. In *Antiepileptic Drugs*, 2nd ed. D.M. Woodbury, J.K. Penry, and C.E. Pippenger, Eds., Raven Press, New York, NY 1981, Ch. 24.
4. Butler, T.C., Some Quantitative Aspects of the Pharmacology of Phenobarbital. In *Antiepileptic Drugs: Quantitative Analysis and Interpretation*. C.E. Pippenger, J.K. Penry, and H. Kutt, Eds., Raven Press, New York, NY 1978, pp 261-271.
5. Porter, R.J., and Penry, J.K., Phenobarbital: Biopharmacology. In *Antiepileptic Drugs: Mechanisms of Action*. G.H. Glaser, J.K. Penry, and D.M. Woodbury, Eds. Raven Press, New York, NY 1980, pp 493-500.
6. Booker, H.E., Phenobarbital: Relation of Plasma Levels to Control of Seizures. In *Antiepileptic Drugs*, 2nd ed. D.M. Woodbury, J.K. Penry, and C.E. Pippenger, Eds., Raven Press, New York, NY 1981, Ch. 27.
7. Schottelius, D.D., Primidone - absorption, distribution and excretion. In *Antiepileptic Drugs*, 2nd ed. D.M. Woodbury, J.K. Penry, and C.E. Pippenger, Eds., Raven Press, New York, NY 1981, Ch. 32.
8. Schottelius, D.D., Primidone - biotransformation. In *Antiepileptic Drugs*, 2nd ed. D.M. Woodbury, J.K. Penry, and C.E. Pippenger, Eds., Raven Press, New York, NY 1981, Ch. 33.
9. Fincham, R.W., Schottelius, D.D., Primidone - relation of plasma concentration to seizure control. In *Antiepileptic Drugs*, 2nd ed. D.M. Woodbury, J.K. Penry, and C.E. Pippenger, Eds., Raven Press, New York, NY 1981, Ch. 35.
10. Fincham, R.W., Schottelius, D.D., Primidone: Interactions with other drugs. In *Antiepileptic Drugs*, 2nd ed. D.M. Woodbury, J.K. Penry, and C.E. Pippenger, Eds., Raven Press, New York, NY 1981, Ch. 34.

# 7

# Combination Phenobarbital/Phenytoin Treatment of Epilepsy

**J. Eric Ahlskog, Ph.D., M.D.**

Medical control of seizure disorders frequently is a difficult problem. Persistence of seizures despite maximal therapeutic doses of a single antiepileptic drug is a fairly common observation. Therefore, a combination drug therapy is often used in treating epilepsy. Undoubtedly, the two anticonvulsants that most commonly are prescribed together are phenobarbital and phenytoin. In combination they are often effective in situations where either alone is not. Here I review combination phenobarbital/phenytoin therapy in clinical practice.

The efficacy of the combined use of phenobarbital and phenytoin is attested to by decades of clinical experience. Phenobarbital was first reported to have anticonvulsant properties by Hauptmann in 1912. He described an epileptic patient who was given phenobarbital for sedation, with a marked reduction in the number of seizures. Phenobarbital was soon in widespread use as an anticonvulsant. Phenytoin was not introduced as an anticonvulsant until the late 1930's, thanks to the pioneering work of Putman and Merritt. They developed an epilepsy model in cats and tested various agents for their anticonvulsant properties. Among the drugs they tested, phenytoin stood out as being particularly effective in elevating the seizure threshold with minimal effects on spontaneous motor activity in the cats. A year later (1938), Merritt and Putnam(*1*) reported the clinical efficacy of phenytoin in the treatment of human epilepsy and it soon became popular as an anticonvulsant. It did not take long for clinicians to discover that epileptic patients who were uncontrolled on maximal doses of either phenobarbital or phenytoin alone often achieved good control with combined used of these agents. It also became apparent that neither drug markedly nor consistently potentiated any of the major side effects of the other. Thus, seizure control with combination therapy could be obtained with an acceptable level of side effects.

## Spectrum of Anticonvulsant Activity

Phenobarbital and phenytoin have a similar spectrum of efficacy but are not effective against all types of seizure disorders. These drugs are most likely

*Dr. Ahlskog is a Fellow in Neurology, Mayo Clinic, Rochester, MN.*

to be useful, both singly and in combination, against generalized motor (grand mal; tonic-clonic) and focal motor seizures. These drugs are frequently used together to treat these types of epilepsy. Complex partial (psychomotor) seizures are less likely to be controlled by therapy with phenobarbital and phenytoin. In fact, some authors consider phenobarbital to be of little value against this type of epilepsy; many clinicians now consider carbamazepine to be the drug of choice. Therefore, the phenobarbital/phenytoin combination is not used in treating most cases of complex partial seizures. Petit mal seizures are notoriously refractory to phenobarbital or phenytoin, or both, and use of these drugs together is almost never seen in treatment of this disorder. Occasionally, treatment of petit mal epilepsy with ethosuximide results in generalized motor seizures, requiring the addition of either phenobarbital or phenytoin, but generally not both.

The phenobarbital/phenytoin combination is occasionally used to treat myoclonic epilepsy of childhood manifested by various types of seizures but in particular atonic-akinetic spells. These latter spells are a major problem because the acute loss of body tone often leads to injury. In most cases the seizures are only poorly controlled by any variety of drug combinations. For physicians treating neonatal and some types of infantile seizures phenobarbital is commonly the drug of choice. However, phenytoin is used much less frequently in this age group because of its side effects, especially the negative cosmetic effects. Consequently, combination therapy with phenobarbital and phenytoin is not common.

In summary, phenobarbital/phenytoin therapy is most likely to be used in treating generalized motor (tonic-clonic) and focal motor seizures. This combination is used in other types of epilepsy but less frequently and with less success.

## Prescribing Practices

Generalized motor (tonic-clonic) convulsions are the most common type of seizure which a physician manages. As noted above, this is the type of seizure disorder that lends itself to combination phenobarbital/phenytoin therapy. Most clinicians would handle it in the manner I have described.

A strong argument can be made for starting with a single drug. First, the likelihood of side effects is less.

Second, in the event of an adverse reaction, the specific offending drug is readily identified and discontinued. In contrast, if a patient receiving two drugs develops a potentially serious reaction, both agents may have to be stopped, and which of the two is responsible may never be discovered.

Whether one starts with phenobarbital or phenytoin is a matter of personal preference, although to some extent it depends on the clinical circumstances. Those who favor initiating treatment with phenobarbital point out its lower incidence of side effects and its lower cost. Phenytoin is preferred by some because it has minimal sedative effects. This latter feature is important in patients whose jobs demand alertness and intact cognitive functioning. However, most patients are not significantly bothered by phenobarbital's sedative effects. Although sedation may be an initial response to this drug, this usually subsides within one to two weeks of continued use. **Age and sex of the patient are also factors affecting** which drug to choose at the start. Most clinicians prefer to avoid the use of phenytoin in young women, because of its adverse cosmetic side effects. Phenobarbital is used cautiously in youngsters who tend to be hyperactive, because the hyperactive behavior is often exacerbated.

A common initial maintenance dose for an adult of average size is 300 mg of phenytoin per day or 90 to 120 mg of phenobarbital per day. Phenobarbital's half-life is about 96 h, and a single daily dose suffices to maintain steady concentrations in the blood. In practice, divided doses are often used to minimize sedative effects. Phenytoin's half-life is about 24 h, but it can be quite variable. One study (2) reported half-lives ranging from 7 to 42 h in human patients (mean = 22 h). Therefore, twice- or even three-times-a-day dosage is required to ensure steady therapeutic concentrations. Once seizures are controlled, less-frequent dosage can be tried if the patient wishes. Measurement of anticonvulsant concentrations in serum can help determine if the frequency of medication is adequate. A serum drug value that is therapeutic a few hours after the anticonvulsant is taken but subtherapeutic just before the next dose **suggests that more frequent dosage may be necessary.**

The clinician's sense of urgency will dictate whether drug loading is used to quickly achieve the desired steady-state concentrations in blood. If loading doses are not used, steady-state values are not approached until after approximately four days with phenytoin or 16 days with phenobarbital. Once the clinician thinks that the steady-state has been achieved and the patient has been on the drug long enough to judge its efficacy, a serum anticonvulsant measurement is indicated. This is useful regardless of the response to the anticonvulsant. In circumstances in which the seizures are not controlled, this provides information regarding: (a) patient compliance; (b) the likelihood that further dose increments will result in toxicity. If concentrations in serum are much lower than would be expected, erratic drug taking may be suspected. Often patients will deny this until confronted with the documented laboratory results. On the other hand, if the patient's seizures are controlled, knowing the attendant anticonvulsant concentration is very useful for future reference. If seizure control is subsequently lost, comparison of the new with the previous serum anticonvulsant values may point to the cause. For example, if a patient is controlled with a given concentration in serum but later develops increased seizures with a significantly smaller concentration, erratic drug taking should be suspected. The alternative possibility is a change in bioavailability or metabolism. However, if the value is essentially unchanged, the patient's anticonvulsant requirements have increased.

Sometimes a patient's seizures may be controlled despite low anticonvulsant concentrations in serum. Doses resulting in subtherapeutic values should be continued as long as the seizures are under control. A low value for a drug is not by itself a sufficient reason for increasing the dose.

Patients on a single drug with persistent seizures should have their dose increased until the concentrations in serum are at the upper end of the therapeutic range. If seizures are still not controlled, then treatment with the other anticonvulsant is begun. The dosages of phenobarbital or phenytoin are the same, whether used together or singly. Anticonvulsant concentrations should be checked after a steady state has been achieved, to help with further dose adjustment. Liver-function tests and a complete blood count should be performed at the same time, as a check on any adverse reactions. Once seizures are controlled, serum anticonvulsant concentrations should be measured about once or twice a year, according to patient and physician preference. Particular attention should be paid to serum levels around the time of puberty since metabolism may change dramatically during this period. The time of the day when the sample is drawn is important. In most circumstances a "trough" concentration, measured just before the next dose, provides the most useful information because it represents the nadir in the daily fluctuation. Also, for comparisons to be most reliable, all samples should be drawn at the same time relative to drug ingestion. When drug toxicity is questioned, information to peak values, those concentrations found 4 to 8 h after dosage with phenobarbital or phenytoin, are most useful. Occasionally, the physician is confronted with a patient in status epilepticus who has been on either phenobarbital or phenytoin alone. In this circumstance, addition of the other drug via a slow intravenous loading dose is an effective treatment of what is potentially an emergency situation. There is little additional risk to loading with one of these medications when the patient has been maintained on the other.

## Mechanisms of Action

Clinical experience indicates that the anticonvulsant effects of phenobarbital and phenytoin tend to be additive. However, whether these drugs work via the same mechanism or via complementary mechanisms is unknown. Various actions have been described for each drug. Which, if any, of these is responsible for the antiepileptic effects has yet to be established.

The initial event in action-potential transmission along an axon is a transient opening of sodium channels. This regenerative event allows propagation distally to the presynaptic terminals. In the terminal region, arrival of the action potential causes a transient influx of calcium which is the trigger for neurotransmitter release into the synapse. In vitro studies have shown that both of these sodium and calcium currents can be blocked by phenytoin or phenobarbital. Phenytoin blocks sodium channels in voltage-clamp experiments with concentrations that are of the same order of magnitude as the usual therapeutic anticonvulsant concentrations. Phenobarbital is also effective, but only in concentrations that are much higher than therapeutic anticonvulsant levels(3). However calcium influx in nerve terminal (synaptosome) preparations is blocked by either drug in therapeutically relevant concentrations(4). Thus, extrapolating to living organisms, one can see that phenytoin probably has effects on both sodium and calcium currents while phenobarbital's influence is mainly confined to calcium conductance. Again, whether either effect is important for anticonvulsant activity is unknown.

Other effects on excitable membranes have been attributed to phenobarbital or phenytoin. Some studies have demonstrated a phenytoin-induced facilitation of the sodium pump ($Na^+K^±ATPase$), which would tend to "stabilize" membranes. However, other studies have produced conflicting results and further investigation is required to sort this out. Recent experiments also indicate that phenobarbital enhances a slow, potassium-dependent outward current, which is thought to lead to adaptation to depolarizing stimuli(5).

Phenobarbital and phenytoin also have prominent effects on synaptic transmission in intact organisms. Several studies have shown that a variety of excitatory postsynaptic potentials (EPSP's) are inhibited while certain inhibitory postsynaptic potentials (IPSP's) are facilitated by each of these drugs. Both drugs are said to facilitate gamma-aminobutyric acid transmission, although the mechanisms involved are not well worked out.

In summary, the precise mechanism of the anticonvulsant activity of phenobarbital and phenytoin are unknown. In vitro studies indicate that phenytoin blocks both sodium and calcium currents. It may also have effects on the sodium pump, but this interaction is complex and information on it is controversial. Phenobarbital appears to block calcium influx in vitro in clinically relevant concentrations; it may also "stabilize" membranes by facilitation of a slow outward potassium current. Studies of synaptic transmission suggest a tendency for both drugs to inhibit some EPSP's and facilitate certain IPSP's.

## Metabolism, Binding, and Interactions

The overall metabolism is approximately the same for both phenobarbital and phenytoin. The major metabolite of each is formed via *para*-hydroxylation by mixed-function oxidase in liver. These metabolic products are without significant anticonvulsant properties. Conjugation of the metabolite to glucuronide, or to a lesser extent sulfate, increases its water solubility; this product is then excreted by the kidneys. Less than 5% of the phenytoin dose and 30 to 60% of the phenobarbital dose is excreted in the urine unmetabolized.

Hepatic metabolism is the major determinant of the half-life of each of these drugs. The pharmacokinetics of phenytoin's elimination has just recently been worked out in detail. Its disappearance is characterized by saturation kinetics. At low concentrations it is eliminated via first-order kinetics; high concentrations obey zero-order relationships. This results in a somewhat variable half-life. As mentioned earlier, half-lives ranging from 7 to 42 h were described in one large series of patients who were taking phenytoin(2). The elimination kinetics of phenobarbital are also not simple and they have not been as well characterized as in the case of phenytoin. The half-life is also somewhat variable and ranges from 53 to 140 h(6).

Both phenytoin and phenobarbital are potent hepatic enzyme inducers. This is a significant consideration when these drugs are used together. Numerous studies have looked at this interaction, with variable results. In vitro, phenytoin metabolism by rat liver microsome preparations is accelerated by pretreatment with phenobarbital. However, phenytoin is a weakly bound substrate for the microsomal enzymes and is easily displaced by adding low concentrations of phenobarbital to the medium(7). These effects may offset each other. Studies in living organisms, including humans, demonstrate that pretreatment with phenobarbital is most likely to decrease the half-life and lower the concentration of phenytoin in blood. However, this is not a consistent finding: some subjects respond to phenobarbital pretreatment with increased phenytoin concentrations and half-lives. Phenytoin tends to have an opposite effect on phenobarbital elimination. Phenobarbital concentrations tend to increase when the two drugs are administered together; the response is attributed to hepatic-enzyme inhibition. This relationship is also inconsistent, and in any given patient the effect of phenytoin on serum phenobarbital values cannot be predicted.

In summary, there is a tendency for phenobarbital to decrease phenytoin's half-life and concentrations in serum, while phenytoin tends to increase phenobarbital concentrations. These interactions are variable, and in any given patient the opposite response may occur. In addition, the magnitude of these responses is usually relatively small; large changes in drug concentrations are uncommon. When therapy with both phenobarbital and phenytoin is begun, the same starting doses are used as when they are used singly. The dose is adjusted later, depending on the clinical response and anticonvulsant concentrations in serum. It is imperative to check the latter when combination phenobarbital/phenytoin therapy is instituted; otherwise inadvertent toxicity or subtherapeutic dosage may result. One additional consequence of this interaction is that the half-life of phenytoin may decrease sufficiently so that patients receiving a single dose of phenytoin may no longer be protected around the clock. Therefore, divided phenytoin doses are especially recommended when combination therapy is used.

Another possible source of interaction of these two drugs is serum binding. Phenytoin is about 90% bound to serum proteins, mainly albumin; phenobarbital is about 40% bound. Available data suggest that phenobarbital and phenytoin do not significantly affect each other's serum binding(8,9). Therefore, the major interaction between these drugs occurs via each influencing the other's rate of metabolism as catalyzed by hepatic enzymes.

## Summary

Combination therapy with phenobarbital/phenytoin is commonly used to treat epilepsy. It is particularly effective in preventing generalized motor seizures. Therapy is initiated with a single drug. The other is added only after it is clear that the first drug was inadequate at maximal therapeutic doses, as documented by measurements of the drug in serum. Each drug affects the metabolism of the other, but the interaction is not consistent from patient to patient and so is not predictable. The magnitude of this interaction is usually not great, but data on serum anticonvulsant concentrations are required to ensure optimal protection against seizures.

## References

1.  Merritt, H.H. and Putnam, T.J., Sodium diphenylhydantoinate in the treatment of convulsive disorders. *J. Am. Med. Assoc.* **111**, 1068-1073 (1938).
2.  Arnold, K., and Garber, N., The rate of decline of diphenylhydantoin in human plasma. *Clin. Pharmacol. Ther.* **11**, 121-134 (1970).
3.  Neumann, R.S., and Frank, G.R., Effects of diphenylhydantoin and phenobarbital on voltage-clamped myelinated nerve. *Can. J. Physiol. Pharmacol.* **55**, 42-47 (1977).
4.  Sohn, R.S., and Ferrendelli. F.A., Anticonvulsant drug mechanisms. *Arch. Neurol.* **33**, 626-629 (1976).
5.  Cote, I.L., Zbicz, K.L., and Wilson, W.A., Barbiturate-induced slow outward currents in aplysia neurones. *Nature* **274**, 594-596 (1978).
6.  Maynert, E.W., Phenobarbital, mephobarbital and metharbital, absorption, distribution and excretion. In: *Antiepileptic Drugs.* D.M. Woodbury, J.K. Penry, and R.P. Schmidt, Eds., Raven Press, New York, N.Y. (1972) pp. 303-310.
7.  Kutt, H. and Fouts, J.R., Diphenylhydantoin metabolism by rat liver microsomes and some of the effects of drug or chemical pretreatment on diphenylhydantoin metabolism by rat liver microsome preparations. *J. Pharmacol. Exp. Ther.* **176**, 11-26 (1971).
8.  Kristensen, M., Hansen, J.M., and Skousted, L., The influence of phenobarbital on the half-life of diphenylhydantoin in man. *Acta Med. Scand.* **185**, 347-350 (1969).
9.  Goldberg, M.A., Phenobarbital binding. In: *Antiepileptic Drugs, Mechanisms of Action; Advances in Neurology,* vol. 27. G.H. Glaser, J.K. Penry, and D.M. Woodbury, Eds., Raven Press, New York, NY, 501-504, (1980).

## Background Reading

*Antiepileptic Drugs.* D.M. Woodbury, J.K. Penry, and R.P. Schmidt, Eds., Raven Press, New York, NY, 1972, pp 103-351.

*Antiepileptic Drugs, Mechanisms of Action; Advances in Neurology,* vol. 27, G.H. Glaser, J.K. Penry, and D.M. Woodbury, Eds., Raven Press, New York, NY, 1980, pp 305-562.

# 8

# Grand Mal Epilepsy
# Case History

**James M. Thornbery, M.D.**
**Robert V. Groover, M.D.**

A 14-year-old female developed the symptoms of an upper respiratory infection and was given aspirin for headache relief. Two days afterwards, she had a grand mal seizure predominantly affecting her left side. She had a similar seizure two days later and was referred to a medical center for evaluation.

Neither the patient nor her immediate family had a history of seizures, though several great aunts had histories of convulsions. The patient was started on phenytoin to prevent further seizures. Computerized axial tomography with intravenous radiopaque contrast media demonstrated a probable vascular malfunction in the right fronto-parietal brain with adjacent hematoma. This vascular malformation was more clearly defined by an arteriogram. Surgery was judged inadvisable because of the increased permanent neurological damage it was likely to cause. Instead, the vascular malformation was treated with 2000 rads radiation in an effort to obliterate the lesion and the patient remained on phenytoin to prevent recurrent seizures.

Six months later she was re-evaluated. No further seizures had occurred in the interim, but there was minimal lateral gaze nystagmus and mild hyperreflexia, both symptoms of possible mild phenytoin toxicity. The serum phenytoin concentration was 25.2 $\mu$g/mL (therapeutic range 10-20 $\mu$g/mL); the phenytoin dosage was accordingly reduced.

Ten months later the patient had brief sensory-motor seizures and three times experienced the aura which had preceded the seizures. When she was seen by her physician, the serum phenytoin was 22 $\mu$g/mL, confirming the patient had been taking the drug when the seizures and aurae occurred. Since increasing her phenytoin dose would likely result in unacceptable side effects, an additional antiepileptic medication, **phenobarbital, was prescribed. Subsequent follow-up** showed serum phenobarbital levels of about 17 $\mu$g/mL (therapeutic range 20-40 $\mu$g/mL) with phenytoin levels

increasing until the phenytoin dose was reduced. The patient has remained seizure-free for two years following the recurrence.

## Discussion

Epilepsy is a disorder of the central nervous system which may be idiopathic in origin or secondary to a defined lesion or trauma. Grand mal seizures, such as this patient had, are characterized by involuntary tonic-clonic muscular movements and may be preceded by a peculiar sensation or "aura." These seizures are usually initially treated with one antiepileptic drug, most commonly phenytoin (Dilantin) or phenobarbital. Often a single drug will provide adequate control, particularly if drug concentrations in plasma are used to assure that generally therapeutic concentrations are achieved before adding a second drug. Similarly, recurrent seizures in a previously well-controlled patient most commonly occur because the patient failed to take his medication. Determination of the drug concentration in plasma allows detection and verification of patient noncompliance.

Therapeutic drug monitoring should curtail the need to follow the traditional approach of adding an additional drug when a single drug seems to fail to control the seizures. The value and scientific basis of such routine polypharmacy has been criticized recently (1), but there is some scientific basis for the combination of phenytoin and phenobarbital. Experimental studies in animals show these drugs differ in their ability to limit the spread of seizure activity versus raising the threshold required to induce seizures. Also, *in vitro* studies indicate the effect of these two drugs on ion transport across nerve cell membranes may be different (2). Finally, the side effects of phenytoin and phenobarbital are different, while their therapeutic effects may be additive.

Blood specimens for routine therapeutic monitoring should be drawn after steady state levels are reached, which occurs at 4-5 times the half-life of the drug. Phenytoin undergoes zero-order elimination; thus its half-life becomes longer as the dose is increased. Ten days may be required for a steady state to be reached. Phenobarbital tends to have a shorter half-life in children than adults. Children will reach steady state

*Dr. Thornbery is a Fellow in Laboratory Medicine at the Mayo Clinic. Dr. Groover is a Consultant in Pediatric Neurology at the Mayo Clinic, Rochester, MN 55905.*

levels in at least 12 days. while adults may take 3 to 4 weeks. Interaction betwwen phenytoin and phenobarbital is variable. So when a second drug is started, the plasma concentration of both drugs should be monitored (2).

Specimens for routine monitoring are "trough" levels drawn just prior to the next drug dose. However, if the reason for TDM is to assess toxic effects of phenytoin, peak concentrations (occurring from 3 to 12 hours after ingestion) may be helpful. A specimen for assessing the etiology of recurrent seizures obviously is best drawn soon after the seizure, before additional drug(s) are administered.

The therapeutic ranges for phenytoin and phenobarbital should be used as guidelines in conjunction with the patients's history and physical findings. Patients with mild seizure disorders may achieve good control at serum drug concentrations somewhat below the therapeutic range. Conversely, patients with severe seizure disorders may tolerate concentrations above the therapeutic range with acceptable side effects.

The need for some flexibility in interpreting the therapeutic range of such antiepileptic drugs stems from the nature of the illness. Epilepsy, in this case **grand mal epilepsy, is not a homogeneous, static** disease; the severity and frequency of seizures vary greatly in individuals. Similarly, the minimal drug concentrations in blood required for the optimal balance of seizure control versus the side effects varies between different individuals.

This variability in the nature of the disease is a major problem in evaluating drug therapy for epilepsy (4). It **is difficult to determine the minimal therapeutic** plasma drug concentration for patients with mild, infrequent seizures unless a large number of patients are followed for a long time. A factor that further complicates any such study is that some patients will spontaneously cease to need any medication. One extensive study found that 5 years after diagnosis, 36% of patients whose epilepsy was of unknown origin did not require medication. The prognosis for patients whose epilepsy is secondary to a defined lesion or trauma was not so favorable (5). Retrospective studies of epileptic patients whose therapy was adjusted prior to the study may even show that patients with higher plasma drug concentrations have more frequent and severe seizures (6, 7). This seems to occur because patients with more frequent, serious seizures are treated more aggressively, in an effort to achieve better, albeit incomplete, seizure control. In summary, a good study of therapeutic plasma drug concentrations should prospectively classify a large number of epileptic patients by type, severity, etiology, and other prognostic factors.

Since 70-90% of plasma total phenytoin is bound to plasma proteins, efforts have been made to measure either plasma unbound ("free") drug concentrations or salivary drug concentrations, in an effort to provide more clinically relevant drug monitoring. It should be noted that only 25 patients were included in the study often cited as establishing that free phenytoin measurements were superior to total phenytoin measurements in non-uremic patients (11). If these patients are classified using a total plasma phenytoin therapeutic range of 10-20 $\mu$g/mL, the total phenytoin concentration in serum identifies correctly 9 of the 12 patients with clinical toxicity. Free phenytoin measurements identified only 8 of the 12. Other studies showing the close correlation of plasma free phenytoin or phenobarbital concentration with plasma total drug concentration make it questionable that free drug levels are significantly more informative in managing most patients (12,13). Patients with renal failure are clearly an exception because the fraction of free phenytoin is doubled with uremia and the therapeutic range for plasma total drug should be reduced accordingly (14,15).

Salivary drug concentrations of phenobarbital, and particularly phenytoin, seem proportional to plasma free drug levels. However, the salivary levels also show good correlations with plasma total drug concentrations (12, 13, 16, 17, 18). Measuring salivary drug concentrations (using commercially available enzyme immunoassays) has one major advantage for treating pediatric patients because parents are more willing to bring a child in for a saliva specimen rather that face the traumatic experience of blood drawing. The result is better patient and parent compliance and more regular medical follow-up (8,9). Specimens also might be collected at home, sent in, and analyzed prior to the clinic visit. Saliva contaminated by recently ingested drugs (both tablet and capsule form) can be a major drawback to such specimens. Precautions include thoroughly rinsing the mouth with water and not ingesting drugs for 3 hours before (10). The low concentrations of these drugs in saliva must also not compromise the accuracy and precision of the assay.

**In summary, epilepsy is a heterogeneous disorder** whose prognosis depends upon a number of factors. Antiepileptic drug assays are particularly helpful to detect failure to take medication, to guide dosage when drugs interact (e.g., phenytoin with phenobarbital, or chloramphenicol with phenytoin), and to limit multiple drug regimens to patients who require such polypharmacy for optimal control. Should toxicity occur in a patient requiring such polypharmacy, plasma drug concentrations help identify the most likely offending drug.

## References

1. Reynolds, E.H., Shorvon S.D., Monotherapy or polytherapy for epilepsy? *Epilepsia* **22**, 1-10 (1981).
2. Woodbury, D.M., Fingl, E., Drugs effective in the therapy of the epilepsies. In *The Pharmocological Basis of Therapeutics* L. Goodman and A. Gilman, Eds., Macmillan Publishing Co., New York, NY, 1975, pp 210-210.
4. Shorvon, S.D., Johnson, A.L., Reynolds, E.H., Statistical and theoretical considerations in the design of anticonvulsant trials. *Adv. in Epileptology: XIIth Epilepsy Int. Sympo.*, 123-128 (1981).
5. Annegers, J.F., Hauser, W.A. Elveback, L.R., Kurland, L.T., Remission and relapse of seizures in epilepsy. *Adv. in Epileptology : Xth Epilepsy Int. Sympo.*, 143-147 (1980).
6. Travers, R.D., Reynolds, E.H., Gallagher, B.B., Variation in response to anticonvulsants in a group of epileptic patients. *Arch. Neurol* **27**, 29-33 (1972).
7. Lund, L., Anticonvulsant effect of diphenylhydantoin relative to plasma levels. *Arch Neurol* **31**, 289-294 (1974).
8. Friedman, I.M., Litt, I.F., Henson, R., Holtzman, D., and Halverson, D., Saliva phenobarbital and phenytoin concentrations in epileptic adolescents. *J. of Peds.* **98**, 564-647 (1981).
9. Zysset, T., Rudeberg, A., Vassella, F., Kupfer, A., and Bircher, J., Phenytoin therapy for epileptic children: Evaluation of salivary and plasma concentrations and of methods of assessing compliance. *Develop. Med. Child Neurol.* **23**, 66-75 (1981).
10. Paxton,J.W., Foote, S., Aberrantly high phenytoin concentrations in saliva. Precaution in monitoring phenytoin concentrations in whole saliva. *Br. J. Clin. Pharm.* **8**, 508-509 (1979).
11. Booker, H.E. and Darcy, B., Serum concentrations of free diphenylhydantoin and their relationship to clinical intoxication. *Epilepsia* **14**, 177-184 (1973).
12. Nishihara. K., Uchino, K., Satioh, Y., Honda, Y., Nakagawa, F., and Tamura, Z., Estimation of plasma unbound phenobarbital concentration by using mixed saliva. *Epilepsia* **20**, 37-45 (1979).
13. Burgmann, G., Kleinau, E., Nolte, R., and Petruch, F., Comparison of phenytoin determinations in plasma, plasma dialysate, and saliva for control of antiepileptic therapy in children. *Klin. Wochenschr.* **57**, 93-94 (1979).
14. Lynn, K., Braithwaite, R., Dawling, S., and Rosser, R., Comparison of the serum protein binding of maprotiline and phenytoin in uraemic patients on haemodialysis, *Eur. J. Clin. Pharmacol.* **19**, 73-77 (1981).
15. Reynolds, F., Ziroyanis, P.N., and Smith, S.E., Salivary phenytoin concentrations in epilepsy and in chronic renal failure. *Lancet II*, 384-386 (1976).
16. Cook, C.E., Amerson, E., Poole, W.K., Lesser, P., and O'Tuama, L., Phenytoin and phenobarbital concentrations in saliva and plasma measured by radioimmunoassay. *Clin. Pharm. and Therap.* **18**, 742-747 (1975).
17. Schmidt, D., and Kupferberg, H.J., Diphenylhydantoin, phenobarbital, and primidone in saliva, plasma, and cerebrospinal fluid. *Epilepsia* **16**, 735-741 (1975).
18. Tondi, M., Mutani, R., Mastropaolo, C., and Monaco, F., Greater reliability of tear versus saliva anticonvulsant levels. *Ann. Neurol.* **4**, 154-155 (1978).

# 9

# Therapy With Antiepileptic Drugs: A Case History

**Dorothy D. Schottelius, Ph.D.**

Current information suggests that between 1 and 2% of our population is afflicted with epilepsy, or "the epilepsies," as symptom complexes. This diagnosis refers to many types of recurrent seizures produced by paroxysms, excessive neuronal discharges in different parts of the brain, which can be related to or caused by a variety of general body or cerebral disorders. The individual so afflicted is usually faced with a lifelong disability and must contend not only with the unpredictable and unexpected physical disability, but also with the embarrassment caused by a public seizure. Because every seizure is potentially dangerous and continuous seizures (status epilepticus) are a medical emergency, every effort must be made to prevent their recurrence by the method most practicable in the individual concerned.

Antiepileptic drugs, alone or in various combinations, are the most frequently used therapeutic measures in the treatment of seizures. Current emphasis is on the development and marketing of drugs that are specific for treatment of a particular type of seizure. New and useful diagnostic aids, along with careful and detailed physical and clinical histories, now enable the clinician to diagnose the type or types of seizures involved and to select the drug most effective for treatment. In many instances more than one drug is used, which adds the problem of drug interaction to an already complicated situation. The case history presented will involve a problem of one example of such a drug interaction with two of the more commonly utilized compounds, phenytoin and primidone.

## Case History

The patient, a 35-year-old man (a truck driver), was first seen by his family physician about one year before admission; his complaints concerned the awareness of a peculiar odor followed by a brief period of unawareness of his surroundings. He was referred to a neurologist and after a complete history and physical examination, an electroencephalogram, and computerized axial tomography, was diagnosed as having partial seizures with complex symptomatology of unknown origin. The patient was placed on primidone with a gradual increase to 250 mg three times per day. Approximately one month later the patient was seen on return follow-up and reported he had not experienced any

*Dr. Schottelius is an Assistant Professor of Neurology at the University of Iowa, Iowa City, IA 52242.*

additional seizures. Laboratory studies revealed normal values for hematological and biochemical studies and drug monitoring gave values of 9.8 mg/L for primidone and 4.5 mg/L of phenobarbital. The patient was returned to the care of his local physician and referred to vocational counseling for assistance in job training. Visits to the local physician were regular and uneventful until approximately one month prior to admission, at which time the patient reported he had been having problems on his job and had intestinal flu. His wife reported he had one seizure which started like the prior ones but also included jerking of the arms and legs and a longer period of unawareness; the patient reported being very tired and sleepy for 3-4 h after this event. Phenytoin, 100 mg three times a day, was prescribed in addition to the previous medication. Drug concentrations were not determined.

Upon admission to the hospital the patient was quite confused and had been brought to the emergency room after being observed to be in a "drunken" state. Nystagmus was noted and laboratory findings revealed no

## Primidone Profile

**Chemical Information**

| | |
|---|---|
| **Trade name:** | Mysoline |
| **Chemical name:** | 5-ethyldihydro-5-phenyl-4,6 (1H, 5H)-pyrimidinedione |
| **Mol Mass:** | 218.25 |
| **Melting point:** | 182°C |
| **Water solubility:** | 600 mg/L at 37°C |

**Absorption and distribution**

| | |
|---|---|
| **Dose absorbed:** | 95% |
| **Peak plasma concentration:** | 2-4 hours |
| **Protein bound:** | 75-80% |
| **Vd:** | 0.6 liter/kg |
| **Excretion:** | primidone, phenylethylmalonamide, phenobarbital and p-hydroxyphenobarbital. First three are active metabolites and can be found in blood. |

| | Adults | Children |
|---|---|---|
| **Half life, h:** | 6-8 | 6 |
| **Steady state, days:** | 2-3 | 2-3 |
| **Effective concentrations, mg/L:** | 6-15 | 6-15 |
| **Toxic concentration, mg/L:** | >15 | >15 |
| **Monitoring methods:** | Gas-liquid and high pressure liquid chromatography and enzyme mediated immunoassay. | |

abnormalities in hematological or biochemical findings. Samples were obtained for drug monitoring and phenytoin intoxication was suspected; drug concentrations requested were alcohol, phenytoin and primidone. The laboratory findings were: blood alcohol 0.0, phenytoin 8.0 mg/L, primidone 5.2 mg/L and, at the laboratory's suggestion, phenobarbital was found to be 52.0 mg/L. Appropriate measures were taken and the patient soon returned to normal. Later the patient was returned to primidone as a singular medication.

## Discussion

Several important points should be noted from this history. There were many possible reasons for the patient's confused state in the emergency room: (a) post-ictal confusion; (b) intoxication as a result of alcohol consumption; or (c) drug intoxication. Only the prompt availability of drug concentrations could rule out the latter two possibilities. The laboratory fortunately requested that phenobarbital be determined and both primidone and phenobarbital concentrations should always be requested when primidone is used in a therapeutic regimen. Not all individuals are aware of the biotransformation of primidone to phenobarbi-

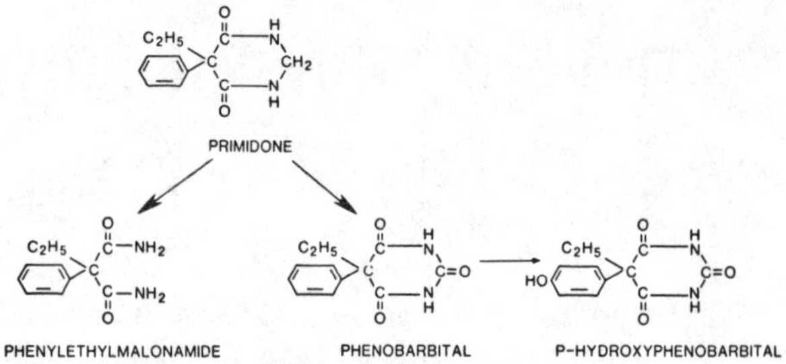

## Fig. 1. Biotransformation of primidone.

tal and even fewer are aware of the fact that phenytoin can markedly enhance this biotransformation. Clearly, the addition of this medication to the patient's regimen in the preceding month had been responsible for intoxication in this patient.

The addition of phenytoin may not have been warranted on the basis of a single complex partial seizure which was secondarily generalized. A single seizure is not sufficient indication for adding an additional drug. The patient should have been more closely monitored following the addition of phenytoin so that proper dose adjustments could have been made.

Phenobarbital accumulates slowly in much the same fashion as if this drug itself were being administered, so that 21 to 30 days would be necessary to achieve the concentration found in this individual. Moreover, one cannot differentiate clinically between signs and symptoms caused by phenytoin and phenobarbital.

As this case illustrates, it is important to make all efforts to control seizures with a single drug and to consider all factors, such as stress and other illness, before abandoning one-drug therapy.

The metabolic conversion of primidone to its active metabolites is illustrated in Figure 1.

## References

1. Schottelius, D.D., Primidone: Biotransformation. In *Antiepileptic Drugs*, 2nd ed., D.M. Woodbury, J.K. Penry, and C.E. Pippenger, Eds., Raven Press, New York, NY, 1981, Ch. 33.
2. Fincham, R.W., and Schottelius, D.D., Primidone: Interactions with other Drugs. In *Antiepileptic Drugs*, 2nd ed., D.M. Woodbury, J.K. Penry, and C.E. Pippenger, Eds., Raven Press, New York, NY, Ch. 34.
3. Pippenger, C.E., Penry, J.K., and Kutt, H., Eds. *Antiepileptic Drugs: Quantitative Analysis and Interpretation*. Raven Press, New York, NY, 1978.
4. Glaser, G.H., Penry, J.K., and Woodbury, D.M., Eds., *Antiepileptic Drugs: Mechanisms of Action*. Raven Press, New York, NY, 1980.
5. Johannessen, S.I., Morselli, P.L., Pippenger, C.E., Richens, A., Schmidt, D., and Meinardi, H., Eds., *Antiepileptic Therapy: Advances in Drug Monitoring*. Raven Press, New York, NY, 1980.

## Phenobarbital Profile

### Chemical information

| | |
|---|---|
| Trade name: | Luminal, etc. |
| Chemical name: | 5-ethyl-5-phenylbarbituric acid |
| pKa: | 7.3 |
| Mol Mass: | 232.23 |
| Melting point: | 176°C |
| Water solubility: | sodium salt freely soluble, acid sparingly |

### Absorption and distribution

| | |
|---|---|
| Dose absorbed: | 80% |
| Peak plasma concentration: | 6-18 hours |
| Protein bound: | 45-50% |
| Vd: | 0.7 liter/kg |
| Excretion: | 15-30% excreted unchanged; variable amount as p-hydroxyphenobarbital |

| | Adults | Children |
|---|---|---|
| Half life, h: | 50-120 | 40-70 |
| Steady state, days: | 14-30 | 10-18 |

| | Adults | Children |
|---|---|---|
| Recommended dose: | 2 mg/kg/day | 4 mg/kg/day |
| Effective concentration, mg/L: | 15-30 | 15-30 |
| Toxic concentration, mg/L: | >40 | >40 |

| | |
|---|---|
| Monitoring methods: | gas-liquid chromatography, high pressure liquid chromatography and enzyme mediated immunoassay. |

# 10

# Methods for Determining Plasma Concentrations of Phenobarbital and Primidone

Dorothy D. Schottelius, Ph.D.

## Introduction

Phenobarbital and primidone (Figure 1) are drugs utilized for the treatment of seizures in adults and children. Phenobarbital is the oldest antiepileptic drug still in use in regular clinical practice. It is a barbituric acid derivative whose efficacy in seizures was first noted in 1912. Generalized seizures, partial seizures and febrile seizures are treated effectively with this agent. Phenobarbital is a weak acid with a $pK_a$ of 7.3; the free acid is sparingly soluble in water but the sodium salt is freely soluble. The partition coefficient (chloroform/water at pH 3.4) is 4.2.

Primidone, a congener of phenobarbital, is a deoxy-barbiturate, introduced into clinical practice in 1954 primarily for treatment of complex partial seizures and their secondary generalization. It is sparingly soluble in water (600 mg/L) and its partition coefficient (chloroform/water at pH 3.4) is 0.7. This compound is biotransformed into two metabolites, phenobarbital and phenylethylmalonamide, in humans and all three compounds may be present in various proportions in the plasma of patients taking this medication. Because phenobarbital is an active anticonvulsant agent, plasma samples should be assayed for both primidone and phenobarbital for the most effective therapeutic utilization of primidone. Since phenylethylmalonamide is present in small quantities and has only weak anticonvulsant properties, it is usually not analyzed in patient's plasma; however it can be quantitated by many of the methods of analysis discussed in this paper.

Accurate measurement of the plasma concentrations of phenobarbital and primidone, along with the other antiepileptic drugs, has provided the clinician the information necessary to provide rational therapy to the epileptic patient. Prior to the availability of such procedures these drugs were often over- or under-utilized with resulting toxicity or poor seizure control. The accurate measurement of these drugs has greatly benefitted the care of the patient, and clinicians have become increasingly aware of the necessity of drug monitoring in these individuals. Drug monitoring of these compounds is especially important because of the lack of dose-plasma correlation and interpatient variability.

Regardless of the method used to determine phenobarbital and primidone, internal and external quality assurance programs are mandatory.

## Methods

### Overview

Procedures for the determination of phenobarbital in biological fluids have employed a variety of techniques; initially the measurements were made spectrophotometrically after separation from other drugs by differential extraction procedures. Chromatographic procedures—first paper and thin-layer and later gas-liquid and high performance liquid—proved to be more suitable. The latter two procedures are also utilized for assay of primidone. Most recently, immunoassay techniques have been introduced for monitoring these drugs.

The older spectrophometric procedures are of little interest or value in today's laboratory because they are time-consuming and inaccurate when other drugs are present—the usual situation in today's patient.

The choice among the three most sensitive and accurate techniques available—gas-liquid and/or high pressure liquid chromatography and immunoassay for the analysis of these drugs will depend on the particular needs of the laboratory and the clinicians involved. At the present time mass fragmentography is the most sensitive and specific method for drug analysis, but the instrumentation is costly and technically difficult, which limits this procedure to the research laboratory. As with the other techniques, future improve-

*Dr. Schottelius is an Assistant Professor of Neurology at the University of Iowa, Iowa City, IA 52242.*

**Fig. 1. Structural formulas for phenobarbital and primidone.**

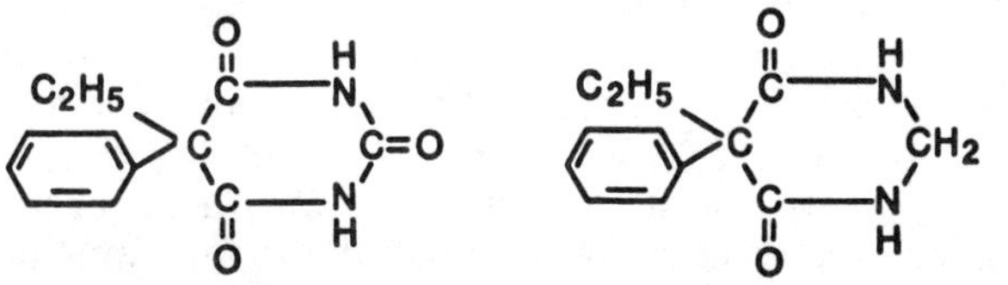

PHENOBARBITAL          PRIMIDONE

Relative mass: phenobarbital 232.23 and primidone 218.25

ments in instrumentation and ease of operation may eventually make this the method of choice.

Several books (*1, 2*) and chapters (*3,4*) present extensive discussions and detailed references for methods of determining phenobarbital and primidone.

**Gas-Liquid Chromatography**

Gas-liquid chromatography (GLC) provides the technology for the sensitive and accurate determination of phenobarbital and primidone, as well as other antiepileptic drugs, and in the past decade more than 80 publications have dealt with procedures for analyzing for these two drugs. A systematic review has recently been published (*5*). Many of the methods are basically the same and most papers have dealt with improvements in gas chromatographs, columns, detectors, or changes in solvents, sample size, derivatizing agents, etc.

When selecting a method, consider that the procedure should have the ability to determine accurately as many of the antiepileptic drugs as possible; and the most frequently used drugs—phenytoin, primidone, and phenobarbital should be easily determined simultaneously. Regardless of the method selected, internal standards must be added; the best procedure is to add as early in the procedure as possible (directly to the biological fluid is best) a compound that is structurally similar to each individual drug.

Sample size should be between 0.5 and 1 mL in most cases, but methods are available for analyzing as little as 20 μL. Various extraction additives have been used to buffer the plasma into the acidic range and extract the drugs into a specific solvent. The volume of the extraction solvent should be kept to a minimum because of cost, effort, glassware requirements, number of simultaneous assays, and environmental consideration. Because the partition coefficients of the individual drugs are considerably different in most solvents, not all drugs will be optimally extracted in a given procedure. This is particularly true of primidone for many solvents.

The solvents used include chloroform, diethyl ether, dichloromethane, acetone, and others. The amount depends on the degree of recovery and the similarity between drugs and internal standard. The appropriate internal standards for phenobarbital and primidone are 5-ethyl-5-*p*-tolylbarbituric acid and 5-ethyl-5-(*p*-tolyl)-hexahydropyrimidine-4-6-dione, respectively. Cleaning an extract with *n*-hexane and aqueous methanol can be eliminated but is useful for removing interfering physiological substances, to prolong the life span of GLC columns and give more reproducible results. The solvent may be removed by a variety of techniques, or the drugs may be re-extracted into a small quantity of derivatization agent if one is to be used. Use of specific columns can give good results without derivatizing (*6*), but most procedures involve on-column methylation with either trimethylphenylammonium hydroxide or tetramethylammonium hydroxide. This step can cause problems with phenobarbital at high concentrations or if the derivatization agent is contaminated with water. Quantitation will

**Fig. 2. Gas chromatogram of on-column methylation method for simultaneous analysis of several drugs utilizing the procedure of Dudley et al.(*7*).**

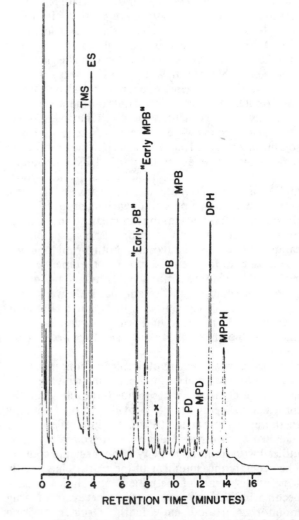

PB, phenobarbital; PD, primidone; MPD, 5-ethyl-5-(*p*-tolyl)-hexahydropyrimidine-4, 6-dione; MPB, 5-ethyl-5-*p*-tolylbarbituric acid; TMS, α, α, β-trimethylsuccinimide; ES, ethosuximide; DPH, phenytoin; MPPH, 5-(*p*-tolyl)-5-phenylhydantoin; x, unknown.

not be a problem if 5-ethyl-5-*p*-tolylbarbituric acid is used as an internal standard. The sample should be injected into the gas chromatograph immediately after adding the derivatization agent. Column supports and stationary phases usually used are acid-washed silanized materials such as Gas Chrom-Q, Chromosorb W, and Supelcoport with OV-17 or SP2110 and SP 2510 in silanized glass columns. Temperature programming is necessary when simultaneous analyses are done. Most methods involve either flame-ionization or nitrogen-selective detectors.

Appropriate standards for each drug to be quantitated must be prepared carefully in plasma or serum in concentrations to cover appropriate ranges expected in patient samples. Calibration data should be obtained with every determination of unknowns. All compounds must be pure and anhydrous. Quantitation can be by either peak height or peak area ratio of drug/

internal standard plotted against concentration of the drug standard and the range should be 0-100 mg/L for phenobarbital and 0-30 mg/L for primidone. Coefficients of variation should be about 5% when the quality control is assessed. An example of a chromatogram from a procedure involving simultaneous determination of several drugs (7) is illustrated in Figure 2.

### High Performance Liquid Chromatography (HPLC)

The basic principles of chromatography apply to both GLC and HPLC. In the first, separations are based on vapor pressure and the mobile phase is a carrier gas; in the second, separations are based on solubility, and the mobile phase is a liquid. Detectors used in HPLC either singly or in series are ultraviolet or visible spectrophotometers, fluorescence monitors, electrochemical detectors, and differential refracto-

## Fig. 3. Daily curve obtained with Syva calibrators for phenobarbital.

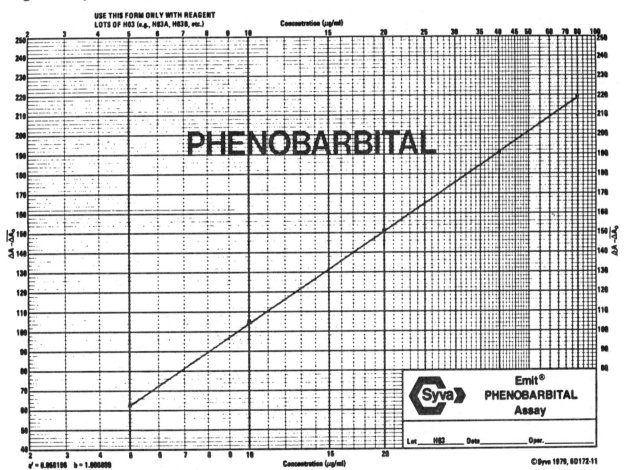

When high concentrations are obtained (above 40 mg/L) the specimen should be diluted with blank plasma and reassayed. Low concentrations (below 5 mg/L) may be determined by modification including dilution of the calibrators.

meters. Recent developments of efficient reversed phase columns (which involve both absorption and partitioning mechanisms), better control of mobile-phase delivery, and improved detectors have made HPLC a highly useful technique. Various methods involving this technique have been published; consult a recent reference (8) for details.

Small samples (25-200 $\mu$L) may be analyzed by HPLC and extraction may or may not be used. Sensitivity of the methods is quite high and good precision and accuracy are possible. Quantitation requires an internal standard and peak-height ratios are usually utilized. No derivatization is necessary and samples can be recovered from the columns. Because total time for analysis is usually about 30 minutes, results can be quickly available to the physician. Interference from either endogenous compounds or other drugs and/or metabolites has not been a significant problem with these methods.

Future improvements involving automation and direct injection of body fluids are undoubtedly coming, which will provide an increasingly important role for this technique in therapeutic drug monitoring and clinical chemistry.

**Immunoassay**

Homogeneous enzyme immunoassay (EMIT, Syva Company, Palo Alto, CA 94304) involves use of an enzyme as a label and the conversion of $NAD^+$ to NADH is measured spectrophotometrically. With this technique the laboratory can rapidly and accurately measure both phenobarbital and primidone in micro-samples; 50 $\mu$L is sufficient for analysis of a single drug. Coefficients of variations of 3 to 5% both within day and between day can be achieved with these reagents (supplied as matched set of two reagents) and appropriate instrumentation. Calibrators are available; examples of the curves obtained are illustrated in Figure 3 and 4. Curves should be prepared daily. The precision and accuracy are best within the therapeutic

### Fig. 4. Daily curve obtained with Syva calibrators for primidone.

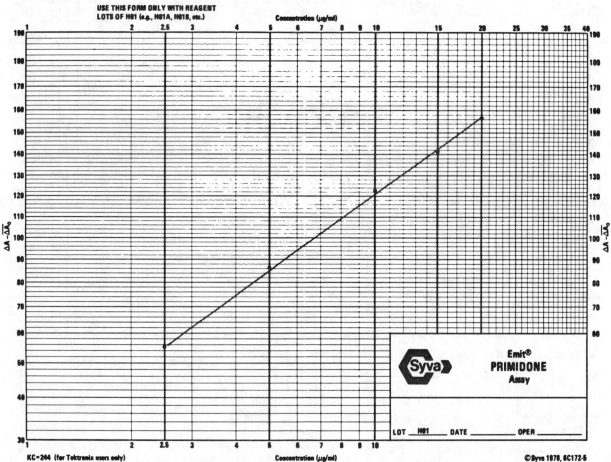

Appropriate modifications for extremely high or low concentrations can be made.

range and appropriate modifications of the method will give excellent results with high or low values (9).

Detailed methods of the procedures and information of cross-reactivity are available in the package insert. Note that the phenobarbital assay is sensitive to mephobarbital and heptobarbital. Cross-reactivity with metabolites or other antiepileptic drugs is not a problem with either phenobarbital or primidone. Problems can arise if the specimen is severely hemolyzed, lipemic, or icteric, and such samples must be analyzed by an alternative method.

Comparison of results of samples analyzed by GLC, EMIT and HPLC have been published (3, 8 and 9). In contrast to the GLC or HPLC procedures, these immunoassay procedures are designed for a specific drug; and screening of a sample is not as convenient and can only be done by repeated assays with specific reagents. This is the most rapid procedure available and results can be obtained within 2 min of obtaining the plasma or serum sample (provided the calibration curves have already been prepared). Future developments may include the ability to measure these drugs even more rapidly and with whole blood.

## Summary

All of the methods possess advantages and disadvantages. GLC and HPLC require preparation of the specimen before analysis, whereas the enzyme procedure does not. The enzyme procedure is very rapid and samples of 50 $\mu$L are sufficient for repeated analysis of a single drug, which is an advantage in continuous monitoring and pediatric patients where finger stick quantities are sufficient.

Technical expertise and experience must be of a higher level in the use of the GLC and HPLC instrumentation. Simultaneous quantitative analysis of samples is possible with GLC and HPLC methods, whereas the enzyme procedure is specific for individual drugs. Metabolites of phenobarbital and primidone may be determined with the GLC and HPLC methods and not with the enzyme. Automation of the enzyme procedure is available and with a large volume of samples is financially feasible; even without automatic equipment the enzyme immunoassay procedure will involve less technical time than the GLC or HPLC methods. Reagent expense is somewhat higher for the enzyme immunoassay procedure than the other two.

With proper attention to calibration curves and methodological details, the GLC, HPLC, or the en-

zyme immunoassay techniques will provide reliable, reproducible, and accurate measurements of phenobarbital and primidone in biological fluids. Choice of the best procedure must be based on the needs of the laboratory.

## References

1. *Antiepileptic Drugs: Quantitative Analysis and Interpretation*, C.E. Pippenger, J.K. Penry, and H. Kutt, Eds., Raven Press, New York, NY 1978.
2. *Antiepileptic Therapy: Advances in Drug Monitoring*, S.I. Johannessen, P.L. Morselli, C.E. Pippenger, A. Richens, D. Schmidt, and H. Menardi, Eds., Raven Press, New York, NY 1980.
3. Johannessen, S.I., Phenobarbital: Chemistry and Methods of Determination. In *Antiepileptic Drugs*, 2nd ed., D.M. Woodbury, J.K. Penry, and C.E. Pippenger, Eds., Raven Press, New York, NY 1981, Ch. 23.
4. Schafer, H., Primidone: Chemistry and Methods of Determination. In *Antiepileptic Drugs*, 2nd ed., D.M. Woodbury, J.K. Penry, and C.E. Pippenger, Eds., Raven Press, New York, NY 1981, Ch. 31.
5. Rambeck, B., and Meijer, J.W.A., Gas Chromatographic Methods for the Determination of Antiepileptic Drugs. *Ther. Drug Monit.* 2, 385-396 (1980).
6. Godolphin, W., and Thoma, J., Quantitation of Anticonvulsant Drugs in Serum by Gas-Chromatography on the Stationary Phase SP-2510. *Clin. Chem.* 24, 483-485 (1977).
7. Dudley, K.H., Buis, D.L., Kraus, B.L., and Boyles, L.W., Gas Chromatographic On-column Methylation Technique for the Simultaneous Determination of Antiepileptic Drugs in Blood. *Epilepsia*, 18, 259-276 (1977).
8. Pesh-Iman, M., Fretthold, D.W., Sunshine, I., Kumar, S., Terrentine, S., and Wallis, C.E., High Pressure Liquid Chromatography for Simultaneous Analysis of Anticonvulsants: Comparison with EMIT System. *Ther. Drug Monit.* 1, 289-329 (1979).
9. Schottelius, D.D., Homogeneous Immunoassay System (EMIT) for Quantitation of Antiepileptic Drugs in Biological Fluids in *Antiepileptic Drugs: Quantitative Analysis and Interpretation*, C.E. Pippenger, J.K. Penry and H. Kutt., Eds., Raven Press, New York, NY 1978, pp 95-108.

# 11

# Pharmacokinetics and Monitoring of Ethosuximide Concentrations in Plasma

## Mario L. Rocci, Jr., Ph.D.

Ethosuximide, an alkylated succinimide derivative, is an effective anticonvulsant agent used in the treatment of petit mal (absence) seizures. This drug was first developed in 1951 in a research effort aimed at designing agents which would prove both safe and effective in the treatment of petit mal seizures (1).

An understanding of the pharmacokinetics of ethosuximide aids in the rational clinical use of this anticonvulsant. There are several reasons for monitoring concentrations of this anticonvulsant in plasma: interpatient variability existing in the relationship between steady-state drug levels in plasma and dose; the need to achieve concentrations in plasma of at least 40 mg/L (285 $\mu$mol/L); and the difficulty in assessing the degree of absence seizure control, particularly in pediatric populations.

In order to effectively use the information gained through the monitoring of ethosuximide concentrations in plasma, the clinician must appreciate several complexities in ethosuximide disposition and their clinical importance. Total clearance of ethosuximide varies as a function of the patient's age, affecting the size of maintenance doses needed to produce adequate seizure control. Ethosuximide has a long half-life in plasma, and in addition, increases in dose can cause disproportionate increases in steady-state concentrations in plasma; these two factors affect both the appropriate time to monitor ethosuximide concentration in plasma and the manner in which dosage alterations are effected. Knowing the effects of concomitant drug therapy on ethosuximide steady-state levels in plasma is important since these effects may produce loss of seizure control or drug toxicity. Finally, appreciating the effects that certain physiologic states such as pregnancy have on ethosuximide pharmacokinetics aids in the rational use of this drug if it is needed during pregnancy.

This review examines the clinical pharmacokinetics of ethosuximide and provides a framework for monitoring ethosuximide concentrations in plasma. Appro-

Dr. Mario L. Rocci Jr. is an Assistant Professor, Department of Pharmacy Practice, Philadelphia College of Pharmacy and Science and an Adjunct Assistant Professor of Medicine, Jefferson Medical College, Philadelphia PA.

priate use of monitoring in conjunction with sound clinical judgement will help optimize therapeutic drug response.

## Pharmacokinetic Characteristics of Ethosuximide

The rate and extent that the body absorbs, distributes, metabolizes and excretes drugs and their metabolites are dictated by various physiologic processes as well as the physicochemical properties of drugs. The rate and extent of each of these processes relative to the others determine the time course of drug concentrations in plasma. Knowing the pharmacokinetic characteristics of ethosuximide is essential to rationally employ ethosuximide concentration monitoring in the clinical setting.

*Absorption.* Ethosuximide is available for oral use in both capsule and syrup formulations. In children given single 500-mg doses in each form (2), the extent of absorption of these preparations are equivalent. Substantial absorption of both preparations occurs by 1 h after ingestion, with peak concentrations in serum occurring anywhere from 3 to 7 h after drug administration. In adults given 500 mg orally, ethosuximide peak concentrations in plasma also occur 3 to 7 h after administration, though the concentrations achieved at this dose are lower than those produced in children since this dose in adults is much smaller on a milligram-per-kilogram basis (3). The rate of absorption of ethosuximide is more rapid from the liquid, though this enhanced rate does not produce clinically significant differences in the time course of concentrations in plasma following a single dose of the drug. (2).

The fraction of orally administered ethosuximide that ultimately gets absorbed from the gastrointestinal tract is not known. The determination of this pharmacokinetic parameter, commonly known as the absolute bioavailability, requires comparison of the time course of ethosuximide concentrations in plasma following oral administration with those obtained following intravenous administration. The lack of a commercially available parenteral ethosuximide preparation prevents this comparison.

*Distribution.* The apparent volume of distribution is a pharmacokinetic parameter which relates the amount of drug in the body to the drug's concentration in plasma (i.e., amount of drug in the body = apparent volume of distribution × drug concentration in plasma). This distribution parameter does not reflect a real physiologic space, but rather represents the hypothetical space into which a drug would distribute if the body (including the plasma) was completely homogeneous. Apparent volume of distribution values for selected drugs that are in the range of real physiologic spaces suggest, though do not indicate, uniform drug distribution within that space, particularly if the physicochemical properties of the drug favor such distribution.

The apparent volume of distribution of ethosuximide in adults and children has been reported to be 0.62 and 0.69 L/kg (2,3). These values are close to 0.7 L/kg which estimates the total body water content of the body suggesting that ethosuximide distributes uniformly throughout the body water (2,3). This is consistent with the physicochemical properties of ethosuximide, which is alkaline with a pKa well above physiologic pH (9.3) (3,4). In addition, ethosuximide is not bound to proteins in plasma (3). The values quoted above for the volume of distribution of ethosuximide assume 100% bioavailability.

Ethosuximide readily distributes into tears, saliva, and cerebrospinal fluid (CSF) with the ratios of the concentrations in tears/plasma, saliva/plasma, and CSF/plasma being 0.86 (±0.61), 0.78 (±0.74), and 0.95 (±0.32) (4). Although the concentrations of ethosuximide in saliva and tears are significantly correlated with those in plasma (4), these correlations are sufficiently variable ($r^2 = 0.55$) (4) to prevent their use in estimating ethosuximide concentrations in plasma from measurements made in tears or saliva.

Ethosuximide has been shown to cross the placenta (5) and also partitions into breast milk with a milk/serum ratio of 0.94 ±0.06 (6). Neonatal exposure to ethosuximide through nursing has been predicted to be 3.6 to 11 mg/kg. The effect of such a dose in a neonate is unknown (6).

*Metabolism and Excretion.* Ethosuximide is eliminated from the body primarily via metabolism. The percent of ethosuximide excreted unchanged in the urine is approximately 17 to 38% (3). The magnitude of the renal clearance of ethosuximide in healthy volunteers is approximately 10 mL/h/kg (6). This value in conjunction with the negligible binding of ethosuximide in plasma indicates substantial renal tubular reabsorption. Although the quantitative metabolic scheme for ethosuximide remains to be elucidated in man, semiquantitative data exist. Data obtained from the urine of a pregnant woman just prior to delivery indicate that ethosuximide is metabolized to four monohydroxy metabolites. These metabolites were present in the plasma of the mother 11 h after her last

dose, and in the plasma of her infant 66 h after the dose, in concentrations exceeding that of ethosuximide. The presence of the metabolites as well as ethosuximide in the infant's plasma confirms that ethosuximide crosses the placenta, and that the metabolites cross the placenta and/or are metabolized by the infant (5).

The apparent total clearance of ethosuximide following single doses of the drug in normal healthy adults is approximately 13 mL/h/kg, assuming complete gastrointestinal absorption of ethosuximide (7). This value is much less than estimates of hepatic blood flow, suggesting that blood flow to the liver is not the rate-determining step involved in the metabolism of ethosuximide. Comparison of clearance values determined following single doses with those obtained at steady state reveals a decrease in the clearance of ethosuximide by the liver at steady state, implying that the high concentrations in plasma attained at steady state may saturate drug-metabolizing enzymes in the liver (7). Since the majority of ethosuximide elimination is metabolic in nature, a disproportionate increase in steady-state concentrations in plasma with increases in dose would be expected. Such a relationship does exist as shown in Figure 1 where steady-state ethosuximide concentrations in plasma are plotted as a function of dose for two patients being treated for absence seizures. The solid line in each panel reflects the relationship one would expect if linear (nonsaturable) clearance of ethosuximide occurred as the lowest dose is increased (7). This figure illustrates that

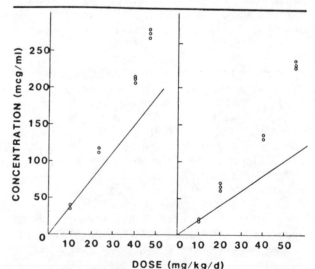

**Fig. 1. Steady-state ethosuximide concentration-dose plot for two patients treated for absence seizures.**

The solid line shows the relationship anticipated from the lowest concentration-dose data pair, assuming linear kinetics. (From Ref. 7).

a doubling of the ethosuximide dose will more than double the resultant steady-state concentration in plasma.

Plasma half-life ($t\frac{1}{2}$) is a pharmacokinetic parameter that expresses the time that it takes for concentrations of a drug in plasma to be reduced by 50%. Half-life measurements are made once drug distribution to tissues are complete.

Half-life can also be expressed as the ratio of the apparent volume of distribution ($V_D$) and the total clearance of a drug ($Cl$) using Eq. 1.

$$t\frac{1}{2} = \frac{0.693 \cdot V_D}{Cl} \qquad (1)$$

The half-life of ethosuximide in plasma appears to be age related, with half-lives in children being on the order of 30 h while those in adults are approximately double that value (53 h) (2,3).

Through the employment of Eq. 1 it is evident that the differences in half-lives between chidren and adults largely reflect differences between these patient populations in the $Cl$ of ethosuximide (which is primarily metabolic in nature) since $V_D$ in these groups are similar. This suggests that children have a greater propensity to metabolize ethosuximide and that this ability is reduced with increasing age..

The $t\frac{1}{2}$ of ethosuximide is likely to be dose-related as well, since higher plasma concentrations (which would result from the administration of larger doses) may saturate drug-metabolizing enzymes in the liver. This would result in a reduced $Cl$ of ethosuximide and as would be expected from Eq. 1, a prolonged half-life.

## Dose vs. Plasma Concentration Relationship

The pharmacokinetic expression relating the dosing rate ($DR$), mean steady-state concentration in plasma ($C_{SS}$), and total clearance ($Cl$) of a drug is presented in Eq. 2.

$$C_{ss} = \frac{DR}{Cl} \qquad (2)$$

where $DR$ is the dose administered (assuming 100% systemic availability of the drug) divided by the dosing interval. This equation also assumes that $Cl$ does not change as a function of dose. While this is not true for ethosuximide, this relationship may be used to semi-quantitatively examine the dose vs. plasma concentration of ethosuximide relationship as a function of age.

As can be seen from Eq. 2, the relationship between the dose and the resultant steady-state drug concentration in plasma will be different for patient populations with different clearances. Thus, the two-fold difference in the half-life of ethosuximide between adults and children, which suggests age-related differences in drug metabolism, implies that the relationship

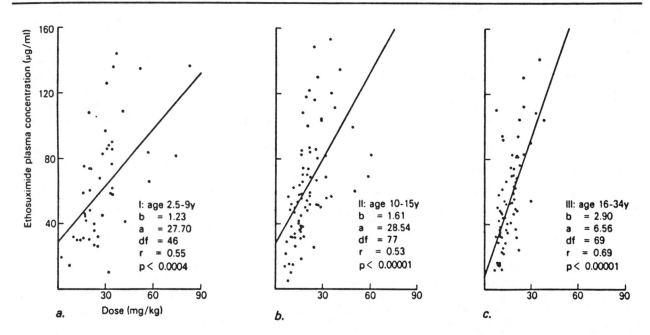

Fig. 2. Linear regressions of ethosuximide plasma concentrations on daily dose as a function of age.
There is a significant correlation between dose and plasma levels in all 3 age groups (p < 0.0004 in group I, p < 0.00001 in groups II and III). The regression of the age groups I and II differs significantly in slope from that of group III (p < 0.05). (From Ref. 8).

between ethosuximide concentrations in plasma and dose will be different as a function of age. The relationship between ethosuximide concentrations in plasma and dose for patients in the 2.5 to 9, 10 to 15, and 16 to 34 year age ranges are presented in Figure 2 (8). A significant correlation exists between ethosuximide dose and level in plasma in each of the age groups, with the relationships in the younger groups differing significantly from the adult group (7). Also evident is the great variability in these relationships at any given age range, making prediction of steady-state serum concentrations for a given dose impossible. Part of this variability may be due to the effects of polytherapy (carbamazepine, phenytoin, primidone, valproic acid, phenobarbital) on ethosuximide clearance since patients on multiple-dose therapy tended to have lower concentrations in plasma for a given dose than patients receiving ethosuximide alone (8).

## Plasma Concentration vs. Clinical Seizure Control

Assessing the relationship between ethosuximide concentrations in plasma and seizure control is complicated by difficulties inherent in assessing the degree of seizure control, particularly for absence seizures, which may often times go undetected. In a study assessing the relationship of drug concentrations in plasma to clinical control, considerable variability in ethosuximide concentrations in plasma was noted both in patients who were clinically controlled as well as those who achieved adequate control. It was further noted that 93% of the patients in the controlled group had ethosuximide concentrations in plasma greater than 40 mg/L (285 $\mu$mol/L) (9). Other studies have confirmed the 40 mg/L range as the minimum effective serum concentration in plasma in the majority of patients and have established a therapeutic range of 40 to 100 mg/L (285 to 710 $\mu$mol/L) for the control of most patients (1).

## Dose vs. Adverse Effects Relationships

A relationship has not been established between adverse effects resulting from ethosuximide therapy and concentration in plasma. Side effects from therapy include several dose-related and nondose-related reactions.

The dose-related side effects from ethosuximide therapy include gastrointestinal effects such as nausea, vomiting, gastric distress, and anorexia as well as central nervous system effects which include dizziness, fatigue, lethargy, headache, hiccups, and euphoria (10). Gastric side effects are the most common, occurring in about 20% of the patients and may be reduced by taking the drug with food. All dose-related adverse effects tend to dissipate with time (1). Reduction in

ethosuximide dosage will also result in amelioration of these effects.

The nondose-related side effects resulting from ethosuximide therapy are generally rare and involve primarily the hematopoietic system and the skin (1,10). Dermatologic reactions include nonspecific rashes, systemic lupus erythematosus, urticaria, and erythema multiforme bullosa (Stevens-Johnson syndrome). Hematologic reactions include eosinophilia, leukopenia, and pancytopenia (10).

Ethosuximide has also been implicated in inducing psychosis and impairing psychometric performance (1). Whether ethosuximide is in fact causative in producing these disturbances is difficult to evaluate.

No definitive conclusions can be made about the teratogenic effects of ethosuximide. Discontinuation of the drug at least one month prior to conception, if possible, has been suggested (1).

## Drug Interactions

The interactions of various drugs with ethosuximide have not been studied in great detail. Existing data suggest, however, that ethosuximide metabolism may be both induced and inhibited by selected drugs that are frequently given in conjunction with ethosuximide. In a study examining the effect of age and concomitant drug therapy on ethosuximide concentrations in plasma, it was noted that lower ethosuximide concentrations resulted for a given dose when patients were receiving other anticonvulsants concomitantly (8). This particular study suggests that phenobarbital and primidone may induce ethosuximide-metabolizing enzymes in the liver, resulting in decreased concentrations in plasma at any given dose. Concomitant carbamazepine administration has also been shown to decrease ethosuximide steady-state concentrations in plasma by 17% through induction of metabolizing enzymes (14).

Conflicting data exist regarding the effect of valproic acid on ethosuximide disposition. In one study conducted in five patients, addition of valproic acid to ethosuximide resulted in an average increase of 53% in ethosuximide concentrations in plasma in four out of five patients with resultant toxicity (12). In another study conducted at steady state in normal volunteers, addition of valproic acid had no effect on ethosuximide concentrations in plasma (7). Until this controversy is resolved, patients receiving both drugs should be monitored closely for changes in plasma concentrations.

## Dosing Guidelines

The choice of a dose for initiating ethosuximide therapy as well as any changes in dose during therapy must take into consideration several factors: age-related changes in the clearance of the drug; the time that is necessary to reach steady state; concomitant drug therapy which may alter the clearance of ethosuximide; and with increases in dose, the disproportionate increases in steady-state concentrations in plasma that may occur due to saturation of drug-metabolizing enzymes.

Daily doses in adults and children of 15 and 20 mg/kg will result in drug levels in plasma of approximately 50 μg/mL, which is above the 40μg/mL therapeutic limit needed for adequate seizure control in most patients (1). The long half-life of ethosuximide in plasma in adults and children suggests that a dosing interval of one day should be acceptable to maintain concentrations in plasma within the therapeutic range. The maximum dosage of ethosuximide employed under normal circumstances is 30 mg/kg/day in adults and 40 mg/kg/day in children (1). These dosage recommendations serve as rough guides to therapy and will not produce therapeutic concentrations in plasma in the 40 to 100 μg/mL range in all patients because of the wide variability in the relationship between steady-state concentrations in plasma and ethosuximide dose (Figure 2). Once therapy is initiated or a dosage change is made it will take four half-lives to be at approximately 95% of steady-state concentrations in plasma. As a result it will take about four or five days in children and eight to nine days in adults to approach steady state. Daily dosage adjustments should only be performed once steady state has been achieved for a given dose and deemed unacceptable due to lack of seizure control. Dosage adjustment may be necessary prior to steady state if excessive accumulation of ethosuximide results in the onset of adverse effects.

Adjustment of therapy should be approached with caution in patients receiving ethosuximide, in light of the potential for saturable metabolism (which reduces the total clearance of the drug) as dose is increased. Incremental increases in the doses of most drugs will produce the same incremental increase in the mean steady-state concentration in plasma (Eq. 1). This does not appear to be true with ethosuximide; an incremental increase in dose may produce disproportionate increases in concentrations in serum, which may predispose the patient to development of any of the dose-related side effects.

The addition, discontinuation, or dosage alteration of drugs which may induce ethosuximide-metabolizing enzymes (carbamazepine, phenobarbital, primidone) or compete with ethosuximide for drug metabolizing enzymes (valproic acid) may necessitate a change in ethosuximide doses. Coadministration of enzyme inducers may increase the clearance and decrease the serum concentrations of ethosuximide in serum so gradually that weeks may be required for their effect to be fully appreciated. In contrast, drugs which may compete with ethosuximide for drug-metabolizing enzymes will do so acutely and may require more immediate dose adjustment.

Finally dosage adjustments of ethosuximide may be necessary during pregnancy and after delivery since concentrations of ethosuximide in plasma have been reported to increase following delivery (1).

## Drug Plasma Concentration Monitoring

*Appropriate Time for Sample Collection.* Monitoring of drug plasma concentration is appropriate when steady-state levels in plasma have been achieved since it is at this time that concentrations in plasma are in equilibrium with drug concentrations in other body tissues including those in which the drug acts. As stated previously, approximately four half-lives of multiple dosing are needed to approach steady state. Blood samples may be taken for monitoring drug concentration in plasma prior to the achivement of steady state, however, to confirm suspected toxicity.

The actual timing of the blood sample collection relative to administration of the dose is relatively unimportant for ethosuximide due to its long half-life; as a result blood samples for monitoring concentrations of ethosuximide in plasma may be taken any time within a dosing interval.

## Indications for Monitoring Ethosuximide Concentration in Plasma

(1) Concentration monitoring can be used in patients apparently unresponsive to the drug to assess compliance.

(2) After the initiation of therapy, measuring concentrations in plasma drug concentrations may be desired once steady state has been attained to confirm the existence of concentrations greater than 40 mg/L. As stated previously, absence seizures easily go undetected, particularly in pediatric patients; thus, confirmation of concentrations of ethosuximide in the therapeutic range may be desirable.

(3) If patients manifest signs of drug toxicity a drug level measurement will help confirm drug-induced toxicity and effect appropriate dosage reduction.

(4) If a dosage adjustment is needed (i.e., onset of seizure activity), measurement of ethosuximide concentrations are warranted to aid in altering the dose, particularly since increases or decreases in dosing rate for ethosuximide may produce disproportionate changes in the steady-state concentrations in plasma; another concentration measurement may be necessary once a new steady state has been established.

(5) If another anticonvulsant that affects ethosuximide disposition is added to the regimen or if the dose of an interacting drug is changed, it is rational to

monitor drug concentrations in plasma to avoid excessive or subtherapeutic levels.

(6) Monitoring ethosuximide concentrations in plasma at regular intervals during pregnancy and after delivery may help to prevent subtherapeutic levels during pregnancy and the accumulation of excessive concentrations after delivery.

(7) Ethosuximide concentrations in plasma should be monitored routinely every six months to a year since gradual reductions in clearance with age may require dosage reduction.

## References

1.  Stoehr, G.P., and Sherwin, A.L., Ethosuximide: Therapeutic use and serum concentration monitoring. In *Individualizing Drug Therapy: Practical Applications of Drug Monitoring*, Vol. 2., A.L. Finn and W.J. Taylor, Eds., Gross, Townsend, Frank, Inc., New York, NY, 1981, pp 1-25.

2.  Buchanan, R.A., Fernandez, L., and Kinkel, A.W., Absorption and elimination of ethosuximide in children. *J. Clin. Pharmacol.* **9**, 393-398 (1969).

3.  Eadie, M.J., Tyrer, J.H., Smith G.A., and McKauge, L., Pharmacokinetics of drugs used for petit mal 'absence' epilepsy. *Clin. Exp. Neurol.* **14**, 172-183 (1977).

4.  Piredda, S., and Monaco, F., Ethosuximide in tears, saliva, and cerebrospinal fluid. *Ther. Drug Monitoring* **3**, 321-323 (1981).

5.  Horning, M.G., Stratton, C., Nowlin, J., Harvey, D.J., and Hill R.M., Metabolism of 2-ethyl-2-methylsuccinimide (ethosuximide) in the rat and human. *Drug Metab. Dispos.* **1**, 569-576 (1973).

6.  Koup, J.R., Rose, J.Q., and Cohen, M.E., Ethosuximide pharmacokinetics in a pregnant patient and her newborn. *Epilepsia* **19**, 535-539 (1978).

7.  Bauer, L.A., Harris, C., Wilensky, A.J., Raisys, V.A., and Levy, R.H., Ethosuximide kinetics: Possible interaction with valproic acid. *Clin. Pharmacol. Ther.* **31**, 741-745 (1982).

8.  Battino, D., Cusi, C., Franceschetti, S., Moise, A., Spina, S., and Avanzini, G., Ethosuximide plasma concentrations: Influence of age and associated concomitant therapy. *Clin. Pharmacokin.* **7**, 176-180 (1982).

9.  Sherwin, A.L., and Robb, J.P., Ethosuximide: Relation of plasma levels to clinical control (continued). In *Antiepileptic Drugs*, Chapter 51, D.M. Woodbury, J.K. Penry, and R.P. Schmidt, Eds. Raven Press, New York, NY, 1972, pp 443-448.

10. Buchanan, R.A., Ethosuximide: Toxicity. In *Antiepileptic Drugs*, Chapter 52, D.M. Woodbury, J.K. Penry, and R.P. Schmidt, Eds. Raven Press, New York, NY, 1972, pp 449-454.

11. Warren Jr., J.W., Benmaman, J.D., Wannamaker, B.B., and Levy, R.H., Kinetics of a carbamazepine-ethosuximide interaction. *Clin. Pharmacol. Ther.* **28**, 646-651 (1980).

12. Mattson, R.H., and Cramer, J.A., Valproic acid and ethosuximide interaction. *Ann. Neurol.* **7**, 583-584 (1979).

# Monitoring of Ethosuximide Plasma Concentrations — A Case Study

**Mario L. Rocci, Jr., Ph.D.**

TM, an eight-year-old white female (32 kg), who was newly diagnosed as having petit mal (absence) epilepsy, was admitted to the outpatient neurology clinic. Her parents complained that the drug that was being used to treat her seizures was not effective. Two days prior to admission, this child had been started on **ethosuximide (Zarontin®) therapy, 250 mg twice daily** for control of her seizures. The parents of the patient were instructed in the clinic to increase her ethosuximide dose to 250 mg three times daily and to return to the clinic in seven days.

One week later the patient had not improved; essentially no decrease in the frequency of absence seizures was noted by her parents. During this clinic visit, a blood sample was obtained (at a time corresponding to 3 h after her last dose) and was analyzed for ethosuximide using an immunoassay technique (Emit®). The ethosuximide concentration in this plasma sample was 35 mg/L (248 µmol/L). Based on the results of this value, the patient was instructed to double her dose to 500 mg of ethosuximide three times daily.

Ten days later the mother of the patient phoned the clinic and indicated that although seizure control was much improved, her daughter was having frequent headaches, appeared lethargic, and complained of dizziness and nausea. The patient was instructed to visit the hospital so that a blood sample could be drawn. Analysis of this sample which was taken 5 h after her last dose revealed an ethosuximide concentration in plasma of 110 mg/L (781 µmol/L).

## Discussion

Several aspects of this case can be used to illustrate how fundamental knowledge of the clinical pharmacokinetics of ethosuximide can be used in conjunction with the patient's clinical status to optimize anticonvulsant therapy.

The initial dosage regimen for this patient was too low based on knowledge of ethosuximide clearance in

*Dr. Mario L. Rocci Jr. is an Assistant Professor, Department of Pharmacy Practice, Philadelphia College of Pharmacy and Science and an Adjunct Assistant Professor of Medicine, Jefferson Medical College, Philadelphia PA.*

children, which is on average twice that observed in adults. This patient's therapy was initiated at a dose which was roughly 15 mg/kg, the dosage recommendation conventionally used in adults (1). An initial dosing rate of 20 mg/kg has been recommended in children (1).

Throughout this case, TM received ethosuximide in divided daily doses. Dividing the dosage is not necessary, because ethosuximide possesses a half-life greater than a day in both children and adults. Once-daily ethosuximide administration has been shown to be an effective alternative to divided doses. Once daily dosing of ethosuximide is advantageous in terms of convenience and potentially increases patient compliance (2).

Assessing the adequacy of the dosing rate of a drug in controlling a clinical condition can only be made once steady state has been attained. Steady state occurs when the dosing rate of a drug matched its rate of elimination from the body. Further accumulation of the drug in plasma and tissues will not occur once steady state has been achieved. As a result, drug concentrations in plasma will be in equilibrium with the concentration of drug in all tissues including those tissues where the drug exerts its pharmacologic effect. It generally takes approximately four half-lives to approach steady state. In light of these considerations, assessment of ethosuximide therapy in this patient after two days of treatment is inappropriate. The half-life of ethosuximide in children is approximately 30 h, indicating that about five days are needed to reach steady state (1). Although it is probable that this dose is inadequate for seizure control in this patient, valid assessments of the effectiveness of this dosage regimen could only be made after five days of therapy.

A dose of 750 mg/day (~23 mg/kg) will result in steady state concentrations in plasma of approximately 50 mg/L (535 µmol/L) in most children. When TM's dose was raised to 750 mg/day, the resulting drug level in plasma was 35 mg/L (248 µmol/L); her case demonstrates the variability that is known to exist in the relationship between dose and resultant steady-state concentration of ethosuximide in plasma among patients of the same age (3). The long half-life of ethosuximide makes monitoring of plasma concentrations at anytime acceptable within a dosing interval at steady state, although plasma concentrations obtained just prior to the next dose are often employed for consistency. The lack of improvement in the clinical status of TM after her first increase in dose is not unusual since studies assessing the relationship between drug levels in plasma and seizure control indicate that ethosuximide concentrations in 93% of patients adequately controlled for seizures were in excess of 40 mg/L (285 $\mu$mol/L) (4). Thus, is appears that the vast majority of patients require concentrations in plasma of at least 40 mg/L (285 $\mu$mol/L) for satisfactory seizure control; some individuals may require substantially greater drug concentrations in plasma.

One cannot rule out partial noncompliance as a potential cause for the low ethosuximide concentrations and lack of clinical control in this patient. In this particular case, TM appeared very willing to comply with any therapy that would help to reduce her seizure frequency. Compliance was further assured through her parents, who were receptive to their child's needs.

The doubling of TM's dose resulted in a disproportionate increase in the resultant steady-state concentration of ethosuximide in plasma, producing a concentration of 110 mg/L (781 $\mu$mol/L), which is slightly above the normal therapeutic concentration of 40 to 100 mg/L (285-710 $\mu$mol/L). The headaches, dizziness, lethargy, and nausea that resulted from the excessive dosage of ethosuximide are signs of dose-related toxicity that commonly occur with excessive concentrations of ethosuximide (5). These dose-related effects ameliorate with a reduction in dose. Although an ethosuximide concentration of 110 mg/L (281 $\mu$mol/L) produced toxicity in TM, it will not for all patients. Occasionally, concentrations in plasma of greater than 100 mg/L (710 $\mu$mol/L) are required for adequate seizure control (1).

Disproportionate increases in ethosuximide concentrations with increases in dose reflect the nonlinearity that exists in ethosuximide clearance presumably due to saturation of hepatic drug-metabolizing enzymes at higher concentrations in plasma (3). As a result, dosage adjustments need to be made cautiously. Increases in dose that would result in therapeutic concentrations for a drug with linear pharmacokinetics may result in toxic concentrations for drugs such as ethosuximide (and phenytoin) that display saturable metabolism. Analogously, dosage reductions of ethosuximide may produce greater than proportionate decreases in concentration in plasma.

The dose of 1500 mg/day which produced the dose-related side effects in TM was reduced to 1000 mg/day; her adverse effects have disappeared and her seizure control is adequate.

## Profile of Ethosuximide

Structure

| | |
|---|---|
| Trade name: | Zarontin® |
| Chemical name: | Ethosuximide (2-ethyl-3-methyl-succinimide) (3-ethyl-3-methyl-2.5-pyrrolidine-dione) |
| $pK_a$: | 9.3 |
| Mol. mass: | 141.2 |
| Melting point, °C: | 64-65 |
| Water solubility: | Freely soluble |
| Dose absorbed: | Not available |
| Peak level in plasma, time, h: | 3-7, depends on dose and frequency |
| Protein bound: | 0% |
| $V_D$: | Children, 0.69 L/kg Adults, 0.62 L/kg |

| Form in urine | Excreted, % | Active | Detectable in blood |
|---|---|---|---|
| Unchanged drug: | 17-38 | Yes | Yes |
| Monohydroxy metabolites | Majority of the dose | na | Yes |

| | Adults | Children |
|---|---|---|
| Half-life, h: | 52 | 30 |
| Steady state, time, h: | 208 | 120 |

| | Adults | Children |
|---|---|---|
| Recommended dose, mg/kg/day: | 15 | 20 |
| Effective levels, mg/L: | 40-100 | 40-100 |
| Toxic levels, mg/L: | >100 | >100 |
| Monitoring Methods | Immunoassay (EMIT®) Gas liquid chromatography | |

## References

1. Stoehr, G.P., and Sherwin, A.L., Ethosuximide: Therapeutic use and serum concentration monitoring. In *Individualizing Drug Therapy: Practical Applications of Drug Monitoring*, Vol. 2., A.L. Finn and W.J. Taylor, Eds., Gross, Townsend, Frank, Inc., New York, NY, 1981, pp 1-25.

2. Buchanan, R.A., Kinkel, A.W., Turner, J.L., and Heffelfinger, J.C., Ethosuximide dosage regimens. *Clin. Pharmacol. Ther.* **19**, 143-147 (1976).

3. Battino, D., Cusi, C., Franceschetti, S., Moise, A., Spina, S., and Avanzini, G., Ethosuximide plasma concentrations: Influence of age and associated concomitant therapy. *Clin. Pharmacokin.* **7**, 176-180 (1982).

4. Sherwin, A.L., and Robb, J.P., Ethosuximide: Relation of plasma levels to clinical control (continued). In *Antiepileptic Drugs*, Chapter 51, D.M. Woodbury, J.K. Penry, and R.P. Schmidt, Eds. Raven Press, New York, NY, 1972, pp 443-448.

5. Buchanan, R.A., Ethosuximide: Toxicity. In *Antiepileptic Drugs*, Chapter 52, D.M. Woodbury, J.K. Penry, and R.P. Schmidt, Eds. Raven Press, New York, NY, 1972, pp 449-454.

# 13

# Therapeutic Drug Monitoring: Carbamazepine

**Janis J. MacKichan, Pharm.D.**

## Introduction

Carbamazepine (CBZ) was approved in 1974 for marketing in the United States as an anticonvulsant agent in adults and is considered the drug of choice for treatment of pain associated with trigeminal neuralgia. Unlike other anticonvulsants, CBZ is an iminostilbine derivative structurally related to the tricyclic antidepressants. It is considered to be as effective as phenytoin, phenobarbital, and primidone in the treatment of generalized tonic-clonic and complex partial seizures and has even been recommended by some as a replacement for these drugs to avoid troublesome side effects such as sedation, hyperactivity, gingival hyperplasia, and hypertrichosis (1). CBZ has been used widely and successfully in children of all ages since 1974, but only recently (1980) was it approved for use in children over 6 years of age.

As with most of the anticonvulsant drugs, therapeutic side effect and administered dosage correlate poorly for CBZ. This can be attributed to interpatient variability in CBZ disposition, which is influenced by factors such as age, weight, pregnancy, and concurrent drug therapy. It is difficult to adjust CBZ dosage based on its therapeutic effect because many epileptics have infrequent seizures–as few as two to three per year. Seizures can have devastating psychological and social effects, and if therapy is monitored purely by clinical effect it could be months before the appropriate dosage is found. A good correlation has been demonstrated between concentrations in plasma and therapeutic effects of CBZ (2). By adjusting the CBZ dose so that concentrations in plasma are within a predetermined therapeutic but nontoxic range, the clinician should be able to minimize the delay in controlling seizure activity.

The range of CBZ plasma conentrations considered (2,3) therapeutic and nontoxic in most patients is 4 to 12 mg/L (17 to 50 $\mu$mol/L). A given individual, however, may demonstrate toxicity of inadequate response to CBZ despite having plasma concentrations within this "therapeutic range." This may be explained in part by factors such as concurrent therapy with other anticonvulsants, the presence of a potentially active metabolite, carbamazepine-10, 11-

*Dr. MacKichan is an Assistant Professor of Pharmacy, Ohio State University, College of Pharmacy, Columbus, OH 43210*

epoxide (CBZ-EP), and considerable variability in plasma protein binding of CBZ and its metabolite. It has been suggested that the value of plasma concentration monitoring of CBZ would be improved by simultaneous measurement of free concentrations of these compounds in plasma –either directly by ultra-filtration or indirectly by measurement in saliva. Of ultimate importance, it must be emphasized that plasma CBZ concentrations are only an aid to dosage regulation and that the best therapeutic results are obtained when clinical judgement is combined with this laboratory information.

## Plasma Concentration vs. Effect Relationships

For most drugs, the intensity of therapeutic and toxic pharmacological effects is directly related to the concentration of drug surrounding the receptors that elicit these effects. Because free drug in plasma is in equilibrium with drug present at these receptor sites, drug concentrations in plasma can serve indirectly as a guide to certain pharmacodynamic effects. Many investigators have attempted to relate plasma CBZ concentrations to its therapeutic and toxic effects. Despite various problems in study design and methodology, these studies (2,3) indicate that in most patients concentrations of at least 4 mg/L (17 $\mu$mol/L) are necessary for effective treatment of seizures. A few patients will benefit from concentrations of less than 4 mg/L; others may not improve with double these concentrations. Plasma CBZ concentrations > 12 mg/L (50 $\mu$mol/L) have been associated with unpleasant neurosensory side effects such as unsteadiness, dizziness, double-vision, and uncoordination in most patients maintained on CBZ alone (4). CBZ concentrations of 9 mg/L (38 $\mu$mol/L) or less may prove toxic in patients who are taking other anticonvulsants, particularly phenytoin (5). Gastrointestinal complaints such as nausea or vomiting occur less frequently but may also be related to the plasma CBZ concentration. Some of the adverse effects to CBZ are not related to its concentration in plasma and most likely are allergic reactions. These rare effects include skin rashes, hematologic abnormalities (thrombocytopenia, aplastic anemia) and hepatic abnormalities (hepatitis, cholestatic and hepatocellular jaundice) (4).

On average, daily maintenance CBZ doses of 200 to 1200 mg in adults will produce steady-state plasma concentrations ranging from 1 to 16 mg/L (4.25 to 50 $\mu$mol/L) (3). At a given dose, however, the resulting

CBZ concentrations in plasma are extremely variable from patient to patient. This is demonstrated in Figure 1 where, for example, average steady-state concentrations in plasma in a group of adult patients taking 1200 mg of CBZ per day are seen to range from 3.8 to 11.8 mg/L (16 to 50 μmol/L) (5). Interpatient variability in rate and extent of absorption, distribution (plasma protein binding), and metabolism of CBZ probably account for most of the variabilities in rate and extent of absorption, given dose. Because of this interpatient variability in CBZ disposition and the fact that plasma concentrations parallel therapeutic effect and toxicity, the concentration of CBZ in plasma is extremely useful for individualization of CBZ dosages.

## Pharmacokinetics

A review of the pharmacokinetics of CBZ is helpful in understanding the sources of interpatient variability in CBZ concentrations in plasma after a given dose. Pharmacokinetics is the mathematical characterization of the time course of drug concentrations in various body tissues and fluids such as plasma. Such data for CBZ in plasma are determined by three physiological processes: absorption, distribution, and metabolism.

*Absorption:* CBZ is commercially available only in oral tablet form (Tegretol®). It is slowly absorbed from the gastrointestinal tract, and absorption is extremely variable. Single-dose studies in normal volunteers have shown that CBZ concentrations in plasma are greatest 6 h on the average after oral administration of the tablet, but the range is 2 to 24 h (4). After reaching a maximum, plasma concentrations typically become constant for 10 to 30 h (4), an effect not seen after administration of CBZ as an alcoholic or propylene glycol solution and probably ascribable to slow dissolution of the tablet owing to the slow solubility of this drug in water (4). Peak plasma concentrations are reached more rapidly (within an average of 3 h) in patients who are chronically treated (4). This may be explained in part by the elimination half-life of CBZ after chronic therapy (see *Metabolism and Elimination*). Because the time required to reach a drug peak concentration in plasma is a function both of rates of absorption and elimination, an increased rate of elimination (decreased half-life) will shorten the interval needed to reach a maximum concentration in plasma. For the same reason, the time to reach peak plasma CBZ concentrations is further reduced in patients who are taking enzyme-inducing drugs concurrently (see *Metabolism and Elimination*).

The fraction of orally administered CBZ that enters the systemic circulation (absolute bioavailability) has not been determined. There are two major causes of decreased bioavailability: decreased absorption and first-pass metabolism by the liver. The absorbed fraction of orally administered CBZ is estimated to be 85 to 90% based on the analytical recovery of 10 to 15% of radiolabeled CBZ in the feces of two normal subjects (6). CBZ is not highly extracted from the circulation by the liver and therefore first-pass metabolism is inconsequential (4). The extent of CBZ absorption is similar in a given patient whether it is given as the commercially available tablet or as a solution or suspension.

*Distribution:* CBZ is a neutral and highly lipophilic compound. Concentrations of CBZ and/or CBZ-EP have been measured in brain tissue, cerebrospinal fluid, and breast milk, and in fetal tissue after placental transport (4). Apparent volumes of distribution of CBZ in epileptic patients who are undergoing chronic treatment range from 0.8 to 1.0 L/kg of body weight (4). These values have been calculated with complete bioavailability of CBZ being assumed; true volumes are probably smaller and less variable.

The degree of plasma protein binding is an important determinant of CBZ distribution as well as efficacy. Only free, unbound drug is available for distribution to the receptors responsible for a drug's effects, yet therapeutic ranges of drug concentrations in plasma are almost always based on total (bound +

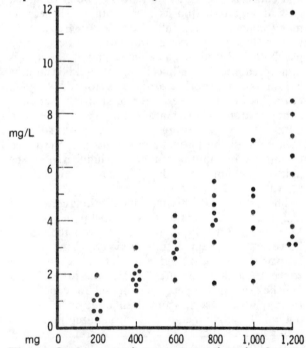

**Fig. 1. Carbamazepine concentrations in plasma of 23 epileptic outpatients on various dosages. From reference 5.**

unbound) drug in plasma. This is because measurement of total drug in plasma is much easier than measurement of free drug only, and most drugs demonstrate little interpatient variability in the fraction of drug in plasma that is in the unbound form. Although the proportion of free CBZ in plasma averages 25% in normal subjects, it ranges from 13 to 33% in epileptic patients (2,7). Likewise, the percentage of CBZ-EP free in plasma is also variable, ranging from 16 to 50% (7). This variability in protein binding may be due in part to interindividual variability in total protein or albumin concentrations (7). Based on these findings, two patients could have total CBZ plasma concentrations of 12 mg/L (50 $\mu$mol/L) but free-drug concentrations of 1.6 mg/L (6.8 $\mu$mol/L) in one and 4 mg/L (17 $\mu$mol/L) in the other. Only the free-drug concentration determines the intensity of both effect and toxicity; thus this difference in free concentration could explain why symptoms of toxicity may appear in one patient but not in another, even though the total drug concentration in the plasma is the same in both. These observations suggest that data on a therapeutic range based on free CBZ concentrations in plasma might improve the predictive nature of CBZ monitoring.

Concentrations of CBZ and CBZ-EP in saliva were found to be strongly related to their respective free concentrations in plasma in a group of 24 epileptic patients (Figure 2) (7). Despite a significant correlation between salivary concentrations and their respective total plasma concentration, salivary concentrations were poor predictors of the corresponding total concentrations (7). In contrast, concentrations in saliva were significantly better predictors of the concentrations of both free CBZ and free CBZ-EP in plasma (7). This may be explained by the fact that CBZ and its metabolites are neutral compunds and thus are completely un-ionized over the pH range of plasma and saliva. The unbound compounds in plasma can therefore passively diffuse into low-protein fluids such as saliva until an equilibrium is attained. Theoretically, concentrations in saliva should be equal to free-drug concentrations in plasma. Hence, measurements of CBZ and CBZ-EP in saliva should provide a better estimate of free-drug in plasma than of total drug, especially when large interindividual differences in protein binding exist. However, in our study, salivary concentrations of both compounds were consistently higher than their respective free plasma concentrations—by 14% for CBZ and 29% for the epoxide metabolite. The reason for this is not known.

*Metabolism and Elimination:* CBZ is almost entirely metabolized by the liver, with only 1 to 2% of a dose excreted unchanged in the urine (4). CBZ may also undergo enterohepatic cycling (3).

The elimination of CBZ can be quantitated by its total body clearance and elimination half-life. Clearance (CL) has units of volume/time or volume/time per body weight and is the proportionality constant relating dose-rate (DR)—i.e.,

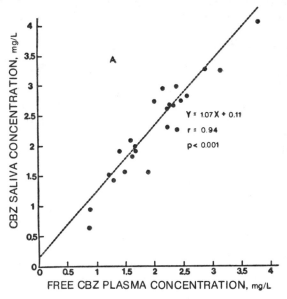

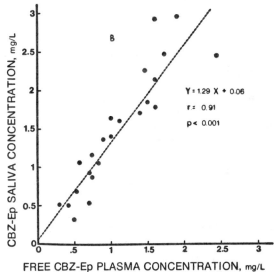

**Fig. 2. Concentration of CBZ (*A*) and CBZ-EP (*B*) in saliva of epileptic patients as a function of concentration in plasma. The dotted lines represent the least-squares regression lines of best fit. *A*) *y* = 1.07*x* + 0.11, *r* = 0.94, *p* < 0.001. *B*) *y* = 1.29*x* + 0.006, *r* = 0.91, *p* < 0.001. From reference 7.**

mg/day–to the resulting average steady-state plasma concentration ($C_{av}^{ss}$)–i.e., mg/day–as shown in the following equation:

$$DR \propto C_{av}^{ss} \times CL \qquad (1)$$

The clearance of CBZ, a reflection of the liver's ability to metabolize this drug, varies from patient to patient. As with volume of distribution, the clearance of CBZ is reported as an apparent value because its bioavailability is unknown but is assumed to be complete. True clearances are probably smaller. Elimination half-life ($t\frac{1}{2}$), the time required to decrease the plasma concentration of CBZ by half after distribution, is determined by both apparent volume of distribution (V) and its apparent clearance according to the following relationship:

$$t\frac{1}{2} = 0.693 \, (V) \, / \, CL \qquad (2)$$

According to equation 2, if the volume of distribution remains constant in a given individual, then half-life will shorten as clearance increases. According to equation 1, if the dose-rate of CBZ is kept constant, then an increase in clearance will result in lower average steady-state plasma concentrations.

After single CBZ doses are administered to normal subjects who have not been previously exposed to CBZ, the biological half-life of the drug averages 35 hours, and apparent clearances range from 11 to 26 mL/h per kg (4). Epileptic patients who take CBZ chronically reportedly have more rapid clearances and shorter half-lives than is the case in single-dose studies. Apparent clearance of 50 to 100 mL/h per kg and half-lives of 5 to 27 h are common in chronically treated patients (4). This observation suggests that CBZ induces its own metabolism and has been termed "autoinduction." This effect was confirmed in a study of three children: the apparent clearance of CBZ increased from an initial average value of 28 mL/h per kg to a maximum average value of 56 mL/h per kg (8). Accordingly, because the dose-rate of CBZ was kept constant in these patients, concentrations in the plasma progressively decreased twofold over the same period. Maximal autoinduction is reported to occur within two to four weeks (4). Autoinduction may also be dose-dependent as it was not observed in adult volunteers who took relatively small CBZ doses, 200 mg/day (4).

CBZ-EP is the most important metabolite of CBZ because it has been shown in rats to possess anticonvulsant properties similar to CBZ (9). This has not yet been confirmed in humans. The ratio of steady-state concentrations of the metabolite to CBZ in plasma is 0.5 on the average but is extremely variable,

ranging from 0.05 to 0.93 (7). This ratio is larger and more variable in patients who are taking the drug with other anticonvulsants than in those who are taking only CBZ (7). This has been attributed to induction by other anticonvulsants of enzymes responsible for biotransformation of CBZ to its epoxide metabolite (4). Accordingly, apparent clearances of CBZ tend to be larger and half-lives shorter in patients treated with other anticonvulsant drugs as compared with those taking CBZ alone (See *Drug Interactions*) (4).

The elimination of CBZ varies as a function of age and pregnancy. Studies have shown apparent clearances of CBZ to be larger and more variable in children who are chronically treated as compared with chronically treated adults (4). The average apparent clearance of CBZ in children is 100 mL/h per kg, with a range of 50 to 200 (4). In newborn infants who acquire CBZ transplacentally, elimination half-lives range from 8 to 28 h, which is similar to half-lives measured in adults after chronic CBZ treatment but shorter than those observed in adults after single doses (4). This indicates a reasonably well-developed metabolic capacity, which may have been induced transplacentally. During pregnancy, the apparent clearance of CBZ increases as much as twofold followed by a gradual decrease to pre-pregnancy values after delivery (10). Concentrations of the epoxide metabolite are increased relative to plasma CBZ concentrations, which suggests an increased rate of metabolism during pregnancy. The potential metabolizing activities of placenta and fetus were excluded as an explanation for these observations; rather it was suggested that high concentrations of circulating estrogens and progesterones in pregnancy may induce certain of the mother's hepatic enzyme systems (10).

## Drug Interactions

The apparent clearance of CBZ frequently increases when other anticonvulsants are added to a patient's regimen. This has been studied for phenytoin and phenobarbital, which presumeably induce the metabolism of CBZ (10). After either phenytoin or phenobarbital was added, average steady-state CBZ concentrations in plasma decreased from 6.7 mg/L to 5.5 and 4.4 mg/L, respectively (11). Administration of both drugs with CBZ tended to increase the apparent clearance of CBZ more than did that of either drug alone, as demonstrated by a decrease in plasma CBZ concentration from 6.7 mg/L to 3.7 mg/L (11). The additional observation that concentrations of CBZ-EP in plasma increased as those of CBZ decreased suggests that the enzymatic pathway responsible for conversion of CBZ to its epoxide metabolite is induced by these anticonvulsants. Clinical observations suggest that primidone, ethosuximide, and sodium valproate may also increase the apparent clearance of CBZ, but prospective studies have not yet been performed to examine the effect of each drug individually (4).

Concentrations of CBZ in plasma were shown to increase by more than 60% during concurrent treatment with propoxyphene, which suggests that the clearance of CBZ is decreased by this drug (4). Propoxyphene is believed to inhibit one of the metabolic pathways of CBZ, although evidently not the one yielding CBZ-EP, because the concentrations of this metabolite in plasma remained constant.

CBZ has been shown to decrease steady-state plasma concentrations of warfarin, clonazepam and phenytoin, and to shorten the half-life of doxycycline (4). The effects are presumeably due to CBZ's ability to induce enzymes that are responsible for metabolism of these drugs. Because of its enzyme-induction capability, there are likely to be many more potential drug interactions involving CBZ that remain to be documented.

## Carbamazepine Dosage Guidelines

*General guidelines.* The proper CBZ maintenance-dosage regimen for a given patient is defined as that which renders optimal seizure control and which maintains average steady-state concentrations in plasma within the therapeutic range for that patient—generally from 4 to 12 mg/L (17 to 50 $\mu$mol/L). A dosage regimen is defined by two variables: the dose-rate and the dosage interval. The dose-rate of oral CBZ necessary to attain a given steady-state concentration in plasma is determined solely by the apparent clearance of CBZ (equation 1). Use of a loading dose on initiating therapy is not advised. Because the clearance of CBZ is initially two to four times lower in a patient previously unexposed to this drug, therapy should be initiated with lower doses than are expected to be needed. A general rule is to give a fourth to a third of the eventually expected maintenance dose-rate initially and increase it weekly during three to four weeks until the final daily maintenance dose-rate is reached. Maximal autoinduction should have occurred by this time. Clinical studies have indicated that many objectionable neurosensory and gastrointestinal side effects are minimized when therapy is initiated gradually, which suggests that many of these side effects are at least in part related to the concentration in plasma (4).

The optimal dosage interval for CBZ is guided by its biological half-life, which shortens as therapy progresses. For most drugs, a dosage interval equal to the half-life of the drug is acceptable, because plasma concentrations will fluctuate only twofold during this period. The shorter the dosage interval, relative to the drug's half-life, the less fluctuation there will be in plasma drug concentrations during that interval. Although CBZ could be given once daily during initiation of therapy when the half-life is relatively long, studies have shown this to be inadequate during maintenance therapy when the half-life is shorter (4). Administration of CBZ as single daily doses during chronic therapy can lead to excessively high peak plasma concentrations, which are associated with side effects. Once-daily therapy may also result in concentrations in plasma that are subtherapeutic for a long period of time near the end of the dosage interval, thus increasing the possibility for "break-through" seizures. More frequent administration of CBZ (same dose-rate, but shorter intervals) helps to avoid side effects that are related to the concentration in plasma and should maintain concentrations above the minimally effective level. CBZ should be given no less frequently than twice daily to adults; children may require three to four daily doses. Adult patients who are taking other anticonvulsants concurrently and for whom CBZ half-lives are shorter as a result may also require more frequent administration of this drug.

*Specific guidelines.* The average maintenance dose-rate of CBZ in adults and children over 12 years of age ranges from 7 to 15 mg/kg per day, or 500 to 1000 mg in the case of a 70-kg person. This range is designed to attain an average CBZ concentration in plasma of about 6 mg/L (25 $\mu$mol/L) in most patients. The manufacturer recommends that daily doses greater than 1200 mg be avoided. The daily CBZ dose should be given in two to four divided doses according to each patient's tolerance to peak-concentration-related side effects.

Based on the higher apparent CBZ clearances reported in children, maintenance dose-rates of 10 to 25 mg/kg per day should provide an average steady-state CBZ concentration of 6 mg/L in the plasma of most children weighing up to 60 kg. This range is consistent with the manufacturer's recommendation for 6 to 12 year old children (400 to 800 mg/day) and with the experience of clinicians who have used CBZ extensively in infants and children (1)(4). The dosage interval may need to be as small as 6 h in children, especially when other anticonvulsants are given concurrently.

Because the apparent clearance of CBZ can increase by as much as twofold during pregnancy, the dose-rate should be increased by the same proportion to maintain the same concentrations that were observed before pregnancy. If the dose-rate is increased during pregnancy to compensate for an increased clearance, it will need to be gradually decreased soon after delivery.

Clearances of CBZ gradually decrease to pre-pregnancy values within two weeks after delivery (*4*).

Little is known about the effect of various disease states on the disposition of CBZ. Because the drug is almost completely metabolized by the liver, its clearance and elimination may be decreased in patients with liver disease, and the dose-rate in patients with liver disease may need to be decreased by the same proportion.

## Concentrations Monitoring in Plasma

*What to measure.* Although it has been suggested that concentrations of both CBZ and its epoxide metabolite in plasma might correlate better with observed therapeutic and toxic effects than measurements of CBZ alone, present knowledge of the activity of this metabolite in humans is minimal. Until more information about the activity of this metabolite is provided, measurements of the parent drug must suffice for clinical monitoring.

In general, only the free-drug in plasma has access to receptor sites that elicit therapeutic and toxic effects. Consequently, when there is a large degree of variability in the protein binding of a drug, the range of total drug concentrations in plasma necessary to accommodate the therapeutic range of unbound drug becomes wider. The relatively large variation among individuals in the percentage of CBZ that is free in plasma implies that the reported therapeutic range of total CBZ concentrations is unnecessarily wide. Studies relating free CBZ concentrations to therapeutic and toxic effects may reveal a narrower therapeutic range. Routine measurements of free CBZ concentrations in plasma by techniques such as equilibrium dialysis are time-consuming and not feasible for a clinical laboratory. Ultrafiltration devices designed for routine determination of unbound plasma concentrations have recently become available for several drugs, including CBZ (Ultra-Free®; Worthington Diagnostics, Freehold, NJ). These systems appear to offer sufficient accuracy but require considerably less time than equilibrium dialysis. Concentrations of CBZ in saliva, which provide reliable estimates of free CBZ concentrations in plasma, may provide an alternative to use of the ultrafiltration devices. Saliva collection has additional advantages in that it is a painless and noninvasive procedure and serial samples can be collected from those patients who cannot tolerate excessive blood loss, specifically pediatric, geriatric, or critically ill patients. Saliva production can be stimulated by the chewing of Parafilm or by putting a citric acid crystal on the tip of the tongue. Based on the average saliva/plasma concentration ratio of 0.27 reported in our study of

epileptic patients (*7*) and the generally accepted therapeutic range of total CBZ concentrations of 4 to 12 mg/L, the initial guideline for a therapeutic range of CBZ in saliva is 1.1 to 3.2 mg/L (4.7 to 13.6 $\mu$mol/L). It must be emphasized that although the importance of monitoring free plasma or salivary CBZ concentrations is still speculative, these measurements may provide more reliable information to the clinician in certain cases.

*When to obtain samples.* As a general guideline, the clinician is advised to obtain the first blood sample for determination of a drug's concentration in plasma after steady-state has been attained. For most drugs this occurs in a time period equal to about four to five half-lives after initiation of therapy. Because of the autoinduction phenomenon, steady-state CBZ concentrations are not achieved for about two to four weeks after therapy is begun. After maximal induction has occurred, plasma concentrations will be at steady-state in three to four days after the final maintenance dose was begun. A concentration measured in plasma at this time best represents the concentrations associated with that dose-rate.

If only one blood or saliva sample is to be obtained, the lowest concentration during the dosage interval may provide the best guide for dosage adjustment. Theoretically, this occurs just before the next dose is to be given, but because of the reported variability in absorption rate of CBZ this may not always be the case. If there is any question, measurement of multiple samples over the dosage interval will reveal the highest and lowest CBZ concentrations.

Saliva samples should always be collected at least 2 h after administration of a CBZ dose. CBZ has been found to linger in the mouth and contaminate the saliva in patients such as children who receive the drug as a suspension or crushed tablet (*7*). Excessively high concentrations in saliva should always be repeated or confirmed by analysis of a serum or plasma sample.

*Indications for monitoring.*

1. At the onset of therapy, after maximal autoinduction has occurred, to see if the patient is within the therapeutic range. If a dose-rate adjustment is necessary because the patient is not within the therapeutic range, is exhibiting toxicities, or is still uncontrolled, the following relationship may be used:

$$\text{new DR} = \text{present DR} \times \frac{\text{desired } C_{av}^{ss}}{\text{present } C_{av}^{ss}} \tag{3}$$

2. When the dose-rate is changed. Measurements taken after a new steady-state has been achieved (three to four days) will most accurately reflect plasma CBZ concentrations associated with the

new dose-rate.

3. If the dose-rate of another anticonvulsant drug has been added, changed or discontinued. It may take one to two weeks for maximal induction or de-induction of hepatic enzymes to occur, and this must be considered when ordering and interpreting CBZ concentrations.

4. When there are toxic symptoms possibly caused by CBZ. Measurement of the plasma CBZ concentration may be the only way to detect intoxication in a comatose or very young patient.

5. If seizure control is lost. Measurement of CBZ in plasma may indicate either a need for an increase in CBZ dose-rate or a lack of patient compliance. Paradoxical seizures may occur with over-doses of CBZ (4) and measurement of the plasma concentration may be the only way to distinguish these seizures from those caused by inadequate therapy.

6. During pregnancy. Little is known about the time-course of clearance changes early in pregnancy; therefore, frequent measurements of plasma CBZ concentrations during this time will provide the best guide for any dosage changes.

## Conclusion

Because CBZ disposition varies with age, pregnancy, and concurrent drug therapy, CBZ concentrations in plasma or saliva are extremely variable in patients taking the same dosages. By combining good clinical judgement with rational plasma concentration monitoring techniques, the physician can maximize therapeutic efficacy and minimize adverse effects due to CBZ. In this regard, clinical laboratory personnel who are involved in therapeutic drug monitoring can be an important resource for the physician. The therapeutic drug monitoring consultant should recognize that plasma CBZ concentrations for some patients may not fall within the usual "therapeutic range" for most patients because of three factors: (1) presence of the potentially active CBZ-EP metabolite; (2) variability in protein binding of CBZ and CBZ-EP; and/or (3) concurrent anticonvulsant therapy. The clinical chemist should assure the specificity of the analytical method used for CBZ with respect to other anticonvulsants and CBZ metabolites. Modification of the method to simultaneously analyze the CBZ-EP metabolite may be considered for the future. The laboratory may want to consider utilization of devices for monitoring the concentration of free-drug in plasma in certain situations. If salivary CBZ concentrations are to be monitored, the laboratory can recommend appropriate procedures for obtaining the specimens.

Lastly, because CBZ concentrations in saliva are approximately one-fourth the concentration in plasma, the assay should be evaluated with respect to sensitivity and precision at these lower concentrations.

## References

1. Wallace, S.J., Carbamazepine in childhood seizures. *Dev. Med. Child. Neurol.* **20**, 223-226, (1978).

2. Bertilsson, L., Clinical pharmacokinetics of carbamazepine. *Clin. Pharmacokin.* **3**, 128-142 (1978).

3. Kutt, H., Clinical pharmacology of carbamazepine. In *Antiepileptic Drugs: Quantitative Analysis and Interpretation,* C.E. Pippenger, J.K. Penry, and H. Kutt, Eds., Raven Press, New York, N.Y., 1978 pp. 297-305.

4. MacKichan J.J., and Kutt, H., Carbamazepine: Therapeutic use and serum concentration monitoring. In *Individualizing Drug Therapy: Practical Applications of Drug Monitoring*, Vol. 2., A.L. Finn and W.J. Taylor, Eds., Gross, Townsend, Frank, Inc., New York, N.Y., 1981, pp. 1-25.

5. Kutt, H., Solomon, G., Wasterlain, G., et al, Carbamazepine in difficult-to-control epileptic outpatients. *Acta Neurol. Scand.*, Suppl. **60**, 27-32 (1975).

6. Faigle, J.W., and Feldman, K.F., Pharmacokinetic data of carbamazepine and its major metabolites in man. In *Clinical Pharmacology of Antiepileptic Drugs*, H. Schneider, et al, Eds., Springer-Verlag, Berlin, 1975, pp. 159-165.

7. MacKichan, J.J., Duffner, P.K., and Cohen, M.E., Salivary concentrations and plasma protein binding of carbamazepine and carbamazepine 10, 11-epoxide in epileptic patients. *Brit. J. Clin. Pharmacol.* **12**, 31-37 (1981).

8. Bertilsson, L., Hojer, B., Tybring, G., et al, Auto-induction of carbamazepine metabolism in children examined by a stable isotope technique. *Clin. Pharmacol. Ther.* **27**, 83-88 (1980).

9. Frigerio, A., Morselli, P.L., Carbamazepine biotransformation, *Adv. Neurol.* **11**, 295-308 (1975).

10. Dam, M., Christiansen, J., Munck, O., and Mygind, K.I., Antiepileptic drugs: Metabolism in pregnancy. *Clin. Pharmacokin.* **4**, 53-62 (1979).

11. Christiansen, J., and Dam, M. Influence of phenobarbital and diphenylhydantoin on plasma carbamazepine levels in patients with epilepsy. *Acta Neurol. Scand.* **49**, 543-546 (1973).

# 14

# Carbamazepine: Two Cases

**Anthony J. Windebank, M.D.**

## Case #1

An 18-year-old girl had suffered from complex partial seizures since the age of 11. She was aware of her seizures, because at the onset she felt a feeling of intense anxiety lasting several seconds, followed by a brief period of confusion. Witnesses reported that during a spell, she would look anxious and then stare blankly ahead; at the same time she smacked her lips and chewed. After about 10 seconds, she would mumble a few unintelligible words and then look around as if confused. Although she never fell, observers noticed that she was unresponsive during this whole 30-second episode. For about one minute after this, she appeared to have difficulty speaking. Interictal electroencephalographic monitoring revealed a focal sharp-wave abnormality over the left temporal lobe which became generalized during her stereotyped seizure behaviour.

These seizures had been well controlled by phenytoin (300 mg/day) and carbamazepine (200 mg three times/day) until early in 1978, when her typical psychomotor seizures began to recur with increasing frequency. When she reported this to her neurologist, he checked blood levels of both drugs and found that the phenytoin level was 18 mg/L (therapeutic range 10—20 mg/L) and carbamazepine level was 8 mg/L (therapeutic range 4—10 mg/L).

These were similar to concentrations measured 6 months previously when seizures were controlled, and he concluded that her disorder had become less sensitive to these medications. He felt that she might benefit by the addition of valproic acid to her drug regime. In order that she should not be on three different drugs, he asked her to reduce phenytoin dosage gradually while increasing the amount of valproic acid.

Four days later she was brought to the emergency room by fellow students who feared she may have taken a drug overdose. They reported that she had been behaving anxiously for several days, and on that evening they had found her in a stupor in her bedroom.

The admitting neurologist found her to be quite normal on examination except for her level of respon-

*Dr. Windebank is Senior Clinical Fellow in Neurology, Mayo Medical School, Mayo Clinic and Mayo Foundation, Rochester, Minnesota 55901.*

siveness. Although apparently awake, she did not respond to any commands or answer any questions. She appeared to be extremely anxious and on occasions would try to speak, although no intelligible words came out.

He suspected that she was suffering from psychomotor status epilepticus and requested blood levels of anticonvulsants and an emergency EEG evaluation. The latter confirmed the clinical diagnosis. Intravenous valium given during the EEG recording aborted the electrical seizure activity.

The following blood levels were found: phenytoin 8 mg/L; carbamazepine undetectable; valproic acid 31 mg/L (therapeutic range 40—100 mg/L). Four hours later, when the patient was able to answer questions, it was determined that the young lady had misinterpreted the neurologist's instructions concerning her medication change. As well as tapering her phenytoin, she had abruptly discontinued taking her carbamazepine. Reinstitution of carbamazepine, together with valproic acid, has kept her seizure-free during the past 12 months.

## Case #2

A 29-year-old married woman had suffered from generalized tonic-clonic seizures since the age of 6. EEG recordings had previously demonstrated multifocal independent sharp waves and spikes over both cerebral hemispheres. This widespread epileptiform abnormality was thought to be the result of perinatal hypoxic injury. Her seizure disorder had always been difficult to treat satisfactorily, but most recently she had been well controlled on a regimen of phenytoin (300 mg/day), phenobarbital (60 mg twice/day) and carbamazepine (400 mg, three times/day).

She came to her neurologist complaining of increasing drowsiness, and a feeling of unsteadiness and incoordination. She took her medication diligently and had not changed the dosage nor added any new drugs during the previous 3 months. On examination, she was dysarthric and had both ataxia of gait and appendicular ataxia. There was prominent horizontal nystagmus on lateral gaze.

She was clearly drug-intoxicated, but there were no

historical clues as to which one of her three anticonvulsants was primarily responsible. Blood levels of the drugs taken at this time were phenobarbital 16 mg/L (therapeutric range 20—40 mg/L), phenytoin 14 mg/L (therapeutic range 10—20 mg/L), and carbamazepine 13 mg/L (therapeutic range 2—10 mg/L), suggesting that the last drug was probably contributing most to her symptoms of overdosage. After admission to the hospital, carbamazepine was discontinued for 2 days and then reinstituted at a lower dosage of 200 mg four times/day.

On this new regimen her seizure frequency increased slightly, but the patient preferred this to the intoxicated state which had prevented her from carrying out her household duties. No cause could be found for her becoming intoxicated without any apparent change in medications.

### Discussion of the Cases

Measurement of drug levels is useful in the management of the epileptic patient, particularly in cases where several different anticonvulsants and used simultaneously. Carbamazepine is rarely used as the drug of first choice in treating seizure disorders. It is therefore frequently used in combination with other agents.

In the first case, two different examples of useful monitoring are illustrated. When the patient came to her neurologist complaining of an increase in seizure frequency, two causes could be considered. Either the seizures had become less responsive to the medication, or the amount of drug reaching the brain had decreased. The blood levels suggested strongly that the former was the case, and the neurologist elected to change medication rather than increase the dosage of the drugs she was taking. At the second presentation, she was in status epilepticus. In previously well controlled epileptics, the most common cause of status epilepticus is a fall in drug levels, leading one to actively seek a reason for such a decrease. In this case, questioning the patient revealed that she had stopped taking her carbamazepine. Thus, the situation could have been adequately managed without measuring blood levels, but the information helped to document the problem. This kind of information is also useful when drug levels fall because of concurrent illness with a resulting change in drug metabolism.

In the second case, a common problem in the management of difficult seizure disorders is illustrated. There is often a fine line between clinical control and overdosage. Use of multiple drugs is often required. Most anticonvulsants produce similar symptoms when given in toxic amounts. Thus, the complaints of

drowsiness and incoordination and the typical constellation of cerebellar signs (dysarthria, ataxia, and nystagmus) could have been produced by any of the three drugs. Since only the carbamazepine was present in a concentration above the accepted therapeutic range, the dosage of this agent was reduced. Adjustment of drugs could have been carried out in the absence of drug-level monitoring, but it may have taken considerably longer to reach a satisfactory result. These cases show that measurement of drug levels is not a substitute for careful clinical management, but it is very helpful in certain situations.

### Other Neurological Disorders Treated With Carbamazepine

Carbamazepine is also used in treating a specific type of severe paroxysmal facial pain known as trigeminal neuralgia. In this condition it is often the drug of first choice and is usually used alone. Blood levels are rarely helpful. Dosage is increased gradually until either the pain is controlled or signs of overdosage become apparent. Raising the dose above 1200 mg/day is unlikely to increase the chance of favorable response.

In other neurological disorders, particularly multiple sclerosis, carbamazepine has been used to treat paroxysmal muscle spasm and pain. In these cases also, clinical usage is based on response and not on drug plasma level.

### Pharmacology and Pharmacokinetics

Carbamazepine was introduced in Europe in the early 1960's for the treatment of epilepsy. It is most effective in treating partial complex (psychomotor seizures) and generalized tonic-clonic seizures. It is structurally related to the tricyclic antidepressants and it has been suggested that this is why it has less sedative effects than the barbiturates or hydantoins. The anticonvulsant mechanism is, at present, not well understood at the physiological or cellular level.

The drug is absorbed relatively slowly from the gastrointestinal tract. Peak plasma levels are reached 6—8 hours after a single oral dose. The plasma half-life is of the order of 15—40 hours in patients taking the drug chronically. In animal models it is distributed throughout all tissues and appears to equilibrate across the blood-brain barrier quite rapidly.

At a constant dosage, steady-state plasma levels are reached in 2—4 days. In most patients, however, the drug is introduced gradually to reduce the incidence of side effects. Carbamazepine is 75% protein-bound in the blood, mainly to albumin. It is metabolized by the liver and excreted by both liver and kidneys. The major metabolite, carbamazepine 10,11-epoxide, is an active antiepileptic, and may reach high concentrations in children. For further discussion of this metabolite, see reference 1.

In adults, daily doses of 200—600 mg carbamazepine produces plasma levels of 1—6 mg/L, while doses of 600—1200 mg produce levels of 3—16 mg/L. Therapeutically effective plasma levels are usually quoted as being in the 2—10 mg/L range.

## Drug Interactions

Carbamazepine may shorten the plasma half-life and hence the time to a steady-state blood level of phenytoin. Therefore, monitoring of blood levels may be particularly useful when carbamazepine is added to a drug regimen including phenytoin. It may cause a decrease in warfarin levels. In spite of the similarity of structure, little interaction has been reported between carbamazepine and the tricyclic antidepressants.

## Side Effects

In general the side effects of the drug may be divided into those that are dose-related and those that are idiosyncratic. Only the most common side effects will be mentioned here.

Dose-related effects are mainly restricted to the gastrointestinal and central nervous system. Nausea and gastric irritation are reported, particularly when the drug is first introduced or the dosage is increased rapidly. Drowsiness, unsteadiness, diplopia, and slurred speech are usually symptoms of intoxication, although they may occur transiently when the drug is first introduced.

Reported rare idiosyncratic side effects include hepatic, cardiac, and renal dysfunction. However, the most frequent adverse reactions are skin and hematologic manifestations. A variety of rashes and the Stevens-Johnson syndrome have been described in association with the use of this drug. They are thought to be a form of hypersensitivity reaction and are indications for discontinuing therapy. The most widely feared side effect is bone-marrow depression. Although this problem is rare, a full blood count should be made both before starting and at regular intervals during treatment. The drug should be withdrawn at the first sign of leukopenia or thrombocytopenia. It must, of course, be remembered that in any epileptic patient, sudden cessation of anticonvulsant medication may precipitate status epilepticus.

In summary, carbamazepine is a drug with proven efficacy in the treatment of certain seizure disorders and trigeminal neuralgia. At all times, dosage should primarily be determined by clinical response and not by plasma levels. However, in certain clinical situations, measurement of blood concentration may be of great value.

## References

Pippenger, C.E., Penry, J.K., and Kutt, H., Eds., Antiepileptic Drugs: Quantitative Analysis and Interpretation, Raven Press, New York, 1978.

Penry, J.K., Ed., Epilepsy: The Eighth International Symposium, Raven Press, New York, 1976.

Laidlaw, J. and Richens, A., Eds., A Text Book of Epilepsy, Churchill Livingstone, 1976.

Rasmussen, P. and Riishede, J., Facial Pain Treated with Carbamazepine, *Acta Neurol. Scand.* **46** 385 (1970).

## CARBAMAZEPINE PROFILE

| | |
|---|---|
| Trade name: | Tegretol |
| pK$_a$: | n/a |
| Mol. wt.: | 236.26 |
| mp, °C: | 204-206 |
| Water solubility: | pract. insol. |
| Chemical name: | 5-H-dibenz(b,f)azepine-5-carboxamide |

Chemical structure:

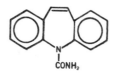

| | |
|---|---|
| Dose absorbed: | 70-80% |
| Peak plasma level, time: | 6-18h |
| Protein bound: | 65-85% |
| V$_d$: | 0.8-1.4 L/kg |

| Form in urine- | % excreted | Active | Detectable in blood |
|---|---|---|---|
| as unchanged drug: | 0.5-1.0 | yes | yes |
| as carbamazepine-10, 11-epoxide: | 12-30 | ? | yes |

| | Adults | Children |
|---|---|---|
| Half life: | 10-30h | 8-19h |
| Steady state, time: | 2-6d | 2-4d |

| | Adults | Children |
|---|---|---|
| Recommended dose: | 10-20 mg/kg/d | 15-30 mg/kg/d |
| Effective levels: | 8-12 µg/mL | same |
| Toxic levels: | <15 µg/mL | same |

| | |
|---|---|
| Monitoring methods: | EMIT, HPLC, GLC |

# 15

# Carbamazepine: Methods for Analysis

### Janis J. MacKichan, Pharm.D.

## Introduction

Carbamazepine (CBZ) is a major antiepileptic drug used to treat generalized and complex partial seizures in adults and children. It is considered as effective as phenytoin or phenobarbital for treating these seizures and may be used in place of these drugs to avoid certain untoward side effects. (1). The utility of plasma CBZ measurements for therapeutic monitoring of patients with seizures has been demonstrated. Optimum seizure control is reported to occur when plasma CBZ concentrations are maintained in the range of 4-12 mg/L (17-50 $\mu$mol/L). Concentrations greater than 12 mg/L are associated with minor and major toxicities (2). Because of the wide interpatient variation in the disposition of CBZ, adjustment of the dosage based on the determination of plasma CBZ concentrations is considered very important.

The relationship between total CBZ plasma concentration and therapeutic effect may be complicated by two factors: 1) the formation of a metabolite, carbamazepine 10, 11-epoxide (CBZ-EP), which has been shown to possess anticonvulsant activity similar to CBZ in the rat (3); and 2) the variability in plasma protein binding of CBZ and CBZ-EP (4). For these reasons it is desirable to use an analytical method that can measure CBZ and CBZ-EP simultaneously and that is sensitive enough to monitor free concentrations of these compounds in plasma. The latter is important because the CBZ free in plasma varies from 13 to 33% of the total plasma concentration. Other desirable characteristics of an assay for CBZ are: 1) absence of interferences from other anticonvulsant or psychotropic agents, since these drugs are likely to be taken concurrently with CBZ; and 2) enough sensitivity to allow analysis in small volumes of plasma or saliva, since this drug is commonly taken by children.

CBZ concentrations in plasma were first measured by a colorimetric technique, and subsequently by fluorometric and spectrophotometric techniques. These methods were nonspecific, insensitive, and unable to quantitate metabolites. Presently, the most common techniques for measuring CBZ and CBZ-EP in biological fluids are gas-liquid chromatography (GLC), high performance liquid chromatography (HPLC) and enzyme immunoassay (EMIT®). Thin-layer chromatographic (TLC) methods are also available but are less commonly used in clinical laboratories.

The choice of a method depends on several factors. Among these are the following: 1) intended application, e.g., research or therapeutic monitoring; 2) specificity, sensitivity and precision requirements; 3) availability of equipment; and 4) cost. The purpose of this article is to present an overview of the most common methods used today for quantitation of CBZ and its epoxide metabolite, with an emphasis on the relative advantages and disadvantages of each method.

## Gas Liquid Chromatography (GLC)

Although it is no longer considered the method of choice, GLC is still widely used in clinical laboratories to analyze CBZ in plasma. Many of the GLC methods allow simultaneous analysis of other major anticonvulsants (phenytoin, phenobarbital and primidone)(5, 6), and the more recent methods also allow quantitation of the CBZ-EP metabolite (7, 8). These methods generally use flame ionization detection and operate at temperatures ranging from 190 to 300° C. They typically have sensitivity limits for CBZ ranging from 0.1-0.25 $\mu$g; thus they allow analysis of CBZ in plasma volumes of 0.2-1 mL. All of the methods use internal standards, usually either cyheptamide or one of the tricyclic antidepressants.

In order for a drug to be analyzed by GLC, it must be volatile and thermally stable. Unfortunately CBZ and CBZ-EP are not stable at high temperatures and also undergo on-column acid-catalyzed degradation and rearrangement to form products which include iminostilbene, 9-methylacridine and 9-acridine carboxaldehyde (9). This is believed to occur partly from contact of CBZ with metallic parts of the injector, from combination of CBZ with residual molecules remaining in the column after previous analyses of other compounds, and from the use of chloride solvents, which may contain trace amounts of acids (8). Because the degree of decomposition varies, systems in which this occurs tend to be less precise.

In spite of these problems, many investigators have developed and successfully applied GLC methods to CBZ analyses. Sheehan and Beam (10) demonstrated

*Dr. MacKichan is an Assistant Professor of Pharmacy, Ohio State University, College of Pharmacy, Columbus, OH 43210.*

that although degradation of underivitized CBZ to iminostilbene was incomplete and variable, the sum of the peak heights of these two compounds was constant. Using more alkaline column conditions, Chambers and Cook (11) were able to completely and reproducibly hydrolyze CBZ to the iminostilbene product, which emerged as a single peak and was quantitated in place of CBZ. This method was subsequently modified to allow simultaneous analysis of the epoxide metabolite (7). Simultaneous analyses of (or interference by) the other anticonvulsants were not possible with this system because they are acidic and are consequently retained by the alkaline column (11).

Other investigators have attempted to minimize on-column thermolysis of CBZ by preparing trimethylsilyl (12, 13) or cyano derivatives (14) or by reacting CBZ with dimethylformamide dimethylacetal (DFDA) (15). Although the precision of CBZ analysis may be improved, sample preparation procedures that require derivitization are usually tedious and time consuming. Moreover, other anticonvulsants are difficult to analyze simultaneously because they differ in derivative formation and stability (12). Of these techniques, reaction with DFDA is considered to be the most precise (16).

On-column methylation techniques (5, 17) have less complex sample preparation procedures. These techniques typically involve a single-step extraction into an organic solvent followed by evaporation and subsequent reconstitution of the residue with a quaternary ammonium hydroxide reagent. This technique has been used for simultaneous GLC analyses of phenobarbital, phenytoin, primidone and CBZ. Good precision was obtained using a single internal standard (5). The precision can be improved by using one internal standard for each anticonvulsant (6).

GLC methods that do not result in decomposition of CBZ have recently been introduced. In the system of Cocks and Dyer (18), negligible hydrolysis of CBZ to iminostilbene during chromatography was demonstrated by comparing the infrared spectra of CBZ, iminostilbene and the column effluent. A method for simultaneous analyses of CBZ and CBZ-EP was developed by Ranise et al. (8) using the structurally similar cyheptamide as an internal standard. The stability of CBZ and CBZ-EP in this method was confirmed by mass-spectral analysis of the column effluent and was attributed by the authors to the use of non-chlorinated column silanizing agents and to the use of direct "on-column" injection techniques. The extraction procedure was simple, and both compounds were completely recovered. Precision and sensitivity of the method were not reported (8).

Interferences with the analysis of CBZ in blood samples collected in Vacutainers® (Bectin-Dickinson, Rutherford, NJ) have been reported in some GLC methods (13, 19). The interfering substance is believed to be the plasticizer present in the rubber stopper of the evacuated tube (19). The possibility of this interference should be considered when developing or initiating a GLC method.

## High Performance Liquid Chromatography (HPLC)

With the recent surge in HPLC technology, this technique is rapidly becoming the method of choice for analyzing CBZ and CBZ-EP. HPLC shares with GLC the advantage of multiple drug analyses, but because it allows separation of compounds at ambient temperature, the problems associated with thermal instability of CBZ and CBZ-EP are avoided. Similarly, time-consuming extraction and derivitization procedures are not necessary. All of the HPLC methods employ UV detection, and the sensitivity of more recent HPLC methods is similar to if not better than the sensitivity of most GLC methods.

Two modes of HPLC have been used for analyzing CBZ. Early HPLC methods used the liquid-solid mode of separation, which uses columns packed with small-particle silica gel and mobile phases composed of organic solvents, such as methylene chloride and n-hexane (20, 21). The liquid-solid chromatographic procedure developed by Westenberg and DeZeeuw (20) uses a variable wavelength UV detector (at 250 nm) and provides excellent sensitivity and specificity. Using a one-step extraction procedure, it is possible to precisely analyze CBZ concentrations as low as 0.5 mg/L using 0.5 mL of plasma. By including an evaporation step and using 1 mL of plasma, as little as 2 μg/L of CBZ can be detected. The authors point out that although a simultaneous analysis of CBZ-EP is possible with their method, the detection limit for the epoxide metabolite is much higher than that for the parent drug (20).

Inherent problems with liquid-solid chromatography have made newer modes of liquid chromatography more popular. Bonded-phase chromatography has several advantages over liquid-solid chromatography. The columns have shorter equilibration times, they are more resistant to damage, and they can be used in the reverse-phase mode with less costly mobile phases composed primarily of water or buffer solutions. One of the first reverse-phase liquid chromatographic methods for analyzing CBZ was introduced by Kabra and Marton (22). Although this method has the advantages of reverse-phase chromatography, the sensitivity for CBZ was inferior to other methods. Using a fixed-wavelength UV detector at 254 nm, only 0.25 mg/L of CBZ could be detected using 2 mL of whole blood. This would not provide the sensitivity needed to monitor CBZ concentrations in children or to measure free CBZ concentrations in plasma. More recent reverse-phase methods have been developed which improve the sensitivity and allow a simultaneous analysis of CBZ-EP. Adams et al. (23) and Milhaly et al. (24) developed methods using columns packed with microparticulate silica that is chemically bonded with octadecyl trichlorosilane (C-18). The mobile phase was acetonitrile in water. Although they used different plasma volumes, both methods provided similar sensitivities. Milhaly was able to detect concentrations of CBZ and CBZ-EP as low as 5 $\mu$g/L and 15 $\mu$g/L, respectively, using 1 mL of plasma and a fixed wavelength UV detector at 254 nm. Adams was able to detect 0.2 mg/L of CBZ and CBZ-EP using only 50 $\mu$L of plasma and a variable wavelength UV detector at 195 nm. Nitrazepam (23) and 10, 11-dihydrocarbamazepine (24) were used as internal standards.

Using a bonded-phase column with an alkylnitrile functionality (CN) and a mobile phase of acetonitrile in water, MacKichan (25) developed a method designed to analyze CBZ and CBZ-EP simultaneously in either plasma or saliva. Using 0.5 mL of plasma or saliva and a fixed wavelength UV detector (254 nm) it was possible to measure CBZ and CBZ-EP concentrations as low as 18 and 15 $\mu$g/L respectively. Because concentrations of the epoxide metabolite may be much smaller than those of the parent drug, particularly after single doses of CBZ, two internal standards were employed in this method to facilitate more reliable quantitation of both compounds simultaneously (25). None of the major anticonvulsants interfered with this method and maximum coefficients of variation at concentrations of 0.5 mg/L were less than 7% for both compounds (25).

In the reverse-phase method developed by Astier and Maury (26), sample extraction was not necessary for quantitation of CBZ and CBZ-EP. Instead, plasma proteins in 200 $\mu$L of plasma were precipitated by the addition of 200 $\mu$L of acetonitrile containing the internal standard, nitrazepam. CBZ and CBZ-EP concentrations as low as 0.2 mg/L could be quantitated by injecting 20 $\mu$L of the clear supernatant onto the column. Although this method was more rapid than those requiring an extraction step, precision was poor at low concentrations, The coefficients of variation were 21% for CBZ and 15% for CBZ-EP at concentrations of 2 mg/L (26). A similar protein precipitation method was used by Kabra et al. (27) for the reverse-phase separation of the major anticonvulsants, including CBZ. With this method, concentrations of phenobarbital, phenytoin, primidone, ethosuximide and CBZ as low as 1 mg/L could be quantitated using only 25 $\mu$L of serum. Precision of this method was good, with the coefficients of variation being 3.9-5% (27). Although these protein precipitation methods of sample preparation provide speed and simplicity in HPLC analysis, continued injections of these non-extracted materials may result in rapid loss of column efficiency or ability to separate compounds. Column-life may be extended somewhat by using "guard" columns installed between the injector and the analytical column. The guard column should be replaced with a fresh column at a frequency determined by the type of sample being analyzed.

## Enzyme Immunoassay (EMIT ®)

The recent development of the homogeneous enzyme immunoassay (EMIT®, Syva Corp., Palo Alto, CA) has been a major advance in analyzing microsamples of antiepileptic drugs rapidly and accurately. This method involves the competition between a drug-enzyme complex and the free drug in serum for an antibody that is specific for the drug. When bound to the antibody, the catalytic activity of the drug-enzyme complex is lost. Unbound drug-enzyme complex is then able to convert the co-factor $NAD^+$ to NADH, which is measured spectrophotometrically. The standard curve relates the rate of this enzymatic reaction to the known drug concentration.

Although this technique does not allow simultaneous analyses of other anticonvulsant drugs or metabolites, it has certain advantages that make it ideal for clinical use. Since no extraction procedure is required, the determination of a single drug in a patient sample requires only about 8 minutes from serum to delivered result, once a standard curve has been established (28). CBZ in the range of 2-20 mg/L can be accurately determined using as little as 50 $\mu$L of serum. Consequently CBZ concentrations can be measured reliably in the pediatric age group using heel- or finger-stick procedures. Cross-reactivity with other anticonvulsants or commonly used psychotropic drugs has not been observed with the EMIT system and results correlate well with those obtained by GLC and HPLC techniques (28). Analysis of CBZ in severely hemolyzed or lipemic samples by the EMIT assay can overestimate CBZ concentrations, and in these situations an alternative technique such as GLC or HPLC should be used (29).

Analysis of CBZ in serum by the EMIT system is only accurate within the range of 2-20 mg/L. Samples of higher concentrations should be appropriately diluted with drug-free serum and reanalyzed (29). Assay sensitivity can be increased by omitting one of the dilution steps normally performed, thus allowing analysis in the 0.2-2 mg/L range. In this situation a new standard curve should be generated using calibrators that have been diluted to the appropriate range with blank serum (29) The EMIT system has been used to measure CBZ in saliva using this procedure (30). A modified enzyme immunoassay technique coupled with a plasma ultrafiltration device is currently under investigation for the routine analysis of free CBZ serum concentrations (Syva Corp., personal communication).

The major disadvantage of the EMIT assay is the cost of reagents. One package of EMIT reagents and calibrators is sufficient to perform 60 determinations using the Syva-Gilford semi-automated spectrophotometer according to the manufacturer's instructions. The number of determinations per package can be increased, however, by adapting the enzyme immunoassay to other detection systems, such as a centrifugal analyzer (31) or a mechanized microliter system (32), and by using smaller volumes and/or more dilute solutions of reagents and calibrators. The cost per analysis can be decreased as much as four-fold in this manner, with only a 20% sacrifice in assay sensitivity (31).

A homogeneous substrate-labeled fluorescent immunoassay has recently been developed (33). This method is based on the same principle as the conventional enzyme immunoassay system except that increasing concentrations of CBZ result in increasing intensity of fluorescence, which is monitored with a conventional fluorometer. Precision and sensitivity of the method are comparable to those of the EMIT assay (33).

### Thin-Layer Chromatography (TLC)

Although TLC was the first technique adapted to multiple anticonvulsant analysis, it is not generally considered as suitable for routine quantitative analyses as are the immunoassay, HPLC or GLC techniques. With the use of automatic plate spotting devices and scanning spectrodensitometers, however, TLC systems can offer advantages over the other chromatographic systems. Like HPLC, the development of a TLC plate is performed at the ambient temperature, so the compounds of interest are not subject to thermal decomposition. TLC systems may further offer the advantage of increased sensitivity. The TLC method developed by Hundt and Clark (34) for simultaneous analyses of CBZ, CBZ-EP and a second metabolite (10, 11-dihydroxycarbamazepine) required that only 1 $\mu$L of serum be directly spotted on the TLC plate for reliable quantitation of concentrations as low as 0.1 mg/L. The plate is treated

to form fluorescent compounds which are then measured using a spectrofluorometer with a TLC scanning attachment. As with other chromatographic methods, the concentration of drug in the original sample is directly related to the peak height measured from the resulting chromatogram. Precision of this method is 9.3% for CBZ at 3 mg/L and 6.4% for CBZ-EP at 0.78 mg/L (34). An internal standard was not used with this method and might be considered to improve reproducibility.

Wad et al (35) have developed a TLC method for simultaneous analyses of CBZ, phenytoin, mephenytoin, phenobarbital and primidone. This technique requires 300 $\mu$L of serum and is able to measure concentrations as low as 1 mg/L for all compounds. Detection is based on diffuse light reflectance from the underivitized drugs, and precision for CBZ at 13 mg/L is 4% (35). No internal standard was incorporated into the method.

### Summary

HPLC is the method of choice for simultaneous analyses of CBZ, CBZ-EP and other anticonvulsants because it can separate compounds at ambient temperatures. Little sample preparation is required before analysis, and concentrations can be analyzed reliably in very small volumes of plasma or saliva. If the clinical laboratory workload is large (i.e., greater than 40 samples per week), then it is worthwhile to invest in a fully automated HPLC system. After the initial investment, the cost per analysis is very low. For laboratories with GLC capabilities, reliable assays for CBZ and CBZ-EP are available. This technique, like HPLC, is more cost-effective in a laboratory with a moderate to heavy workload.

Although it does not provide simultaneous analyses of other anticonvulsants, the EMIT system is simple to operate, provides rapid and precise results and requires only a small sample of serum. In addition to CBZ, analyses for phenobarbital, phenytoin, primidone and ethosuximide, as well as the major antiarrhythmic drugs are available. Because the reagents are costly, this assay is probably more cost-effective in a laboratory that does a variety of drug analyses less frequently. The cost can be significantly decreased, however, by appropriate modifications.

### References

1.  Cereghino, J.J., Brock, J.T., Van Meter, J.C., Penry, J.K., Smith, L.D., and White, B.G., Carbamazepine for epilepsy. *Neurology* (Minneap.) **24**, 404-410 (1974).
2.  MacKichan, J.J., and Kutt, H., Carbamazepine:

Therapeutic use and serum concentration monitoring. In *Individualizing Drug Therapy: Practical Applications of Drug Monitoring*, Vol. 2, A. Finn and W. Taylow, Eds., Gross, Townsend, Frank, Inc., New York, N.Y., 1981, pp. 1-25.

3. Frigerio, A., and Morselli, P.L., Carbamazepine biotransformation. In *Advances in Neurology*, Vol. 11, J.K. Penry and D.D. Daly, Eds., Raven Press, N.Y., (1975), pp. 295-308.

4. MacKichan, J.J., Duffner, P.K., and Cohen, M.E., Salivary concentrations and plasma protein binding of carbamazepine and carbamazepine 10, 11-epoxide in epileptic patients. *Brit. J. Clin. Pharmacol.* **12**, 31-37 (1981).

5. Abraham, C.V., and Joslin, H.D., Simultaneous gas-chromatographic analysis for phenobarbital, diphenylhydantoin, carbamazepine and primidone in serum. *Clin. Chem.* **22**, 769-771 (1976).

6. Kumps, A., and Mardens, Y., Improved gas-liquid chromatographic method for the simultaneous determination of phenobarbital, phenytoin, carbamazepine and primidone in biological fluids. *J. Chromatogr. Biomed. Appl.* **182**, 116-120 (1980).

7. Chambers, R.E., Simultaneous determination by gas-liquid chromatography of carbamazepine and carbamazepine 10, 11-epoxide in plasma. *J. Chromatogr.* **154**, 272-274 (1978).

8. Ranise, A., Benassi, E., and Besio, G., Rapid gas-chromatographic method for the determination of carbamazepine and unrearranged carbamazepine 10, 11-epoxide in human plasma. *J. Chromatogr. Biomed. Appl.* **222**, 120-124 (1980).

9. Frigerio, A., Baker, K.M., and Morselli, P.M., Gas chromatographic-mass spectrometric studies on carbamazepine. *Adv. Biochem. Psychopharmacol.* **7**, 125-134 (1973).

10. Sheehan, M., and Beam, R.E., GLC determination of underivitized carbamazepine in whole blood. *J. Pharm. Sci.* **64**, 2004-2006 (1975).

11. Chambers, R.E., and Cook, M., Simple and reliable gas chromatographic assay for the determination of carbamazepine in plasma. *J. Chromatogr.* **144**, 257-262 (1977).

12. Kupferberg, H.J., GLC determination of carbamazepine in plasma. *J. Pharm. Sci.* **61**, 284-286 (1972).

13. Lensmeyer, G.I., Isothermal gas-chromatographic method for the rapid determination of carbamazepine ("Tegretol") as its TMS derivitive. *Clin. Toxicol.* **11**, 443-454 (1977).

14. Gerardin, A., Abadie, F., and Laffont, J., GLC determination of carbamazepine suitable for

pharmacokinetic studies. *J. Pharm. Sci.* **64**, 1940-1942 (1975).

15. Perchalski, R.J., Andresen, B.D., and Wilder, B.J., Reaction of carbamazepine with dimethylformamide dimethylacetal (for gas chromatography). (Letter) *Clin. Chem.* **22**, 1229-1230 (1976).

16. Perchalski, R.J., and Wilder, B.J., GLC analysis of carbamazepine. (Letter) *Ther. Drug Monitoring* **2**, 289 (1980).

17. Drummer, O., Morris, P. and Vajda, F., Plasma carbamazepine determinations: a simple gas chromatographic method. *Clin. Exp. Pharmacol. Physiol.* **3**, 497-501 (1976).

18. Cocks, D.A., and Dyer, T.F., Simple and rapid gas-liquid chromatographic method for estimating carbamazepine in serum. *J. Chromatogr. Biomed. Appl.* **222**, 496-500 (1981).

19. Missen, A.., and Dickson, S.J., Contamination of blood samples by plasticizer in evacuated tubes. *Clin. Chem.* **20**, 1247 (1974).

20. Westenberg, H.G.M., and DeZeeuw, R.A., Rapid and sensitive liquid chromatographic determination of carbamazepine suitable for use in monitoring multiple drug anticonvulsant therapy. *J. Chromatogr.* **118**, 217-224 (1976).

21. Eichelbaum, M., and Bertilsson, L., Determination of carbamazepine and its epoxide metabolite in plasma by high-speed chromatography. *J. Chromatogr.* **103**, 135-140 (1975).

22. Kabra, P.M., and Marton, L.J., Determination of carbamazepine in blood or plasma by high pressure liquid chromatography. *Clin. Chem.* **22**, 1070-1072 (1976).

23. Adams, R.F., Schmidt, G.J., and Vandemark, F.L., A micromethod for the determination of carbamazepine and its 10, 11-epoxide metabolite in serum and urine by reverse-phase liquid chromatography. *Chromatogr. Newslett.* **5**, 11-13 (1977).

24. Milhaly, G.W., Phillips, J.A., Louis, W.J., and Vajda, F.J., Measurement of carbamazepine and its epoxide metabolite by high-performance liquid chromatography, and a comparison of assay techniques for the analysis of carbamazepine. *Clin. Chem.* **23**, 2283-2287 (1977).

25. MacKichan, J.J., Simultaneous liquid chromatographic analysis for carbamazepine and carbamazepine 10, 11-epoxide in plasma and saliva by use of double internal standardization. *J. Chromatogr. Biomed. Appl.* **181**, 373-383 (1980).

26. Astier, A., and Maury, M., Simultaneous rapid high performance liquid chromatographic microanalysis of plasma carbamazepine and its 10, 11-epoxide metabolite. *J. Chromatogr. Biomed.*

*Appl.* **164**, 235-240 (1979).

27. Kabra, P.M., Stafford, B.E., and Marton, L.J., Simultaneous measurement of phenobarbital, phenytoin, primidone, ethosuximide and carbamazepine in serum by high-pressure liquid chromatography. *Clin. Chem.* **23**, 1284-1288 (1977).

28. Schottelius, D.D., Homogeneous immunoassay system (EMIT®) for quantitation of antiepileptic drugs in biological fluids. In *Antiepileptic Drugs: Quantitative Analysis and Interpretation,* C.E Pippenger, J.K. Penry, and H. Kutt, Eds., Raven Press, New York, N.Y., (1978) pp. 95-108.

29. Pippenger, C.E., and Kutt, H., Common errors in the analysis of antiepileptic drugs. In *Antiepileptic Drugs: Quantitative Analysis and Interpretation,* C.E. Pippenger, J.K. Penry and H. Kutt, Eds., Raven Press, New York, N.Y., (1979) pp. 199-208.

30. Bartels, H., Oldigs, H., and Gunther, E., Use of saliva in monitoring carbamazepine medication in epileptic children. *Eur. J. Pediat.* **126**, 37-44 (1977).

31. Lacher, D.A., Valdes, R., and Savory, J., Enzyme immunoassay of carbamazepine with a centrifugal analyzer. *Clin. Chem.* **25**, 295-298 (1979).

32. Kleine, T.O., Lowering the cost of the enzyme immunoassay (EMIT®) for carbamazepine by its adaptation to a mechanized microliter system. *Clin. Chim. Acta* **82**, 193-195 (1978).

33. Miller, J.E., Li, T.M., Krausz, L.M., Wong, R.C., and Burd, J.F., Substrate-labeled fluorescent immunoassay (SLFIA) for carbamazepine in serum. (Abstract) *Clin. Chem.* **26**, 1002 (1980).

34. Hundt, H.K.L., and Clark, E.C., Thin-layer chromatographic method for determining carbamazepine and two of its metabolites in serum. *J. Chromatogr.* **107**, 149-154 (1975).

35. Wad, N., and Rosenmund, H., Rapid quantitative method for simultaneous determination of carbamazepine 10, 11-epoxide, diphenylhydantoin, mephenytoin, phenobarbital and primidone in serum by thin-layer chromatography. *J. Chromatogr.* **146**, 167-168 (1978).

# 16

# Valproic Acid:
# Physical and Pharmacological Properties

Roger L. Boeckx, Ph.D

## Clinical Pharmacology

The correlation between therapeutic dosage and the resulting concentration in serum is poor for valproic acid. Although the manufacturer recommends a maximum dose of 30 mg/kg per day, several studies have shown that this does not result in therapeutic concentrations. The recommended approach is to begin at a relatively low dosage (10-15 mg/kg per day) and increase this slowly until therapeutic effect is noted. One study of 25 patients reported a mean initial dose of 11 mg/kg per day and a final dose of 39 mg/kg per day. On this regimen, most patient demonstrated marked to moderate improvement and had concentrations of 55-100 mg/L in the serum.

The biological half-life of valproate has been variously reported as from 6 to 15 h. Adult epileptics show the longest half-life (10-12 h) and children with epilepsy can occasionally show shorter half-lifes (8-15 h).

If a mean half-life of 11 h is assumed steady-state would be reached after about 2 to 2½ days. A steady-state concentration of 55–100 mg/L should be produced by the administration of about 40 mg/kg per day, divided into three doses taken at 8-h intervals.

Concentrations of valproic acid over 200 $\mu$g/mL have been associated with hemorrhagic abnormalities. When found in conjunction with anticoagulants such as aspirin or warfarin, inhibition of the secondary phase of platelet aggregation has been observed.

Only limited experience with overdose has been reported and no information on toxic concentrations is available.

## Mechanism and Site of Action

The exact mechanism of anticonvulsant action is unknown. Also, it is unclear at present whether

*Dr. Boeckx is the Assistant Director of Clinical Chemistry at Childrens Hospital, National Medical Center, 111 Michigan Avenue, N.W., Washington, D.C. 20010.*

valproic acid itself or some active metabolite(s) is responsible for the anticonvulsant action.

In animal studies, valproic acid has been shown to raise brain (and specifically cerebellar) concentrations of $\gamma$-aminobutyric acid (GABA) while lowering the concentration of cyclic guanosine monophosphate (cGMP).

Numerous effect of valproic acid on GABA metabolism have been reported.

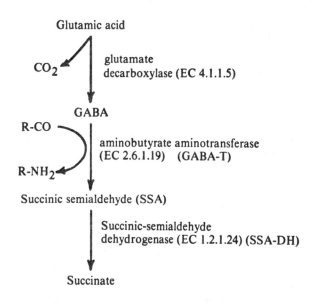

Some workers have reported that valproic acid acts as an inhibitor of GABA-T, while others suggest that valproate inhibits SSA-DH more than GABA-T. Still others have hypothesized that valproate increases GABA concentrations by inhibiting the uptake of GABA by glial cells.

## Drug-Drug Interactions

Several interactions between valproate and other anticonvulsants have been reported.

## (a) Phenobarbital -

Several studies have shown increased phenobarbital concentrations after valproate administration, necessitating significant decreases in phenobarbital dosages to prevent over-sedation. The mechanism of the interaction is unclear, but may be related to altered renal excretion of phenobarbital.

## (b) Phenytoin -

There are conflicting reports describing the effect of valproate on phenytoin concentrations. Therapeutic valproate concentrations have been shown competitively to displace phenytoin from its binding site on albumin, resulting in a transient increase in free phenytoin concentration. This free phenytoin is more available for liver hydroxylation, resulting in increased excretion of hydroxylated phenytoin, and lowered concentrations in plasma. On the other hand, other workers have reported a dose-dependent increase in phenytoin concentrations when valproate was administered.

## (c) Other anticonvulsants -

There are also conflicting reports regarding interaction between valproate and clonazepam and between valproate and primidone. Patients receiving anticonvulsants in additon to valproic acid should have the concentrations of those anticonvulsants in their plasma monitored and adjusted if necessary.

## Side Effects

Liver dysfunction has been reported in some patients. A fatal case of Reye-like syndrome in a 12-year-old girl and some fatal and non-fatal cases of hepatic necrosis have been reported. Routine monitoring of liver function during the course of valproate therapy is recommended. Transient nausea, vomiting, and indigestion can occur at the start of therapy. Diarrhea and abdominal cramps have been reported. Some transient increased hair loss has been reported.

Various psychiatric symptoms have been occasionally reported, including emotional upset, depression, psychosis, aggression, hyperactivity, and behavioral deterioration.

## Sample Type, Storage, Stability

Serum or plasma can be analyzed. The samples are stable if stored refrigerated or frozen if analysis is to be delayed.

## VALPROIC ACID PROFILE

| | |
|---|---|
| Generic name: | Valproic acid |
| Chemical name: | n-dipropylacetic acid, 2-propylpentanoic acid, 2-propylvaleric |

Chemical structure:

$$CH_3-CH_2-CH_2$$
$$CH_3-CH_2-CH_2 \quad CH-C \overset{O}{\underset{OH}{}}$$

| | |
|---|---|
| Trade name*: | Sodium salt: Depakine, Depakin, Epilim, Ergenyl, Eurekene, Labazene, Convulex, Orfiril. Magnesium salt: Atemperator. |
| Molecular weight: | 144.2 (free acid) |
| Boiling point, °C: | 166.2 (sodium salt) 128-130 |
| Solubility in water, mg/mL: | 1.3 (9.0 mmol/L) |
| $pK_a$: | 4.95 |
| Partition coefficient: | not available |
| Dose absorption – time to peak plasma conc., h: | 0.5-1.5 (fasting)   2-8 (non-fasting) |
| percentage dose absorbed: | 85-100 |
| Protein binding – percentage bound: | 85-95 |
| percentage free: | 5-15 |
| Tissue distribution, $V_d$ , L/kg: | 0.15-0.4 (higher in children) |
| CSF/plasma: | 0.1 |
| Brain/plasma: | 0.3 |
| Urinary excretion, % daily dose – as unchanged drug: | 3-7 |
| as glucuronide conjugate: | 80 |
| as 4-hydroxyvalproic acid, 3-hydroxyvalproic acid. | 13-17 |

### CLINICAL PHARMACOLOGY

| | Adults | Children |
|---|---|---|
| Recommended dose, mg/kg/d: | 30-60 | 30-60 |
| Half-life, h: | 10-12 | 6-15 |
| Time to steady state, h: | 2-2 1/2 | 2-2 1/2 |
| Effective levels, $\mu$g/mL: | 55-100 | 55-100 |
| Toxic levels, $\mu$g/mL: | not available | not available |
| Steady-state level expected from 1 mg/kg/d, $\mu$g/mL: | 1.5 | 1-1.5 |
| Methodologies available for analysis: | gas - liquid chromatography | |

*Sodium valproate is the most commonly administered form. In the stomach this is quickly converted to valproic acid.

Peak values can be obtained by sampling 2-4 h after last dose. Values are lowest for samples collected just before the next dose.

## Analytical Techniques

Various gas-chromatographic approaches are available. Care must be taken to avoid loss of the highly volatile free acid. Concentration by evaporation of extraction solvents should be avoided unless the drug is first converted to a sodium or potassium salt.

Valproate can be analyzed directly in acidified plasma or serum; directly after extraction into chloroform, hexane, carbon disulfide, or toluene; as methyl or butyl derivatives produced by pre-column or on-column derivatization of extracts. Some direct (non-derivatization) methods suffer from interference. Direct extraction of acidified serum or plasma can be complicated by the formation of thick emulsions. Methods involving direct injection of acidified plasma or serum result in extensive column contamination.

The most successful current methods involve extraction of acidified serum or plasma, pre-column methylation or butylation and chromatography on column packing materials of intermediate polarity, such as OV-17. Octanoic acid, heptanoic acid, or cyclohexane carboxylic acid can be used as internal standards.

## References

Hulshoff, A., and Roseboom, H. Determination of valproic acid (di-*n*-propylacetic acid) in plasma by gas-liquid chromatography with pre-column butylation. *Clin. Chim. Acta* **93** 9-13 (1979).

Gyllehaal, O., and Albinsson, A., Gas chromatographic determination of valproate in minute serum samples after extractive methylation, *J. Chromatogr.* **161** 343-346 (1978).

Vajda, F., Drummer, O., Morris, P., et al., Gas chromatographic measurement of plasma levels of sodium valproate: Tentative therapeutic range of a new anticonvulsant in the treatment of refractory epileptics. *Clin. Exp. Pharmacol. Therap.* **5** 67-73 (1978).

# II. Cardioactive Drugs

# 17

# Digitalis Glycosides

John F. Bresnahan, M.D.

Ronald E. Vlietstra, M.B., Ch.B., F.A.C.C.

*Reprinted from Mayo Clin Proc 54, 675-684, 1979*

*The digitalis glycosides number among the most commonly used cardiovascular drugs. Despite 200 years of investigation, much new information regarding their mechanisms of action and clinical use continues to be developed. Clinicians dispensing these potent drugs need to be aware of these advances if they are to make the best possible therapeutic decisions.*

In his "An Account of the Foxglove, and Some of Its Medical Uses," published in 1785, Withering[1] recognized that digitalis "has a power over the heart to a degree yet unobserved in any other medicine." He emphasized that great care was needed for its proper clinical use and that "knowledge of a remedy to counteract its effects would be a desirable thing." Intensive investigations and widespread clinical use of digitalis glycosides have repeatedly confirmed Withering's original statements.

In this review, we propose to emphasize the most commonly used digitalis glycoside, digoxin — its physiologic actions, pharmacology, and clinical use. Anticipating that most readers already have experience with the drug, we plan to give greatest emphasis to pertinent recent developments in its understanding.

## SUBCELLULAR ASPECTS OF DIGITALIS INOTROPY

The cardiac cycle can be divided into three parts: excitation, contraction, and relaxation. Excitation is the electrophysiologic event that initiates the cycle. It depends on a steep electrochemical gradient across the cell membrane (sarcolemma), produced and maintained in large part by the "sodium pump." This "pump" provides an exchange mechanism whereby intracellular sodium ions ($Na^+$) are exchanged for extracellular potassium ions ($K^+$), with the utilization of ATP.

The major site of action of the digitalis glycosides appears to be on the "sodium pump" by way of inhibition of $Na^+,K^+$-ATPase, an enzyme integral in the pump's function.[2] Experiments have demonstrated that the degree of positive inotropic effect produced by digitalis generally correlates directly with the

Dr. Vlietstra is the Assistant Professor of Medicine and Dr. Bresnahan is a resident in Cardiovascular Diseases, Mayo Medical School, Rochester, Minn.

degree of sarcolemmal $Na^+,K^+$-ATPase inhibition. Derivatives of digitalis that do not inhibit $Na^+,K^+$-ATPase lack inotropic effects. Cardiac glycosides appear to bind reversibly to the $Na^+,K^+$-ATPase on the outer cell membrane and induce conformational changes that prevent the binding of substrate, ATP, and thus inactivate the pump.[2]

The steps that link $Na^+, K^+$-ATPase inhibition to increased inotropy have been extensively investigated. The digitalis effects cannot be ascribed only to decreased myocardial $K^+$, increased intracellular $Na^+$, or changes in energy metabolism. Changes in calcium ion ($Ca^{++}$) turnover, however, have been documented, and they may be responsible for the inotropic effects.[3]

Calcium ions play a central role in the regulation of muscle contraction (Fig. 1). In the resting myocardial cell, interaction of the contractile proteins (actin and myosin) is inhibited by a set of regulatory proteins (troponin and tropomyosin). Following an action potential, there is an increase in the intracellular concentration of free $Ca^{++}$. This $Ca^{++}$, by combining with and altering the regulatory proteins, facilitates actin-myosin interaction and initiates contraction.[4] The amount of $Ca^{++}$ available to the contractile proteins affects the total number of actin-myosin interactions and, therefore, the maximum tension produced. Digitalis results in increased availability of $Ca^{++}$ and, thus, enhances the contractile response. This has been illustrated in experiments involving frog heart muscle cells injected with a $Ca^{++}$-sensitive bioluminescent protein (aequorin). Acetylstrophanthidin (a cardiotonic steroid) increased both the light intensity and the tension associated with contraction, and these changes are consistent with the hypothesis that an increase in $Ca^{++}$ mediates the digitalis effect.[5]

The way in which digitalis affects movements of $Ca^{++}$ in heart muscle is not fully understood. In skeletal muscle, which is little affected by the cardiac glycosides, $Ca^{++}$ dynamics have been fairly well worked out. Calcium is stored within the sarcoplasmic reticulum, an intracellular membranous network that surrounds the myofilaments. Upon stimulation of the skeletal muscle cell, $Ca^{++}$ is released from the sarcoplasmic reticulum to react with the contractile apparatus. In myocardial cells, however, handling of $Ca^{++}$ is different. First, the sarcoplasmic reticulum is not as extensive as in skeletal muscle. Second, extracellular $Ca^{++}$ is very important in myocardial contraction, as evidenced by the pronounced changes in contractile force brought about by changes in extracellular concentration of $Ca^{++}$. Thus, an increase in intracellular $Ca^{++}$ can be effected either by an increase in $Ca^{++}$ influx from the extracellular environment[6] or by enhanced release of bound intracellular $Ca^{++}$ from sites such as the sarcoplasmic reticulum.[7] The relative contribution of these two mechanisms is the subject of active investigation.

A number of theories have been proposed in order to explain how digitalis-induced inhibition of $Na^+,K^+$-ATPase produces an increase in available $Ca^{++}$. Langer[8] proposed that, in addition to the $Na^+,K^+$ pump, a $Na^+,Ca^{++}$ exchange exists in which $Na^+$ efflux is linked to $Ca^{++}$ influx. Digitalis inhibition of the $Na^+,K^+$ pump results in increased intracellular $Na^+$, which then stimulates $Na^+,Ca^{++}$ exchange and thereby produces extrusion of $Na^+$ coupled with an electrically neutral influx of $Ca^{++}$ (Fig. 1). Conversely, Reuter[9] suggested that the increased intracellular $Na^+$ diminishes the $Na^+$ gradient across the membrane. Because this $Na^+$ gradient is the energy source for $Ca^{++}$ extrusion, the result is less $Ca^{++}$ efflux and a net gain in intracellular $Ca^{++}$. Another theory proposes that digitalis-induced conformational changes in $Na^+,K^+$-ATPase allow intracellular $Ca^{++}$ to bind to the complex and then to be released upon depolarization of the membrane.[10] Morad and Greenspan,[11] noting the shortening of the repolarization period induced by digitalis, have suggested that $Ca^{++}$ influx is coupled with $K^+$ efflux. Finally, it is also possible that the inhibition of the $Na^+,K^+$ pump and the increases in intracellular free $Ca^{++}$ are not related as cause and effect but rather are the result of digitalis action on two separate membrane systems.[12]

### Electrophysiologic Effects

The resting myocardial cell has a transmembrane potential difference of about —90mV (Fig. 2). Potassium concentration is greater inside the cell, whereas sodium concentration is greater outside. The resting myocardial cell membrane is quite permeable to $K^+$ but scarcely so to $Na^+$. Some cells (pacemaker cells) exhibit a spontaneous decay of the transmembrane potential difference during diastole (phase 4, Fig. 2), whereas others (nonpacemaker cells) maintain a steady transmembrane potential difference unless electrically stimulated by a conducted impulse.

When the membrane potential reaches the "threshold potential" in the resting myocardial cell, $Na^+$ permeability increases abruptly and $Na^+$ influx occurs. The transmembrane potential rapidly becomes positive (phase 0). This increase in permeability to $Na^+$ is

only transient, and the transmembrane potential soon starts to recover (phase 1). Cardiac muscle is unusual in that full repolarization is delayed. An inward calcium ion current appears to have the greatest responsibility for this plateau phase (phase 2). Finally, the action potential is completed by an outward $K^+$ current (phase 3), and the transmembrane potential returns to its initial value

Although most myocardial cells rely on a transient increase in $Na^+$ conductance for depolarization (that is, they are $Na^+$-dependent or "fast fibers"), some depend on calcium. These $Ca^{++}$-dependent fibers manifest a slower action potential upstroke and operate at a less negative transmembrane potential (approximately -60 to -70mV). They also conduct impulses more slowly—hence the name "slow fibers."

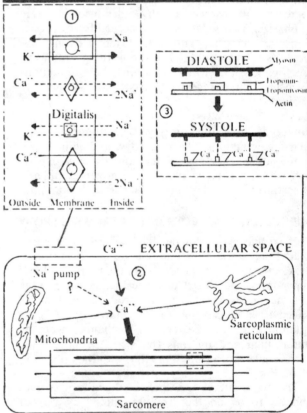

Fig. 1. Schematic diagram of myocardial cell, illustrating proposed mechanism of digitalis-induced inotropy. 1, Upper portion of diagram depicts predominance of $Na^+,K^+$-ATPase pump over $Na^+,Ca^{++}$ pump in undigitalized state. Lower portion shows change in relative activity of two systems after administration of digitalis. 2, Sources of intracellular $Ca^{++}$ available for interaction with contractile proteins. 3, $Ca^{++}$ combines with troponin-tropomyosin complex; this releases inhibition of actin-myosin interaction. (See text for further details.)

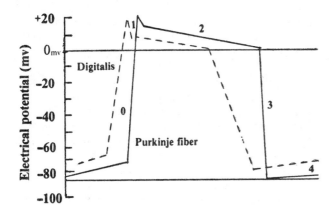

**Fig. 2.** Effects of digitalis on transmembrane action potential of specialized cardiac conduction tissue. (See text.)

These slow fibers make up the pacemaker tissue in the sinoatrial and atrioventricular nodes.

With low doses of digitalis, the resting membrane potential and the rapid inward $Na^+$ current are unchanged, and thus the slope of phase 0 is unchanged. With higher and with toxic doses, however, both the resting potential and the slope of phase 0 are decreased (Fig. 2)—events that have been linked to $Na^+,K^+$-ATPase inhibition. In "fast fibers" exhibiting spontaneous diastolic depolarization (for example, Purkinje fibers), the rate at which the membrane potential decreases (slope of phase 4) is increased.

Repolarization changes appear to vary not only with dose but also with stimulation rate. At low doses and low stimulation rates (for example, 30 per minute), the action potential duration increases, primarily because of an increase in the duration of phase 3. At higher rates of stimulation, as well as at higher doses of digitalis, the action potential duration decreases. The shortening results from a decrease in the duration of the plateau, or phase 2; phase 3 remains relatively prolonged.[13]

From the above changes in the action potential, a number of observations can be made with respect to the electrophysiologic properties of excitability, automaticity, and refractoriness. The reduction in transmembrane potential makes it possible for stimuli that otherwise would be unable to achieve threshold to do so. In toxic doses, however, with pronounced lowering of the membrane potential, excitability may decrease as a result of $Na^+$ channel inactivation. In tissues having spontaneous diastolic depolarization, the increased slope of phase 4 depolarization leads to enhanced automaticity. The decreased slope of phase 0 likely underlies the decrease in conduction velocity

associated with digitalis. Finally, shortening of the effective refractory period appears to result from shortening of the action potential duration.

In addition to these direct effects, digitalis has important effects on the autonomic nervous system. Increased impulse traffic in the vagal fibers to the heart has been demonstrated after administration of digitalis. This change is due, in part, to glycoside sensitization of carotid sinus baroreceptors, and it leads both to an increase in vagal output and a withdrawal of sympathetic tone. Increased central parasympathetic activity has been noted as well. Digitalis appears to have a dose-dependent, biphasic effect on sympathetic activity. In low doses there is a reduction in sympathetic activity as a result of baroreceptor sensitization. In higher doses, however, there is an increase in sympathetic outflow, primarily as a result of hypothalamic and brainstem stimulation.[14] This increased sympathetic activity may contribute to the pathogenesis of digitalis-induced arrhythmias.

The direct and indirect actions of digitalis glycosides combine to produce different effects in atrial, atrioventricular nodal, and ventricular tissues. Atrial muscle shows no appreciable change in membrane potential or excitability. However, vagal effects produce a shortening of the refractory period, which accounts for the increased atrial rates sometimes observed in atrial flutter.

The effects of digitalis on the atrioventricular node represent a most important clinical action of the drug. Neural effects produce prolongation of the effective refractory period and slowing of intranodal conduction. Studies in heart transplant patients, who are devoid of cardiac autonomic innervation, have also demonstrated a direct depressant effect of digitalis on atrioventricular nodal conduction.[15] In patients with sinus rhythm, these effects on the atrioventricular node are commonly manifested as a prolongation of the P-R interval. In patients with atrial flutter and fibrillation, slowing of the ventricular rate is due not only to the increased refractoriness of the atrioventricular node but also to more "concealed conduction."

Effects on ventricular muscle and the Purkinje system are, for the most part, predicted by the changes produced in the action potential. In addition to enhanced diastolic depolarization, Purkinje fibers may also show a greater propensity to "triggered automaticity." Both mechanisms may be of importance in the pathogenesis of digitalis-induced ventricular arrhythmias. Furthermore, studies with intracellular electrodes have shown functional heterogeneity in the degree of impaired conduction produced[16]—a situation favoring the development of reentry.

## Effects on Hemodynamics

Although salutary effects of digitalis in congestive heart failure have long been recognized, evidence for inotropic effects in the normal heart has been acquired only recently. Although digitalis does not produce an increase in cardiac output in the normal heart, studies of the effects of digitalis on isolated myocardial muscle strips and on the intact nonfailing heart clearly demonstrate an increase in the contractile force.[17] In order that this increase in contractility can be reconciled with the lack of significant change in cardiac output, peripheral actions of digitalis must be implicated. These peripheral effects include an increase in peripheral arteriolar resistance and a decrease in venous return.

In the failing heart, the net result on the peripheral circulation is different. An increase in sympathetic nervous system activity accompanies congestive heart failure. Administration of digitalis, with its subsequent increase in myocardial contractility, causes an increase in cardiac output and brings about a reversal of this compensatory mechanism. Therefore, whereas in normal subjects digitalis produces an increase in overall peripheral vascular tone, in patients with congestive heart failure it results in a net decrease in vascular tone.

The net effects of digitalis on myocardial oxygen consumption also depend on whether the heart is normal or abnormal. Myocardial oxygen consumption is determined by myocardial wall tension, contractility, heart rate, and afterload. Myocardial wall tension is a major determinant of myocardial oxygen consumption and, according to Laplace's law, is directly proportional to the radius of the ventricle and the filling pressure. In the normal heart, with low myocardial wall tension, digitalis increases myocardial oxygen consumption by increasing contractility and afterload. In the failing heart, however, the compensatory mechanisms of dilatation and increased sympathetic activity greatly increase myocardial oxygen consumption. Digitalis decreases the intraventricular volume and filling pressure and reduces sympathetic tone and so produces a net reduction in myocardial oxygen consumption.[18]

This effect of digitalis has relevance in its use for treatment of patients with angina pectoris. Many patients with coronary artery disease manifest normal resting hemodynamics but experience abnormal hemodynamics with exercise. Studies in these patients have shown that digitalis often results in improved exercise hemodynamics.[19,20] Clinical improvement of angina might, however, be expected only in those patients in whom a beneficial hemodynamic effect of digitalis on myocardial oxygen consumption outweighed a deleterious effect on myocardial oxygen consumption as a result of increased contractility.

## Pharmacokinetics

The amount of digoxin available for binding to $Na^+,K^+$-ATPase is influenced by a number of factors. First of all, the bioavailability of the preparation and the completeness of absorption determine the net amount of drug made available to the body. Next, the distribution of the drug and its binding to various body tissues affect the concentration that reaches the desired site of action. Finally, the rate of elimination influences both the magnitude and the duration of the effect.

*Bioavailability and Absorption.*—In the early 1970's, it was discovered that tablets of similar indicated strengths produced by different manufacturers resulted in markedly different steady-state plasma concentrations of digoxin.[21] On further investigation, it became apparent that these variations were due to differences in tablet formulation, which produced a wide range of "bioavailability" (a measure of the extent to which a drug reaches the general circulation). Digoxin bioavailability is markedly influenced by the dissolution rate of the digoxin tablets. Those with low dissolution rates have significantly lower bioavailability than faster-dissolving ones. Food and Drug Administration standards have now been set to minimize these differences in bioavailability.[22] As a result of these FDA regulations, much of this bioavailability problem appears to have been settled, at least for the present. Because of this, it is likely that the bioavailability of generic drugs will be equivalent to that of brand-name preparations.

The oral bioavailability of tablet digoxin is less than 100% (usually 70%) also because it is incompletely absorbed from the gastrointestinal tract. Investigators comparing digoxin given orally in solution with that given by intravenous administration have shown that gastrointestinal absorption is approximately 75 to 85% complete. Disease states or drugs that affect gastrointestinal motility further affect absorption. Malabsorption syndromes characterized by hypermotility may decrease absorption of digoxin tablets.[23] Drugs such as metoclopramide, which increase gastrointestinal motility, also decrease absorption. On the other hand, drugs that retard gastrointestinal motility, for example, anticholinergics, tend to increase absorption.[24] A number of drugs have been shown to bind digoxin in the gut and, thus, hinder absorption. Magnesium trisilicate-containing antacids, kaolin-pectin antidiarrheal compounds, cholestyramine, colestipol, neomycin, and activated charcoal have all been shown to have inhibitory effects on absorption.[25] Taking digoxin with meals does not affect the total amount of digoxin absorbed; however, it does retard the rate of absorption.[36]

*Distribution and Excretion.*—For clinical purposes, the distribution of digoxin in the body can be approximated by the use of a two-compartment model. This model consists of a central compartment corresponding to the plasma and extracellular fluid space, where digoxin reaches a rapid equilibrium, and a larger peripheral compartment corresponding to tissues such as muscle and skin, where equilibrium is achieved much more slowly (Fig. 3). For such a model, the "apparent volume of distribution" can be defined as "the volume of body water which would be required to contain the amount of drug in the body if it were uniformly present in the same concentration in which it is in blood."[27] For digoxin, the "apparent volume of distribution" is very high—approximately 7 liters/kg in patients with normal renal function.[28] It can be markedly altered by factors that alter digoxin tissue binding.

After the administration of digoxin tablets, peak serum levels are reached in 1 to 1-1/2 hours, whereas with intravenous injections, peak levels are obtained almost immediately. There is subsequently a rapid decline in the serum digoxin concentration, for the most part due to uptake of digoxin by the organs constituting the "peripheral" compartment. After approximately 8 hours, the distribution phase is completed and the central and peripheral compartments are in equilibrium. There is then a gradual decay in the digoxin content of both compartments due to excretion (Fig. 4). It can be seen from Figure 4 that after the distribution phase, the slopes of the central and peripheral digoxin concentrations are essentially the same; this

finding indicates a close correlation between plasma and tissue digoxin levels during the elimination phase.

The kidney is a major route of excretion for digoxin; in persons with normal renal function, approximately 60 to 80% of an intravenous dose is eliminated unchanged in the urine. The primary mechanism of clearance is by glomerular filtration, and tubular secretion accounts for a small additional amount. Hepatic metabolism accounts for the remaining elimination and does not appear to be affected by mild to moderate liver disease or by drugs that promote induction of hepatic microsomal enzymes. There have been rare cases reported, however, of the ability to convert large quantities of digoxin to a less active metabolite, dihydrodigoxin.[29] A small enterohepatic circulation has also been shown to exist.[30]

In addition to bioavailability, various conditions are known to result in significant alteration of digoxin pharmacokinetics, the clinically most important of which is impairment of renal function. As the glomerular filtration rate decreases, so does the digoxin excretion rate, and thus the plasma half-life is prolonged. Tissue binding is also altered in severe renal failure, the result being a decrease in the volume of distribution of up to 30 to 50%.[28] Hyperkalemia decreases $Na^+,K^+$-ATPase binding; hypokalemia, conversely, increases binding. Hyperthyroidism has been associated with low serum digoxin levels; whether this is result of an increased volume of distribution, malabsorption, or enhanced renal clearance is unsettled. Hypothyroidism has been associated with elevated serum digoxin levels, and the opposite mechanisms have been proposed.[31] A recent significant finding is that quinidine increases serum digoxin levels, possibly as a result of alteration of tissue binding.[32] This drug interaction may be of great importance in terms of producing digitalis toxicity.

*Use of Pharmacokinetic Principles in Designing a Digoxin Treatment Program.*—Knowledge of the pharmacokinetic properties of digoxin and the conditions that alter them is of clinical importance, for they help the practitioner make rational decisions regarding dosage. Consideration of the factors that affect the parameters of bioavailability, volume of distribution, and excretion, along with judicious use of digoxin levels, will not only allow improved treatment programs but will also aid in trouble-shooting situations in which there is a discrepancy between dosage and response or in cases of suspected toxicity.

The aim of such a clinical pharmacokinetic approach is to design a practical dosage schedule that produces and maintains an optimum amount of di-

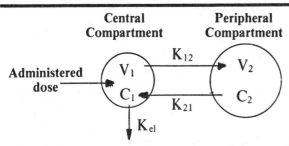

**Fig. 3.** Conceptual diagram of two-compartment pharmacokinetic model. $V_1$, $V_2$ = apparent volumes of the central and peripheral compartments; $C_1$, $C_2$ = drug concentrations in two compartments; $k_{12}$, $k_{21}$ = first order rate constants for intercompartmental drug movement; $k_{el}$ = rate constant for elimination.

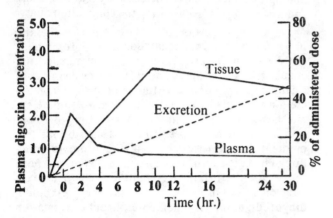

**Fig. 4.** Relative distribution of digoxin after oral dose of 0.5 mg. Close correlation exists between plasma and tissue compartments after absorption and distribution are complete (approximately 8 to 10 hours).

goxin in the body. The success of the approach may be judged by the patient's heart failure response, control of ventricular rate in atrial fibrillation, achievement of therapeutic plasma digoxin levels (approximately 1.0 to 2.0 ng/mL), and absence of symptoms or signs of toxicity.

After administration of maintenance doses of digoxin, steady-state levels will be achieved after five half-lives. For a person with normal renal function, and a half-life of 1.5 days, this would therefore be after about 7 days. However, for the anuric patient, with a half-life of 4 days, steady-state levels would not be reached until 3 weeks. Because the risk of toxicity is increased with loading doses, initiation of therapy with maintenance doses is preferable if the clinical situation permits. A formula for predicting the daily maintenance dose of digoxin which employs pharmacokinetic principles has been derived[33] and is as follows:

$$D = \frac{Cp \ Vd \ T}{1.44F \ t\frac{1}{2} \ \beta}$$

where D = dosage, Cp = mean plasma concentration, Vd = volume of distribution, T = dosing interval, F = bioavailability, and $t\frac{1}{2} \ \beta$ = half-life for excretion. Therefore, for a 70-kg patient with normal renal function, the daily dosage required to produce a level of 1 ng/mL might be calculated as

$$D = \frac{1 \ ng/mL \times 7 \ liters/ \ kg \times 70 \ kg \times 24 \ h}{1.44 \times 0.7 \times 36 \ h}$$

= 0.32 mg daily

where Vd is assumed to be 7 liters/kg, F is 0.7, and the $t\frac{1}{2}\beta$ is assumed to be 36 hours. This could be given as 0.25 mg on one day, alternating with 0.375 mg on the next.

For a 70-kg patient with markedly impaired renal function, for example, a creatinine clearance of 10 mL/min (where Vd=4 liters/kg and $t\frac{1}{2} \ \beta$=96 h),

$$D = \frac{1 \ ng/mL \times 4 \ liters/kg \times 70 \ kg \times 24 \ h}{1.44 \times 0.7 \times 96 \ h}$$

= 0.07 mg daily

This could be given as 0.125 mg every second day.

It must be pointed out that these calculations represent only guidelines for therapy and should be interpreted cautiously. Individual variations in absorption, volume of distribution, metabolism, and excretion are impossible to predict with precision, and they reduce the accuracy of the determinations. The "therapeutic level" for digoxin might also differ in disease states, such as renal failure, in which specific drug-receptor binding might be altered. Careful observation of the individual patient's response remains most important.

## Clinical Use

The clinical usefulness of the digitalis glycosides depends on their ability to increase the force of cardiac contraction and to decrease conduction through the atrioventricular node. Congestive heart failure and supraventricular tachycardias are, therefore, the major clinical indications for the use of digitalis.

*Congestive Heart Failure.*—Digitalis therapy may produce beneficial effects when used in low-output heart failure. Those forms of heart failure characterized by high cardiac output, such as thyrotoxicosis, beriberi heart disease, arteriovenous fistula, and anemia generally respond less well. Heart failure produced by coronary artery disease, valvular heart disease (with the exception of mitral stenosis and normal sinus rhythm), systemic hypertension, and congenital heart disease often respond favorably with increased cardiac output, lower end-diastolic pressure, and decreased pulmonary congestion. In diffuse myocardial disease a favorable response may be seen, but in idiopathic hypertrophic subaortic stenosis, the increased contractile force produced by digitalis may aggravate left ventricular outflow obstruction.

The primary role of digitalis glycosides in heart failure therapy has been challenged in recent years. By decreasing the work of the heart, diuretics and vasodilators can significantly improve patients with heart failure. The future use of digitalis glycosides will depend, to a large extent, on the success of these alternative measures.

*Supraventricular Tachycardias.*—Cardiac glycosides effect a slowing of the ventricular rate in atrial fibrillation and atrial flutter by increasing refractoriness of the atrioventricular node. In paroxysmal supraventricular tachycardia due to atrioventricular node reentry, digitalis prolongs the refractory period and slows the conduction velocity in the antegrade limb of the reentrant circuit, while having little or no effect on the retrograde pathway.[34] This change alters the critical relationships of refractory periods and conduction velocities necessary to produce reentry and thereby makes initiation of tachycardia more difficult. Although the beneficial electrophysiologic changes seen in atrioventricular node reentrant paroxysmal supraventricular tachycardia also apply in Wolff-Parkinson-White syndrome, patients in whom atrial fibrillation develops may have an accelerated ventricular response as a result of a decreased refractory period in the bypass tract. In these circumstances, digitalis may precipitate ventricular fibrillation. For this reason, it has been suggested that patients with Wolff-Parkinson-White syndrome be challenged with digitalis during electrophysiologic study before institution of long-term therapy.[35]

*Cautions.*—There are several clinical situations in which cardiac glycosides should be used with extra caution: namely, myocardial infarction, sick sinus syndrome, and electrical cardioversion.

Experimental studies have shown that although the use of digitalis in acute infarction does increase contractility, its use in the nonfailing heart can increase infarct size.[36] In addition, it has been stated that the freshly infarcted heart is more likely to develop toxic dysrhythmias with digitalis. This last observation has recently been challenged.[37] In view of these potential problems, it would seem safest in the setting of acute myocardial infarction to withhold digitalis unless atrial fibrillation with rapid ventricular response or congestive heart failure unresponsive to diuretics and vasodilators is present.

Although its use is not absolutely contraindicated in patients with sick sinus syndrome, cardiac glycoside therapy should be monitored very closely, for serious bradyarrhythmias can result. Prophylactic permanent pacing should be considered in patients who require digitalis for inotropic support but who manifest significant bradycardia on normal doses of digitalis.

Electrical cardioversion is associated with a higher incidence of ventricular tachydysrhythmia in digitalized patients, and hence the cardiac glycosides should be withdrawn several days before elective cardioversion. If this is not clinically feasible, the risk of dysrhythmia can be reduced by using low-energy DC shock or by covering the period of cardioversion with intravenous phenytoin.[38] Cardioversion is contraindicated in cases of digitalis toxicity unless a life-threatening ventricular dysrhythmia exists.

## Digitalis Toxicity

Digitalis toxicity remains a common and serious clinical problem. In prospective studies of hospitalized patients over the last decade, the reported incidence of digitalis toxicity ranged from 13 to 29%.[39,40] Mortality in these patients was also significant; some series reported deaths in up to 39% of patients with toxicity.[41] In view of the number of factors that can interact to produce alterations in both pharmacokinetic handling and patient sensitivity to digoxin, it is not surprising that toxicity remains a problem. Encouraging reports from several centers over the last few years have shown, however, that through patient and physician education the incidence of digitalis intoxication can be significantly reduced.[42,43]

*Factors Affecting Myocardial Sensitivity to Digitalis.*—It has been observed that some patients experience toxic manifestations at low or "therapeutic" levels, whereas others fail to show optimal clinical effect despite high or "toxic" levels. A number of conditions that have been identified as being associated with altered myocardial sensitivity are listed in Table 1. Electrolyte abnormalities account for some instances of increased sensitivity and are the most readily amenable to correction. Hypokalemia allows increased glycoside binding to the $Na^+,K^+$-ATPase enzyme system and so increases the digitalis effect. Hypomagnesemia and hypercalcemia also enhance the effect of digitalis.[44,45] Widespread use of diuretics for treatment of congestive heart failure may be responsible for many of these electrolyte abnormalities. The presence of organic heart disease, most notably ischemic heart disease, predisposes the patient to the formation of ectopic impulses, and both in vivo and in vitro studies have demonstrated ventricular tachydysrhythmias much lower doses of digitalis in diseased as opposed to normal myocardium.[46,47] Whether hypoxia significantly increases the sensitivity of the heart to the toxic effects of the cardiac glycosides is controversial; however, patients with pulmonary disease have been reported to have a higher incidence of digitalis toxicity.[48] Decreased sensitivity of the atrioventricular node to digoxin is seen in some supraventricular tachycardias, especially when they are precipitated by an acute event such as pericarditis, thoracotomy, or pulmonary embolus.[49] The apparent sensitivity to digoxin in hypothyroidism and resistance in hyperthyroidism may result from changes in activity of the $Na^+$ pump, pharmacokinetics, or sympathetic nervous system activity.[31]

*Use of Digoxin Levels in the Diagnosis of Digitalis Toxicity.*—Although most studies demonstrate elevated digoxin levels (more than 2 ng/mL) in patients with digitalis toxicity, a considerable number of patients with apparent toxicity have levels in the "therapeutic range." Ingelfinger and Goldman[50] evaluated the literature on this subject and concluded that digoxin levels are of limited usefulness in diagnosing toxicity. Although the likelihood of toxicity increases with increasing concentrations, there is no precise value that clearly separates toxic from nontoxic levels. Therefore, the serum digoxin level is not, in itself, sufficient for the diagnosis of digoxin toxicity.

*Manifestations and Mechanisms. Cardiac.*—Cardiac dysrhythmias are the most important toxic manifestations of digitalis. The most common dysrhythmias stem from increased automaticity, especially in Purkinje fibers, and result in ventricular ectopy manifested by multiform premature ventricular contractions, ventricular bigeminy, ventricular tachycardia, and ventricular fibrillation. Digitalis may also depress sinus node function and atrioventricular node conduction. Combinations of decreased conduction and increased automaticity can result in paroxysmal atrial tachycardia with block and nonparoxysmal junctional tachycardia.

The underlying mechanism for the enhanced ventricular ectopy associated with digitalis toxicity has been explained on the basis of reentry or by increased diastolic depolarization in the Purkinje fibers. Recent work, however, suggests that glycoside-induced ventricular automaticity is due to transient oscillations in diastolic membrane potential, commonly referred to as oscillatory after-potentials.[51] With increasing degrees of toxicity, these oscillations increase in amplitude and reach threshold, and they thereby propagate action potentials. Furthermore, subthreshold oscillatory after-potentials can reduce membrane excitability and produce conduction defects. In vitro studies have reproduced automatic activity occurring singly, in bigeminy, and in sustained runs. In addition, intermittent conduction block also has been demonstrated. Evidence to date suggests that oscillatory after-potentials are produced by slow inward fluxes of $Ca^{++}$; varying the extracellular $Ca^{++}$ concentration directly affects the amplitude of oscillatory after-potentials, and calcium-blocking agents (for example, verapamil) may abolish them completely.

The central nervous system also plays a significant role in the pathogenesis of digitalis toxicity. Cardiac glycosides have an excitatory effect on the brainstem, and increased activity in both sympathetic and parasympathetic cardiac nerves has been documented in association with toxicity. Experiments that exclude the central nervous system influence (for example, spinal transection) have demonstrated that much larger amounts of digitalis are needed to induce toxic dysrhythmias than when the central nervous system is intact.[52] Exactly how autonomic stimulation predisposes to intoxication is not entirely clear; however, it is known that norepinephrine can produce oscillatory after-potentials, and it is possible that increased sympathetic activity in the ventricle facilitates production of oscillatory after-potentials and augments their amplitude.

*Noncardiac.*—In addition to the cardiac manifestations, other organ systems, particularly the central nervous system, demonstrate abnormal function in response to toxic amounts of digitalis. A unique insight into these reactions was obtained a number of years ago in the Netherlands following the discovery that tablets labeled as 0.25 mg of digoxin actually contained 0.05 mg of digoxin and 0.2 mg of digitoxin (approximately 2½ times the prescribed dose).[53] In these patients, 95% complained of acute fatigue, 85% complained of gastrointestinal symptoms such as anorexia, nausea, and abdominal discomfort, and 95% were noted to have visual disturbances in the form of hazy vision, photophobia, spots, and red-green color blindness. Interestingly, 55% of patients noted psychic disturbances in the form of agitation, nervousness, pseudohallucinations, and even psychoses. Unfortunately, the extracardiac manifestations are not very specific, do not always precede the cardiac abnormalities, and do not correlate well with serum glycoside levels.[40] Nevertheless, the physician should be aware of these symptoms, for in a significant number of cases extracardiac manifestations appear first,

**Table 1.—Factors Affecting Myocardial Sensitivity to Digitalis**

Electrolyte disturbances
    Hypokalemia
    Hyperkalemia
    Hypercalcemia
    Hypomagnesemia
Organic heart Disease
Pulmonary disease
Hyperthroidism and Hypothyroidism
Autonomic nervous system status

and recognition of them may prevent severe toxicity.

*Treatment.*—Management of digitalis toxicity is dictated by the clinical setting and the mode of expression. Initial therapy in situations of acute overdosage is quite different from that of patients who are on long-term therapy and should include measures aimed at retarding further absorption of the drug by the use of activated charcoal, cathartics, or nonabsorbable binding resins such as cholestyramine or colestipol.[54] Patients who are on long-term therapy, on the other hand, should be evaluated for electrolyte imbalance such as hypokalemia or hypomagnesemia or for a recent change in renal function. Obviously, digitalis therapy should be discontinued.

Although many cases of intoxication can be treated by simply discontinuing use of the drug and observing the patient, some dysrhythmias represent an immediate threat to life and should be treated accordingly. Mild degrees of atrioventricular block or sinus node depression can be treated with atropine. Patients exhibiting complete heart block or Mobitz II block should have a temporary pacemaker inserted. Ventricular ectopy is best treated initially with lidocaine because this drug has little or no effect on atrioventricular nodal conduction, has a rapid onset of action, and is easily titratable. Potassium can also be used as an initial agent in the treatment of ectopy, particularly when hypokalemia exists.[55] Potassium should be used with caution, however, and is contraindicated in advanced atrioventricular block because its action to prolong the refractory period of the atrioventricular node may result in complete heart block. Phenytoin is also useful for ectopy, particularly when atrioventricular block is present, for it rarely depresses atrioventricular nodal conduction. Propranolol may be effective in controlling both atrial and ventricular tachydysrhythmias but may prolong atrioventricular conduction. Quinidine and procainamide, although effective in controlling ventricular ectopy, have even greater potential for prolonging atrioventricular conduction. The newer calcium-antagonist drugs (for example, verapamil), which have been shown to inhibit oscillatory after-potentials in vitro, may be of future benefit.

The goals of management of digitalis toxicity at this time remain supportive until the body stores of digitalis have been metabolized or excreted. Hemodialysis is relatively ineffective in hastening removal of glycoside from the body because of the high degree of tissue binding.[56] Progress has been made, however, by use of the Fab portion of digoxin-specific antibodies. Experimental studies in animals have shown that digoxin Fab binding rapidly reverses the toxic and pharmacologic effects of the cardiac glycosides.[57] Recently, Smith and associates[58] published the first report of successful reversal of digitalis toxicity in a human by the use of Fab antibody fragments. With this method we may be close to meeting Withering's desire to have an agent that specifically counteracts the effects of digitalis glycosides.

In closing, one might consider how very appropriate Withering's comments still are when he wrote,[1]

"It is now about ten years since I first began to use this medicine. Experience and cautious attention gradually taught me how to use it. For the last two years I have not had occasion to alter the modes of management; but I am still far from thinking them perfect."

## References

1. Withering W: An Account of the Foxglove, and Some of Its Medical Uses: With Practical Remarks on Dropsy and Other Diseases. London, C.G.J. and J. Robinson, 1785
2. Akera T, Brody TM: The role of $Na^+$, $K^+$-ATPase in the inotropic action of digitalis. Pharmacol Rev 29:187-220, 1977
3. Lee KS, Klaus W: The subcellular basis for the mechanism of inotropic action of cardiac glycosides. Pharmacol Rev 23:193-261, 1971
4. Katz AM, Brady AJ: Mechanical and biochemical correlates of cardiac contraction. Mod Concepts Cardiovasc Dis 40:45-48, 1971
5. Allen DG, Blinks, JR: Calcium transients in aequorin-injected frog cardiac muscle. Nature 273:509-513, 1978
6. Langer GA: Ionic basis of myocardial contractility. Annu Rev Med 28:13-20, 1977
7. Klaus W, Lee KS: Influence of cardiac glycosides on calcium binding in muscle subcellular components. J Pharmacol Exp Ther 166:68-76, 1969
8. Langer GA: Effects of digitalis on myocardial exchange. Circulation 46:180-187, 1972
9. Reuter H: Exchange of calcium ions in the mammalian myocardium: mechanisms and physiological significance. Circ Res 34:599-605, 1974
10. Schwartz A: Is the cell membrane $Na^+$,$K^+$-ATP enzyme system the pharmacological receptor for digitalis? Circ Res 39:2-7, 1976
11. Morad M, Greenspan AM: Excitation-contraction coupling as a possible site for the action of digitalis on heart muscle. *In* Cardiac Arrhythmias: The Twenty-Fifth Hahnemann Symposium. Edited by LS Dreifus, W Likoff, New York, Grune & Stratton, 1973, pp 479-489

12. Okita GT: Dissociation of Na⁺, K⁺-ATP inhibition from digitalis inotropy. Fed Proc 36:2225-2230, 1977

13. Hoffman BF: Effects of digitalis on electrical activity of cardiac fibers. *In* Digitalis. Edited by C Fisch, B Surawicz. New York, Grune & Stratton, 1969, pp 93-109

14. Gillis RA, Pearle DL, Levitt B: Digitalis: a neuro-excitatory drug (editorial). Circulation 52:739-742, 1975

15. Ricci DR, Orlick AE, Reitz BA, Mason JW, Stinson EB, Harrison DC: Depressant effect of digoxin on atrioventricular conduction in man. Circulation 57:898-903, 1978

16. Moe GK, Mendez R: The action of several cardiac glycosides on conduction velocity and ventricular excitability in the dog heart. Circulation 4:729-734, 1951

17. Selzer A, Kelly JJ Jr: Action of digitalis upon the nonfailing heart: a critical review. Prog Cardiovasc Dis 7:273-283, 1964

18. Covell JW, Braunwald E, Ross J Jr, Sonnenblick EH: Studies on digitalis. XVI. Effects on myocardial oxygen consumption. J Clin Invest 45:1535-1542, 1966

19. Glancy DL, Higgs LM, O'Brien KP, Epstein SE: Effects of ouabain on the left ventricular response to exercise in patients with angina pectoris. Circulation 43: 45-57, 1971.

20. Sharma B, Majid PA, Meeran MK, Whitaker W, Taylor SH: Clinical, electrocardiographic, and haemodynamic effects of digitalis (ouabain) in angina pectoris. Br Heart J 34:631-637, 1972

21. Lindenbaum J, Mellow MH, Blackstone MO, Butler VP Jr: Variation in biologic availability of digoxin from four preparations. N Engl J Med 285:1344-1347, 1971

22. Harter JG: Comments from the Food and Drug Administration. Am J Med 58:477-478, 1975

23. Heizer WD, Smith TW, Goldfinger SE: Absorption of digoxin in patients with malabsorption syndromes. N Engl J Med 285:257-259, 1971

24. Manninen V, Melin J, Apajalahti A, Karesoja M: Altered absorption of digoxin in patients given propantheline and metoclopramide. Lancet 1:398-400, 1973

25. Shaw TRD: Clinical pharmacokinetics of digitalis. Recent Adv Cardiol 7:425-445, 1977

26. White RJ, Chamberlain DA, Howard M, Smith TW: Plasma concentrations of digoxin after oral administration in the fasting and postprandial state. Br Med J 1:380-381, 1971

27. Notari RE: Biopharmaceutics and Pharmaco-kinetics: An Introduction. Second edition. New York, Marcel Dekker, 1975, p 53

28. Reuning RH, Sams RA, Notari RE: Role of Pharmacokinetics in drug dosage adjustment. I. Pharmacologic effect kinetics and apparent volume of distribution of digoxin. J Clin Pharmacol 13: 127-141, 1973

29. Luchi RJ, Gruber JW: Unusually large digitalis requirements: a study of altered digoxin metabolism. Am J Med 45:322-328, 1968

30. Doherty JE, Flanigan WJ, Murphy ML, Bulloch RT, Dalrymple GL, Beard OW, Perkins WH: Tritiated digoxin, XIV. Enterohepatic circulation, absorption, and excretion studies in human volunteers. Circulation 42:867-873, 1970

31. Lawrence JR, Sumner DJ, Kalk WJ, Ratcliffe WA, Whiting B, Gray K, Lindsay M: Digoxin kinetics in patients with thyroid dysfunction. Clin Pharmacol Ther 22:7-13, 1977

32. Ejvinsson G: Effect of quinidine on plasma concentrations of digoxin. Br Med J 1:279-280, 1978

33. Jusko WJ: Clinical pharmacokinetics of digoxin, *In* Clinical Pharmacokinetics: A Symposium. Edited by G Levy. American Pharmaceutical Association, Academy of Pharmaceutical Sciences, 1974, pp 31-43

34. Wellens HJJ, Duren DR, Liem KL, Lie KI: Effect digitalis in patients with paroxysmal atrioventricular nodal tachycardia. Circulation 52:779-788, 1975

35. Sellers TD, Bashore TM, Gallagher JJ: Digitalis in pre-excitation syndrome: analysis during atrial fibrillation. Circulation 56:260-267, 1977

36. Maroko PR, Kjekshus JK, Sobel BE, Watanabe T, Covell JW, Ross J Jr, Braunwald E: Factors influencing infarct size following experimental coronary artery occlusions. Circulation 43:67-82, 1971

37. Reicansky I, Conradson T-B, Holmberg S, Ryden L, Waldenstrom A, Wennerblom B: The effect of intravenous digoxin on the occurrence of ventricular tachyarrhythmias in acute myocardial infarction in man. Am Heart J 91:705-711, 1976

38. Kleiger R, Lown B: Cardioversion and digitalis. II. Clinical studies. Circulation 33:878-887, 1966

39. Carruthers SG, Kelly JG, McDevitt DG: Plasma digoxin concentrations in patients on admission to hospital. Br Heart J 36:707-712, 1974

40. Beller GA, Smith TW, Abelmann WH, Haber E, Hood WB Jr: Digitalis intoxication: a prospective clinical study with serum level correlations. N Engl J Med 284:989-997, 1971

41. Fogelman AM, La Mont JT, Finkelstein S, Rado

E, Pearce ML: Fallibility of plasma-digoxin in differentiating toxic from non-toxic patients. Lancet 2:727-729, 1971

42. Jelliffe RW, Buell J, Kalaba R: Reduction of digitalis toxicity by computer-assisted glycoside dosage regimens. Ann Intern Med 77:891-906, 1972

43. Ogilvie RI, Ruedy J: An educational program in digitalis therapy. JAMA 222:50-55, 1972

44. Seller RH, Cangiano J, Kim KE, Mendelssohn S, Brest AN, Swartz C: Digitalis toxicity and hypomagnesemia. Am Heart J 79:57-68, 1970

45. Nola GT, Pope S, Harrison DC: Assessment of the synergistic relationship between serum calcium and digitalis. Am Heart J 79:499-507, 1970

46. Smith TW: Contribution of quantitative assay technics to the understanding of the clinical pharmacology of digitalis. Circulation 46:188-199, 1972

47. Rosen MR, Gelband H, Merker C, Hoffman BF: Mechanisms of digitalis toxicity: effects of ouabain on phase four of canine Purkinje fiber transmembrane potentials. Circulation 47:681-689, 1973

48. Green LH, Smith TW: Factors influencing individual sensitivity to cardiac glycosides. Adv Man Clin Heart Dis 3:161-187, 1978

49. Goldman S. Probst P, Selzer A, Cohn K: Inefficacy of "therapeutic" serum levels of digoxin in controlling the ventricular rate in atrial fibrillation. Am J Cardiol 35:651-655, 1975

50. Ingelfinger JA, Goldman P: The serum digitalis concentration—does it diagnose digitalis toxicity? N Engl J Med 294:867-870, 1976

51. Ferrier GR: Digitalis arrhythmias: role of oscillatory afterpotentials. Prog Cardiovasc Dis 19: 459-474, 1977

52. Gillis RA, Raines A, Sohn YJ, Levitt B, Standaert FG: Neuroexcitatory effects of digitalis and their role in the development of cardiac arrhythmias. J Pharmacol Exp Ther 183:154-168, 1972

53. Lely AH, van Enter CHJ: Non-cardiac symptoms of digitalis intoxication. Am Heart J 83:149-152, 1972

54. Ekins BR, Watanabe AS: Acute digoxin poisonings: review of therapy. Am J Hosp Pharm 35: 268-277, 1978

55. Mason DT, Zelis R, Lee G, Hughes JL, Spann JF Jr, Amsterdam EA: Current concepts and treatment of digitalis toxicity. Am J Cardiol 27:546-559, 1971

56. Ackerman GL, Doherty JE, Flanigan WJ: Peritoneal dialysis and hemodialysis of tritiated digoxin. Ann Intern Med 67:718-723, 1967

57. Smith TW, Haber E: Digitalis. N Engl J Med 289: 1125-1129, 1973

58. Smith TW, Haber E, Yeatman L, Butler VP Jr: Reversal of advanced digoxin intoxication with FAB fragments of digoxin-specific antibodies. N Engl J Med 294:797-800, 1976

# 18

# Understanding and Using Data on Serum Digoxin Concentrations in Clinical Practice: A Case Study

**John F. Bresnahan, M.D.**

The development of the radioimmunoassay for determining serum digoxin has significantly advanced the understanding of digoxin pharmacokinetics. A case of digitalis intoxication is described, with emphasis on the contribution of data on serum digoxin to the patient's management. Such data can be very useful to the clinician when they are interpreted with an understanding of digoxin pharmacokinetics.

The digitalis glycosides are the oldest of the cardioactive drugs in common use today. The beneficial effects of digitalis in the treatment of congestive heart failure and certain rhythm disturbances have been recognized for centuries. Digoxin, because of its rapid onset and intermediate duration of action, is the most commonly used digitalis preparation in this country.

Just over a decade ago, the radioimmunoassay technique for determining serum digoxin concentrations was introduced, and as a result the understanding of digoxin pharmacokinetics has increased dramatically. While there is no absolute concentration that clearly separates subtherapeutic from therapeutic or therapeutic from toxic, experience has shown that serum digoxin concentrations between 1 and 2 $\mu g/L$ are usually associated with optimum clinical effect. The following case illustrates how serum digoxin concentrations can be used to aid the physician in the clinical decision-making and management of a patient with digitalis intoxication.

## Case History

A 35-year-old man was in good health until April 1980, when he developed a flu-like syndrome with migrating joint and muscle pains. He was treated with salicylates by his local physician, but his symptoms did not improve. The following July he developed severe hypertension with blood pressures of 210/120 mmHg, loss of appetite (anorexia), episodes of fever to 104°F, and excruciating abdominal pain. He was hospitalized and, after an extensive work-up, an exploratory laparotomy was performed. Tissue removed at the time of surgery revealed vascular changes compatible with polyarteritis nodosa (PAN), a multisystem inflam-

matory disease that results in destruction of medium-size and small arteries.

Postoperatively the patient's blood pressure was poorly controlled despite large doses of antihypertensives, and he developed congestive heart failure with pulmonary edema. Digoxin and diuretics were administered with prompt relief of the pulmonary edema, and as the values for the patient's serum creatinine and electrolytes were normal, a maintenance digoxin dose of 0.25 mg per day was prescribed. Additionally, corticosteroids in large doses were given for treatment of the patient's underlying PAN. He responded well to this therapy with rapid improvement in his symptoms. His hypertension, which was felt to be due to renal involvement with PAN, was also easier to control.

The patient remained stable until January 1981, when he developed progressive nausea, anorexia, and dizziness, along with right testicular pain. Examination at the time of admission to the hospital revealed a bradycardia with a rate of 44 beats per minute and a tender, inflamed right testicle. An electrocardiogram demonstrated complete heart block and the remaining initial laboratory data were unremarkable, except for a markedly above-normal value for serum creatinine, 42 mg/L. The initial diagnosis was reactivation of PAN, with either myocardial involvement or superimposed digitalis toxicity. The serum digoxin concentration was significantly high: 3.8 $\mu g/L$. Digoxin therapy was withdrawn and during the next several days the patient's rhythm returned to normal and his anorexia and nausea improved. When serum digoxin was measured four days later, when the patient had returned to normal sinus rhythm, it was 1.6 $\mu g/L$. Aggressive treatment of the patient's PAN was begun with Cytoxan and high-dose corticosteroids, and his creatinine gradually decreased and stabilized at 18 mg/L. Digoxin therapy was restarted with alternating doses of 0.125 and 0.25 mg per day, with the aim of acheiving a serum concentration just under 1.6 $\mu g/L$. A subsequent steady-state digoxin concentration of 1.2 $\mu g/L$ was attained. The patient's creatinine has remained stable, and he has had no further rhythm disturbances.

## Discussion

The goal of digoxin therapy is to deliver to the myocardial cells an adequate concentration of drug to produce the desired clinical effect without inducing toxicity. The amount of digoxin that ultimately reaches the

*Dr. Bresnahan is in the Department of Cardiovascular Diseases at Mayo Clinic, Rochester, MN 55901.*

myocardium after an oral dose is affected by several factors. Absorption of digoxin by the gastrointestinal tract controls the total amount of drug made available for use by the body. Distribution and differential uptake by various organ systems further influences the net concentration of digoxin that reaches the myocardium. Lastly, the rate of inactivation and excretion affects both the magnitude and duration of the digoxin concentration in both the plasma and the tissues. Several investigations have demonstrated close correlation between the steady-state concentration in serum and the myocardial concentration of digoxin. Furthermore, there also appears to be good correlation between serum concentrations and physiological effects (1). An understanding of digoxin pharmacokinetics and the factors that produce altered pharmacokinetic states, such as observed in this patient, is thus necessary for the proper interpretation and use of data on serum digoxin.

The bioavailability of digoxin tablets (that fraction of the administered dose that reaches the systemic circulation) is about 70%. Most of the digoxin is absorbed in the upper portion of the small intestine, and incompleteness of absorption accounts for most of the low bioavailability. Several years ago it became apparent that bioavailability was also subject to the dissolution rate of the digoxin tablet (2). Owing to marked differences in dissolution rates among tablets supplied by various manufacturers, the bioavailability of digoxin tablets ranged from 40 to 70%. Currently, regulations for tablet dissolution rates are in effect and minimize inter-manufacturer differences in bioavailability.

The alterations in bioavailability that arise clinically are related primarily to disturbances in gut motility, either disease or drug-induced, or to drugs that bind to digoxin, thereby making it unavailable for absorption. In general, drugs or disease states that increase small-bowel motility decrease absorption of digoxin; conversely, factors that reduce motility (e.g., anticholinergics) enhance absorption. Compounds known to bind digoxin in the gut include magnesium trisilicate-containing antacids and kaolin-pectin antidiarrheal compounds among those most commonly encountered clinically.

Absorption is rapid under normal circumstances and peak serum values usually are attained within 90 min. Distribution of digoxin within the body is a two-phase process. The first phase occurs rapidly and involves equilibrium of digoxin with the plasma and extracellular fluids. The second phase occurs much slower and is produced by the uptake of digoxin by the various organ systems, including the heart. It requires about 8 h for both phases of distribution to be completed and the fluid and tissue compartments to be in equilibrium. During the distribution process, serum digoxin concentrations do not correlate with the myocardial digoxin concentration and thus assay values obtained during this period are misleading.

After the distribution phase, the amount of digoxin in the serum and the tissue compartments gradually decreases as a result of metabolism and excretion. Excretion takes place mainly in the kidney by virtue of glomerular filtration; about 80% of a given dose is excreted unchanged in the urine. Hepatic metabolism accounts for approximately 10 to 15% of overall excretion, and current evidence suggests that hepatic metabolism is not altered by drugs that promote enzyme induction or by liver disease unless it is severe (3).

## DIGOXIN PROFILE

| | |
|---|---|
| Trade name: | Lanoxin |
| pk$_a$: | n/a |
| Mol. mass: | 780.92 |
| Melting Point, °C: | n/a |
| Water Solubility: | insoluble |

Chemical Structure:

| | |
|---|---|
| Dose Absorbed: | 60-75% |
| Peak plasma level, time: | 1.5-5.0 h |
| Protein bound: | 20-40% |
| V$_d$: | 5.0-10.0 L/kg |

| FORM IN URINE | % excreted | Active | Detectable in blood |
|---|---|---|---|
| unchanged drug: | 80-90 | yes | yes |

| | Adults | Children |
|---|---|---|
| Half-life (h): | 36-51 | 11-50 |
| Steady state, time (d): | 7-11 | 2-10 |

| | Adults | Children |
|---|---|---|
| Recommended dose ($\mu$g/kg/d): | 3-5 | 10-15* |
| Effective levels (ng/mL): | 0.8-2.0 | same |
| Toxic level (mg/mL): | >2.4 | same |

*age dependent

| | |
|---|---|
| Monitoring methods: | RIA EMIT |

Reduction in the renal excretion of digoxin, such as observed in the patient presented here, represents the most important clinical alteration of digoxin kinetics. In patients with normal renal function, the serum half-life of digoxin is approximately 36 h, whereas in patients with severe renal failure the half-life is over four days. It is easy to see how a decrease in renal function without a corresponding decrease in digoxin dose can lead to increased body stores of digoxin and result in toxicity. Another clinically important situation is the recently recognized increase in serum digoxin concentrations produced by quinidine (4). Evidence thus far suggests that quinidine interferes with the renal clearance of digoxin. As quinidine and digoxin are commonly used concurrently, this drug interaction may play an important role in the production of digitalis intoxication.

The preceding case illustrates two of the three major clinical situations where information on digoxin concentrations is of assistance in patient management. First of all, the markedly increased digoxin concentration served to support the clinical impression of digitalis toxicity. Therapy was appropriately discontinued, with ultimate resolution of the rhythm disturbance. In this instance the diagnosis of digitalis toxicity was clear cut: the rhythm disturbance was highly suggestive of digitalis intoxication and the concentration in serum was significantly high. Although as a general rule the risk of toxicity increases as the serum digoxin concentration increases, as noted above there is no clearly definable concentration that separates therapeutic from toxic. Unfortunately, in a substantial number of patients with clinically suspected digitalis toxicity, the concentration in serum falls within the "therapeutic" range (5). One review of the literature several years ago addressed the question of serum digoxin concentrations in the diagnosis of digitalis toxicity and concluded that in view of the significant overlap of toxic and therapeutic concentrations, digoxin measurements are of little diagnostic value (6). Digitalis toxicity is—and will most likely remain—a clinical diagnosis. Perhaps the proper perspective in this regard would be to view digoxin concentrations as a piece of corroborative information, either supporting or detracting from the diagnosis rather than as a definitive test. The other major application of digoxin concentrations demonstrated by this case is in assisting dosage schedules. In patients with abnormal digoxin pharmacokinetics such as seen with renal disease or bioavailability problems, the ability accurately to predict serum digoxin concentrations is poor. In these situations, the use of data on drug concentrations can give valuable feedback and guide future dosage adjustments to achieve optimum therapeutic effect. Additionally, in those patients who become toxic at "therapeutic" concentrations, defining the concentration at which toxicity occurs may be of value so that subsequent adjustments in dose can be made to achieve a lower drug concentration.

The final situation where information on digoxin concentrations may be helpful is in troubleshooting those cases showing an inadequate clinical response, despite seemingly appropriate dosage. Alterations in bioavailability owing to malabsorption or drug interactions can be uncovered, as can the problem of patient noncompliance with prescribed dosage.

In conclusion, a few instances deserve mention in which digoxin measurements are of little or no clinical use. As noted above, it takes approximately 8 h after an oral dose before there is equilibrium between the fluid and tissue compartments. Concentrations measured in serum during the distribution phase do not correlate with those in myocardial tissue, which can lead to erroneous conclusions (7). It is also rarely necessary to measure digoxin for the purpose of monitoring therapy in patients of normal size with normal renal function who are receiving 0.25 mg or less of dioxin per day. The likelihood of finding abnormally high values in such patients is very low.

## References

1. Chamberlain, D.A., White, R.J., Howard, M.R., and Smith, T.W., Plasma digoxin concentrations in patients with atrial fibrillation. *Br. Med. J.* 3, 429-432 (1970).
2. Lindenbaum, J., Mellow, M.H., and Blackstone, M.D., Variation in biologic activity from four preparations. *N. Engl. J. Med.* 285, 1344-1347 (1971).
3. Shaw, T.R.D., Clinical pharmacokinetics of digitalis. *Recent Adv. Cardiol.* 7, 425-445 (1977).
4. Ejvinsson, G., Effect of quinidine on plasma concentrations of digoxin. *Br. Med. J.* 1, 278-280 (1978).
5. Beller, G.A., Smith, T.W., Abelman, W.H., et al., Digitalis intoxication. A prospective clinical study with serum level correlations. *N. Engl. J. Med.* 284, 989-997 (1971).
6. Inglefinger, J.A., and Goldman, P., The serum digitalis concentration—does it diagnose digitalis toxicity? *N. Engl. J. Med.* 294, 867-870 (1976).
7. Doherty, J.E., How and when to use the digitalis serum levels. *JAMA* 239, 2594-2596 (1978).

## Suggested Reading

Bresnahan, J.F., and Vlietstra, R.E., Digitalis glycosides. *Mayo Clin. Proc.* 54, 675-684 (1979). Review.

# 19

# Digoxin-Quinidine Interactions

**Carl Ludvigsen, Ph.D.**
**Larry D. Bowers, Ph.D.**

The use of drugs has significantly increased in recent years to the point where an average patient on a medical service may receive 14 drugs during his stay. The incidence of simultaneous multiple drug regimens has also increased. With the rate of adverse reactions reported to be between 2 and 30%, it is important for the laboratory to recognize potentially dangerous drug interactions. One such interaction is that between digoxin and quinidine. The interaction was first noted in 1932 by Gold (1). He later expressed his concern about the potential danger of this interaction by stating that the drugs should never be given together (2).

## Case Study

A 36-year-old white male was admitted in October 1981 for electrocardioversion. He has had long-standing recurrent atrial flutter and fibrillation. On admission, he had a supraventricular arrhythmia, nausea, emesis, and altered sensorium. Laboratory examination revealed a pH of 7.39, $P_{CO_2}$ of 41 mm Hg, $P_{O_2}$ of 42 mm Hg, and a $HCO_3$ of 24 mmol/L. Renal function tests had results of 300 mg/L for blood urea nitrogen and 19 mg/L for creatinine. The patient had a trough digoxin concentration of 3.7 $\mu$g/L and a quinidine concentration of 3.5 mg/L. Digoxin was discontinued immediately (day 1) and the patient was taken off quinidine the following day (day 2).

**Past history.** This patient was born with a single ventricle, transposition of the great veins, and an atrial septal defect. He underwent several surgical procedures to correct the congenital defects in 1963. He has continuing cyanotic heart disease. He had experienced numerous episodes of atrial flutter and fibrillation requiring five cardioversions in the year preceding this reported admission. The patient was receiving digoxin (0.25 mg/day) and quinidine (325 mg three times a day) in an effort to control his arrhythmias. In August of 1981 he had experienced extreme discomfort, headaches, nausea, and vomiting due to atrial fibrillation and severe dyspnea on

exertion. He was electrocardioverted. The quinidine dose was increased to 650 mg/three times a day on day 7 of this prior admission to control his supraventricular arrhythmias (see Table 1). Apparently no drug concentration was measured after increasing the dose prior to his release.

**Patient follow-up.** The patient was observed for several days after the described admission in the absence of any drug administration. He was successfully cardioverted on day 7. He was subsequently discharged on 0.25 mg/day of digoxin. He continues to have recurrent atrial flutter/fibrillation.

## Mechanism and Site of Action

Digoxin is the drug of choice for congestive heart failure and atrial fibrillation or flutter. In the former case, the positive inotropic effect of the drug on ventricular function is important, although other interactions with the sympathetic nervous system also have a role in mediating its therapeutic effect. The increased contractility of the heart appears to be due to inhibition of the membrane $Na^+$, $K^+$ - ATPase which results in an increase in intracellular $Na^+$ and a decrease in intracellular $K^+$. An increased $Ca^{++}$ concentration in the sarcoplasm, due to a $Na^+$ - $Ca^{++}$ exchange via an alternate $Na^+$ pump, results in an increase in the force of myocardial contraction with subsequent beneficial effects for the patient. In atrial flutter or fibrillation (the clinical dilemma in the case presented here) digoxin is used to slow ventricular rate. This slowing occurs because of blockade of a larger than normal fraction of atrial impulses through the A-V junction resulting in an increase in the effective refractory period. These effects are predominantly due to the increased efferent vagal activity and a decreased sensitivity to sympathetic

*Dr. Ludvigsen is a Clinical Chemistry Fellow and Dr. Bowers is Director of the Drug Analysis Section, Department of Laboratory Medicine and Pathology, University of Minnesota, Minneapolis, MN 55414.*

## Table 1. Drug Concentrations During Most Recent Admissions

|  | Prior Admission | | | Present Admission | | | | |
|---|---|---|---|---|---|---|---|---|
|  | Day 1 | Day 4 | Day 7 | Day 1 | Day 2 | Day 3 | Day 4 | Day 5 |
| Digoxin ($\mu$g/L) | 2.1 | 2.3 | 2.4 | 3.7 | 3.7 | 2.7 | 1.9 | 1.2 |
| Quinidine (mg/L) | 1.2 | 1.4 | 1.7 | 3.5 | - | 0.6 | - | - |

activity. There are also direct effects of digoxin on cardiac electrical activity. It should be noted that since the mechanism of drug action is mediated by changes in intra- and extracellular cation concentrations, toxicity can be exacerbated in either treatment regimen by changes in the concentrations of potassium, calcium, and sodium (toxicity more apparent when calcium concentration is increased or either sodium or potassium concentration is decreased).

Because digoxin does not affect atrial fibrillation, quinidine or the other Class I antiarrhythmic agents can be used to control supraventricular rhythm (either naturally occurring or digoxin induced). Quinidine acts to increase the effective refractory period in atrial, ventricular, and Purkinje cells as well as to decrease spontaneous phase - 4 depolarization in these cells. As a result, both formation and conduction of premature depolarizations are suppressed. In many cases sinus rhythm can be restored. The mechanism of action of quinidine is not fully understood, although there is evidence that $Na^+$, $K^+$ - ATPase is not the active binding site. It is clear that the membrane transport of cations is involved in the drug action. The pharmacological effect of quinidine is strongly affected by tissue $K^+$ concentrations. Quinidine also has an indirect effect due to inhibition of the vagal nerve which facilitates A-V node conduction. This effect is apparently overridden by the action of digoxin during coadministration.

## Clinical Side Effects

Digitalis and quinidine toxicity exhibit similar extracardiac symptoms including anorexia, nausea, vomiting, diarrhea, and abdominal pain. Digoxin intoxication is also associated with neuromuscular symptoms and visual disturbances such as blurry or hazy vision, photophobia, and abnormal color perception. Cardiac toxicity frequently occurs and may present as an arrhythmia of virtually any type. Digitalis-induced arrhythmias may cause death.

The cardiac toxicity associated with quinidine includes atrioventricular block, ventricular tachyarrhythmias, and depressed myocardial contractility. The first two usually are associated with an increased QRS interval which may be helpful in diagnosis of quinidine overdose. These arrhythmias, a part of the clinical syndrome "quinidine syncope", can cause sudden death.

## Drug-Drug Interaction

Since the first documentation of the quinidine-digoxin interaction (1), a number of clinical reports of the interaction have appeared (3-11). In several of these studies, the overall rate of combined quinidine-digoxin therapy in cardiac care patients was between 2 and 11%, so the problem is not trivial. A second common finding was a mean increase of digoxin concentration by two-fold. Bigger (12) has suggested that 90% of the patients on digoxin and quinidine exhibit this increase. It was interesting that this increase was observed even in patients who had recently discontinued digoxin therapy (8). A similar observation was made in anuric patients (10). Leahey et al. (3) reported that 16 of 27 patients developed anorexia, nausea or vomiting and ventricular arrhythmias developed or worsened during co-administration of the drugs. Pedersen (9) reported ECG changes consistent with digoxin intoxication. Decreasing the dose of digoxin almost invariably improved the symptomatology although the mean value of the digoxin concentration in symptomatic and asymptomatic populations was not significantly different. This is not surprising in that digoxin intoxication can be observed at a rather wide range of values, depending on other physiological factors and idiosyncratic sensitivity.

One explanation of the digoxin quinidine interaction is explained by an apparent decrease in the volume of distribution. Under normal circumstances, digoxin has a volume of distribution ($V_d$) of 5-8 L/kg. There is a 5 to 15-fold concentration difference between skeletal muscle and serum digoxin, and about twice that differential in cardiac tissue. Because of the mass of skeletal muscle, about 60% of the total body dose is located there. Several studies indicate that displacement of digoxin from low affinity non-$Na^+$, $K^+$ - ATPase sites in peripheral tissues results in the observed decrease in the volume of distribution (13-15). The protein bound fraction makes a minimal contribution to the $V_d$ and does not change during co-administrative of other antiarrhythmics (10).

The second pharmacokinetic factor involved in the increased serum digoxin concentration is a decreased renal (5, 7, 10, 16) and total body (7, 17) clearance of digoxin in the presence of quinidine. The degree of this decrease has been reported up to three-fold. Normally 40-70% of a digoxin dose is cleared in unaltered form by glomerular filtration, although active tubular secretion and passive tubular reabsorption have been shown to occur. By definition, clearance of a drug is the product of $V_d$ and the elimination rate constant. Thus a decrease in the volume of distribution, an increase in half-life, or a combination of both would be observed as a decreased clearance. Ochs et al. (17) have observed both a decrease in $V_d$ and an increase in $t_{1/2}$ as well as a significant decrease in total body clearance. Renal clearance, which is the product of fractional excretion in urine and the total clearance, decreased concomitantly since fractional excretion was constant. The observed reduction in renal clearance was observed in conjunction with an unaltered creatinine clearance. Thus the change in $V_d$ may explain the observed decrease in renal clearance.

The increase in serum digoxin concentration begins shortly after administration of the quinidine. There appears to be a consensus that for 3-5 days after initiating or adjusting quinidine therapy the serum digoxin concentration should be monitored. If the levels increase to the toxic range, the digoxin dosage should be decreased 2 to 2.5 fold. In the case presented here, the patient's digoxin concentration continued to increase, and continued monitoring would have been efficacious. It also appeared that the increase in dosage was not followed by monitoring. Holding the digoxin dose during the toxic episode resulted in a decrease in blood concentration at a rate consistent with a normal elimination half-life. Symptoms of toxicity disappeared upon return to a therapeutic concentration of digoxin.

It is apparent from a number of studies that the magnitude of the interaction is dependent on the serum concentration of quinidine. This issue is clouded somewhat by the unknown role of quinidine metabolites in the interaction and their contribution to the measured concentration of quinidine. Quinidine is metabolized in the liver to (3S)-3-hydroxyquinidine, and O-desmethylquinidine. Hydroxylation is increased by drugs which induce the microsomal hydroxylases, such as phenobarbital and dilantin. No such induction effect has been observed for digoxin. A recent case report indicated onset of digitalis toxicity in a patient receiving digoxin, quinidine, and pentobarbital only after discontinuation of the pentobarbital (18). This may imply that only quinidine is involved in the digoxin interaction.

## References

1. Gold, H., Modell, W., Price, L., Combined actions of quinidine and digitalis on the heart. *Arch. Int. Med.* **50**, 766-796 (1932).

2. Gold, H., *Quinidine in Disorders of the Heart,* Hoeber, New York, NY, 1950, pp 85-92.

3. Leahey, E.B., Jr., Reiffel, J.A., Drusin, R.E., Heissenbuttel, R.H., Lovejoy, W.P., and Bigger, J.T., Jr., Interaction between quinidine and digoxin. *J. Am. Med. Assoc.* **240**, 533-534 (1978).

4. Ejvinsson, G., Effect of quinidine on plasma concentrations of digoxin. *Br. Med. J.* **1**, 279-280 (1978).

5. Hooymans, P.M., and Merkus, F.W.H.M., Effect of quinidine on plasma concentration of digoxin. *Br. Med. J.* **1**, 1022 (1978).

6. Burke, W.S., and Matke, G.R., Effect of quinidine on serum digoxin concentrations. *Am. J. Hosp. Pharm.* **36**, 968-971 (1979).

7. Hager, W.D., Fenster, P., Mayersohn, M., Perrier, D., Graves, P., Marcus, F.I., and Goldman, S., Digoxin-quinidine interaction. *N. Engl. J. Med.* **305**, 1238-1241 (1979).

8. Dahlqvist, R., Ejvinsson, G., and Schenk-Gustafsson, K., Effect of quinidine on plasma concentration and renal clearance of digoxin. *Br. J. Clin. Pharmac.* **9**, 413-418 (1980).

9. Pedersen, K.E., Clinical aspects of the digoxin quinidine interaction. *Dan. Med. Bull.* **28**, 128-131 (1981).

10. Doering, W., Fichtl, B., Hermann, M., and Besenfelderr, E., Quinidine-digoxin interaction: Evidence for involvement of extrarenal mechanism. *Eur. J. Clin. Pharmacol.* **21**, 281-285 (1982).

11. Doering, W., Quinidine-digoxin interaction: Pharmacokinetics, underlying mechanism, and clinical implications. *N. Engl. J. Med.* **301**, 400-404 (1979).

12. Bigger, J.T., The quinidine-digoxin interaction: What do we know about it? *N. Engl. J. Med.* **301**, 779-781 (1979).

13. Doherty, J.E., Straub, K.D., Murphy, M.L., de Soyza, N., Bisset, J.K., and Kane, J.J., Digoxin-quinidine interaction. *Am. J. Cardiol.* **45**, 1196-1200 (1980).

14. Schenk-Gustafsson, K., Jogestrand, T., Norlander, R., and Dahlqvist, R., Effect of quinidine on digoxin concentration in skeletal muscle and serum in patients with atrial fibrillation. *N. Engl. J. Med.* **305**, 209-211 (1981).

15. Kim, D.-H., Akera, T., and Brody, T.M., Tissue binding sites involved in quinidine-cardiac glycoside interactions. *J. Pharmacol. Exp. Ther.* **218**, 357-362 (1981).

16. Straub, K.D., Kane, J.J., and Bissett, J.K., Alteration of digitalis binding by quinidine: a mechanism of digitalis-quinidine interaction. *Circulation* **58** (Suppl. 2), 11-58 (1978).

17. Ochs, H.R., Bodem, G., and Greenblatt, D.S., Impairment of digoxin clearance by coadministration of quinidine. *J. Clin. Pharmacol.* **21**, 396-400 (1981).

18. Chaperon, D.J., Mumford, D., and Pitegoff, G., Apparent quinidine-induced digoxin toxicity after withdrawal of pentobarbital. *Arch. Int. Med.* **139**, 363-365 (1979).

# 20

# Clinical Evaluation of Antiarrhythmic Drug Therapy

**Dan M. Roden M.D.,**
**Raymond L. Woosley, M.D., Ph.D.**

The margin between effective and toxic drug concentrations in plasma is particularly narrow for the antiarrhythmic agents. It is for this reason that therapy is best guided by a sound knowledge of their clinical pharmacokinetics. Treatment based on pharmacokinetic principles will increase the effectiveness of therapy and decrease the incidence of toxicity. Monitoring concentrations of these potent drugs in plasma provides an invaluable tool to further optimize therapy. To make the best use of drug concentration monitoring in plasma, physicians should incorporate it into their routine approach to patients on antiarrhythmic drugs. Routine plasma samples can help establish a minimal effective concentration; should the patient's underlying status change (e.g., renal failure develops), such data can be invaluable in guiding therapy. Drug concentration monitoring in plasma can also help detect poor compliance and help confirm (or rule out) a clinical suspicion of drug toxicity.

Drugs are only one part of the approach to a patient **with a disturbance of cardiac rhythm. Life-threatening arrhythmias (ventricular fibrillation, most ventricular tachycardia, supraventricular arrhythmias with hemodynamic compromise) require emergency DC-countershock. Rhythm disturbances due to an underlying** metabolic or homeostatic derangement (e.g., hypoxia, hypercapnia, hypokalemia, hyperthyroidism) may respond very poorly to antiarrhythmic drugs; the primary cause must be treated. Finally, arrhythmias may themselves be provoked by drug therapy. Theophylline, thioridazine, and tricyclic antidepressants are all examples. More importantly cardioactive drugs (including digitalis, exogenous catecholamines, and the antiarrhythmic agents themselves) are notorious for precipitating rhythm disturbances when used in excess **or inappropriately. A list of reversible causes of arrhythmias is shown in Table 1.**

*This work was supported by grants from the General Clinical Research Center Program of The Division of Research Resources (5 M01 RR-95) and the United States Public Health Service GM15431 and GM07569.*

*Dr. Roden is Assistant Professor of Medicine and Pharmacology, and Dr. Woosley is Associate Professor of Medicine and Pharmacology, Vanderbilt University Medical Center, Nashville, TN 37232.*

## Lidocaine (Xylocaine®)

Lidocaine is the drug of choice for the acute treatment of ventricular arrhythmias. While it has been administered intramuscularly (e.g., by paramedics out-of-hospital), the intravenous route is preferable, Prophylactic lidocaine therapy is also widely used to prevent primary ventricular fibrillation during the first 48-72 h following acute myocardial infarction. Because of very poor bioavailablity (due to avid hepatic metabolism), lidocaine is not used orally. It is important to recognize that therapeutic and occasionally even toxic concentrations can be achieved with the use of lidocaine as a local anesthetic, especially following accidental intravascular administration. Central nervous system symptoms (dysarthria, tremor, changes in hearing, and, at higher concentrations, confusion and seizures) are the major side effects of lidocaine therapy. Cardiac symptoms are more unusual and tend to occur in patients with underlying heart disorders. These include accelerated AV conduction during atrial flutter, asystole, or bradycardia in patients with conduction system disease and depression of myocardial contractility in patients with heart failure.

## Table 1. Reversible Causes of Arrhythmias

Myocardial ischemia
Acid-base disturbances
Electrolyte disturbances
Operative manipulation (e.g., intubation)
Passage of intracardiac catheters
Drugs
    Digitalis
    Catecholamines
    Antiarrhythmic agents
    Anesthetic agents
    Tricyclic antidepressants
    Phenothiazines
    Over-the-counter drugs (anorexiants, decongestants)
Thyrotoxicosis
Respiratory failure
Tetanus
**Cerebrovascular injury**

*Pharmacokinetics:* Lidocaine concentrations follow a two-compartment open model after intravenous administration. The half-life of the initial phase is short ($t_{1/2}\alpha = 8$ min) and corresponds to the distribution of lidocaine from the small central compartment (which includes plasma, myocardium, and CNS) to the peripheral compartment. The terminal half-life is longer ($t_{1/2}\beta = 120$ min) and corresponds to the elimination of drug primarily by hepatic metabolism. Thus, the effect following an initial bolus will be very transient (because of rapid distribution). However, once steady-state conditions are achieved, changes in plasma concentrations are governed by the longer elimination half-life: once a maintenance dosage (see below) is changed, four to five half-lives (6-10 h) must elapse until a new steady state is achieved. This also holds true when lidocaine therapy is stopped.

*Administration.* Since lidocaine is usually used for acute rhythm disturbances, prompt attainment of **therapeutic concentrations is desirable. The usual** 100-mg bolus administered to a normal patient will achieve such concentrations only very transiently (until distribution occurs). A larger single bolus is likely to produce severe toxicity (seizures, asystole). The most appropriate loading regimen consists of a series of boluses separated by 5-10 min (as long as side effects are absent); 100 mg initially, followed by three 50-mg bolluses at 8-min intervals is one approach. The total loading dose of 3-4 mg/kg can also be given as a single 100-mg bolus followed by 8 mg/min for 20 min. Following lidocaine loading, an infusion of 20-60 µg/kg/min (1-4 mg/min) should be started to maintain therapeutic plasma concentrations.

*Modification of Dosages.* Lidocaine dosages given above are appropriate for patients with normal cardiac and hepatic function. The magnitude of the loading dose is a function of volume of distribution, which is markedly reduced in heart failure. Thus, the loading dose should be smaller (e.g., by 50%) in patients with ventricular dysfunction.

Clearance, on the other hand, is the major determinant of the eventual steady-state concentration (steady-state concentration = infusion rate/clearance). Lidocaine clearance is a function of liver blood flow which is reduced in both heart failure and liver disease. Thus, in both these states, the maintenance infusion rate should be reduced. (Propranolol may also elevate lidocaine levels by decreasing liver blood flow.) Clearance is also reduced (for uncertain reasons) during prolonged lidocaine administration. **Maintenance infusion rates should be adjusted downward** after plasma concentration determinations during prolonged therapy.

The time required to attain the eventual steady-state concentration is determined by the elimination half-life, which itself varies directly as the volume of distribution and inversely as the clearance. In heart failure, half-life may be little altered (since both clearance and volume of distribution are reduced) while half-life may be markedly prolonged in liver disease. Lidocaine administration is not altered by renal disease.

*Drug Concentration Monitoring in Plasma.* Because rapid turnaround is essential to optimally guide therapy, the enzyme immunoassay is probably the preferred method for clinical use. Therapeutic effects occur at concentrations greater than 1.5 µg/mL, and increasing side effects are noted above 5 µg/mL. Some patients may reguire 5-9 µg/mL for arrhythmia suppression, but the incidence of side effects rises rapidly in this range. Since steady-state conditions are approached only after four to five elimination half-lives (regardless of the loading regimen), drug concentration monitoring in plasma may be especially helpful in a number of situations late after the start of therapy. First, should the steady-state concentration be too low, the arrhythmia my recur. In **this setting, a drug concentration in plasma may help** rule out other causes such as recurrent myocardial ischemia. A small bolus (e.g., 25-50 mg) should be administered and the maintenance infusion rate increased. (Recall that if the infusion rate alone is increased, four to five half-lives—up to 10 h—will elapse before the new steady state is attained.) Second, should the steady-state concentration be too high, side effects may occur hours after the institution of seemingly optimal therapy. Side effects may include confusion (often misdiagnosed as "ICU psychosis"), seizures, and heart failure (which decreases clearance and thus further elevates lidocaine concentation in plasma).

## Procainamide (Pronestyl®)

Procainamide is the drug of choice for the acute **treatment of lidocaine-resistant ventricular arrhythmias, although some authorities prefer bretylium in this setting. Procainamide can also be given orally for the chronic treatment of ventricular** arrhythmias and has also been used for acute and chronic therapy of some supraventricular arrhythmias. Intravenous procainamide can produce hypotension (possibly related to ganglionic blockade). Gastrointestinal symptoms are the major dose-related side effect of chronic procainamide therapy. These can be avoided by decreasing the peak drug levels in plasma (i.e., by giving smaller doses more often). In addition, chronic therapy with procainamide regularly produces a lupus erythematosus type picture:

arthralgias and fever are the most common symptoms but more serious manifestations such as arthritis and pericarditis with tamponade can occur, This symptom complex occurs more often and earlier during chronic therapy in those patients who are genetically slow acetylators. Antinuclear antibodies are common during therapy and while they presage the development of the lupus syndrome, they are not an indication to stop therapy in the absence of symptoms. Procainamide, quinidine, and disopyramide may cause excessive QT prolongation and torsades des pointes (a polymorphic ventricular tachycardia). In addition, these agents may accelerate the ventricular rate during atrial flutter, both by slowing the flutter rate and enhancing AV conduction; patients with atrial flutter should therefore be digitalized prior to receiving these drugs. Depression of myocardial function can also occur, especially in patients with pre-existing heart failure.

*Pharmacokinetics.* Procainamide is well absorbed with peak concentrations 0.5-4 h after a dose. It is rapidly eliminated ($t_{1/2}$ 3-4 h) both by renal excretion of unchanged drug and by hepatic conjugation to *N*-acetylprocainamide (trademarked NAPA). This metabolite does have some antiarrhythmic activity, does not induce lupus, and has a longer half-life than the parent drug. Unfortunately, antiarrhythmic dosages regularly produce gastrointestinal side effects so it is not likely to be useful as a drug in its own right.

*Administration.* Like lidocaine, intravenous procainamide should be started with a loading regimen. A dose of 5-15 mg/kg administered slowly (e.g., 100 mg/5 min or 250-300 µg/kg/min) over 30 min is usually sufficient. If side effects are absent and the blood pressure and ECG are unchanged, further loading doses (up to an additional 5 mg/kg) can be given. The maintenance intravenous dosage is 20-60 µg/kg/min and steady-state conditions are approached only after 12-20 h (four to five elimination half-lives).

Oral therapy usually starts with 250-500 mg every 3-4 h. Once steady-state is achieved (2 days), the dose can be increased if arrhythmia is still present and side effects are absent. Once an antiarrhythmic dosage is found, therapy on a 6-hourly basis can be tried; unless elimination is slightly impaired by renal disease, this is usually not successful. A slow-release form (Procan-SR®) has recently been marketed but its place in therapy remains to be well defined.

In general, loading doses are only used in ill patients who require intravenous therapy. Procainamide can also be given intramuscularly, but the indications are rare. Conversion from intravenous to oral therapy is best accomplished by stopping the maintenance infusion, waiting 2-3 h, and then starting oral therapy.

*Modification of Dosages.* Because of a decrease in volume of distribution, the loading dosage of procainamide should be reduced in heart failure. Since elimination of both parent drug and its active metabolite are impaired in renal disease, dosages and dosing intervals should be adjusted (e.g., 250-500 mg every 8-12 h). Adjustments required in liver disease have not been studied.

*Drug Concentration Monitoring in Plasma.* Antiarrhythmic effects occur above 4 µg/mL, while the incidence of side effects rises above 10 µg/mL. Some investigators have used dosages producing concentrations well above 20 µg/mL but side effects (particularly the lupus syndrome, which is probably related to cumulative dose) are very common. Studies following the administration of *N*-acetylprocainamide to man showed antiarrhythmic effects above 9 µg/mL and side effects commonly above 19 µg/mL. While no generalization can be made on what combination of procainamide and *N*-acetylprocainamide concentrations is optimal, both should be routinely measured. Thus, an unexpected therapeutic or toxic effect, particularly in renal failure, could be due to accumulation of metabolite. Alternatively, lack of an antiarrhythmic effect could be due to drug resistance (high concentrations) or inadequate dosages (low concentrations).

## Quinidine

Quinidine is widely used for the oral treatment of ventricular arrhythmias and maintenance of sinus rhythm following conversion of atrial flutter or fibrillation. While an intravenous form is available, it often causes hypotension and is therefore seldom used. Intramuscular adminstration causes pain and erratic absorption and is rarely used. Side effects (mainly diarrhea and tinnitus) are the reason that up to 50% of patients cannot tolerate chronic therapy. Cardiovascular side effects are described under procainamide above. Quinidine can also induce thrombocytopenia or hepatitis. Patients who have experienced these immunologic reactions should not be rechallenged with quinidine or quinine (contained in tonic water).

*Pharmacokinetics.* Quinidine sulfate is well absorbed following oral administration. It is metabolized by the liver, and some of the metabolites may be active. Its mean elimination half-life is 6 h, but is highly variable (4-19 h) in normal subjects. The bioavailability of other salts (e.g., gluconate, polygalacturonate) has not been as widely studied.

*Administration.* As with chronic therapy with other antiarrhythmic agents, dosages should start low (e.g., 200-300 mg 6-hourly). Some authorities recommend a "screening dose" of 100 mg to detect patients at risk for

QT prolongation. However, multiple doses are often required to produce major QT prolongation in those at risk and so institution of therapy ideally should be carried out in a hospital under monitored conditions. If, after steady-state is achieved, arrhythmias persist and side effects are absent, the dose can be increased. The final dosage is highly variable (200-600 mg 4-6 hourly).

*Modification of Dosages.* The elderly require smaller doses. There are no known consistent dosage adjustments in heart failure or liver or kidney disease. Induction of hepatic mixed-function oxidase (by phenytoin and phenobarbital) causes a marked rise in quinidine requirements. It is important to recall that quinidine causes a rise in digitalis concentrations in the digitalis patient.

*Drug Concentration Monitoring in Plasma.* Older methods which failed to exclude inactive metabolites generally gave higher results than the now-accepted double extraction method of Cramer and Isaakson. Therapeutic effects occur above 1.5-2.0 $\mu$g/mL, while the incidence of toxic effects rises above 5 $\mu$g/mL. Arrhythmic exacerbation after the first few doses is occasionally accompanied by low levels, suggesting enhanced myocardial sensitivity or an active metabolite. Trough concentrations are most useful in establishing the minimal effective level. Peak concentrations, widely recommended, will help only to confirm a clinical suspicion of toxicity.

## Phenytoin (Diphenylhydantoin, Dilantin®)

This widely prescribed anticonvulsant has also been useful in the treatment of some ventricular arrhythmias, notably those due to digitalis intoxication. It can also be used chronically, especially in combination with other agents such as procainamide or propranolol. Side effects include bradyarrhythmias and hypotension during intravenous use and nystagmus, ataxia, gingival hypertrophy, lymphoid hyperplasia, macrocytic anemia, and teratogenicity with chronic therapy.

*Pharmacokinetics.* The drug should be administered by syringe to avoid crystallization in intravenous lines. Similarly, intramuscular administration is not recommended since crystallization in tissues can occur, with resulting erratic absorption. Elimination is by hepatic metabolism; this process is saturable so small increases in doses can cause marked increases in drug concentrations in plasma. The elimination half-life is long (16-24 h). Protein binding, normally 90%, can vary in disease (see plasma concentration monitoring).

*Administration.* Intravenous loading can be accomplished by giving 10-15 mg/kg, no faster than 50 mg/min under continuous ECG and blood pressure monitoring. Alternatively, the load can be given orally in three divided doses over 12 h. Because elimination is so slow, intravenous maintenance doses are not used. The usual oral maintenance regimen is 5 mg/kg/day, administered in divided doses one to three times daily. There is much variability in the final dose required, and because of saturable elimination, dosage adjustments should be made only by small increments.

*Modification of Dosages.* Renal, liver, and heart disease are not accompanied by consistent alterations in phenytoin requirements. A number of drugs can inhibit phenytoin metabolism, resulting in lower dosage requirements: these include barbiturates, isoniazid, sulfonamides, carbamazepine, chloramphenicol, and disulfiram. Phenytoin will result in increased requirements of quinidine or disopyramide.

*Drug Concentration Monitoring in Plasma.* Antiarrhythmic effects occur at free drug concentrations above 1 $\mu$g/mL, while toxicity is noted above 2 $\mu$g/mL. This corresponds to total phenytoin concentrations of 10-20 $\mu$g/mL. However, in uremia and hyperbilirubinemia, binding is decreased from 90 to 80% and monitoring of free phenytoin concentration is thus mandatory. In addition, because of the variable dosages required for effect, trough phenytoin concentrations should be routinely measured.

## Drugs Whose Plasma Concentrations Are Not Routinely Measured

*Disopyramide (Norpace®, Rhythmodan®).* This drug, used orally for atrial and ventricular arrhythmias, shares electrophysiologic effects and toxicity with quindine and procainamide. It is also a potent myocardial depressant and has anticholinergic properties which can cause urinary retention or can precipitate glaucoma. It is metabolized in the liver and excreted by the kidneys. Dosages are 100-300 mg three or four times daily; high doses should be used with caution. Dosages should be adjusted downward in renal or liver disease, and the drug should be used with great caution, if at all, in heart failure. The therapeutic range is 2-5 $\mu$g/mL, but protein binding is variable and free drug concentrations may in the future be a better guide to therapy.

*Propranolol (Inderal®).* Propranolol had been used successfully in the treatment of supraventricular and ventricular arrhythmias. Some patients require drug concentrations in plasma considerably in excess of those producing substantial beta blockade (i.e., > 100 ng/mL). Plasma concentration monitoring may therefore be useful in following such patients.

*Bretylium (Bretylol®).* This agent is used in the treatment of recurrent ventricular tachycardia or

## Table 2. Characteristics of Antiarrhythmic Drugs

| Drug | Dose | Range of Therapeutic Concentrations ($\mu$g/mL) | Indication | States Requiring Dosage Adjustment | Major Side Effects |
|---|---|---|---|---|---|
| Lidocaine | Load: 3-4 mg/kg (IV) Maintenance: 20-60 $\mu$g/kg/min (IV) | 1.5-5 | V (acute) | Heart failure Liver disease | CNS |
| Procainamide | Load: 10-15 mg/kg (IV) Maintenance: 20-60 $\mu$g/kg/min (IV) Oral: 250-750 mg q4h | 4-8 | SV,V | Renal disease | Lupus syndrome |
| Quinidine | 200-600mg q4-6h | 2-5 | SV,V | Age Phenytoin Phenobarbital | Cardiac GI Immunologic |
| Phenytoin | 50-150 mg q8h | 10-20 (1-2 free) | V | Inhibition of metabolism (many drugs) | CNS Cardiac (IV) |
| Disopyramide | 100-300 mg q6-8h | 2-5 | (SV),V | Renal disease Liver disease Phenytoin | Cardiac Urinary retention |
| Propranolol | 80-640 mg/day (q6-12h) | ? | SV,V | Liver disease | Cardiac |
| Bretylium | Load: 5-30 mg/kg (IV) Maintenance: 1-4 mg/min (IV) | ? | V (acute) | ?Renal disease | Adrenergic |
| Verapamil | I.V. 1-10 mg *p.o. 40-120 mg q8h | ?.1-.3 | SV | ? | AV block Hypotension |
| Mexiletine* | 100-300 mg q6-8h | .5-2 | V | ? | GI (nausea) CNS (tremor) |
| Tocainide* | 200-800 mg q6-12h | 3-10 | V | ? | GI (nausea) CNS (tremor) Allergy |
| Aprindine* | 100-300 mg/day (q8-24h) | .5-2 | SV,V | ? | CNS (tremor) Hematologic (1/500 aplastic anemia) |
| Amiodarone* | 200-600 mg once daily | ? | SV,V | ? | Corneal micro deposits Skin discoloration Pulmonary fibrosis Abnormal liver function Sinus bradycardia |
| Encainide* | 50-300 mg/day (q4-12h) | ? | (SV?),V | ? | Arrhythmia exacerbation Blurred vision Conduction disturbance |

V = ventricular

SV = supraventricular

The range of therapeutic concentrations is bounded below by the concentration likely to produce an antiarrhythmic effect and above by that likely to produce side effects.

* Investigational in U.S.A.

fibrillation. As with lidocaine, a loading regimen is required (5-30 mg/kg) followed by a maintenance infusion (1-4 mg/kg). Transient hypertension **followed by orthostatic hypotension is usual during** bretylium therapy. The therapeutic range and dosage adjustments in disease remain to be evaluated.

*Verapamil (Isoptin®, Calan®).* This calcium channel blocker has recently been marketed in the U.S.A. It will usually convert paroxysmal supraventricular tachycardia to sinus rhythm following 1-10 mg intravenously. It is also useful in controlling the ventricular response in atrial fibrillation or flutter. It undergoes extensive first pass hepatic metabolism and so oral dosages (40-120 mg three times daily) are higher than intravenous dosages. A tentative therapeutic range of 100-300 ng/mL has been suggested.

*Other Agents.* A number of investigational agents are available in the U.S.A. and tentative dosing schedules and therapeutic ranges are listed in Table 2.

## Selected References

1.  Anderson, J.L., Harrison, D.C., Mefflin, P.J. and Winkle, R.A., Antiarrhythmic drugs: Clinical pharmacology and therapeutic uses. *Drugs* **15,** 271-309, 1978.

2.  Collingsworth, K.A. Sumner, M.K. and Harrison, D.C., The clinical pharmacology of lidocaine as an antiarrhythmic drug. *Circulation* **50,** 1217, 1974.

3.  Woosley, R.L., and Shand, D.G., Pharmacokinetics of antiarrhythmic drugs. *Am J. Cardiol.* **51,** 986-99, 1978.

4.  Zipes, D.P., and Troup, P.J., New antiarrhythmic agents: Amiodarone, aprindine, disopyramide, ethmoszin, mexiletine, tocainide, verapamil. *Am. J. Cardiol.* **41,** 1005-1024, 1978.

# 21

# Antiarrhythmic Drug Therapy

**Ronald E. Vlietstra, M.B., Ch.B., F.A.C.C.**
**Jacob Federman, M.B., B.S., F.R.A.C.P.**

*Reprinted from Mayo Clin Proc 54, 531-542, 1979*

*The selection of appropriate antiarrhythmic drug therapy depends on a knowledge of the drugs available, their spectrum of action, their pharmacokinetics, and their major side effects. It is important to know how the pharmacokinetics of a drug vary with different disease states so that appropriate adjustments to dosage can be made. Drugs with similar actions can be assigned into groups, and five different groups can be identified. The commonly used antiarrhythmic drugs are reviewed, and some of the newer drugs are discussed.*

The use of antiarrhythmic drugs dates back to 1749, when Jean Baptiste de Senac used cinchona for the treatment of "rebellious palpitation."[1] Despite more than 200 years of use, we still have a lot to learn about how antiarrhythmic agents work, which ones to use, and what dosage to give. Decision-making in this area is less secure than it is in many more recently developed fields of pharmacology, for example, antibiotic therapy. Selection of antibiotics is determined by identification of the organism and sensitivity testing; effectiveness is easily checked by means of simple clinical and laboratory end points. As we learn more about antiarrhythmic agents, we can hope that they, too, can be administered on the same rational basis.

Over recent years, an increasing number of antiarrhythmic agents have been developed. Many of these are still undergoing preliminary evaluation and are not available for routine clinical use. Some will be mentioned to illustrate how new approaches may solve old problems.

## Classification of Antiarrhythmic Drugs (Table 1)

A variety of different classifications of antiarrhythmic drugs have been proposed.[2] Ideally, the classification should be linked to the key electrophysiologic abnormalities that underlie various arrhythmias. However, our limited knowledge of these precise abnormalities does not permit classification on this basis. As a framework for discussion, much of our current understanding can be characterized by a classification that defines five different groups.[3]

*Dr. Vlietstra is the Assistant Professor of Medicine and Dr. Federman is a resident in Cardiovascular Disease, Mayo Medical School, Rochester, Minn.*

**Group I.**—Group I drugs appear to act by depressing $Na^+$ conductance.[4] In doing so they slow the action potential upstroke in phase 0, a feature associated with slowing of conduction velocity. They prolong the action potential and the refractoriness. Finally, they decrease automaticity by decreasing the slope of phase 4 depolarization.

They act in supraventricular and ventricular arrhythmias that are due to either an automatic focus or a reentry circuit. With reentry arrhythmias, they increase the refractoriness of one or more components of the circuit. They directly suppress atrioventricular node conduction, His bundle conduction, and intraventricular conduction.[5] This tends to prolong the P-R interval, QRS duration, H-V interval, and Q-T interval. Complete heart block may result, and the sup-

**Table 1.—Classification of Antiarrhythmic Drugs**

| Group | Agent |
| --- | --- |
| I | Quinidine |
| | Procainamide |
| | Disopyramide |
| II | Lidocaine |
| | Phenytoin |
| | Mexiletine* |
| | Tocainide* |
| III | Propranolol |
| | Metoprolol |
| IV | Bretylium |
| V | Verapamil |
| | Nifedipine |

*Not currently available for routine clinical use.

pression of lower pacemakers may result in asystole. However, some drugs in this group also manifest an atropine-like effect, which tends to counter the direct action on atrioventricular node conduction. Occasionally, the net effect may be to accelerate atrioventricular conduction.

**Group II.**—These drugs have little influence on the conduction velocity of normal tissues. Previous work had suggested that they increased conduction in injured fibers and thereby exerted their effect in ventricular arrhythmias by removing the unidirectional block to the reentry loop.[6,7] More recently, El-Sherif and associates[8,9] have shown a selective decrease in conduction in ischemic myocardium with both lidocaine and phenytoin. This suggests that their action in reentry ventricular arrhythmias associated with myocardial infarction is to increase further the conduction block in the reentry loop. Lidocaine has little effect on atrial tissue and is relatively ineffective against supraventricular arrhythmias.

**Group III.**—In addition to beta-adrenergic blockade, group III drugs have group I[10] and group II[11] effects. Accordingly, they are effective in supraventricular and ventricular arrhythmias. In high doses they may occasionally cause atrioventricular nodal block and may suppress lower pacemaker foci, with resulting asystole. They have little effect on the H-V interval.

**Group IV.**—Originally, the antiarrhythmic effects of bretylium were thought to be related to its effects on the adrenergic neuron.[12] However, recent work has suggested that its antiarrhythmic properties may be related, in large part, to its quaternary ammonium structure. For example, it had been shown to reduce the disparity in duration of action potential between normal and ischemic zones,[13] a property shared by other quaternary ammonium compounds such as dimethylpropranolol and methyllidocaine.[14]

**Group V.**—This group acts by blocking the slow inward channel that is largely carried by $Ca^{2+}$ ions.[15] These drugs have been shown to act in supraventricular and ventricular arrhythmias and in cases resistant to group I, II, and III drugs.[3]

Although it is convenient to assign drugs into separate groups, there is still much to be learned about the exact mechanism of each drug's action in specific arrhythmias. This is exemplified by recent changes in the theories of how lidocaine and bretylium may exert their antiarrhythmic actions in myocardial ischemia.[8,9,13]

## Pharmacokinetic Principles

In selecting the optimal dosage schedule for antiarrhythmic drugs, it is important to be aware of factors that may importantly influence their distribution in the body. "Pharmacokinetics" is the name given to such a study. A number of recent review articles[16-19] are available for the reader who wishes to learn more of this new aproach to therapy.

Fundamental to the pharmacokinetic approach is the observation that drugs differ markedly in their absorption, distribution, metabolism, and excretion. The extent to which an orally administered drug reaches the systemic circulation is referred to as the "oral bioavailability." It is high for quinidine (approximately 80%), but because of avid metabolism on first passage through the liver it is quite low (approximately 30%) for both lidocaine and propranolol. In general, the lower the bioavailability, the more interindividual variation there is in requirements for oral dosage of the drug.

The apparent distribution volume of the drug will influence its blood levels. In low cardiac output states, it is usual for the distribution volume to be decreased. Therefore, the same drug dose will produce higher blood levels. It is partly for this reason that requirements for lidocaine are less in heart failure.

The half-life of an antiarrhythmic drug is the time for the level of drug in the body to decrease to half its original level. This is determined primarily by the combined rates of its liver metabolism and its renal excretion. Drugs that rely heavily on liver metabolism (for example, lidocaine) may persist much longer in body when liver function is impaired or liver perfusion is compromised (as in shock). Similarly, drugs that rely on renal excretion (for example, procainamide and its N-acetylated metabolite) will be retained if renal function is abnormal. Knowledge of the half-life of a drug allows prediction of whether or not intermittent oral therapy is practical and approximately what dosage intervals should be used. At least four half-lives of therapy are required for more than 90% of steady-state blood levels to be reached.

Because of interindividual differences in drug kinetics, plasma drug levels usually provide a better index of adequate therapy than does drug dosage alone. It is reasonable, therefore, to measure drug blood levels for antiarrhythmic drugs given for antiarrhythmic prophylaxis. Blood levels are also useful in identifying problems of poor compliance and dose-related side effects.

Various formulas are available that allow more accurate prediction of dosage requirements.[16]/Increasingly, computer application of these predictive models is being used in hospital pharmacies and intensive care units in an effort at more precise definition of drug requirements in patients with abnormal drug kinetics.

## Specific Drugs

**Quinidine**—As expected for a group I drug, quinidine has direct depressant effects on excitability, conduction velocity, and contractility in the heart as well as indirect anticholinergic actions. The effective refractory period is increased in atrial, ventricular, and Purkinje fibers, with a lesser increase in action potential duration, so that the ratio of effective refractory period to action potential duration is increased. The direct effect of quinidine on the atrioventricular node is to increase the refractory period, but its anticholinergic action opposes this and usually predominates. In peripheral blood vessels there is an antiadrenergic effect.

*Therapeutic Application*—Quinidine is often effective in premature atrial and ventricular contractions. Paroxysmal supraventricular tachycardia due to an ectopic pacemaker is suppressed, probably by a reduction in the slope of diastolic depolarizatrion. In paroxysmal supraventricular tachycardia or ventricular tachycardia due to a reentrant arrhythmia, quinidine acts by increasing refractoriness in one or both limbs of the reentrant loop. Quinidine is effective in the Wolff-Parkinson-White syndrome, either by suppressing the initiating beats or by interfering with the sustaining reentry mechanism.[20] In that syndrome the effectiveness of quinidine in prolonging the refractory period of the accessory pathway is related to the initial length of the refractory period.[21] Effectiveness is greatest when the refractory period is already long; in a sense, therefore, patients with the greatest need for lengthening the refractory period of their accessory pathways are least likely to benefit. Quinidine prolongs the atrial effective refractory period by direct and antivagal effects and is sometimes effective in the conversion of atrial fibrillation or atrial flutter to sinus rhythm. In atrial flutter, quinidine may slow the flutter rate and increase atrioventricular node conduction by its anticholinergic effect. This may result in a 1:1 atrioventricular node conduction, so that prior digitalization is advisable before the use of quinidine.

Because quinidine may slow ventricular pacemakers, its use should be avoided in patients who have heart block. Similarly, it should be avoided in circumstances in which the risk that heart block will develop is high (for example, digitalis toxicity).

*Pharmacokinetics (Table 2)*— Quinidine is metabolized predominantly in the liver. Its metabolism yields hydroxylated derivatives that have minimal pharmacologic activity but that may interfere significantly with measurements of plasma quinidine.[17] Quinidine is well absorbed, and the bioavailability varies from 70 to 90%. With oral administration the onset of action begins within 30 minutes, and a peak effect is reached in 2 to 3 hours. The duration of action of quinidine can be increased by the use of slow-release oral preparations. Approximately 20% of a quinidine dose is excreted unchanged in the urine.

Several different techniques are available to measure the serum level of quinidine. The older protein-precipitation and double-extraction methods suffer from a lack of specificity. A recently developed high-pressure liquid chromatography technique promises greater specificity with less interference by metabolites and impurities.[22]

Renal disease has little effect on the distribution and metabolism of quinidine, although plasma concentrations of metabolites may be elevated.[17] In congestive heart failure there is a decreased volume of distribution for quinidine but little change in clearance or half-life. In liver disease, protein binding may be reduced, and plasma levels may then underestimate the amount of active quinidine present. It has been noted that warfarin-type anticoagulants may reduce steady-state plasma levels of quinidine by hepatic enzyme induction of quinidine metabolism.

*Side Effects*—Side effects are common with quinidine, and they prompt cessation of therapy in up to one-third of patients.[23] Gastrointestinal intolerance with nausea, vomiting, and diarrhea is common. Hypersensitivity phenomena occur and include hemolytic anemia, thrombocytopenia, skin rash, hepatic **granulomas, and angioneurotic edema.**[24] With overdose, cinchonism and respiratory depression may occur. Quinidine suppresses the synthesis of vitamin K-dependent clotting factors, and concomitant use of anticoagulants may produce profound hypoprothrombinemia and hemorrhage.[25]

Cardiac reactions include sinoatrial depression, sinus arrest, sinoatrial block, atrioventricular block, H-V prolongation, ventricular tachycardia, ventricular fibrillation, and sudden death. Although usually seen only with high doses, these ill effects may occur with normal doses. Ventricular dysrhythmias appear to result from the depressant effects of quinidine on conduction or refractoriness, leading to unmasking of a reentry pathway. Hypotension may occur (alphareceptor blockade), and reduced myocardial contractility may aggravate cardiac failure.

Recently it has been reported that serum levels of digoxin are increased in patients who are taking quinidine. Not only are the digoxin levels increased, but the manifestations of digitalis toxicity may occur.[26]

*Dosage*—Dosage requirements vary widely. The dosage of quinidine sulfate usually ranges from 200 to 600 mg three or four times daily. Longer-acting quinidine preparations may be given on a twice-daily program.[18] Blood levels of quinidine may help in the clinical judgment of how much drug should be given.

**Procainamide**—The electrophysiologic actions of procainamide and its mechanism of action in the suppression of arrhythmia are essentially the same as those for quinidine. Its clinical use is also similar, although the most favorable results are seen in ventricular arrhythmias.

*Pharmacokinetics (Table 2)*—Procainamide is me-

Table 2.—Pharmacokinetics of Selected Antiarrhythmic Drugs

| Drug | Route of administration | Oral bioavailability (%) | Total volume distribution, liters/kg | Half-life (h) | Routes of excretion | Active metabolites | Therapeutic levels |
|---|---|---|---|---|---|---|---|
| Quinidine | Oral and rarely parenteral | 70-90 | 2-3 | 6-7 | Liver, 10-30% unchanged in urine | Dihydroquinidine | 2.3-5 $\mu$g/ml |
| Procainamide (Pronestyl) | Oral and parenteral | 85 | 2.0 | PCA*3.5 NAPA* 6 | Liver, 50% unchanged in urine | N-acetyl procainamide | 4-8 $\mu$g/ml (PCA)* 8-16 $\mu$g/ml (PCA + NAPA)* |
| Disopyramide (Norpace) | Oral and parenteral | 70-85 | 1.3 | 6-7 | Liver, 50-60% unchanged in urine | N-dealkylated metabolite | 3-8 $\mu$g/ml |
| Lidocaine | Parenteral | Poor | 1.3 | 100 min | Liver, <% unchanged in urine | Monoethylglycine-xylidide, glycine-xylidide | 2-5 $\mu$g/ml |
| Propranolol (Inderal) | Oral and parenteral | 20-50 | 3.5 | 4-6 | Liver, 1% unchanged in urine | 4-hydroxypropranolol | 40-100 ng/ml (occasionally up to 300 ng/ml) |
| Bretylium (Bretylol) | Oral and parenteral | Variable 15-20 | ... | 5-10 | Little metabolism, 50% of dose in urine in first 24 h | ... | ... |
| Verapamil (Isoptin) | Oral and parenteral | 10-22 | ... | 3-7 | Liver, 80% urine in 5 days | ... | 50-200 ng/ml |

*PCA = procainamide; NAPA = N-acetyl procainamide.

tabolized in the liver to N-acetyl procainamide, which is an equipotent active metabolite. The enzyme involved is N-acetyltransferase, and the rate of acetylation depends on whether the patient is a fast or slow acetylator.[27] In rapid acetylators the plasma levels of N-acetyl procainamide usually exceed those of procainamide, whereas the reverse is true in slow acetylators. Accordingly, measurement of both procainamide and N-acetyl procainamide is essential if plasma levels are to be interpreted meaningfully. Procainamide is approximately 15% protein bound, and 50% of an oral dose is excreted in the urine unchanged, with 7 to 24% as N-acetyl procainamide.[28]

Procainamide has an oral bioavailability of 85% and a half-life of 3.5 hours (this also varies with the acetylator status). The half-life of N-acetyl procainamide in normals is about 6 hours, and the substance is excreted predominantly in the urine.[29] The therapeutic level of procainamide is 4 to 8 $\mu$g ml and for procainamide plus N-acetyl procainamide it is 8 to 16 $\mu$g/ml. More than 16 to 20 $\mu$g ml for the combined level is often associated with toxicity. With renal failure, the volume of distribution is reduced and the half-lives of procainamide and N-acetyl procainamide are prolonged. In this setting, it is important to monitor levels of N-acetyl procainamide as well as those of procainamide, for the level of N-acetyl procainamide may be markedly increased without a similar increase in that of procainamide.[30] If the patient has cardiac failure, the volume of distribution is decreased and the half-life is increased, so that lower dosage may be required. In the early postinfarction period there may be erratic gastrointestinal absorption, and plasma levels may again be useful.

*Side Effects*—Procainamide has serious toxic effects if given rapidly intravenously, including asystole, ventricular fibrillation, myocardial depression, and hypotension. At high blood levels, procainamide may prolong atrioventricular and His-Purkinje conduction and thus result in heart block or widening of the QRS. In patients who are on long-term procainamide therapy (up to 6 months), approximately 50% will have antinuclear antibody.[31] More than 20% may show clinical evidence of the lupus syndrome.[32] This syndrome does not result in renal or neurologic problems, and although there is no antibody to native DNA, antibodies to heat-denatured DNA can be demonstrated.[31] It occurs more often in patients who are slow acetylators.[33]

Cross-sensitivity of procainamide with related drugs such as procaine can occur. Procainamide may produce nausea, anorexia, vomiting, diarrhea, and skin rash. Agranulocytosis has also been reported.[34]

*Dosage and Administration*—Procainamide may be given orally or parenterally. The total oral daily maintenance dose is approximately 50 mg/kg. This is given in divided doses at intervals of 4 to 6 hours (usually doses of 250 to 500 mg).

During intravenous administration, procainamide should be given slowly (never more than 50 mg per minute) with electrocardiographic and blood pressure monitoring. For rapid control of arrhythmia, procainamide should be given as 100 mg slowly intravenously every 5 minutes until side effects develop, the arrhythmia is controlled, or a total dose of 1 g is reached. Procainamide given intramuscularly has a peak action at 15 minutes to 1 hour; this method of administration has little advantage over oral dosage.

**Disopyramide**—This group I drug has electrophysiologic properties similar to those of quinidine and has a similar spectrum of clinical use. Its vagolytic action may also be important in some of its antiarrhythmic actions.

*Pharmacokinetics (Table 2)*—Disopyramide is metabolized in the liver, with about 50 to 60% of an oral dose being eliminated unchanged in the urine.[35] The N-dealkylated metabolite of disopyramide also has mild antiarrhythmic properties.[36]. Disopyramide is well absorbed and has a bioavailability of 70 to 85%[37]; its half-life is 6 to 7 hours.[35] The pharmacokinetics of disopyramide are nonlinear; the percentage that is plasma protein bound varies with the serum concentration. With increasing serum concentration the plasma protein binding decreases.[38]

The therapeutic range for disopyramide is 3 to 8 $\mu$g ml; atrial arrhythmias are controlled at lower levels than those required for ventricular arrhythmias.[39] In renal disease and heart failure, the half-life is increased and the volume of distribution is decreased, so that lower dosages may be required. In patients who have had myocardial infarction there is reduced oral absorption and consequently serum levels are lower. However, in these patients, clearance of the drug is also decreased.[40]

*Side Effects*—Disopyramide is well tolerated generally, but it has significant side effects related to its anticholinergic action. These are seen particularly in elderly males, in whom urinary retention may be a problem. Other effects are dry mouth, constipation, blurred vision, and worsening of glaucoma.[37]

**Disopyramide can depress myocardial function, and cardiac decompensation may be seen. Psychosis has been reported, and vomiting and diarrhea may occur.**

*Dosage and Administration*—The usual oral dosage is 200 to 300 mg as a loading dose, then 100 to 200 mg every 6 hours. With decreasing clearance of creatinine, the interval between doses should be increased.

**Lidocaine**—Lidocaine reduces the action potential duration in normal myocardial cells. It also reduces the effective refractory period but less so, and so the ratio of effective refractory period to action potential duration is, in fact, increased.[41] Lidocaine has also been shown to depress automaticity in Purkinje fibers by retarding phase 4 depolarization.[41] In normal tissues the membrane responsiveness and conduction velocity are unaffected. However, recently it has been shown that the effect of lidocaine in ischemic tissues may be markedly different. For example, as opposed to its negligible effect on conduction velocity in normal fibers, lidocaine slows conduction in the His-Purkinje system and in the ventricular myocardium when the fibers are depressed by acute ischemia.[42,43]

Lidocaine usually has little effect on atrioventricular conduction. However, occasionally it may enhance conduction, with a resulting accelerated ventricular rate in atrial tachyarrhythmias.[44] Conversely, rare cases of heart block have been reported.[45]

*Clinical Application*—Lidocaine is effective against both ectopic and reentrant ventricular dysrhythmias. It is of little use in supraventricular arrhythmias.[46] It is particularly useful in the coronary care unit for management of ventricular arrhythmias associated with acute myocardial infarction. It is also useful in the management of digitalis-induced ventricular arrhythmias.

*Pharmacokinetics (Table 2)*—Lidocaine is rapidly metabolized in the liver, with 70% being metabolized on the first passage through.[47] This leads to poor bioavailability, and it is of little use orally. Lidocaine is metabolized to monoethylglycinexylidide and glycinexylidide, which are active metabolites. Both potentiate the toxic effects of lidocaine; monoethylglycinexylidide also has antiarrhythmic properties. Less than 3% of the administered lidocaine dose is excreted unchanged in the urine. The half-life of lidocaine is about 100 minutes.[48]

Because of the high rate of liver metabolism, the clearance of lidocaine shows a direct relationship with hepatic blood flow. Thus, in the setting of reduced cardiac output as seen in cardiac failure and in acute myocardial infarction, there is reduced plasma clearance of lidocaine. The half-life may be markedly prolonged, and toxicity is more often seen.[49] The volume of distribution is also reduced in these circumstances. Therefore, lower doses of lidocaine should be used in order to avoid toxicity. In liver disease, the half-life may be increased markedly as a result of reduced clearance, and this reduces the required dosage. In

renal failure there is little effect on lidocaine levels, for only a small percentage of the drug is excreted in the urine.[49] The therapeutic range of lidocaine is 2 to 5 $\mu$g/ml; in this range, up to 70% is bound to plasma protein, but this decreases at higher levels. Toxic effects are seen at levels above 6 to 10 $\mu$g/ml.

In a group of 26 patients in whom plasma levels of lidocaine were monitored in the coronary care unit, we found high levels (more than 6 $\mu$g/ml) in 7 patients (27%). Two patients had markedly elevated levels of monoethylglycinexylidide (more than 5 $\mu$g/ml); in both this was associated with elevated levels of lidocaine and both had pronounced central nervous system toxicity. High levels of lidocaine were seen more commonly in patients who had reduced cardiac output, hypotension (systolic blood pressure less than 90 mm Hg), and liver dysfunction.

*Side Effects*—The major side effects of lidocaine are related to the central nervous system. In toxic doses, dizziness, drowsiness, excitement, psychosis, euphoria, paresthesias, nausea, vomiting, and seizures may occur. The seizure threshold is reduced by respiratory acidosis and alkalosis. At high levels, respiratory arrest may occur. In therapeutic doses, lidocaine exerts minimal or no cardiac depressant effects, but occasional episodes of sinoatrial arrest and heart block have been reported.[48]

*Dosage*—For a prompt therapeutic effect, an initial loading dose of 1 to 1.5 mg/kg of lidocaine should be given intravenously; then a continuous infusion of 1 to 4 mg/min should be started. Because body size is related to the volume of distribution of the drug, some adjustment of dosage should be made for very large or very small patients. As a general rule, an infusion rate of 10 $\mu$g/kg per minute will produce a steady-state blood level of 1 $\mu$g/ml. Because of an initial rapid distribution phase, the blood level of lidocaine often decreases to below therapeutic levels before the constant infusion is able to return the level to the therapeutic range (Fig. 1 A). This can be avoided by giving half the loading dose as a further bolus dose after 10 minutes (Fig. 1 B). To minimize central nervous system toxicity, one should give each lidocaine bolus over 1 to 2 minutes.

Lidocaine may also be given intramuscularly. This approach has been used in prehospital prophylaxis against ventricular arrhythmias associated with acute myocardial infarction. Whether or not this intramuscular mode of therapy is effective has not yet been resolved.[50] On the other hand, effective prophylaxis seems to be afforded by the intravenous use of lidocaine in hospitalized patients.[51]

Because of its high hepatic extraction, lidocaine is of

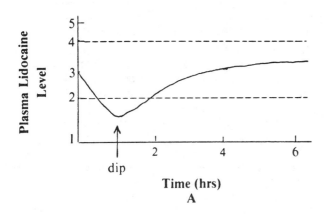

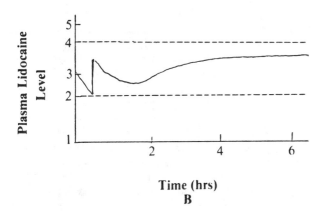

**Fig. 1.** Representation of plasma lidocaine levels versus time. A, Single intravenous bolus given as constant infusion was started. Early subtherapeutic 'dip' is seen. B, Additional small intravenous bolus provides sustained therapeutic levels.

little use as an oral agent. Congeners of lidocaine have been developed which undergo much less rapid hepatic metabolism and have higher oral bioavailability (Fig. 2). Two of these, tocainide and mexiletine, are orally effective antiarrhythmic agents that have effects similar to those of lidocaine; they are presently undergoing clinical evaluation.[52,53] Consistent with their slower hepatic metabolism, they have longer half-lives (approximately 12 hours).

**Propranolol** Propranolol is a competitive beta-adrenergic receptor blocker; it also has group I and group II actions.[3] The beta-adrenergic blockade results in reduction of heart rate, cardiac output, and myocardial contractility at rest and even more on exercise. Unlike some other beta blockers, it has no intrinsic sympathomimetic activity.

Propranolol reduces the velocity of the upstroke of the action potential and suppresses phase 4 depolarization.[10] The action potential duration of ventricular muscle is unchanged, but there is an increased rate of repolarization of Purkinje fibers with reduction in the effective refractory period. The ratio of effective refractory period to action potential duration is increased.[10] Propranolol reduces excitability, membrane responsiveness, and conduction velocity.[54] Although it has a direct negative inotropic action on isolated cardiac muscle, this is seen only at extremely high concentrations. Its clinically important nega-

Lidocaine

Tocainide

Mexiletine

**Fig. 2.** Chemical structure of lidocaine and two of its analogues, tocainide and mexiletine.

tive inotropic effect is likely due to its blockade of cardiac sympathetic nervous system effects.

*Clinical Application*—Propranolol is useful in the management of atrial and ventricular premature beats and in ectopic and reentrant supraventricular and ventricular tachycardia.[3] It is particularly useful in the management of digitalis-induced tachyarrhythmias. In atrial flutter and fibrillation, propranolol acts on the atrioventricular node to reduce the rate of the ventricular response.

*Pharmacokinetics (Table 2)*—Propranolol is predominantly metabolized in the liver, with only 1% being excreted unchanged in the urine. There are numerous metabolites, but the predominant one is 4-hydroxypropranolol, which has sympathomimetic, membrane-stabilizing, and beta-blocking activity.[55] Propranolol has a high hepatic extraction, so that after a single oral dosage up to 80% is removed in the liver (first-pass effect). With long-term therapy there is some saturation of liver-binding sites so that the extraction ratio decreases to about 65%.[56] There are individual differences in oral bioavailability, which varies from 20 to 50%. The half-life with chronic oral dosage is 4 to 6 hours, but it is less for a single intravenous dose. Protein binding is 91 to 95%, and the plasma therapeutic range is 40 to 100 ng/ml. Occasionally, higher plasma levels are required to suppress ventricular arrhythmias, and increasing effectiveness with levels up to 300 ng/ml has been demonstrated.[57] After prolonged use, it may take up to 48 hours for all propranolol activity to disappear.[58]

In hepatic dysfunction there is reduced plasma clearance, and this results in prolongation of the half-life of propranolol. On the other hand, in patients with portacaval shunts, there is a reduced hepatic first-pass effect, with higher plasma levels resulting.

*Side Effects*—Propranolol may cause cardiac failure by blocking sympathetic nervous system support for the failing ventricle. With high doses, severe bradycardia and heart block may be seen, with suppression of lower escape foci and consequent asystole. In patients with angina pectoris, sudden withdrawal of propranolol may result in exacerbation of angina and even myocardial infarction. Although there are several theories as to why this should occur, the exact mechanism is still undefined.[59]

Because of beta-receptor blockade, propranolol may precipitate acute bronchospasm in patients who have asthma or chronic obstructive pulmonary disease. Peripheral vascular insufficiency may be aggravated,[60] and in diabetic patients the symptoms of hypoglycemia may be masked. Propranolol may produce fatigue, depression, bad dreams, impotence,

alopecia, nausea, and vomiting.

*Dosage*—There is wide interindividual variation in oral dosage requirements for propranolol. The usual oral dosage is 40 to 360 mg per day given in three or four divided doses. Occasionally, higher dosage may be required in resistant cases.

The intravenous dosage is approximately 0.15 mg/kg given slowly at a rate not greater than 1 mg/min. The usual dosage is 5 to 10 mg intravenously.

**Metoprolol**—Cardiac beta-adrenergic receptors appear to differ from beta-adrenergic receptors in many other sites, for example bronchi and peripheral blood vessels. The former have been called beta$_1$ receptors and the latter, beta$_2$.[61] Metoprolol is one of a number of compounds that show a greater affinity for the beta$_1$ receptor. Preliminary clinical evidence suggests that the use of metoprolol is associated with less bronchospasm than is seen with propranolol.[62] However, great caution should be exercised in using any beta blocker in patients who are susceptible to bronchospasm.

In most respects other than beta$_1$-receptor affinity, metoprolol resembles propranolol. Although the drug is well absorbed in the gut, a major hepatic first-pass effect reduces its bioavailability to about 30%. Its half-life is about 4 hours, with most elimination being due to hepatic metabolism. Therapeutic plasma levels range from 20 to 100 ng/ml.

Clinical studies have shown it to be effective in hypertension, and it is for this use that FDA approval has recently been given. Its use as an antiarrythmic drug is less well defined but looks promising.[63] Oral dosages of 50 to 100 mg two to three times a day appear to be effective in supraventricular and ventricular arrhythmias.

By antagonizing the effect of the sympathetic nervous system on the heart, metoprolol may precipitate heart failure in patients who have impaired myocardial function. Like propranolol, it may produce depression and fatigue.

An early beta$_1$ blocker, practolol, which never reached the United States market, was found to cause a syndrome of polyserositis. No ill effects of this type has been reported for metoprolol.

**Bretylium**—This drug initially causes release of norepinephrine from postganglionic adrenergic nerve terminals and is then taken up by the nerve terminal; it inhibits the release of norepinephrine in response to nerve stimulation.[64] Bretylium also appears to have direct actions, which have not been fully elucidated. These may be related to its quaternary ammonium structure, for a structural analogue, M-360, is a quaternary ammonium compound with no sympatholytic action but pronounced antifibrillatory effects.[65] The overall effect of bretylium may be a combination of its direct and indirect effects.

In animal experiments it has been shown that, at low doses, the release of catecholamines produces an increase in conduction velocity, spontaneous rate, and maximum stimulation frequency and a decrease in voltage necessary for stimulation. At high doses, the electrical threshold is increased and there is reduction in conduction velocity, spontaneous and maximal stimulation frequencies, and rate of increase of the action potential.[66]

Bretylium causes an increase in action potential duration and effective refractory period without affecting their ratio. In myocardial injury the rate of increase of the action potential is slowed, the amplitude is reduced and the resting membrane potential is lowered. Bretylium restores the values for these parameters toward normal, although it has little effect on these parameters in the normal myocardium. Bretylium has been shown to prolong the action potential duration throughout the left ventricular conduction system, but this is greater in normal myocardium than in ischemic zones. Because the action potential duration in ischemic areas is already prolonged, this tends to reduce the disparity between the two regions. This may be an important factor in its antifibrillatory action.[13]

*Clinical Application*—The major use of bretylium is in the suppression of ventricular premature beats, ventricular tachycardia, and ventricular fibrillation in patients who are resistant to other medications.[67] Experience with this drug in the United States is limited, but it can be expected to increase now that the drug has been released for clinical use.

*Pharmacokinetics (Table 2)*—Bretylium has variable gastrointestinal absorption, but usually only 15 to 20% is absorbed. Approximately 50% of an intravenous dose is excreted in the urine in 24 hours. There is little metabolism in the body, and a small amount is passed in the feces. The half-life is 5 to 10 hours.

*Side Effects*—With the release of norepinephrine there may be transient hypotension and an increase in arrhythmias. With adrenergic blockade, hypotension secondary to vasodilatation may result. Other side effects include bradycardia, nausea, vomiting, diarrhea, erythematous macular rash, flushing, hyperthermia, renal dysfunction, and psychosis.

*Dosage*—In the acute management of ventricular fibrillation, bretylium is given intravenously in a dosage of 5 to 10 mg/kg, with the dosage being repeated up to a total dose of 30 mg kg. Doses are given at intervals of 15 to 30 minutes. For long-term manage-

ment, the dosage is 5 to 10 mg. kg. given at intervals of 6 to 8 hours. Bretylium ampules of 500 mg are diluted in 50 to 100 ml of 5% dextrose in water or sodium chloride and given over 10 to 20 minutes. The alternative is to give bretylium as a constant intravenous infusion of 1 to 2 mg/min.

The intramuscular dose of bretylium is 5 to 10 mg/kg initially, repeated in 1 to 2 hours if necessary, and then at intervals of 6 to 8 hours.

The oral dosage is 200 to 400 mg every 8 hours. Usually this approach is avoided, for it is often associated with nausea.

**Verapamil**—Verapamil is a papaverine derivative that appears to exert its antiarrhythmic action by blocking the inward calcium current in cardiac muscle cells. It is also thought to inhibit a slow channel for sodium.[15] Because it blocks these slow channels, its antiarrhythmic actions are different from those of other groups. It depresses activity in the sinoatrial node, atrioventricular node, and diseased myocardial fibers with slow channel-dependent properties. The conduction time in the sinoatrial and atrioventricular nodes is increased, as are the effective and functional refractory periods of the atrioventricular node.[52,68] The sinus rate is slowed, but sympathetic reflexes secondary to a verapamil-induced hypotension may modify this response. Verapamil also has a negative inotropic effect, which results from its calcium antagonist property.

A number of other calcium-blocking agents have been developed (for example, nifedipine and diltiazem). Their antiarrhythmic effects appear to be less than those for verapamil.

*Clinical Application* — Verapamil is used in the management of supraventricular arrhythmias, particularly reentrant paroxysmal supraventricular tachycardia involving the sinoatrial or atrioventricular node. There has been some success in the reversion of atrial flutter and atrial fibrillation to sinus rhythm, but more commonly there is a slowing of the ventricular response. Verapamil also appears to be effective in the management of ventricular premature beats and ventricular tachycardia.[69,70] Benefit has also been described in a patient with variant angina who had recurrent ventricular tachycardia and fibrillation.[71] In that case, the coronary vasodilator properties of verapamil appeared to be responsible for the clinical improvement.

*Pharmacokinetics (Table 2)*—Varapamil is rapidly metabolized in the liver, and the metabolites are thought to be only weakly active. It is well absorbed from the gastrointestinal tract, but the oral bioavailability is low (10 to 22%) because of a pronounced first-pass hepatic effect. The half-life is 3 to 7 hours, and 80% of an intravenous dose appears in the urine or feces within 5 days.[72] It is highly protein bound in plasma (about 90%).

*Side Effects*—Verapamil is usually well tolerated and has few side effects. Cardiovascular side effects are related to its depressant effects and include hypotension, cardiac failure, bradycardia, heart block, asystole, and disturbances in rhythm. The use of a beta blocker with verapamil is contraindicated, because the cardiac depressant effects of these two types of agents are additive and severe depression of cellular activity in the myocardium and conduction tissue may result.[52] Verapamil should be used with caution in sick sinus node syndrome, for it may depress sinoatrial node automaticity. Other reported side effects include nausea, constipation, dyspnea, skin reactions, headache, and dizziness.

*Dosage and Administration*—The usual dosage for management of an acute arrhythmia is 5 to 10 mg intravenously (0.1 mg/kg). The usual oral dosage of verapamil is 40 to 80 mg three or four times daily.

## Selection of Antiarrhythmic Drugs

Fundamental to the drug management of dysrhythmias is the accurate diagnosis of the underlying disturbance in rhythm. This diagnosis can often be made on clinical grounds, but an electrophysiologic study may be required in difficult clinical cases. It is important to distinguish atrial from ventricular dysrhythmias, and the therapy for an ectopic dysrhythmia may be quite different from that for a reentrant tachycardia. If an underlying metabolic defect is present—for example, thyrotoxicosis, hypokalemia, or acid-base imbalance—then correction of the defect is fundamental to any therapeutic intervention.

Atrial dysrhythmias are currently best treated by group I and group III drugs, whereas ventricular dysrhythmias may be managed by drugs from all groups. As an initial parenteral drug in ventricular arrhythmias, lidocaine is the first choice, whereas for oral therapy quinidine, procainamide, disopyramide, and propranolol may all be of use. Although drugs within each group have similar actions, they are not identical in their actions, and success may be obtained with one drug in a group in cases in which other agents of the same group have failed. When combination drug therapy is used, it is a good principle to select drugs from different groups rather than drugs from the same group.[3]

The age of the patient, desired length of therapy, and clinical state of the patient may all influence the selection of a drug. An elderly man with prostatism may experience acute urinary retention with disopyramide, and a patient with colitis may not tolerate quinidine. In any given patient, these factors will influence not only the drug selected but also the route of administration and dosage required.

The development of simple long-term electrocardiographic monitoring methods has led to the recognition of considerable "spontaneous" variation in the frequency of arrhythmias.[53] Caution should therefore be exercised in ascribing apparent benefits to the drugs that have been used. Whenever practical, evaluation of the effectiveness of an antiarrhythmic drug should be based on relatively more objective assessments (intensive-care unit monitoring, Holter monitoring, treadmill exercise testing), preferably done sequentially with the patient both on and off the drug.[53] For some very serious arrhythmias, invasive electrophysiologic studies of drug response may be therapeutically helpful.[73]

Of course, not all arrhythmias need treatment. For example, unifocal premature ventricular complexes occurring in a patient who has no heart disease do not appear to carry any prognostic disadvantage. Even in patients with heart disease, it seems that premature ventricular complexes need to be multiform, to be bigeminal, to interrupt the preceding T wave, or to occur in runs of two or more before a significant ill effect on prognosis is observed.[74] To what extent these premature ventricular complexes should be suppressed and whether or not such suppression improves survival are matters yet to be resolved.

## Conclusions

Appropriate antiarrhythmic drug selection depends on an accurate initial diagnosis of the patient's illness and of the disturbance in rhythm. If the use of antiarrhythmic drugs is indicated, one must select the drug that is most likely to control the arrhythmia but least likely to produce side effects. It is important to understand the mechanism of action, pharmacokinetics, clinical application, and potential side effects of the various agents. With this knowledge, a suitable trial drug dosage can be selected, which may need to be modified according to the patient's response. At times plasma drug levels may be needed to achieve optimal dosage, particularly if cardiac failure, renal impairment, or liver disease is present. The assignment of drugs with similar mechanisms of action into groups is helpful in that drugs within each group have a similar spectrum of clinical effectiveness. Much remains to be learned, however, regarding the precise mode of action of these drugs in specific cardiac arrhythmias.

## REFERENCES

1. Moe GK, Abildskov JA: Antiarrhythmic drugs. *In* The Pharmacological Basis of Therapeutics. Fifth edition. Edited by LS Goodman, A Gilman. New York, Macmillan Publishing Company, 1975, pp 683-704

2. Gettes LS: On the classification of antiarrhythmic drugs. Mod Concepts Cardiovasc Dis 48:13-18, 1979

3. Arnsdorf MF: Electrophysiologic properties of antidysrhythmic drugs as a rational basis for therapy. Med Clin North Am 60:213-232, 1976

4. Johnson EA: The effects of quinidine, procainamide and pyrilamine on the membrane resting and action potential of guinea pig ventricular muscle fibers. J Pharmacol Exp Ther 117:237-244, 1956

5. Bigger JT Jr, Heissenbuttel RH: Clinical use of antiarrhythmic drugs. Postgrad Med 47:119-125, January, 1970

6. Bigger JT Jr, Bassett AL, Hoffman BF: Electrophysiological effects of diphenylhydantoin on canine Purkinje fibers. Circ Res 22:221-236, 1968

7. Bigger JT Jr, Mandel WJ: Effect of lidocaine on conduction in canine Purkinje fibers and at the ventricular muscle-Purkinje fiber junction. J Pharmacol Exp Ther 172:239-254, 1970

8. El-Sherif N, Scherlag BJ, Lazzara R, Hope RR: Re-entrant ventricular arrhythmias in the late myocardial infarction period. 4. Mechanism of action of lidocaine. Circulation 56:395-402, 1977

9. El-Sherif N, Lazzara R: Re-entrant ventricular arrhythmias in the late myocardial infarction period. 5. Mechanism of action of diphenylhydantoin. Circulation 57:465-472, 1978

10. David LD, Temte JV: Effects of propranolol on transmembrane potentials of ventricular muscle and Purkinje fibers of the dog. Circ Res 22:661-677, 1968

11. Stagg AL, Wallace AG: The effect of propranolol on membrane conductance in canine cardiac Purkinje fibers (abstract). Circulation 49-50, Suppl 3:145, 1974

12. Bigger JT Jr, Jaffe CC: The effect of bretylium tosylate on the electrophysiologic properties of ventricular muscle and Purkinje fibers. Am J Cardiol 27:82-92, 1971

13. Cardinal R, Sasyniuk BI: Electrophysiological effects of bretylium tosylate on subendocardial Purkinje fibers from infarcted canine hearts. J Pharmacol Exp Ther 204:159-174, 1978

14. Lucchesi BR: Antiarrhythmic drugs. *In* Cardiovascular Pharmacology. Edited by MJ Antonaccio. New York, Raven Press, 1977, pp 269-335.

15. Shigenobu K, Schneider JA, Sperelakis N: Verapamil blockade of slow $Na^+$ and $Ca^{++}$ responses in myocardial cells. J Pharmacol Exp Ther 190:280-288, 1974

16. Greenblatt DJ, Koch-Weser J: Clinical pharmacokinetics. N Engl J Med 293:702-705; 964-970, 1975

17. Harrison DC, Meffin PJ, Winkle RA: Clinical pharmacokinetics of antiarrhythmic drugs. Prog Cardiovasc Dis 20:217-242, 1977

18. Woosley, RL, Shand DG: Pharmacokinetics of antiarrhythmic drugs. Am J Cardiol 41:986-995, 1978

19. Vlietstra RE: Pharmacokinetics of cardiovascular drugs. Cardiovasc Clin (in press)

20. Sellers TD Jr, Campbell RWF, Bashore TM, Gallagher JJ: Effects of procainamide and quinidine sulfate in the Wolff-Parkinson-White syndrome. Circulation 55:15-22, 1977

21. Wellens HJ, Bar FW, Gorgels AP: Effect of drugs in WPW syndrome: importance of initial length of effective refractory period of accessory pathway (abstract). Am J Cardiol 41:372, 1978

22. Drayer DE, Restivo K, Reidenberg MM: Specific determination of guinidine and (3S)-3-hydroxyquinidine in human serum by high-pressure liquid chromatography. J Lab Clin Med 90:816-822, 1977

23. Lown B, Wolf M: Approaches to sudden death from coronary heart disease. Circulation 44:130-142, 1971

24. Cohen IS, Jick H, Cohen SI: Adverse reactions to quinidine in hospitalized patients: findings on data from the Boston Collaborative Drug Surveillance Program. Prog Cardiovasc Dis 20:151-163, 1977

25. Koch-Weser J: Quinidine-induced hypoprothrombinemic hemorrhage in patients on chronic warfarin therapy. Ann Intern Med 68:511-517, 1968

26. Ejvinsson G: Effect of quinidine on plasma concentrations of digoxin. Br Med J 1:279-280, 1978

27. Reidenberg MM, Drayer DE, Levy M, Warner H: Polymorphic acetylation of procainamide in man. Clin Pharmacol Ther 17:722-730, 1975

28. Giardina EGV, Dreyfuss J, Bigger JT Jr, Shaw JM, Schreiber EC: Metabolism of procainamide in normal and cardiac subjects. Clin Pharmacol Ther 19:339-351, 1976

29. Strong JM, Dutcher JS, Lee W-K, Atkinson AJ Jr: Pharmacokinetics in man of the N-acetylated

metabolite of procainamide. J Pharmacokinet Biopharm 3:223-235, 1975

30. Drayer DE, Lowenthal DT, Woosley RL, Nies AS, Schwartz A, Reidenberg MM: Cumulation of N-acetylprocainamide, an active metabolite of procainamide, in patients with impaired renal function. Clin Pharmacol Ther 22:63-69, 1977

31. Blomgren SE, Condemi JJ, Vaughan JH: Procainamide-induced lupus erythematosus: clinical and laboratory observations. Am J Med 52:338-348, 1972

32. Condemi JJ, Blomgren SE, Vaughan JH: The procainamide-induced lupus syndrome. Bull Rheum Dis 20:604-608, 1970

33. Woosley RL, Drayer DE, Reidenberg MM, Nies AS, Carr K, Oates JA: Effect of acetylator phenotype on the rate at which procainamide induces antinuclear antibodies and the lupus syndrome. N Engl J Med 298:1157-1159, 1978

34. Konttinen YP, Tuominen L: Reversible procainamide-induced agranulocytosis twice in one patient (letter to the editor). Lancet 2:925, 1971

35. Ranney RE, Dean RR, Karim A, Radzialowski FM: Disopyramide phosphate: pharmacokinetic and pharmacologic relationships of a new antiarrhythmic agent. Arch Int Pharmacodyn Ther 191: 162-188, 1971

36. Baines MW, Davies JE, Kellett DN, Munt PL: Some pharmacological effects of disopyramide and a metabolite. J Int Med Res 4 Suppl 1:5-7, 1976

37. Heel RC, Brogden RN, Speight TM, Avery GS: Disopyramide: a review of its pharmacological properties and therapeutic uses in treating cardiac arrhythmias. Drugs 15:331-368, 1978

38. Hinderling PH, Bres J, Garrett ER: Protein binding and erythrocyte partitioning of disopyramide and its monodealkylated metabolite. J Pharm Sci 63:1684-1690, 1974

39. Niarchos AP: Disopyramide: serum level and arrhythmia conversion. Am Heart J 92:57-64, 1976

40. Rangno RE, Warnica W, Ogilvie RI, Kreeft J, Bridger E: Correlation of disopyramide pharmacokinetics with efficacy in ventricular tachyarrhythmia. J Int Med Res 4 Suppl 1:54-58, 1976

41. Bigger JT Jr, Mandel WJ: Effect of lidocaine on the electrophysiological properties of ventricular muscle and Purkinje fibers. J Clin Invest 49:63-77, 1970

42. Gerstenblith G, Scherlag BJ, Hope RR, Lazzara R: Effect of lidocaine on conduction in the ischemic His-Purkinje system of dogs. Am J Car-

diol 42:587-591, 1978

43. Allen JD, Brennan FJ, Wit AL: Actions of lidocaine on transmembrane potentials of subendocardial Purkinje fibers surviving in infarcted canine hearts. Circ Res 43:470-481, 1978

44. Klein HO, Di Segni E, Kaplinsky E: Paradoxic acceleration of ventricular rate after therapy with lidocaine and ajmaline: findings in two patients with supraventricular tachyarrhythmia. Chest 71: 531-533, 1977

45. Lichstein E, Chadda KD, Gupta PK: Atrioventricular block with lidocaine therapy. Am J Cardiol 31:277-281, 1973

46. Bigger JT Jr, Heissenbuttel RH: The use of procaine amide and lidocaine in the treatment of cardiac arrhythmias. Prog Cardiovasc Dis 11:515-534, 1969

47. Stenson RE, Constantino RT, Harrison DC: Interrelationships of hepatic blood flow, cardiac output, and blood levels of lidocaine in man. Circulation 43:205-211, 1971

48. Benowitz NL: Clinical applications of the pharmacokinetics of lidocaine. Cardiovasc Clin 6 No. 2:77-101, 1974

49. Thompson PD, Melmon KL, Richardson JA, Cohn K, Steinbrunn W, Cudihee R, Rowland M: Lidocaine pharmacokinetics in advanced heart failure, liver disease, and renal failure in humans. Ann Intern Med 78:499-508, 1973

50. Lie KI, Liem KL, Louridtz WJ, Janse MJ, Willebrands AF, Durrer D: Efficacy of lidocaine in preventing primary ventricular fibrillation within 1 hour after a 300 mg intramuscular injection: a double-blind, randomized study of 300 hospitalized patients with acute myocardial infarction. Am J Cardiol 42:486-488, 1978

51. Lie KI, Wellens HJ, von Capelle FJ, Durrer D: Lidocaine in the prevention of primary ventricular fibrillation: a double-blind randomized study of 212 consecutive patients. N Engl J Med 291-1324-1326, 1974

52. Zipes DP, Troup PJ: New antiarrhythmic agents: amiodarone, aprindine, disopyramide, ethmozin, mexiletine, tocainide, verapamil. Am J Cardiol 41:1005-1024, 1978

53. Winkle RA, Meffin PJ, Harrison DC: Long-term tocainide therapy for ventricular arrhythmias. Circulation 57:1008-1016, 1978

54. Vaughan Williams EM: Mode of action of beta receptor antagonists on cardiac muscle. Am J Cardiol 18:399-405, 1966

55. Fitzgerald JD, O'Donnell SR: Pharmacology of 4-hydroxy-propranolol, a metabolite of propran-

olol. Br J Pharmacol 43:222-235, 1971

56. Evans GH, Shand DG: Disposition of propranolol. V. Drug accumulation and steady-state concentrations during chronic oral administration in man. Clin Pharmacol Ther 14:487-493, 1973

57. Woosley RL, Shand DG, Kornhauser D, Nies AS Oates JA: Relation of plasma concentration and dose of propranolol to its effect on resistant ventricular arrhythmias (abstract). Clin Res 25:262A, 1977

58. Faulkner SL, Hopkins JT, Boerth RC, Young JL Jr, Jellett LB, Nies AS, Bender HW, Shand DG: Time required for complete recovery from chronic propranolol therapy. N Engl J Med 289:607-609, 1973

59. Shand DG, Wood AJJ: Propranolol withdrawal syndrome—why? (editorial). Circulation 58:202-203, 1978

60. Frohlich ED, Tarazi RC, Duston HP: Peripheral arterial insufficiency: a complication of beta-adrenergic blocking therapy. JAMA 208:2471-2472 1969

61. Lands AM, Arnold A, McAuliff JP, Luduena FP, Brown TG Jr: Differentiation of receptor systems activated by sympathomimetic amines. Nature 214:597-598, 1967

62. Skinner C, Gaddie J, Palmer KNV: Comparison of effects of metoprolol and propranolol on asthmatic airway obstruction. Br Med J 1:504, 1976

63. Wasin HS, Mahapatra RK, Bhatia ML, Roy SB, Sannerstedt R: Metoprolol—a new cardioselective β-adrenoceptor blocking agent for treatment of tachyarrhythmias. Br Heart J 39:834-838, 1977

64. Boura ALA, Green AF: The actions of bretylium: adrenergic neurone blocking and other effects. Br J Pharmacol 14:536-548, 1959

65. Kniffen FJ, Lomas TE, Counsel RE, Lucchesi BR: The antiarrhythmic and antifibrillatory actions of bretylium and its o-iodobenzyl trimethylammonium analog. UM-360. J Pharmacol Exp Ther 192:120-128, 1975

66. Papp JG, Vaughan Williams EM: The effect of bretylium on intracellular cardiac action potentials in relation to its anti-arrhythmic and local anaesthetic activity. Br J Pharmacol 37:380-390, 1969

67. Bernstein JG, Koch-Weser J: Effectiveness of bretylium tosylate against refractory ventricular arrhythmias. Circulation 45:1024-1034, 1972

68. Wellens HJJ, Tan SL, Bär FWH, Düren DR, Lie KI, Dohmen HM: Effect of verapamil studied by programmed electrical stimulation of the heart in patients with paroxysmal re-entrant supraventricular tachycardia. Br Heart J 39:1058-1066, 1977

69. Krikler D: Verapamil in cardiology. Eur J Cardiol 2:3-10, 1974

70. Rosen MR, Wit AL, Hoffman BF: Electrophysiology and pharmacology of cardiac arrhythmias. VI. Cardiac effects of verapamil. Am Heart J 89: 665-673, 1975

71. Solberg LE, Nissen RG, Vlietstra RE, Callahan JA: Prinzmetal's variant angina—response to verapamil. Mayo Clin Proc 53:256-259, 1978

72. Schomerus M, Spiegelhalder B, Stieren B, Eichelbaum M: Physiological disposition of verapamil in man. Cardiovasc Res 10:605-612, 1976

73. Fisher JD: Ventricular tachycardia: practical and provocative electrophysiology (editorial). Circulation 58:1000-1001, 1978

74. Ruberman W, Weinblatt E, Goldberg JD, Frank CW, Shapiro S: Ventricular premature beats and mortality after myocardiol infarction. N Engl J Med 297:750-757, 1977

# 22

# Lidocaine: A Case Study

**Wayne Stargel, Pharm. D.**

## Introduction

Lidocaine is presently the most commonly used drug in the acute management of ventricular arrhythmias following myocardial infarction. Recently, the recommendation of administering lidocaine prophylactically to prevent primary ventricular fibrillation in patients with suspected myocardial infarction has generated new interest in therapeutic drug monitoring of lidocaine plasma concentrations (*1*). Since clinical effectiveness of lidocaine prophylaxis can only be measured retrospectively, the only measurable clinical endpoint is drug toxicity, which may be serious. Therefore, therapeutic monitoring of lidocaine plasma concentration may be valuable in maintaining an adequate drug concentration while avoiding severe drug toxicity. The following case illustrates the use and limitations of plasma lidocaine concentration in a patient admitted with myocardial infarction.

## Case

A 53-year-old man was in excellent health until two days prior to admission, when he noticed a heavy sensation in the precordium that was not related to exertion. He thought that the chest discomfort was caused by indigestion, and he did obtain some relief from antacids. Just prior to admission, the patient went to bed after dinner, only to wake up an hour later with severe substernal chest pain, which radiated into the neck and jaw. Pain was severe for more than an hour and was only relieved by morphine in the emergency room.

On arrival at the coronary care unit, his physical examination was unremarkable. The patient had no previous history of heart disease, paroxysmal nocturnal dyspnea, or edema. He had a ten-year history of hypertension, which was well controlled on 50 mg/day of hydrochlorothiazide. Clinical lab values were within normal limits. The diagnosis of acute anterior myocardial infarction was made by the electrocardiogram and later substantiated by serial cardiac enzyme studies.

Lidocaine prophylaxis was initiated with a loading

*Dr. Stargel is the clinical pharmacist for the Coronary Care Unit of Duke University Medical Center, Durham, NC 27710.*

dose of 225 mg over 20 min, administered as a 75 mg priming dose over 2 min, followed by three 50 mg injections given over 1 min at 7, 13, and 19 min. This was followed by a maintenance infusion of 2 mg/min. Measurements of plasma lidocaine concentrations, free lidocaine concentrations, and alpha-1-acid glycoprotein (AAG) were measured by protocol at 1, 12, 24, 36, 48, and 72 h. Results are illustrated in Table 1. The patient experienced no toxicity throughout the 72 h continuous infusion, even on direct questioning for minor central nervous system toxicity. Lidocaine was discontinued after 72 h, and the patient remained in the coronary care unit for 5 days without complications.

## Pharmacology and Pharmacokinetics

Clinical studies indicate that plasma lidocaine concentrations of 0.6-2 mg/L are the minimum needed to suppress premature ventricular contractions (*2*). However, some patients may require much higher concentrations (i.e., 8 mg/L) in order to control arrhythmias. Other patients may experience toxicity with plasma lidocaine concentrations within the therapeutic range (i.e., 3 mg/L). Therefore, wide overlap exists between therapeutic and toxic plasma concentrations, with a therapeutic range of 1.5-5 mg/L generally accepted in clinical practice. This case illustrates some of the problems encountered in measuring total plasma lidocaine concentrations and examines altered drug disposition in myocardial infarction.

Lidocaine, with a distribution volume of approximately 130 liters, is widely distributed throughout body tissue. The protein binding of lidocaine varies greatly among individuals with approximately 70% of lidocaine being protein bound within the therapeutic range. Protein binding is concentration dependent, with higher plasma concentrations demonstrating a higher unbound lidocaine concentration. Binding occurs predominantly to AAG (approximately 70% of total binding) and albumin (approximately 30% of total binding).

Several studies have reported that lidocaine plasma concentrations continue to increase over time in patients with myocardial infarction so that a steady state is apparently never obtained (*3*). We have recently reported that plasma AAG increases in patients with myocardial infarction, but remains unchanged in patients with chest pain who show no objective evidence of cardiac damage (4). This increased protein binding causes the total plasma lidocaine concentration to increase, but the increase in unbound (free lidocaine concentration) is attenuated due to increased protein binding. This patient illustrates that AAG increases following myocardial infarction and that is associated with increased plasma binding and an elevation of total plasma lidocaine concentration. Although total plasma lidocaine concentration is increased 118%, from 3.8 mg/L at 12 h to 8.3 mg/L after 72 h the corresponding free drug concentration increased by only 48%, from 0.7 to 1.04 mg/L. Since the free drug concentration is responsible for the pharmacological effects of a drug, the increased plasma binding may help explain why this patient had no toxicity with a total plasma concentration at 72 h of 8.3 mg/L. Recommendations to decrease the lidocaine infusion based on the total plasma concentration may cause the free concentration to fall below the therapeutic range.

However, using the loading regimen of 225 mg over 20 min followed by a constant infusion of 2 mg/min enables the use of the 1 h plasma lidocaine concentration for therapeutic drug monitoring. The 1 h plasma concentration is a good predictor of both 12 and 24 h plasma concentrations with the latter being approximately 50% higher (5). Due to the AAG increase on the second day of therapy in patients with myocardial infarction, the only adequate measures of toxicity are clinical diagnosis and possibly the free lidocaine concentration. Clearly, further studies are needed to establish the therapeutic and toxic ranges of free lidocaine concentrations.

Lidocaine is primarily metabolized by the liver to monoethylglycinexylidide (MEGX) and glycinexylidide (GX) with a maximum of 10% excreted as unchanged drug at low urinary pH. Both major metabolites (MEGX, GX) have shown some antiarrhythmic and convulsant activity in animal studies. It has been estimated in animals that MEGX has an antiarrhythmic potency similar to lidocaine, while GX has an antiarrhythmic potency around 25% of lidocaine's. Both metabolites are further metabolized by the liver with GX also being excreted in the urine. These major metabolites (MEGX, GX) are generally found in low concentrations in comparison to lidocaine, but accumulation has been reported in some patients. Accumulation of these active metabolites may contribute to the therapeutic/ toxic effects, but more work is needed to clarify their contribution.

## Factors Affecting Lidocaine Disposition

Lidocaine is a drug which is normally efficiently metabolized by the liver. The plasma clearance of lidocaine is generally dependent upon liver blood flow, although hepatic enzyme activity may influence clearance in certain disease states (i.e., hepatocellular liver disease). Drugs, such as propranolol or norepinephrine, or diseases, such as congestive heart failure which can decrease hepatic blood flow, have been reported to decrease the clearance of lidocaine in animals and man. Drugs which can increase hepatic blood flow, e.g. isoproterenol, may increase the clearance of lidocaine. The clinical significance of these drug interactions, however, requires further investigation.

## Adverse Effects

The adverse effects of lidocaine primarily involve the central nervous system and consist of drowsiness, paraesthesiae, dizziness, euphoria, confusion, dysarthria, coma, and epileptic seizures. Other side effects include hypotension, asystole, muscle twitching, and respiratory depression. The relationship of toxicity to plasma concentration is still not entirely clear. Convulsions and coma generally occur at concentrations greater than 6 mg/L. However, the rate of plasma concentration change may be an important factor in toxicity development. For example, minor central nervous system toxicity is relatively common after an initial bolus of 75-100 mg given over 30 s even though the plasma concentration may be in the therapeutic range. Therefore plasma concentrations during the continuous infusion appear to relate better to toxicity and may not be reliable during bolus doses. Recent evidence suggests that the free lidocaine concentration is a better index of toxicity because of the known changes in plasma

**TABLE 1. Serial Lidocaine and Alpha-1-acid glycoprotein concentrations in an individual patient over 72 h following acute myocardial infarction.**

| Time, (h) | Total Lidocaine conc., mg/L | Free Lidocaine conc., mg/L | Alpha-1-acid glycoprotein mg/L |
|---|---|---|---|
| 1 | 2.7 | 0.52 | 1550 |
| 12 | 3.9 | 0.70 | 1570 |
| 24 | 4.9 | 0.86 | 1740 |
| 48 | 6.0 | 0.94 | 2240 |
| 72 | 8.3 | 1.04 | 2500 |

binding via elevation of AAG (6). Adverse effects generally occur more frequently in older patients and those with congestive heart failure, myocardial infarction, or low body weight.

The method of collecting samples may also interfere with the determination of lidocaine concentrations. We recently reported that spuriously low values can occur when several commercial, rubber-stoppered collection tubes are used (7). This is due to the displacement of lidocaine from alpha-1-acid glycoprotein and subsequent redistribution into red cells caused by a plasticizer in the rubber stopper. We recommend the use of an all-glass collecting tube or thorough testing of any commercial collection tube.

## References

1. Noneman, J.W., and Rogers, J.F., Lidocaine prophylaxis in acute myocardial infarction. *Medicine* **57**, 501-515 (1978).

2. Benowitz, N.L., and Meister, W., Clinical pharmacokinetics of lignocaine. *Clin. Pharmacokin.* **3**, 177-201 (1978).

3. Prescott, L.F., Adejepon-Yamoah, K.K., and Talbot, R.G., Imparied lignocaine metabolism in patients with myocardial infarction and cardiac failure. *Brit. Med. J.* **1**, 939-941 (1976).

4. Routledge, P.A., Stargel, W.W., Wagner, G.S. and Shand, D.G., Increased alpha-1-acid glycoprotein and lidocaine disposition in myocardial infarction. *Ann. Intern. Med.* **93**, 701-704 (1980).

5. Stargel, W.W., Shand, D.G., Wagner, G.S., and Routledge, P.A., Therapeutic monitoring of lidocaine concentrations. *Clin. Pharmacol. Ther.* **29**, 284 (1981).

6. Pieper, J.A., Wyman, M.G., Goldreyer, B.N., Cannom, D.S., Slaughter, R.L., and Lalka, D., Lidocaine toxicity: Effects of total versus free lidocaine concentrations. *Circulation* **62**, 181 (1980).

7. Stargel, W.W., Roe, C.R., Routledge, P.A., and Shand, D.G., Importance of blood-collection tubes in plasma lidocaine determinations. *Clin. Chem.* **25**, 617-619 (1979).

## Lidocaine Profile

Generic Name: Lidocaine HCl
Chemical Name: 2-(Diethylamino)-$N$-(2,6-dimethylphenyl) acetamide
Chemical Structure:

Trade Name: Xylocaine® (Astra)
pKa: 7.85
Molecular Mass: 234.33
Melting Point: 68-69°C
Solubility in Water: Lidocaine Base: insoluble
Lidocaine HCl: freely soluble
Absorption: Percent absorbed: Oral-100%
Intravenous-100%
Intramuscular-100%
Bioavailability: Oral*-25-50%
Intravenous-100%
Intramuscular-100%
*oral route not recommended
Time to peak plasma conc.
after intramuscular injection: deltoid- 10-20 min
vastus lateralis- } 30-45 min
gluteus maximus- }
Protein bound: 70% { Albumin-30% of total binding
{ Alpha-1-acid glycoprotein-70% of total binding
(concentration dependent)
Volume of
Distribution: ~130 liters
(decreased in congestive heart failure)

| form in urine | % excreted | active? | detect in blood? |
|---|---|---|---|
| unchanged: | 5-10 | yes | yes |
| monoethylglycinexylidide (MEGX): | 3-4 | ? | yes |
| glycinexylidide (GX): | 1-3 | ? | yes |

| | Adults | Children |
|---|---|---|
| Half-life: | Normals: 74-140 min | N/A |
| Steady State, time: | 6-12 h | N/A |

(prolonged in congestive heart failure and cirrhosis)

| Dosage: | Adults-Normals* | Children |
|---|---|---|
| intravenous load: | 200-300 mg at a rate not exceeding 50 mg/min | Not available |

maintenance
infusion: 1-4 mg/min continuous infusion
*loading dose should be decreased in congestive heart failure.
(maintenance infusion should be decreased in cirrhosis and congestive heart failure)
Effective levels: 1.5-5 mg/L
Toxic levels: >6 mg/L
Monitoring
Methods: GLC, HPLC, and immunoenzymatic (EMIT®) assay.

# 23

# Therapeutic Monitoring of Procainamide Levels: Clinical Correlation

**Mark R. Wick, M.D.**
**Thomas P. Moyer, Ph.D.**

Following an observation by Mautz in 1936 (*1*) that procaine elevated the threshold of myocardial muscle to electrical stimulation, research on congeners of this agent was undertaken in an attempt to identify those with antiarrhythmic properties. This work resulted in the clinical introduction of procainamide in 1951 (*2*); since then, it has enjoyed wide application for the treatment of ventricular ectopy and tachyarrhythmias. The case to be presented illustrates the advantages of therapeutic drug monitoring in correlating clinical cardiac function with levels of procainamide in plasma.

## Case Report

A 66-year-old white man had a syncopal episode in November 1980 and was admitted to the hospital through the emergency room. He had had two near-syncopal attacks in April and September of the same year, accompanied by chest pain. However, electrocardiographic and enzymatic evidence had been insufficient on both occasions to diagnose myocardial infarction. During the past two months, he had experienced increasing dyspnea. On the day of his admission, paramedics had been summoned to his aid after his syncope; they found the patient to be in sinus tachycardia with occasional premature ventricular contractions (PVC's).

In the emergency room, physical examination showed the patient to be unresponsive, with a blood pressure of 100/60 mmHg, a respiratory rate of 40/min, a rectal temperature of 38°C, and a pulse rate of 110/min with occasional PVC's. Increased jugular venous pressure, bibasilar pulmonary rales, and diminished peripheral pulses were noted. No cardiac murmurs or gallop sounds were heard. The remainder of the examination was unremarkable.

Admitting laboratory data included electrocardiographic evidence of left bundle branch block, with sinus tachycardia and one to three PVC's per minute. ST segments were depressed in precordial leads $V_4$

*Drs. Wick and Moyer are associated with the Departments of Laboratory Medicine and Clinical Chemistry, Mayo Clinic and Mayo Foundation, Rochester, MN 55905.*

through $V_6$, and there was poor R wave progression across the precordium. Results of a complete blood count and a serum electrolyte determination were normal. Plasma glucose measured 246 mg/dL. Creatine kinase was measured at 44 U/L (normal less than 90), but 5% MB isoenzyme fraction was present. Blood lactate measured 11.3 mmol/L (normal 0.93-1.65 mmol/L). Chest radiographs disclosed cardiomegaly and pulmonary venous congestion.

A diagnosis of left ventricular failure and cardiogenic shock was made, and the patient was treated with oxygen by nasal cannulae, with furosemide, and with intravenous bicarbonate and dopamine. A Swan-Ganz catheter was placed, showing a cardiac output of 4.3 L/min (normal 4.5-6.5 L/min), with a pulmonary arterial pressure of 43/22 torr and a peripheral capillary wedge pressure of 22 torr. Intravenous lidocaine was given at a rate of 2 mg/min.

Seven hours after admission, the patient developed ventricular tachycardia, which responded to electroconversion. Dobutamine was given by intravenous drip. Repeated cardiac enzyme profiles showed a creatine kinase level of 145 U/L with a 5% MB fraction; lactate dehydrogenase measured 199 U/L, with 23% $LD_1$ and 17% $LD_2$, consistent with myocardial infarction.

The following day, procainamide therapy was initiated intravenously at a rate of 4 mg/min; lidocaine administration was maintained as well. On day 3, two runs of self-limited ventricular tachycardia were noted. The procainamide (PA) level was 17.5 mg/L; N-acetylprocainamide (NAPA) measured 13.6 mg/L. Lidocaine measured 13.5 mg/L.

Over the next four days, the patient remained dopamine-dependent referable to support of his cardiac output. Because of the possibility that antiarrhythmic drug treatment had a negative influence on ventricular function, lidocaine was discontinued, and an attempt was made to progressively wean him from PA infusion (see Table 1). From day 4 through day 7 of the hospital course, dysrhythmias were not problematic.

However, on day 8 another episode of self-limited ventricular tachycardia occurred. PA was administered orally (250 mg oral loading dose and 375 mg every 6 h) and continued for the remainder of the hospital course.

### Table 1. Procainamide and NAPA Levels in Plasma During Hospital Course

| Day of hospitalization | Procainamide/NAPA levels (mg/L) | |
|---|---|---|
| 3 | 17.5/13.6 | |
| 4 | 11.6/16.4 | Poor cardiac output |
| 5 | 10.2/19.7 | |
| 6 | 4.2/17.2 | Procainamide |
| 7 | 0.8/9.2 | tapered |
| 8 | 0/4.4 | Oral therapy begun |
| 9 | 5.1/5.7 | |
| 10 | 4.9/10.0 | |
| 11 | 2.2/7.5 | |
| 12 | - - - | |
| 13 | 1.5/5.2 | Oral therapy |
| 14 | 3.7/8.7 | continued |
| 15 | 5.4/9.9 | |
| 16 | - - - | |
| 17 | - - - | |
| 18 | 4.8/9.5 | |

On day 13, a murmur of mitral regurgitation was noted, and diffuse left ventricular hypokinesia with paradoxical septal movement was seen on M-mode cardiac sector scanning. Nonetheless, the patient felt well, and was able to become increasingly ambulatory. Over the next 12 days, his clinical status progressively improved, and he was dismissed 25 days after admission. Discharge medications included digoxin (0.25 mg/day), furosemide, hydralazine, and procainamide S-R (500 mg four times a day).

## Discussion

*Physiological Effects of Procainamide.* Pharmacologically, procainamide is qualitatively similar to procaine with respect to sites and mechanisms of activity. Quantitatively, however, the former drug has a much more specific effect on the myocardium, with relatively little influence on the central nervous system when used in therapeutic dosages (2). Also, as an amide, it is not readily hydrolyzed by plasma esterases and thereby possesses a longer duration of action. Finally, procainamide is efficacious following oral administration, whereas procaine is not.

The sites of action of procainamide within the myocardium are several, including the atrial and ventricular muscle and the Purkinje cells of the cardiac conduction system. Physiologically, this drug (and its primary metabolite N-acetylprocainamide) decrease the excitability of these tissues by elevating their threshold potentials. Also, although the action potential duration of the muscle and conduction system is modestly increased, the effective refractory period is more markedly prolonged, such that the myocardium remains refractory to electrical stimuli for a significant period, even after restoration of the resting membrane potential. Regarding the latter effect, atrial muscle seems to be primarily affected; however, the elevation of the effective refractory period to action potential duration ratio both there and in the ventricles accounts for the utility of procainamide in suppressing atrial and ventricular ectopy alike. Finally, the conduction of impulses through the atrioventricular node is substantially diminished by this agent, and high doses may cause complete AV block (3).

All of these mechanisms of action are essentially identical to those of quinidine and overlap significantly with those of lidocaine; thus, procainamide and the latter drugs should be used in combination only cautiously, to avoid unwanted additive toxicity. In addition, procainamide is not recommended for the treatment of digitalis-induced arrhythmias, because of the unpredictable effects on myocardial electrophysiology resulting from the combined actions of these medications (4).

*Pharmacokinetics.* Pharmacokinetically, intravenously administered procainamide follows two-compartment kinetics and attains a large final volume of distribution of 2 L/kg body weight (lower in patients with decreased cardiac output) (5,6). For the latter reason, substantial loading doses are required. The elimination half-life of this drug is 2.5 to 4.7 h (average 3.5) and its systemic clearance is 500 ml/min in individuals with normal renal and hepatic function (7). After oral administration, absorption from the gastrointestinal tract is rapid and from 75 to 90% complete. However, since both absorption and elimination are rapid, concentrations in plasma can fluctuate by a factor of two to three times over the usual dose interval of 3 to 4 h. In addition, concentrations in plasma show up to a 10-fold variability when the same dose is compared among a group of patients (5). Approximately 15% of procainamide in plasma is bound to proteins.

Procainamide is metabolized by hepatic N-acetyltransferase, an enzyme whose activity is genetically determined and polymorphous in expression (8). Roughly one-half of American and European patients show slow acetylation rates, whereas 90% of Orientals are rapid acetylators (9). The latter group may have higher concentrations in plasma of the principal metabolite of procainamide, NAPA, than of the parent drug (10). Approximately 15 to 30% of a given dose of procainamide is acetylated, reflecting the individual metabolic variation mentioned above, and a small **fraction may be hydrolyzed to *p*-aminobenzoic acid.** NAPA is primarily excreted by the kidneys, with an elimination half-life of 6 to 8 h (*11*). In addition, 40 to 55% of procainamide is secreted unchanged into the urine. As one might expect, patients with renal failure manifest decreased elimination of both agents (*12*).

*Dose and Administration of Procainamide.* Since procainamide is usually used in the therapy of ventricular arrhythmias only after lidocaine has already been administered, the former drug must be employed cautiously, and with close clinical and pharmacologic monitoring, to avoid additive toxicity (*13*). When using intravenous treatment, loading infusions (25-50 mg/min) are necessary to obtain therapeutic drug levels in plasma within a reasonably short time. Giardina and colleagues have advocated giving sequential doses of 100 mg over 2 min every 5 min to a total dose of 1 g (*14*), but this practice is regarded as controversial. Once pharmacologic efficacy has been achieved, the infusion rate should be slowed to 2-4 mg/min. Patients with decreased ventricular function and/or renal failure should receive lower loading and maintenance infusion rates (*12*).

When converting from intravenous to oral therapy, infusion of the drug should be stopped from 1 to 3 h before the first oral dose. Since levels in plasma decline slowly and gastrointestinal tract absorption is rapid, the initial oral doses should be relatively small to avoid toxicity (*7*).

*Adverse Reactions to Procainamide.* Untoward effects of procainamide include anorexia, nausea, vomiting, diarrhea, fatigue, and psychiatric disturbances, even when the drug is given in therapeutic dosage (*15*). Similarly, hypersensitivity reactions, manifested by angioedema, urticaria, and exanthematous skin rash, a serum sickness-like illness, thrombocytopenia, hemolytic anemia, and agranulocytosis have been documented (*6*). Perhaps the most well known among the idiosyncratic reactions to this drug is the appearance of a syndrome mimicking systemic lupus erythematosus (*16*). This problem presents a particular risk to those patients maintained on long-term therapy with procainamide, and the duration of treatment should thus be as short as possible. Individual metabolism of the drug correlates with the likelihood that a lupus-like syndrome will appear, with rapid acetylators being at primary risk (*17*). It is of interest that patients given NAPA for prolonged periods in the absence of procainamide have shown good control of dysrhythmias and have had no laboratory or clinical evidence of this syndrome (*18*). Furthermore, some individuals who had developed antinuclear antibodies while taking procainamide lost them when NAPA was substituted for the parent drug (*19*).

More directly related to levels of procainamide and NAPA in plasma are manifestations of toxicity such as hypotension, depression of cardiac contractility and cardiac output, and paradoxic worsening of electrical impulse conduction within the myocardium, resulting in bradycardia, asystole, or ventricular fibrillation (*20*). These effects are predominantly seen with intravenous administration of procainamide (but not exclusively so) and usually appear only after concentrations in plasma of greater than 10-12 mg/L for the parent drug and/or 18-20 mg/L for NAPA have been attained.

## Indications for Therapeutic Drug Monitoring of Procainamide and N-Acetylprocainamide

Because of the marked individual variation in concentrations of procainamide and NAPA in plasma due to differing rates of metabolism or absorption, and a relatively narrow range of therapeutic efficacy (4-12 mg/L for procainamide and 10-18 mg/L for NAPA), monitoring the level of these drugs in plasma is a particularly desirable procedure attending their use. In view of the fact that the manifestations of PA and NAPA toxicity overlap those of the primary disorders they are used to treat, and bearing in mind the large doses required by some individuals to attain therapeutic levels in plasma, therapeutic drug monitoring affords an objective means of separating overdosage from noncompliance and of titrating dosage to meet individual patient needs. Rapid acetylation and the contribution of NAPA levels to possible toxic symptoms and signs will only be possible if both the parent drug and this metabolite are assessed concurrently. Lastly, patients with renal insufficiency represent a subgroup in whom proper dosage titration is extremely difficult without the use of drug level determinations of procainamide and NAPA in plasma.

## Specimen Collection and Handling

Specimens for procainamide and NAPA levels in plasma may be collected in any variety of commercial venipuncture tubes. If frozen, plasma samples yield reliable procainamide and NAPA values for several weeks; unless the determination of such is to be done within 12 h after specimen collection, freezing is recommended. The most reliable time for drug level measurement in plasma is just before the next dose, i.e., at the trough level.

## Methodology

Several methods are available for procainamide and NAPA measurement, including colorimetric (*21,22*), spectrophotometric (*23*), thin layer chromatographic (*24*), gas chromatographic (*25*), high performance liquid chromatographic (*26*), and enzyme immunoassay (EMIT) techniques (*27*). In general, only EMIT and

HPLC are both sensitive and specific, and are rapid enough for practical clinical use. Specifically, EMIT kits allow quick analysis (15 to 30 min) of small samples. However, these are expensive, and most labs receiving samples of sufficient quantity have employed HPLC techniques with good results.

## Comment

The case presented in this exercise illustrates several of the points made in the foregoing discussion. Possibly because the patient experienced decreased renal perfusion and clearance, procainamide and NAPA levels early in the course of treatment were measured in the toxic range. With concomitant lidocaine administration, this situation very probably further compromised the patient's cardiac output and may have stimulated, rather than suppressed, the ventricu-

lar dysrhythmias which were observed. This deduction, and the subsequent attenuation of intravenous dosage, would not have been possible without regular monitoring of drug levels in plasma. Similarly, the response to oral procainamide was optimized late in the hospital course by therapeutic drug monitoring. Clinical cardiac stability was correlated with PA/NAPA levels in the therapeutic range at the time of dismissal, allowing for greater confidence on the part of the clinician that the treatment protocol was indeed efficacious.

Unfortunately, though the patient remained in stable condition, with therapeutic procainamide and NAPA levels and freedom from dysrhythmias for one month after discharge from the hospital, he was lost to followup at our institution after that time.

## Procainamide Profile

| Trade name: | Pronestyl® (Squibb) |
| Chemical name: | Procainamide HCl |
| pKa: | 9.23 |
| Mol. mass: | 271.8 Dalton |
| Melting point, °C: | 165-169 |
| Water solubility: | 1g/0.05 L |
| | |
| Dose absorbed: | oral 75-90% |
| Peak plasma level, time: | IV: 15-60 min after infusion |
| | Oral: 1 h after ingestion |
| Protein bound: | 15% |
| $V_d$: | 2 L/kg |

Structure:

$$NH_2 - C_6H_4 - CONHCH_2CH_2N(C_2H_5)_2$$

| Form in urine | % excreted | Active | Detectable in blood |
|---|---|---|---|
| Procainamide (unchanged) | 40-55 | yes | yes |
| N-acetylprocainamide | 15-30 | yes | yes |

| | Adults | Children |
|---|---|---|
| Half-life: | average 3.5 h | n/a |
| Steady state, time: | 5-7 half-lives (IV) | n/a |
| Recommended dose: | IV: Loading, 25-50 mg/min | |
| | Maintenance, 2-4 mg/min | |
| | Oral: Loading, 1 g | |
| | Maintenance, 250-500 ng q 3 h | |
| | weight dependent | |
| Effective levels: | 4-12 μg/mL | |
| Toxic levels: | >12 μg/mL | |
| Monitoring methods: | HPLC, EMIT | |

## References

1. Mautz, F.R., The reduction of cardiac irritability by the epicardial and systemic administration of drugs as a protection in cardiac surgery. *J. Thorac. Surg.* **5**, 612-628 (1936).
2. Mark, L.C., Kayden, J.J., Steele, J.M., et al., The physiologic disposition and cardiac effects of procainamide. *J. Pharmacol. Exp. Ther.* **102**, 5-15 (1951).
3. Woske, H., Belford, J., Fastier, F.N., et al., The effect of procainamide on excitability, refractoriness, and conduction in the mammalian heart. *J. Pharmacol. Exp. Ther.* **107**, 134-140 (1953).
4. Zapata-Diaz, J., Cabrera, C.E., and Mendez, R., An experimental and clinical study on the effects of procainamide on the heart. *Am. Heart J.* **43**, 854-870 (1952).
5. Koch-Weser, J., Pharmacokinetics of procainamide in man. *Ann. N.Y. Acad. Sci.* **179**, 370-382 (1971).
6. Baer, D.M., and Dito, W.R., *Interpretation in Therapeutic Drug Monitoring*, American Society of Clinical Pathology, Chicago, IL, pp 39-42 (1981).
7. Koch-Weser, J., and Klein, S.W., Procainamide dosage schedules, plasma concentrations, and clinical effects. *JAMA* **215**, 1454-1460 (1971).
8. Weber, W.W., Acetylating, deacetylating, and amino acid conjugating enzymes. In *Concepts of Biochemical Pharmacology, Handbook of Experimental Pharmacology, Vol. 28*, B.B. Brodie and J.R. Gillette, Eds., Springer-Verlag, New York, NY (1971).
9. Ellard, G.A., Variations between individuals and populations in the acetylation of isoniazid and its significance for the treatment of pulmonary tuberculosis. *Clin. Pharmacol. Ther.* **19**, 610-625 (1976).

10. Elson, J., Strong, J.M., Lee, W-K, et al., Anti-arrhythmic potency of N-acetylprocainamide *Clin. Pharmacol. Ther.* **17**, 134-140 (1975).

11. Dutcher, J.S., Strong, J.M., Lucas, S.V., et al., Procainamide and N-acetyl-procainamide kinetics investigated simultaneously with stable isotope methodology. *Clin. Pharmacol. Ther.* **22**, 447-457 (1977).

12. Drayer, D.E., Lowenthal, D.T., Woosley, R.L., et al., Cumulation of N-acetylprocainamide, an active metabolite of procainamide, in patients with impaired renal function. *Clin. Pharmacol. Ther.* **22**, 63-69 (1977).

13. Cote, P., Harrison, D.C., Basile, J., et al., Hemo-dynamic interaction of procainamide and lidocaine after experimental myocardial infarction. *Am. J. Cardiol.* **32**, 937-942 (1973).

14. Giardina, E.G.V., Heissenbuttel, R.H., and Bigger, J.T., Intermittent intravenous procaina-mide to treat ventricular arrhythmias. *Ann. Intern. Med.* **78**, 183-193 (1973).

15. Lima, J.J., Goldfarb, A.L., Conti, D.R., et al., Safety and efficacy of procainamide infusions. *Am. J. Cardiol.* **43**, 98-105 (1979).

16. Kosowsky, B.D., Taylor, J., Lown, B., et al., Long-term use of procainamide following acute myocardial infarction. *Circulation* **47**, 1204-1210 (1973).

17. Woosley, R.L., Drayer, D.E., Reidenberg, M.M., et al., Effect of acetylator phenotype on the rate at which procainamide induces antinuclear antibodies and the lupus syndrome. *N. Engl. J. Med.* **298**, 1157-1159 (1978).

18. Kluger, J., Drayer, D.E., Reidenberg, M.M., et al., The clinical pharmacology and antiarrhythmic efficacy of acetylprocainamide in patients with arrhythmias. *Am. J. Cardiol.* **45**, 1250-1257 (1980).

19. Kluger, J., Drayer, D.E., Reidenberg, M.M., et al., Acetylprocainamide therapy in patients with previous procainamide-induced lupus syndrome. *Ann. Intern. Med.* **95**, 18-23 (1981).

20. Koch-Weser, J., Clinical applications of the phar-macokinetics of procainamide. *Cardiovasc. Clin.* **6**, 63-75 (1974).

21. Gey, G.O., Levy, R.H., Fisher, L., Plasma concentrations of procainamide and prevalence of exertional arrhythmias. *Ann. Intern. Med.* **80**, 718-722 (1974).

22. **Dreyfuss, J., Bigger, J.T., et al., Metabolism of procainamide in rhesus monkey and man. *Clin. Pharmacol. Ther.* 13, 366-371 (1972).**

23. Ambler, P.K., and Masarei, J.R.L., A new fluorometric method for procainamide. *Clin. Chim. Acta.* **70**, 379-383 (1976).

24. Reidenberg, M.M., Drayer, D.E., Levy, M., et al., Plasma concentration and renal clearance of procainamide and its acetylated metabolite in man. *Clin. Res.* **23**, 223A (1975).

25. Simons, K.J., and Levy, R.H., GLC determination of procainamide in biological fluids. *J. Pharm. Sci.* **64**, 1967-1970 (1975).

26. Gadalla, M.A.F., Peng, G.W., and Chiou, W.L., Rapid and macro high-pressure liquid chroma-tographic method for simultaneous determination of procainamide and N-acetylprocainamide in plasma. *J. Pharm. Sci.* **677**, 869-871 (1978).

27. Fanciullo, R.A., Huber, N., Izutsu, A., et al., Homogenous enzyme immunoassay for PCA in serum. *Clin. Chem.* **24**, 1056 (1978).

# 24

# Procainamide: A Case Study

Henry J. Duff, M.D., F.R.C.P.(c)
Raymond L. Woosley, M.D., Ph.D.

Procainamide has long been recognized to be effective in treatment of ventricular arrhythmias. A relation between procainamide concentration in plasma and the extent of suppression of ventricular extrasystoles has been documented (1). The therapeutic range of procainamide, in which ventricular extrasystoles are suppressed with the least incidence of toxicity is reportedly 4-8 mg/L (2), but recent studies (2) indicate that higher plasma concentrations (mean 12.3±3.0 mg/L), achieved during intravenous infusions, were well tolerated, and indeed may be required for effective treatment of patients with documented ventricular tachyarrhythmias (3,4). However, during oral therapy with procainamide, if similar procainamide concentrations are attained in plasma, the major metabolite of procainamide, N-acetylprocainamide, may accumulate.

Here we present a case that illustrates that the toxic manifestation of oral procainamide therapy may be related to the combined electrophysiologic and toxic properties of both procainamide and acecainide (generally known as N-acetylprocainamide).

## Case Report

This 58-year-old man presented with chest pain and unifocal ventricular ectopic depolarizations four years after coronary bypass surgery. Serial antiarrhythmic-drug evaluations including procainamide, quinidine, and propranolol did not control the patient's ventricular arrhythmia. Oral disopyramide effectively suppressed the arrhythmia and he was discharged on this medication.

The patient was asymptomatic until the day of his admission, when he was hospitalized with an acute inferolateral myocardial infarction. On the third hospital day, despite oral disopyramide (200 mg every 6 h) and a maintenance lidocaine infusion of 2 mg/min, the patient had two episodes of ventricular fibrillation requiring electrical defibrillation. Oral disopyramide and intravenous lidocaine were continued, but recurrent bursts of ventricular tachycardia persisted. On the 10th hospital day the patient was transferred to the Nashville Veterans Administration Hospital.

*Dr. Duff is in the Division of Clinical Pharmacology and Dr. Woosley is Associate Prof. of Med. and Clin. Pharmacology, School of Medicine, Vanderbilt University.*

On arrival there, his blood presure was 90/60 mm Hg, his temperature 37.8°C, his respiration rate 32/min, and his pulse rate 88/min and irregular. Jugular venous distention was evident 4 cm above the clavicle with patient positioned at 45°. On auscultation, rales were heard throughout both lung fields to the mid-scapular level. A grade II systolic murmur was audible along the left sternal border and apex and S₃ gallop was present. The liver and spleen were not enlarged. There was no presacral or peripheral edema.

## Hospital Course

The congestive heart failure was managed with digoxin, diuretics, and nitrates. Oral disopyramide was continued. On the 11th hospital day, increasingly frequent unifocal ventricular ectopic depolarization appeared. Because of increasing signs and symptoms of congestive heart failure, disopyramide was discontinued on the 14th hospital day, and oral procainamide (375 mg every 4 h) was started. As illustrated in Table 1, high frequency ventricular arrhythmia continued. Oral procainamide dosage was increased to 500 mg every 4 h in an attempt to gain better control of the ventricular arrhythmia. In addition, the digoxin dosage was increased to 0.25 mg alternating with 0.375 mg every other day. Table 1 illustrates the electrocardiographic and antiarrhythmic response to this dosage of procainamide. High frequency ventricular arrhythmias and episodic ventricular tachycardia continued. The oral procainamide dosage was increased to 750 mg every 4 h. On the 37th hospital day trough drug concentrations in the plasma were: digoxin 1.7 μg/L, procainamide 9.6 mg/L and acecainide 21.1 mg/L. Table 1 demonstrates the progressive prolongation of the $QT_c$ interval with increasing dosage.

On this regimen and without preceding cardiac symptoms, the patient sustained a cardiac arrest. The initial ECG rhythm strip showed coarse ventricular fibrillation. After repeated defibrillations and a 500 mg intravenous bolus of bretylium, the patient converted to sinus rhythm. The remainder of the patient's hospitalization was complicated by pulmonary edema, and a pulmonary embolus.

On the 93rd hospital day the patient developed a recurrence of chest pain, became hypotensive, and died. Postmortem examination showed a grossly dilated left ventricle with evidence of a recent (less than 48 h) myocardial infarction in the lateral wall of the left ventricle.

## Discussion

By spectrophotometry, which does not measure acecainide, the upper limit of the therapeutic range for procainamide in the past has been established to be 8-10 mg/L (2), and clinicians seldom increase the dosage of oral procainamide above this range because they anticipate side effects such as hypotension, conduction disturbances, and gastrointestinal disturbances. Nevertheless, in more recent studies higher doses of intravenous procainamide (mean concentration in plasma 12.3±3.0 mg/L) not only were well tolerated but also provided effective ventricular arrhythmia control, whereas lower concentrations within the previously accepted therapeutic range had failed to do so (3,4).

During an acute infusion of procainamide little acecainide is generated; thus any antiarrhythmic or toxic effects must be attributed to procainamide itself. However, during prolonged oral procainamide therapy, high concentrations of acecainide may accumulate, as was the case in this patient. The electrophysiological properties of acecainide are very different from those of procainamide. The major effect of acecainide is to prolong the duration of the action potential. The changes in phase 0 and phase 4 produced by procainamide (5) have not been observed with acecainide. During prolonged oral therapy with procainamide the combined electrophysiological actions of these two antiarrhythmic agents may be either synergistic or antagonistic, and additive toxic effects may be possible.

A therapeutic range for acecainide has not been clearly established. Roden et al. (6) demonstrated that during the administration of oral acecainide alone, the mean acecainide concentration in plasma associated with antiarrhythmic efficacy was 14.3 mg/L (range 9.4-19.5) and the mean concentration associated with side effects (primarily gastrointestinal) was 22.5 mg/L.

A recent study by Kluger et al.(7) found antiarrhythmic activity at plasma concentrations of 10-30 mg/L but toxicity was also seen at concentrations ranging from 11 to 20 mg/L. Other investigators have reported that acecainide concentrations as high as 41 mg/L were well tolerated, with no electrocardiographic or hemodynamic signs of toxicity. The maximal antiarrhythmic effect of acecainide, administered alone, was achieved at a mean concentration in plasma of 30 mg/L.

This case illustrates a major potential problem in the clinical use of chronic oral procainamide for the treatment of ventricular arrhythmias. In this patient the oral procainamide dosage was progressively increased, the finally attained concentration in plasma being in excess of the generally accepted therapeutic range, with a simultaneous acecainide concentration of 21.1 mg/L. Given the results obtained during intravenous infusions (3,4), this procainamide concentration would not have been expected to cause severe cardiac toxicity. However, as reported in patients with renal disease (8), the combined effects of acecainide and procainamide may have resulted in additive toxicity and precipitation of ventricular fibrillation in this individual. Large interindividual differences preclude accurate prediction of circulating concentration that will be achieved from a given dose of procainamide; therefore, measurements in plasma of both acecainide and procainamide are essential. In the presence of plasma acecainide concentrations in excess of 20 mg/L, a concentration of procainamide in the high therapeutic range (6-10 mg/L) may be associated with toxicity (8).

Prolongation of the QT$_c$ interval is known to have several etiologies; electrolyte disorders, drug therapy, a sequel to myocardial infarction, and the inherited "prolonged QT syndrome." The incidence of life-threatening ventricular arrhythmias and sudden death

**Table 1. Therapeutic and Clinical Data**

| Doses of procainamide | Procainamide concn (mg/L) | Acecainide concn (mg/L) | QRS duration | QTC duration | Ventricular arrhythmia characteristics |
|---|---|---|---|---|---|
| Baseline (during disopyramide withdrawal) | | | 0.08 | 0.46 | recurrent nonsustained ventricular tachycardia multifocal VEDs* - 10-400/h |
| 375 mg every 4 h | 3.2 | 6.0 | 0.08 | 0.48 | single episode of sustained ventricular tachycardia multifocal VEDs* - 50-500/h |
| 500 mg every 4 h | 5.8 | 12.8 | 0.08 | 0.50 | single episode of nonsustained ventricular tachycardia unifocal VEDs* - 10-400/h |
| 750 mg every 4 h | 9.6 | 21.1 | 0.08 | 0.70 | ventricular fibrillation |

*VED: ventricular ectopic depolarization

### N-Acetylprocainamide Profile

$$CH_3-\overset{O}{\underset{}{C}}-NH-\underset{}{\bigcirc}-\overset{}{\underset{O}{C}}-NH-CH_2-CH_2-N\overset{C_2H_5}{\underset{C_2H_5}{}}$$

| | |
|---|---|
| Trade name: | NAPA®, Acecainide |
| pK$_a$: | 8.3 |
| Rel. Mol. mass: | 313.8 |
| mp, °C: | |
| Water solubility: | Freely soluble |
| Alcohol solubility: | Freely soluble |

| | |
|---|---|
| Dose absorbed: | 85% |
| Peak plasma level, time: | 45 - 90 min |
| Protein bound: | 11% |
| V$_d$: | 1.2 - 1.7 L/kg |

| Form in Urine | % Excreted | Active | Detectable in blood |
|---|---|---|---|
| unchanged drug: | 80% | unknown | Yes |

| | Adults | Children |
|---|---|---|
| Half-life: | 3.1 - 11.4 h  (depends on | n/a |
| Steady state, time: | 15.5 - 57.5 h renal function) | |

| | Adults | Children |
|---|---|---|
| Recommended dose: | 0.75-2.5g orally each 8 h | n/a |
| Effective levels: | 10-30 mg/L | |
| Toxic levels: | highly variable, when procainamide is 6 mg/L, acecainide levels >20 mg/L may be toxic. When procainamide <2 mg/L, acecainide 35 mg/L may be toxic. | |

**Monitoring methods:**  HPLC and immunoenzymatic (EMIT®)

### Procainamide Profile

$$NH_2-\underset{}{\bigcirc}-\overset{}{\underset{O}{C}}-NH-CH_2-CH_2-N\overset{C_2H_5}{\underset{C_2H_5}{}}$$

| | |
|---|---|
| Trade name: | Procainamide HCl, Pronestyl® |
| pK$_a$: | 9.2 |
| Rel. Mol. mass: | 272 |
| mp, °C: | 165-169 |
| Water solubility: | Freely soluble |

| | |
|---|---|
| Dose absorbed: | 75-90%, but varies widely |
| Peak plasma level, time: | 1-2 h |
| Protein bound: | 15% |
| V$_d$: | 1.7-2.2 L/kg, |
| | but decreased in congestive heart failure |

| Form in Urine | % excreted | Active | Detectable in blood |
|---|---|---|---|
| unchanged drug: | 45-65% | N-acetyl procainamide | Yes |

| | Adults | Children |
|---|---|---|
| Half-life: | 2.5 - 4.7 h  (depends on | n/a |
| Steady state, time: | 12.5 - 23.5 h renal function)· | |

| | Adults | Children |
|---|---|---|
| Recommended dose: | I.V.: Load 275 µg/kg per minute constant infusion over 20 min - monitoring BP and rhythm. maintenance: 20-60 mg/kg per minute oral therapy: 250-750 q 3-6 h | n/a |
| Effective levels: | 4 - 8 mg/L | |
| Toxic levels: | >12.0 mg/L | |

**Monitoring methods:**  HPLC and immunoenzymatic (EMIT®) assay

is increased in patients with this finding. In the patient presented in this case report, the QT$_c$ interval appeared to be prolonged even in the absence of therapy with antiarrhythmic agents. The administration of either procainamide or acecainide could be expected to further prolong the QT$_c$ interval and increase the chance of life threatening arrhythmias.

Careful monitoring of plasma concentration and electrocardiographic intervals is essential during dosage adjustment of antiarrhythmic drug therapy. When using plasma concentration data, one must consider the presence of other drugs or metabolites and their potential pharmacological actions and interactions.

## References

1. Giardina, E.V., Heissenbuttel, R.H., and Bigger, J.T., Correlation of plasma concentration with effect on arrhythmias, electrocardiogram and blood pressure. *Ann. Intern. Med.* **78**, 183-193 (1973).
2. Koch-Weser, J., and Klein, S.W. Procainamide: Dosage schedules, plasma concentrations, and clinical effects. *J. Am. Med. Assoc.* **215**, 1454 (1971).
3. Greenspan, A.M., Josephson, M.E., Farshidi, A., et al., High dose procainamide for malignant ventricular arrhythmia. *Circulation* Vol **87**, Supp. II, 965 (1978).
4. Horowitz, L.N., Josephson, M.E., Farshidi, A., et al., Recurrent sustained ventricular tachycardia. 3. Role of electrophysiologic study in selection of antiarrhythmic regimens. *Circulation* **58**, 986 (1978).
5. Dangman, K.H., and Hoffman, B.F. Effects of N-acetylprocainamide on cardiac Purkinje fibers. *Pharmacologist* **20**, No. 3, 27 (1979).
6. Roden, D.M., Reele, S.B., Higgins, S.B., et al., Antiarrhythmic efficacy, pharmacokinetics and safety of N-acetylprocainamide in man: Comparison to procainamide. *Am. J. Cardiol.*, in press.
7. Kluger, J., Drayer, D., Reidenburg, M., et al., The clinical pharmacology and antiarrhythmia efficacy of acetylprocainamide in patients with arrhythmias. *Am. J. Cardiol.* **45**, 1250-1257 (1980).
8. Drayer, D., Lowenthal, D., Woosley, R.L., et al., Cumulation of N-acetylprocainamide, an active metabolite of procainamide, in patients with impaired renal function. *Clin. Pharmacol. Ther.* **22**, 63-69 (1977).

# 25

# Quinidine: A Case History

**H. William Kelly, Pharm. D.**
**William H. Jeffery, Pharm.D.**

### Introduction

Quinidine, the dextro isomer of quinine, is a naturally occurring alkaloid found in cinchona bark. Quinidine has electrophysiologic properties which are similar to those of procainamide in that both agents reduce cardiac automaticity, decrease atrioventricular and intraventricular conduction velocity, and increase action potential duration, which prolongs the refractory period. In addition, quinidine possesses a vagolytic effect and dilates peripheral vessels, which may produce hypotension.

Many quinidine preparations contain an impurity, dihydroquinidine, which has pharmacologic and pharmacokinetic properties essentially identical to those of quinidine. Both dihydroquinidine and quinidine are assayed by extraction-fluorescence techniques. However, more specific assay techniques such as HPLC, GLC, and GLC-MS permit quantitation of each drug separately.

The major route of elimination of quinidine is through hydroxylation by the hepatic mixed-function oxidase system, with about 20% of the drug excreted unchanged in the urine. Drugs which induce hepatic microsomal enzymes, such as phenobarbital and phenytoin, can significantly increase the clearance rate and decrease the half-life of quinidine. Pathologic conditions such as hepatic failure in hepatic cirrhosis will decrease the clearance of quinidine, and patients with these diseases should be monitored closely with serum drug level determinations. It has also been demonstrated that older healthy volunteers have a lower intrinsic clearance of the drug than young healthy volunteers. Renal failure and congestive heart failure do not significantly alter plasma levels and elimination half-life of quinidine. Quinidine kinetics appear to be dose-dependent, and any increase in dosage should be done in small increments while utilizing plasma drug determinations to document the magnitude of the increases.

Quinidine is completely absorbed from the gastrointestinal tract, but first-pass metabolism in the liver

*Dr. Kelly is Assistant Professor of Pharmacy, College of Pharmacy and Clinical Assistant Professor of Pediatrics, School of Medicine, University of New Mexico, Albuquerque, New Mexico. Dr. Jeffery is Associate Professor of Pharmacy, University of New Mexico.*

accounts for its decreased oral bioavailability. There are a number of sustained-release (SR) preparations available. However only a few have been adequately studied for bioavailability. In general, all preparations demonstrate first-order absorption, with the SR preparations having more prolonged absorption half-lives.

The extensive protein binding of quinidine probably underlies the considerable variability and overlap in "therapeutic" and "toxic" serum levels. There is a significant interpatient variability in protein binding. The use of salivary measurements, which better reflect unbound or pharmacologically active drug, may provide a more accurate assessment of the therapeutic range. Protein binding also may play a part in drug interactions such as the increased hypoprothrombinemic effect produced with warfarin.

Routine monitoring of plasma quinidine levels is a necessary adjunct to therapy because of the wide range in clearance rates and distribution volumes between patients. The variability in absorption characteristics of different preparations and between patients with the same preparation is also a reason for monitoring plasma levels.

### Case History

This case illustrates several clinical problems associated with the use of quinidine. There are very few drugs available for outpatient treatment of supraventricular and ventricular arrhythmias. Quinidine is the drug of choice. However, intolerance to side effects frequently requires substitution of another antiarrhythmic agent. The interaction of quinidine with digoxin requires careful monitoring of the plasma levels and effects of both agents when they are used concurrently. Compliance with complex drug regimens may improve when patients are hospitalized. This compliance may result in unexpected increases in plasma levels and thus, drug toxicity.

### Case Presentation

A 70-year-old white male was admitted to the hospital complaining of increased shortness of breath, nervousness, and nausea. His problem list included chronic obstructive pulmonary disease, congestive heart failure, and suspected recurrent pulmonary embolus. Prior to this admission he noticed increasing shortness of breath, dyspnea on exertion, three pillow orthopnea, paroxysmal nocturnal dyspnea, and a constant productive cough. He had a history of myocardial infarction and multifocal premature ventricular contractions. At the time of admission he was taking isosorbide dinitrate 10 mg *qid*, digoxin 0.25 mg daily, furosemide 120 mg daily, triamterene 100 mg *bid*, terbutaline 2.5 mg *qid*, long-acting theophylline 250 mg *tid*, and quinidine sulfate 200 mg *qid*. On physical examination there was increased anterior-posterior diameter of the chest and hyperresonance, increased expiratory phase with moist rales to the tips of both scapulae, and decreased breath sounds. Gynecomastia was noted. Examination of the heart revealed an $S_3$ and a grade III/IV harsh holosystolic murmur at the apex. There was no jugular venous distension, hepatojugular reflux, or pedal edema, and peripheral pulses were normal.

The patient's congestive heart failure improved with vigorous diuresis. On the fourth hospital day he complained of severe nausea, vomiting, and diarrhea. Quinidine toxicity was suspected. The quinidine level proved to be 7.2 mg/L (therapeutic 3-6 mg/L). The following day quinidine was discontinued because of continued nausea, vomiting, and diarrhea, and disopyramide 100 mg *qid* was started. The nausea, vomiting, and diarrhea continued, and digoxin toxictiy was considered. The digoxin level was found to be 2.5 $\mu$g/L (therapeutic 0.9-2.4 $\mu$g/L). Soon after disopyramide was started, the patient's cardiac function acutely deteriorated. A Swan-Ganz catheter was placed and dopamine was infused to maintain blood pressure and renal perfusion. He recovered, and was discharged with prescriptions for long-acting theophylline 250 mg *bid*, hydralazine 25 mg *q* 6 h, digoxin 0.25 mg daily, warfarin 7.5 mg daily, and quinidine gluconate 330 mg *bid*.

## Discussion

This case illustrates several problems associated with quinidine therapy. The patient's compliance with his complicated medication regimen probably improved after admission to the hospital. His digoxin level on admission was 0.9$\mu$g/L. Five days later it was 2.5 $\mu$g/L, on the same daily dose of digoxin and quinidine as at admission. He developed severe nausea, vomiting, and diarrhea, which could have

been due to either quinidine or digoxin. Quinidine was most suspect, and was replaced with disopyramide. Acute decompensation of congestive heart failure and cardiogenic shock followed the change to disopyramide. The temporal relationship between disopyramide and cardiogenic shock was very suggestive of a drug-induced event, which has been reported recently by Story et al. (1979). In retrospect, the patient's nausea, vomiting, and diarrhea might have been treated by reducing the dose of both quinidine and digoxin.

A second problem illustrated by this case is the interaction between quinidine and digoxin. It is well documented that quinidine causes an increase in digoxin plasma levels (Ochs et al., 1980). An increase in digoxin effect has also been demonstrated. The mechanism of this interaction appears to be a quinidine-induced reduction in both the volume of distribution and the renal clearance of digoxin. The current recommendation is to reduce the digoxin dosage by 30-50% when quinidine is given concurrently, and to monitor digoxin plasma levels closely.

A third potential problem illustrated by this case is the interaction between quinidine and warfarin. Quinidine administration appears to have resulted in hemorrhage in a few patients taking warfarin (Hansten, 1979). The mechanism appears to be additive hypoprothrombinemic effects of quinidine and coumarin anticoagulants, and the clinical significance is undetermined.

## Bibliography

Ochs, H.R., Greenblatt, D.J., and Woo, E., Clinical pharmacokinetics of quinidine. *Clinical Pharmacokinetics* **5,**150-168 (1980).

Hansten, Philip D., *Drug Interactions*. 4th ed. Philadelphia, Lea & Febiger, 1979.

Melmon, Kenneth L., and Morrelli, Howard F., *Clinical Pharmacology*. 2nd ed. New York, Macmillan, 1978.

Story, J.R., Abdulla, A.M., and Frank, M.J., Cardiogenic shock and disopyramide phosphate; *JAMA* **242,** 654-6555 (1979).

# Quinidine Profile

**Trade name:** Quinaglute, Quinora, Quinidex

**Chemical structure:**

| | | |
|---|---|---|
| **Molecular weight:** | 746.93(sulfate) | |
| **Melting point, °C:** | 174-175 | |
| **Solubility in water, g/mL:** | .01 (sulfate) | |
| **pK$_a$:** | 8.57 | |

| | rapid release | sustained release |
|---|---|---|
| **Time to peak plasma conc., h:** | 1 - 2 | 2 - 8 |
| **Percentage dose absorbed:** | 60 - 100 | 40 - 95 |

| | |
|---|---|
| **% protein bound:** | 60 - 96 |
| **Tissue distribution (V$_d$, L/kg):** | 1.4 - 4.0 |

| Form in urine: | % excreted | active | detectable in blood |
|---|---|---|---|
| unchanged drug: | 15 - 40 | yes | yes |
| 3-hydroxyquinidine: | 40 - 50 | yes | yes |
| 2'-oxo-quinidinone: | ? | no | yes |
| 0-desmethylquinidine: | ? | no | yes |

| | Adults |
|---|---|
| **Recommended dose (mg/kg/d):** | 10 - 20 |
| **Half-life, h:** | 3 - 14 |
| **Time to steady state, h:** | 15 - 60 |
| **Effective levels ($\mu$g/mL):** | 2 - 6 |
| **Toxic levels ($\mu$g/mL):** | > 10 |
| **Monitoring methods:** | EMIT, HPLC, GLC |

# 26

## Quinidine: Apparent Alteration in Half-Life Associated with Phenobarbital in A Patient with Ventricular Tachycardia

### Philip R. Reid, M.D.

### Case History

In 1976, a 16-month-old boy was transferred to the Johns Hopkins Hospital when an electrocardiogram demonstrated ventricular tachycardia after an irregular pulse was noted during a routine visit to the patient's physician.

The patient was the product of a normal pregnancy and uncomplicated vaginal delivery. His earlier growth and development had been unremarkable. The patient did not take any regular medication. The mother denied the possible ingestion of any cardioactive drugs by the patient; the only medications kept in the home were vitamins, aspirin, and dextropropoxyphene. Although other potentially toxic agents such as cleaning materials were available, their location prevented access by the child.

The family history revealed that the 28-year-old mother and 37-year-old father were in good health, had no known chronic illnesses, and took no regular medications. The patient had three siblings (ages 6 years, 5 years, and 4 months) who were in good health. Although a maternal uncle died of a "heart attack" in childhood (age 2) the details were lacking and there was no other family history of sudden cardiac death at an early age.

Results of the physical examination were unremarkable except for an irregular pulse. Results of routine laboratory blood studies were within normal limits and a toxicology screen reported no evidence of barbiturates, narcotics, salicylates, acetaminophen, or tricyclic antidepressants. Results of other laboratory studies such as chest radiograph, echocardiogram, and electroencephalogram were within normal limits. The electrocardiogram demonstrated sinus rhythm with ventricular bigeminy, trigeminy, and long runs of ventricular tachycardia at rates of 180 beats/min but the blood pressure was normal.

The patient was placed on continuous electrocardiographic monitoring and switched to quinidine gluconate after lidocaine or propranolol or both failed to suppress the arrhythmia. The initial dose of quinidine gluconate was 2.5 mg/kg per day intravenously every

Dr. Reid is Associate Professor of Medicine, Departments of Medicine and Pharmacology at the Johns Hopkins Hospital, Baltimore, Maryland 21205.

4 h. Because the quinidine was administered intravenously, several post-dose samples were collected, permitting the biological half-life to be calculated: it was 4.3 h. The immediate pre-dose concentration in serum was 2.1 mg/L. The arrhythmia was somewhat improved but spontaneous episodes of ventricular tachycardia continued. Therefore, the quinidine dose was gradually increased to 5.0 mg/kg per day, given in six divided doses per day. At this quinidine dose there was no evidence of toxicity, the pre-dose concentration was 4.3 mg/L and the ventricular tachycardia appeared to be suppressed, although single premature contractions were occasionally noted.

At this time one of the physicians caring for the patient noted that nearly all ectopy was absent during sleeping hours. Therefore, he instituted phenobarbital (4.8 mg/kg per day) in an attempt to sedate the patient lightly and further reduce the ventricular ectopy.

About 12 days later and with the patient receiving the same dose of quinidine, ventricular tachycardia was again noted. Repeat blood samples showed quinidine concentration to be 2.6 mg/L, and the half-life decreased to 2.8 h. The quinidine dose was temporarily increased to suppress the ventricular tachycardia, and the phenobarbital was discontinued.

Fourteen days later, the quinidine half-life was remeasured and found to be 4.5 h with a pre-dose concentration of 4.4 mg/L on a quinidine dose of 5.0 mg/kg per day. Thereafter, the patient was discharged, to receive quinidine in a daily dose of 5 mg/kg per day and is doing well 3 years later.

### Mechanism of Action

Quinidine produces a slowing of impulse transmission in nearly all parts of the cardiac conduction system, an increase in the effective refractory period, and a depression of phase-4 spontaneous depolarization in Purkinje fibers. These effects tend to reduce the discharge potential of ectopic pacemakers in either the atrium or ventricle. As a reflection of the effects, the routine electrocardiogram will show a prolongation of the QRS and QT intervals, which can be used to assess its use clinically. In addition to these effects, quinidine exerts an indirect antivagal action which may, paradoxically, enhance conduction through the A-V node.

These electrophysiological features are shared by

other antiarrhythmic agents such as procainamide and disopyramide. Thus a classification system has been developed based on the mechanism of action which places these drugs in Class I. The effects of Class I drugs are in contrast to other antiarrhythmic agents such as lidocaine and phenytoin (Class II), which do not tend to slow intracardiac impulse transmission.

## Site of Action

Quinidine and other Class I drugs directly affect the myocardial cell, apparently by altering membrane conductance to specific cations such as sodium, potassium, and calcium. It is the movement of these cations that determines the conduction velocity during depolarization and cell refractoriness which follows.

In addition to this direct cardiac effect, quinidine also has an indirect effect: partial inhibition of the vagus nerve. Because the A-V node is heavily innervated with vagal fibers, inhibition tends to facilitate A-V node impulse transmission and offset, to some extent, the direct effect described above. With higher quinidine doses the direct effect appears to predominate.

## Drug-Drug Interaction

Quinidine, like many other drugs that undergo extensive hepatic metabolism, may have its elimination rate accelerated by known enzyme inducers such as phenobarbital. While this potential drug-drug interaction is not widely appreciated, the case presented suggests that it may have clinical importance. Since other drugs such as birth-control pills, chlorinated hydrocarbons, and alcohol may also produce hepatic enzyme induction, unexpected results with quinidine therapy should cause one to examine the clinical picture for this potential interaction.

Recently it has been recognized that quinidine can displace digoxin from its extravascular protein binding sites and decrease renal digoxin clearance. This results in increased serum digoxin concentrations, which may result in digitalis toxicity. Because these two drugs are frequently used together in clinical therapy, many cases of toxicity after the addition of quinidine to previously stable digoxin doses may have been ascribable to digitalis rather than direct quinidine toxicity. A similar mechanism may account for the increases in prothrombin time when quinidine is added to stable doses of the anticoagulant warfarin.

Because similar electrophysiological properties are shared by quinidine, procainamide, and disopyramide, combined clinical use of these drugs should be cautiously undertaken. Measurement of only one of these agents in the blood when their use is combined may result in underestimation of the total electrophys-

iological effect of the Class I drugs.

## Side Effects

Many side effects are described for quinidine, but the most common, perhaps in 20% of patients, are anorexia, nausea, vomiting, and diarrhea. These gastrointestinal side effects often limit its use clinically. At times, switching from the most frequently used salt, quinidine sulfate, to quinidine gluconate may reduce the gastrointestinal side effects.

Other, less common, side effects include thrombocytopenia, skin rash, hemolytic anemia, and hepatitis. Some patients may have their ventricular arrhythmias worsened to produce a clinical picture described as "quinidine syncope." This infrequent result may occur with therapeutic doses and is one of the reasons why initiation of quinidine therapy is recommended while the patient is in the hospital.

Toxic doses of quinidine may produce a clinical picture called "cinchonism." This includes nausea, vomiting, lethargy, tinnitus, visual disturbances, parasthesias, hypotension, and cyanosis. Cinchonism may quickly lead to death unless it is recognized and the quinidine stopped. Until recovery, the patients usually require general supportive measures such as fluids, vasopressors and, possibly, over-drive ventricular pacing.

## Specimen Collection, Storage, Transport and Stability

Either plasma or serum may be used as the sample source. Quinidine concentrations may be measured by a wide variety of methods, which include spectrophotofluorometry, gas-liquid chromatography, and radioimmunoassay. Because of its simplicity, spectrophotofluorometry has been one of the most popular techniques.

Depending on the extraction technique used, variable amounts of the water-soluble metabolites may be included in the finally measured value, the cardiac effects of which are not yet completely certain. It is important to recognize that different assay techniques may give different results for this reason. For example, quinidine undergoes ring hydroxylation and then renal elimination. While the cardiac activity of the hydroxylated metabolite is less than the parent compound, this metabolite will be measured as "quinidine" if the assay employed extracts the water soluble metabolites. These results may be particularly confusing when renal function, and thus the rate of metabolite elimination, is changing.

The quinidine compounds commercially available contain a variable percent of dihydroquinidine. This is not a metabolite but a compound very similar to quinidine, difficult to separate since it differs only by a molecular mass of 2 and is formed by hydrogen saturation of the quinidine double bond. Although there are very few studies of this compound, it appears very similar to quinidine in cardiac activity and apparent metabolism. The standard assay techniques readily measure dihydroquinidine and, in consideration of clinical use, it does not appear necessary for the clinicians to need independent assay of this compound.

Therapeutic concentrations are based upon determinations on samples obtained immediately before the next dose. For quinidine the dosing interval is usually 6 hours and sampling at this time provides a "predose" serum level. If it becomes necessary to determine the half-life ($t_{1/2}$), this can be easily done by collection of at least three timed specimens 30-60 minutes apart. These results are displayed as a log-concentration versus time plot and the $t_{1/2}$ determined directly. A somewhat more erudite means would divide 0.693 by the slope of the plotted regression line (the rate constant of elimination). If the dose has been administered orally, specimen collection should be delayed for 2-3 hours so as to allow for gastrointestinal absorption. If this is not taken into consideration the apparent quinidine $t_{1/2}$ will be longer due to continued addition of absorbed quinidine to systemic circulation.

## Clinical Pharmacology

Quinidine is used in the clinical management of both atrial and ventricular arrhythmias. It is most commonly used to atrial fibrillation, atrial flutter, and ventricular premature beats, including ventricular tachycardia. Although it is generally used to suppress the ventricular arrhythmias, quinidine also has been used to pharmacologically cardiovert both atrial fibrillation and flutter, and then to suppress their recurrence.

When quinidine is used in the treatment of atrial arrhythmias it is usually given after digitalis or propranolol, to avoid the "paradoxical" response described above, which may accelerate the ventricular response. Digitalis remains the classical agent used with quinidine in the treatment of atrial arrhythmias, and the clinician may consider having digoxin measured in serum also.

The usual adult dosage of quinidine sulfate is 800 to 3000 mg per day, given in four equally divided doses. It should be remembered that the active component of the quinidine molecule is the "base" form of the drug, which represents about 83% of the molecular mass for quinidine sulfate. Most laboratories report the plasma or serum concentration in terms of the base. These considerations become important if the physician elects to switch from one salt form to another. For example, if a patient is taking 800 mg of quinidine sulfate per day and is switched to 800 mg of quinidine gluconate (approximately 62% quinidine base) per day, the patient would be receiving nearly 20% less quinidine base. The laboratory may not know which quinidine salt is being used, so it is important for the prescribing physician to be familiar with these aspects of quinidine therapy.

Quinidine is well absorbed after oral administration and reaches peak concentrations in the blood within 60-90 min. Its elimination half-life averages 6 h. The major route of quinidine detoxification appears to be through ring hydroxylation and glucuronide formation. This metabolite is excreted through the kidney. Only about 10% of the parent compound may appear unchanged in the urine.

Quinidine may be administered parenterally, but this should be done cautiously. In addition to its cardiac effects, quinidine also produces peripheral vasodilation. This effect appears to be at least partly mediated through alpha-adrenergic blockade and severe hypotension may result. Thus, if it is necessary to use quinidine parenterally, blood pressure should be carefully monitored and fluids and vasopressors should be ready for use in the event of hypotension. While quinidine has some negative inotropic effect on the heart, the major contribution to the hypotension is probably related to its peripheral vascular effects.

Despite the potential for side effects, quinidine stands as one of the most effective agents available in the treatment of cardiac arrhythmias. The physician using quinidine can do so quite safely when proper attention is given to the pharmacology of this drug and its potential for drug-drug interaction.

## References

1. Kessler, K.M., Lowenthal, D.T., et al., Quinidine elimination in patients with congestive heart failure or poor renal function. *N. Engl. J. Med.* **290**, 706-709 (1974).

2. Ueda, C.T., Williamson, B.J., et al., Absolute quinidine bioavailability. *Clin. Pharmacol. Therap.* **20**, 260-265, (1975).

3. Wosilait, W.D., A theoretical analysis of the distribution of quinidine in the plasma: The relationship between protein binding and therapeutic drug levels. *Res. Commun. Clin. Pathol. Pharmacol.* **12**, 147-154, (1975).

4. Hoffman, B.F., Rosen, M.R., et al., Electrophysiology and pharmacology of cardiac arrhythmias VII. Cardiac effects of quinidine and procainamide. *Am. Heart J.* **89**, 804-808 (1975).

# 27

# Disopyramide: Two Case Histories

Edward W. Bermes, Jr., Ph.D.
Leonas G. Bekeris, M.D.

Disopyramide is an effective type I antiarrhythmic agent that, although structurally different from quinidine, elicits similar qualitative, electro-physiologic, and electrocardiographic responses, and is usually better tolerated than this drug. It was reported for the first time in 1962, was approved by the Food and Drug Administration in 1978, and since then has gained wide acceptance in the United States.

## Case 1

A 52-year-old white man was admitted to the hospital with a prolonged history of atrial fibrillation. During the last 18 months he had been hospitalized at least five times for his arrhythmia, which had been refractory to cardioversion, usually reappearing several days after discharge. For the last eight to nine months the patient had suffered several syncopal episodes, apparently associated with the arrhythmia, and at the time of his admission he was taking diazide, digoxin (0.25 mg/day), disopyramide phosphate (150 mg every 6 h), allopurinol, phenylbutazone and theophylline.

Physical examination of this markedly obese (141 kg) man showed arrhythmia and moderate hypertension. An electrocardiogram confirmed the presence of atrial fibrillation with a fast ventricular response of 120 to 150 per minute. Results of routine laboratory tests were within normal limits.

Blood samples were drawn for assay of digoxin and disopyramide, with the following results: digoxin: 0.5 $\mu$g/L (therapeutic range 0.9 - 2.0 $\mu$g/L), disopyramide: 1.6 mg/L (therapeutic range 2-5 mg/L).

In view of these results, non-compliance was suspected and all medications were stopped. The patient was placed on telemetry and was given intravenous digoxin. After a total of 1 mg injected over 24 hours he converted to normal sinus rhythm. At this time it was decided not to restart the patient on disopyramide and he was discharged on a daily dose of 0.375 mg of digoxin, plus diazide, Inderal and allopurinol.

*Dr. Bermes is Professor, Departments of Pathology and Biochemistry and Director of Clinical Chemistry, and Dr. Berkeris is Assistant Professor, Department of Pathology and Clinical Pathologist, Loyola University Medical Center, Maywood, IL 60153.*

Several weeks after discharge the patient was found to be again in atrial fibrillation. The dosage of digoxin and Inderal were adjusted during visits to the outpatient clinic, but no improvement was observed. Two months after discharge, although he was supposed to be taking 0.25 mg of digoxin twice a day, serum concentrations of digoxin were below therapeutic range (0.7 mg/L).

The patient was rehospitalized and chemical cardioversion was obtained again in less than 24 hours.

## Case 2

This 54-year-old white man was hospitalized for aorto-coronary bypass surgery. He had been in relatively good health until a month before this admission, when he suffered an acute myocardial infarction. Cardiac catheterization revealed severe blockage of the left anterior coronary artery and its branches.

Results of physical examination at the time of admission were unremarkable, except for moderate diastolic hypertension. The electrocardiogram showed sinus bradycardia with nonspecific S-T segment abnormalities. Results of routine laboratory tests were within normal limits.

A triple aorto-coronary bypass was performed. It was complicated by atrioventricular blocks, atrial arrhythmias, and a small peri-operative myocardial infarction, which was confirmed by electrocardiogram, serial enzyme determinations, and nuclear medicine studies.

Shortly after surgery, he developed supraventricular tachycardia which responded adequately to digitalization, but during the following four days occasional premature atrial contractions (PAC's) and premature ventricular contractions (PVC's) were recorded. Six days after surgery, atrial bigeminy was observed and the patient was placed on quinidine.

While on a low dose of quinidine, he developed marked diarrhea and increase in PVC's. At this stage, he was switched to disopyramide phosphate; an initial dose of 300 mg was administered, followed by 150 mg every 6 h, as recommended by the manufacturer. Twenty-four hours later, PVC's were still frequent, with runs of bigeminy and aberrant conduction.

Because it was believed that, in spite of the arrhythmia, the ventricular function was good, the dose of

# DISOPYRAMIDE PROFILE

## (NORPACE)

**Generic name**  Disopyramide
**Chemical name**  4-(Diisopropylamino)-2-phenyl-2-(2-pyridyl)butyramide
**Chemical structure**

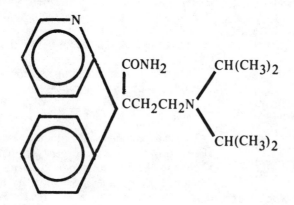

**Trade name(s)**  Norpace (Searle, U.S.)
                   Rhythmodan (Roussel, Europe)
**Molecular mass**  339.47
**Melting point, °C**  94.5 - 95
**Solubility in H$_2$O**  1 g/L
**pKa**  8.34
**Dose absorption:**
   **Time to peak plasma concn, h**  0.5 - 3.0

   **% dose absorbed**  80
**Protein binding:**
   **% bound**  10-80  (Concn. dependent)
   **% free**  20-90
**Volume distribution**  0.8 L/kg

| **Urinary excretion, % daily dose** | % | Active | Detected in blood |
|---|---|---|---|
| Unchanged | 50-55 | yes | yes |
| N-desisopropyl disopyramide | 20-30 | yes | yes |

|  | Adults | Children |
|---|---|---|
| **Recommended dose** | 8.6 mg/kg/d | N/A |
| **Effective concns.** | 2-5 mg/L | N/A |
| **Toxic concns.** | >7 mg/L | N/A |
| **Time to steady state, h** | 25-30 | N/A |

disopyramide was increased to 300 mg every 6 h. By the evening of the same day the arrhythmias had disappeared, eventually allowing the patient to be discharged from the Intensive Care Unit.

Serum sampled 36 h after the change in dose contained 5.3 mg of disopyramide per liter. The patient continued to improve and was discharged 11 days after surgery, free of arrhythmia, on 300 mg of disopyramide phosphate every 6 h, plus digoxin, Inderal, and prednisone.

### Discussion of the Cases

Since the mean disopyramide concentration in responders and non-responders is identical, some believe the only reason to measure the drug in serum is to confirm compliance (Pennock). This is illustrated by our first case, where low concentrations of both digoxin and disopyramide made the cardiologist suspect that the patient was not taking the drugs as instructed, and the therapeutic strategy was changed with fast and adequate temporary responses.

Disopyramide is a promising agent for prophylaxis of arrhythmias associated with acute myocardial infarction. Long-term oral therapy for refractory ventricular arrhythmias may require larger doses of disopyramide (up to 300 mg every 6 h), which increase the incidence of side effects.

The second case illustrates a patient with intolerance to quinidine, who needs high doses of disopyramide, but on whom any drug toxicity could have devastating effects during his stormy postoperative period. The results obtained, after waiting an adequate time for the drug to reach a steady state, allowed the cardiologist to continue a treatment, which had proved to be effective.

### Pharmacology and Pharmacodynamics

Disopyramide is an effective antiarrhythmic agent. It seems to be a promising agent in the treatment of acute and chronic ventricular and atrial arrhythmia of various etiologies, in the prophylaxis of arrhythmias associated with acute myocardial infarction, and in preventing recurrence of atrial fibrillations.

As with other antiarrhythmic drugs, the mechanism of action of disopyramide is not entirely understood. Transmembrane action potential studies in animals have shown that it decreases the rate of diastolic depolarization in cells with augmented automaticity, decreases the upstroke velocity, and increases the action potential duration of normal cardiac cells.

Disopyramide and its metabolites have anticholinergic activity, which for disopyramide is about 1200-fold less than atropine, while the N-mono-dealkylated metabolite is about 50-fold less active than atropine.

After oral administration, 80% of the oral dose is absorbed, reaching peak plasma concentrations by 0.5 to 3 h. Disopyramide does not undergo significant hepatic first-pass metabolism. The degree of protein binding shows wide variation between patients and is concentration dependent, with an increased proportion of unbound drug at higher total drug concentration in plasma.

Studies in rats with radiolabeled disopyramide showed wide distribution to most organs, except the central nervous system. The concentration in the myocardium was similar to that in the plasma, but fat, liver, and spleen contained 7-15 times the radioactivity found in plasma. Conceivably, in obese patients, a large part of the dose would be "lost" in the adipose tissue. Thus, determination of disopyramide in such patients not only helps assure that the patient has ingested the drug, but also helps in adjusting the dosage so that therapeutic circulating concentrations are obtained before the drug is considered ineffective. Animal studies also show that the drug transfers readily to placenta and breast milk.

The major metabolic pathway of disopyramide is via N-dealkylation to form N-desisopropyl disopyramide, which has some antiarrhythmic activity. About 55% of a single dose is excreted unchanged in the urine independently of urine flow and urinary pH, 25% appears as the N-dealkylated metabolite, and 10% as minor metabolites. The remaining drug is excreted in the feces.

The mean elimination half life is 8.9 h. This time is markedly increased in patients with renal dysfunction and may be prolonged during ventricular tachycardia and in the presence of ventricular ectopic beats.

Concentrations in plasma between 2 and 7.4 mg/L control arrhythmias; those exceeding 7 mg/L are considered toxic.

### Drug Interactions

Intravenous administration of disopyramide along with a β-blocker (acetabutol) significantly increases the atrioventricular node and His-Purkinje conduction times. Administration of this combination to patients with coronary artery disease also produces a more profound negative inotropic effect than would have been expected with either drug alone.

Disopyramide has been reported to potentiate the action of warfarin. The mechanism of this action is unknown; in vitro enzyme induction studies did not significantly affect the metabolism of bishydroxycoumarin. In human volunteers there is no evidence of stimulation of hepatic microsomal drug-metabolizing enzymes.

Other antiarrhythmic drugs (e.g., quinidine, procainamide, lidocaine, propranolol) have occasionally been used concurrently with disopyramide, but no specific drug interaction studies have been conducted. Such use may produce serious negative inotropic effects or may excessively prolong conduction.

## Side Effects and Toxicity

Disopyramide's adverse reactions are usually due to the anticholinergic properties of the drug. Urinary retention, although uncommon (2%), is the most serious effect, but dry mouth (40%), urinary hesitancy (10-20%), constipation, blurred vision, dry nose, eyes, or throat, urinary frequency, nausea and vomiting, and other reactions associated with the drug's atropinic activity have been reported.

Severe hypotension after disopyramide has been observed in patients with primary cardiomyopathy or inadequately compensated congestive heart failure. Cardiac decompensation may worsen in patients with poorly compensated or uncompensated heart failure, or who have a history of heart failure. This drug should not be administered to these patients unless there is evidence that the heart failure is secondary to arrhythmia. Cardiac failure has also occurred in patients without previous history of decompensation who are on long-term oral disopyramide treatment.

Less common side effects include various situations ranging from severe allergic reactions to neurologic and psychiatric complications.

In several cases of documented self-inflicted overdosage, the individuals presented with early loss of conciousness after an apneic episode. There was an initial response to resuscitation and antiarrhythmic therapy, followed by rapid deterioration complicated by cardiac arrhythmias and loss of spontaneous respiration.

No specific antidote for disopyramide has been identified. Treatment of overdosage is largely supportive and may include administration of isoproterenol, dopamine, hemoperfusion with charcoal, hemodialysis, intra-aortic balloon counterpulsation and mechanically assisted respiration. In vitro studies have demonstrated good dialyzability for disopyramide.

Gas-liquid chromatography and "high-pressure" liquid chromatography are used to determine disopyramide in serum. A successful liquid-chromatographic method involves use of p-chlorodisopyramide as an internal standard and chloroform to extract the drug from serum. The residue after evaporation of the extract is dissolved in methanol and a portion is injected into a liquid chromatographic column with an absorbance detector at 254 mn and C18 (P/N 27324) reversed phase column. A new method using EMIT technology is also available now for the determination of disopyramide. If analysis cannot be performed within 24 h, the specimen should be stored at -20°C.

## References

Heel, R.C., Brogden, R.N., Speight, T.M., and Avery, G.S., Disopyramide: A review of its pharmacological properties and therapeutic use in treating cardiac arrhythmias. *Drugs* **15**, 331-368 (1978).

Koch-Weser, J., Disopyramide. *N. Engl. J. Med.* **300**, 957-960 (1979).

Ankier, S.I., Carmichael, D.J.S., and Kider, P.H. Disopyramide - a review. *Scot. Med. J.* **300**, 957-960 (1977).

Anderson, J.L., Harrison, D.C., Meffin, P.J., and Winkle, R.A., Antiarrhythmic drugs: Clinical pharmacology and therapy uses. *Drugs* **15**, 271-309 (1978).

Pennock, R.S., How useful are serum levels of cardiac drugs? *Am. Fam. Physician* **17**, 194-196 (1978).

Podrid, P.J., Schoenberger, A., and Lown, B., Congestive heart failure caused by oral disopyramide, *N. Engl. J. Med.* **302**, 614-617 (1980).

Hayler, A.M., Holt, D.W., and Volans, G.N., Fatal overdosage with disopyramide. *Lancet* **1**, 968-9 (May 1978).

Hutsell, T.C., and Stachelski, S.J., Determination of disopyramide and its mono-*N*-dealkylated metabolite in blood serum and urine. *J. Chromatog.* **106**, 151-158 (1975).

Meffin, P.J., Harapat, S.R., and Harrison, D.C., High pressure liquid chromatographic analysis of drugs in biological fluids. III. Analyis of disopyramide and its mono-*N*-dealkylated metabolite in plasma and urine. *J. Chromatog.* **123**, 503-510 (1977).

# 28

# Propranolol: Pharmacokinetics and Pharmacology

C.E. Pippenger, Ph.D.

Propanolol is a beta-adrenergic receptor blocking agent. It is not specific for cardiac tissue, but affects a wide variety of organs. It is the most thoroughly studied of the beta blockers and consequently more pharmocokinetic information is available on propranolol than other beta blockers.

## Pharmacology

Propranolol elicits several pharmacological effects. Sinus bradycardia are produced by the blocking of beta-adernergic receptors. The A-V nodal transmission, stimulated by beta receptors, is slowed. The rate of rise in membrane potential is decreased, membrane responsiveness depressed and decremental conduction in the His-Purkinje is blocked. These effects account for propranolol's antiarrhythmic properties. Cardiac sympathetic nerve stimulation of circulating catecholamines is also prevented by propanolol. This beta blockade of the positive inotropic and chronotropic actions and suppression of renin release by the kidneys render propranolol useful as a antihypertensive drug. Propranolol will produce hemodynamic effects such as lower cardiac output, decreased mean arterial blood flow, depressed ventricular stroke work and maximal oxygen uptake.

Propranolol therapy is indicated in symptomatic sinus tachycardia associated with pheochromocytoma or thyrotoxicosis where its effect will decrease the sinus rate; in paroxysmal atrial flutter or atrial fibrillation to slow the A-V node; in supraventricular and ventricular arrhythmias associated with digitalis intoxication also to slow A-V nodal transmission; and in hypertension to decrease cardiac output without altering total peripheral resistance. Propranolol is the only beta blocker which will not alter total peripheral resistance.

The side effects commonly associated with propranolol are related to its beta-adernergic blocking

---

*Dr. Pippenger is an Assistant Professor of Neuropharmacology in the Department of Neurology at the College of Physicians and Surgeons of Columbia University in New York.*

---

properties. Potentially severe but infrequent side effects include cardiac depression, heart failure, cardiac conduction disturbances, and bronchial constriction. The most commonly encountered side effects of propranolol are nausea, vomiting, diarrhea, insomnia, and weakness.

## Pharmacokinetics

When administered orally plasma concentrations of propranolol are significantly lower than from intravenous administration. This occurs with drugs which are completely absorbed by the gastrointestinal tract and is referred to as the first pass effect. When a drug is absorbed from the gastrointestinal tract it enters the venous circulation and is transported via the hepatic portal system directly to the liver where it is rapidly metabolized. When the drug reaches the systemic circulation via gastrointestinal absorption it appears as metabolites. The level of propranolol in plasma when administered orally may be only 10-25% of the total dose; however, the major metabolite of propranolol, 4-hydroxypropranolol, also displays beta blockade. Therefore, oral administration of propranolol is just as effective as intravenous administration. And it may be established that routine monitoring of 4-hydroxypropranolol might be clinically significant.

Less than 1% of propranolol is excreted unchanged in urine; 1-4% in feces. The remainder (84-92%) is excreted as metabolites. Twelve metabolites, including the active beta blocker 4-hydroxypropanolol, have been identified: 1) *N*-desisopropyl propanolol; 2) a proposed aldehyde intermediate; 3) propanolol glycol; 40 naphthoxyl acetic acid; 5) naphthoxy hydroxy acetic acid; 6) 4-hydroxypropanolol glycol; 7) alpha-naphthol; 8) 1,4-dihydroxy-naphthalene; 9) isopropylamine; 10) 4-hydroxy-*N*-desisopropylpropanolol; 11) 4-hydroxynaphthoxyl acetic acid.

## Concentrations and Effects

Peak levels of propranolol are usually observed 60-120 minutes after oral administration. There is a tendency towards higher peak concentrations with higher dosages, but peak levels do not appear to be strictly dose related. There may be a 20- to 30-fold difference in the peak plasma levels of propranolol in a group of patients who are receiving the same ng/kg dose. There is a linear relationship between dose and plasma concentration for an individual patient, however. Either pharmacogenetic or drug absorption patterns play a major role in determining the individual's observed steady state propranolol plasma concentrations.

There appears to be no correlation between the toxic effects of propranolol and plasma concentration; however, the toxic effects have not been rigidly established. Since propranolol is highly protein bound (90-96%) pharmacologic effects may correlate more closely with free rather than total plasma concentration. Therefore, particular care should be taken in the interpretation of total plasma propranolol concentrations in uremic patients or patients with low serum albumin levels (geriatric patients). Concomitant drug therapy can also precipitate undesirable side effects.

The relationships between propranolol plasma concentrations and beta-adrenergic blockade are well documented. Plasma levels of 50-100 ng/mL are effective in inhibiting exercise tachycardia, and suppressing ventricular ectopic beats: 20 ng/mL will cause a complete suppression of PAF; 30-60 ng/mL are required for a significant reduction of heart rate; and 100 ng/mL are required to treat high to moderately severe hypertension.

Propranolol is a widely utilized antiarrhythmic agent in pediatrics. While the number of clinical pediatric studies with pharmacokinetic data is limited, the clearance and half-life of propranolol in children (1.5-4 h) is faster than in adults (4-6 h).

## Conclusions

The clinical pharmacokinetics and the correlation between plasma concentration and therapeutic effect of propranolol are just now becoming established. At the present time propranolol monitoring is done primarily by research laboratories studying various aspects of propranolol clinical pharmacology. But over the next two to three years monitoring of propranolol concentrations will probably become routine as the technologies become available. Propranolol can be dosed empirically since there are clear-cut physiological guidelines to the effectiveness of the agent for the abolishment of an arrhythmia or a

### PROPRANOLOL PROFILE

| | |
|---|---|
| Generic name: | Propranolol, Inderol |
| Chemical name: | 1-(Isopropylamino-3-Cl-naphthyl-oxy)-2-propanol |
| Chemical structure: | |

$$O-CH_2-CH-CH_2-NH-CH-(CH_3)_2$$
$$\quad\quad\quad |$$
$$\quad\quad\quad OH$$

| | |
|---|---|
| Molecular weight: | 259.34 |
| Melting point, °C: | 163-164 |
| Solubility in water, mg/mL: | very soluble |
| $pK_a$: | 9.45 |
| Dose absorption— | |
| time to peak plasma conc., h: | 1-2 |
| percentage dose absorbed: | 100 |
| Protein binding— | |
| percentage bound: | 90-96 |
| percentage free: | 4-10 |
| Tissue distribution, $V_d$, L/kg: | 3.6-4.6 |

| Urinary excretion, % daily dose— | | Active | Detectable in Blood |
|---|---|---|---|
| as unchanged drug: | 1 | yes | yes |
| as 4 hydroxypropranolol and others: | 84-92 | yes | yes |

| Recommended dose, mg/kg/d: | | Adults | Children |
|---|---|---|---|
| | Oral | 1-2 | 1-2 |
| | IV | 0.15/6 h | |

| | Adults | Children |
|---|---|---|
| Half-life, h: | 4-6 | 1.5-4 |
| Time to steady state, h: | 48 | 48 |
| Effective levels, ng/mL: | 50-100 | 50-100 |
| Toxic levels, $\mu$g/mL: | variable | variable |

decrease in blood pressure. But since propranolol exhibits wide individual variability in steady state concentrations on fixed dosage regimens, concentrations should be routinely monitored once the optimal therapeutic concentrations have been established, to check on compliance, in the development of an associated disease state, or other change in the patient's clinical status. The clinical utility of propranolol monitoring will be in this rapid plasma level assessment and consequent adjustments in individual dosage regimens. The value of rapid individualization of drug therapy will assure propranolol as one of the routinely monitored antiarrhythmic agents.

### References

Avery, G.S., *Drug Treatment—Principles and Practice of Clinical Pharmacology and Therapeutics,* Adis Press, Sydney, 1976.

Melmon, K.L. and Morrelli, H.F. (Ed) *Clinical Pharmacology—Basic Principles in Therapeutics* (second edition) Little, Brown and Company, Boston, 1978.

Morselli, P. (Ed) *Drug Disposition During Development: An Overview,* Spectrum Publications, Inc. New York, 1977.

# III. Antimicrobial Drugs

# 29

# How the Clinician Chooses an Antibiotic

Margan J. Chang, M.D.

Antibiotic choice is the result of many complex decisions which take place in the frontal lobes of the clinician caring for the patient. Many people are vitally interested in the result of this complex decision-making process: these include the patient himself, the physician who makes the decision, the nurses, the pharmacist, the clinical laboratories, and the pharmaceutical companies and their representatives. The patient's interest is in a cure, and secondarily he desires no side effects relating to the proposed antibiotic. The physician making the antibiotic choice also desires to cure the patient of his presumed infectious disease. Further, he hopes for minimal side effects, primarily for the sake of the patient but also for the benefit of his malpractice insurance carrier. The nurses are interested primarily in the route and ease of administration of the chosen drug, whereas the pharmacist is concerned with the drug's availability, cost, concentration, and amenability to unit dosing. The clinical laboratory's involvement with antibiotic choice revolves around the ability to monitor therapeutic (and occasionally toxic) drug concentrations as well as other laboratory abnormalities associated with administration of the drug. The pharmaceutical company is interested in the antibiotic choice made, principally from the economic point of view.

Pressures from each of these sources influence the physician's choice of antibiotic. Some of these pressures are appropriate; others are not. Some pressures are well thought out and considered; others exert their influence subconsciously. It is my intent to examine some of the factors that influence the antibiotic choice. It is appropriate, therefore, to address first the magnitude of antibiotic use.

## Magnitude of Antibiotic Use

Collection of data on the number of prescriptions dispensed (compiled from the National Prescription Audit) and the quantity of injectable antibiotics

Dr. Chang is Attending in Infectious Diseases, and Associate Director, Clinical Microbiology and Serology at Children's Hospital National Medical Center, Washington, D.C. and Assistant Professor, Department of Child Health and Development, The George Washington University School of Medicine and Health Sciences, Washington, D.C.

certified by the FDA provides a relatively simple way of measuring antibiotic use in the United States. In 1977, 43 million prescriptions for tetracycline were dispensed by pharmacies across the United States. Thirty-three million were dispensed for erythromycin and 32 million for ampicillin. In the same year, 41 million doses of cephalosporins and 24 million doses of gentamicin were certified by the FDA for use in hospitals across the country. (1)

Antibiotic use is extensive at most hospitals and accounts for a significant proportion of total pharmacy costs. (2) Antibiotics are administered to between 23 and 38% of hospitalized patients; these drugs represent 20-35% of total pharmacy costs. The use of these drugs has increased significantly in recent years. Craig et al (2) reviewed the cost and total grams of antibiotics used in 19 hospitals (10 community hospitals and 9 VA hospitals) throughout the United States. In their study the mean hospital antibiotic cost was $1.03 per patient day, with considerable variation from hospital to hospital. The total cost of antibiotic agents at these 19 hospitals amounted to $2,158,530 or 29% of total pharmacy drug costs.

Kass (3) conducted a study of antibiotics used in 20 general hospitals in Pennsylvania. He found that 28% of the patients reviewed in the study received at least one antibiotic during their hospitalization. In 60% of the patients, the drugs were given for the treatment of infectious disease; in 30% they were given for prophylaxis of a surgical or non-surgical procedure. When antibiotics were given for prophylaxis of surgical procedures, they were given for more than 48 hours in 60% of cases, despite the fact that prophylaxis is generally felt to be ineffective after 48 h. Kass estimated that discontinuing prophylaxis 48 hours after a surgical procedure would decrease all antibiotic use by about 20% and would result in a nationwide saving of $100 million annually.

Thus it is apparent that the magnitude of antibiotic use is enormous. Furthermore, it is clear that patterns of antibiotic choice are very significant, not only from the perspective of the patient, nurse, the doctor, and the pharmacist, but also from the point of view of health care planners and government funding agencies. Patterns of antibiotic use will come under scrutiny. It is to be hoped that this will be through a process of judicious peer review; if not accomplished, it is likely to happen through pressure from a federal regulatory agency.

## Factors Influencing the Clinician in His Choice of Antibiotic

The factors influencing the clinician in his choice of antibiotics fall into two categories: appropriate and inappropriate. Appropriateness is determined primarily by consensus among the infectious disease community. Generally this subspecialty group has the greatest experience with drug efficacy and pharmacokinetics and is expected to be current with regard to newer antibiotics. Controversies do occasionally arise within this community; they are virtually always resolved with time or so trivial as to be of no consequence to patient or doctor.

## Appropriate Factors

*The nature of the suspected or proven infectious disease.* The nature of the suspected or proven infectious disease is probably the most important factor governing the appropriate choice of an antibiotic. The clinician must mentally answer the following questions sequentially: "Is this proven or suspected infection bacterial or likely to be bacterial in etiology?" If the answer to this question is yes, then antibiotic therapy may be indicated. If the answer is no, then no antibiotic is generally indicated. (*Pneumocystis carinii* infection is a protozoan infection that responds to the commonly used antibiotic trimethoprim-sulfamethoxazole. Hence this infection is an exception.) Antibiotics are *not* indicated in the treatment of common viral infections.

If the answer to the question is "yes, this infection is likely to be bacterial in origin," then the clinician asks the next mental question, "Which bacterial organisms are likely to cause the disease entity which I wish to treat?" If the clinician is unable to answer this question, he must search the textbooks or literature for this information. "Broad spectrum" antibiotic coverage should not be administered in a decerebrate fashion. Rarely, "broad spectrum" coverage is administered after the possible etiologic agents have been carefully considered and found to be so diverse in their collective antibiotic sensitivities as to justify the administration of broad antibiotic coverage. Blind "broad spectrum coverage" is never justified with the possible exception of the patient whose disease process is unknown and who appears to be near death.

If an infectious process is suspected but not yet proven, the clinician must ask himself, "What cultures should I obtain to determine the precise nature of the bacterial infection?" If the clinician fails to ask himself this question, fails to obtain appropriate cultures, and initiates antibiotic coverage on the basis of his conjecture regarding etiology, he is headed for difficulty. A situation such as that which follows occurs all too commonly.

Patient X is admitted to the hospital with a fever and is believed to be suffering from disease Y. He is placed on antibiotics A and B, one of which is invariably a cephalosporin. No cultures are obtained. Seven days later he is still spiking fevers and has developed a side effect, possibly from antibiotic B. In addition he has had a tube placed in every orifice, has a phlebitis from his IV line, a urinary tract infection from his indwelling Foley catheter, and is growing mixed bacterial and fungal flora from his endotracheal tube. At this point the following questions are asked:

1. Was patient X suffering from disease Y in the first place?
2. What was the etiology of disease Y?
3. Why is patient X still febrile?
4. Is the side effect from which patient is suffering due to antibiotic A, B, or to the other invasive procedures which patient X has suffered in the hospital?
5. Is his fever from the phlebitis?
6. What is the etiology of his urinary tract infection? (By now urine cultures have been obtained and they are negative on antibiotics A B).
7. What is the significance of the mixed bacterial and fungal flora in his endotracheal tube?
8. What antibiotics are indicated now?

It is apparent that answering these questions is now very difficult and that had cultures been obtained initially many of these questions would not have arisen. Appropriate cultures are essential *before* choosing an antibiotic!

After appropriate cultures have been obtained and are positive for a bacterial agent, antibiotic therapy may need to be changed, depending upon the specific sensitivity pattern of the bacterium isolated. Antibiotic sensitivities whether by the Kirby-Bauer method or minimum inhibitory concentration (MIC) method must be checked when they become available.

*The age and physiological state of the patient.* The age of the patient is a major factor to consider in choosing an antibiotic. For example, gastric pH is higher in children under three years of age and the **prevalence of achlorhydria increases with advancing** age. Oral absorption of some antibiotics, especially penicillins, is enhanced by achlorhydria or high gastric pH.

Tetracyclines are contraindicated in children younger than seven or eight years because they produce grey-brown staining of the teeth; they may be used if otherwise indicated in older children when crown formation of the permanent teeth has already taken place.

Elderly patients are more at risk for adverse effects of a variety of antibiotics. Hepatotoxicity associated with isoniazid (INH) administration clearly increases with age. Hepatotoxicity due to INH is rare in patients under 20 years of age but the incidence rises to 2.3% in patients over 50 who ingest INH (4).

Many nephrotoxic or ototoxic effects of antibiotics occur with increased frequency among the elderly. Antibiotics included in this category are the cephalosporins, colistin, and the aminoglycosides.

Finally, hypersensitivity reactions are more common among the aged, due primarily to a greater likelihood of prior exposure to the offending antibiotic.

At the opposite end of the age spectrum, many drugs cannot be used or must be used with extreme care in the neonate. Sulfonamides compete with bilirubin for binding sites on serum albumin. When given to neonates, sulfonamides increase the concentration of unbound bilirubin in the serum, placing the child at risk for kernicterus. For this reason sulfonamides must not be given to neonates.

Renal and hepatic function are often unpredictably immature in neonates. Drugs such as the penicillins and the aminoglycosides that are cleared through the kidney cannot be administered to neonates in standard pediatric dose but the dosage must be reduced or the dosage intervals extended, to accommodate immature renal function.

Chloramphenicol is metabolized in the liver by conjugation to the glucuronide form. In the neonate, hepatic glucuronyltransferase is relatively deficient. Hence unconjugated chloramphenicol may accumulate, reach toxic concentrations, and may produce the "gray baby" syndrome of infancy, a syndrome characterized by the sudden onset of shock, cardiovascular collapse, and death. If it is necessary to administer this drug to the neonate, the dosage must be adjusted according to the child's age and degree of prematurity.

Not only is age a significant factor in choosing an antibiotic but the patient's physiological state is equally important. If the patient who is to receive the antibiotic is pregnant, the potential of the proposed antibiotic for teratogenicity must be assessed. If the patient who is to receive the antibiotic is lactating, the potential for the appearance in the breast milk of the antibiotic or its metabolites must be assessed. Other physiological factors that may significantly alter the choice of an antibiotic include the history of a previous drug reaction, the presence of glucose-6-phosphate dehydrogenase deficiency, an underlying chronic or immunodeficiency disease, chronic steroid therapy, the presence of neutropenia, diabetes, or shock, or any known compromise in renal or hepatic function.

compromise in renal or hepatic function.

*Adverse effects of antibiotics: the risk-benefit analysis.* No antibiotic is without adverse effects. The clinician choosing an antibiotic must consider the question; "Do the risks that may be incurred by use of this antibiotic outweigh the risk to the patient of not using it?" He must also mentally answer the question, "Is there another, equally efficacious antibiotic whose potential side effects are less serious?" Thus the risk of each drug must be weighed against the risks of the patient's disease and also against other equally efficacious antibiotics. Certain antibiotics are notorious for their adverse effects. Chloramphenicol is, in the words of Shulman (5) an "exasperatingly good" antibiotic, "exasperating" because of the ominous potential (1:24000-1:200000) for irreversible bone marrow aplasia unrelated to dose, duration of therapy, or route of administration (6) and "good" because of its excellent spectrum of bacterial susceptibility and its superb ability to diffuse rapidly throughout the body, achieving respectable concentrations in liver, kidney, blood, brain, CSF, saliva, semen, and the eye.

Aminoglycoside antibiotics, including kanamycin, gentamicin, tobramycin, and amikacin, are a family of antibiotics whose use must be weighed carefully against their adverse effects. The nephrotoxicity and ototoxicity of these drugs are dose-related and cumulative. The frequency of gentamicin nephrotoxicity ranges from 2 to 10%. The clinical prevalence of gentamicin ototoxicity is 2 to 3%. The rates of both nephrotoxicity and ototoxicity are increased in groups of high risk patients, particularly those with pre-existing renal impairment. (7) Unfortunately, the patients who are most likely to need aminoglycoside antibiotic therapy are the very patients most likely to have disease states that predispose them to aminoglycoside toxicity. Aminoglycoside antibiotics are among the most commonly used antibiotics in the hospitalized population, yet their therapeutic index is among the narrowest of any antibiotics commonly in use.

Clindamycin is another excellent example of an antibiotic whose efficacy and risks must be carefully assessed. If one were treating staphylococcal sepsis in an elderly patient one could choose either a semi-synthetic penicillin such as oxacillin or methicillin, or clindamycin, a drug with excellent antistaphylococcal efficacy. In this example clindamycin would not be an appropriate choice. Clindamycin is associated with a 2 to 10% incidence of psuedomembranous colitis, a potentially life threatening complication which occurs more commonly in the older patient (8,9). On the other hand a semi-synthetic penicillin carrying the remote risk (1 in 50,000) of death due to anaphylaxis and a modest incidence of reversible nephrotoxicity, would be the drug of choice (*10*).

*Pharmacokinetic considerations.* The pharmacokinetics of an antibiotic refers to the absorption, the distribution of the drug among various body tissues, the excretion of the drug, and the various rates at which these all take place. In choosing an antibiotic appropriately, the clinician does not need to be aware of the pharmacokinetic intricacies of all the antibiotics he contemplates using. On the other hand, he should be aware of a few basic facts that will allow him to choose more wisely.

1. Some antibiotics are absorbed poorly or not at all by the oral route. These include the aminoglycosides (kanamycin, gentamicin, tobramycin, neomycin) and vancomycin. For this reason these antibiotics are not usually given by the oral route to treat systemic infection.

2. Some antibiotics do not penetrate the central nervous system well, despite administration by the intravenous route. These include the entire family of traditional cephalosporins, clindamycin, and the aminoglycosides. Appropriate antibiotics for the treatment of central nervous system infection include the penicillins and chloramphenicol. The penetration of penicillins into the central nervous system ranges between 5-18% of concomitant serum concentrations, depending on the degree of inflammation of the meninges (*11*). Chloramphenicol concentrations in the cerebrospinal fluid are approximately 50% of concomitant serum, and are independent of meningeal inflammation (*6*).

3. Antibiotics that are excreted by the kidneys, penicillins, aminoglycosides, cephalosporins, sulfonamides, tetracyclines, vancomycin, and rifampin are concentrated manyfold in the urine, implying that when the target organism is in the urine, large doses of antibiotic are not necessary to eradicate the organism.

4. As already mentioned, chloramphenicol penetrates most tissues in therapeutic amounts with one outstanding exception. In bile, most of the drug is conjugated and hence inactive, thus chloramphenicol is not an optimal drug for use in treating biliary tract infections.

5. Current dosage schedules for common antibiotics are arrived at empirically. The in vitro activity of the drug against a number of microorganisms is matched with achievable concentrations of the drug in blood or urine. An attempt is made to maintain the antibiotic concentration in serum or urine well above the minimum inhibitory concentration of the target organism at all times. The major limiting factors are the frequency of administration, the cost of the drug, and the development of toxicity. If the drug is a relatively safe one, the dosage schedule is often adjusted upward to assure efficacy. If the therapeutic index is thought to be narrow, the dosage schedule is more conservative. Minimum inhibitory, minimum bactericidal and serum bactericidal concentrations have been the cornerstones of careful antibiotic therapy for several decades. However, these parameters are at best an extremely crude approximation of the complex and dynamic in vivo variables.

*The cost of antibiotic therapy.* "Antibiotics are among the most frequently prescribed drugs in this country, exceeded only by the psychoactive drugs" (Sen. Gaylor Nelson, Sub-Committee on Monopoly of the Select Committee on Small Business, Washington, D.C., 1972). The collective cost of this use is staggering. Accordingly, the cost of antibiotic therapy is an appropriate factor to consider in making a choice. For example, cefaclor is a new oral cephalosporin, identical to cephalexin except for the substitution of a chlorine atom for a methyl group, which is currently being promoted for infections of the urinary tract, skin and soft tissue, and respiratory tract, as well as for otitis media. Cefaclor has been shown to be effective for otitis media caused by susceptible organisms including *S. pneumoniae*, *H. influenza*, and *S. pyogenes*. A 10-day course of treatment for otitis media in a 10-kg child currently costs the pharmacist $2.01 for genetic amoxicillin. A similar course of treatment with trimethoprin-sulfamethoxazole (Septra) or erythromycin plus sulfisoxazole costs $2.13 or $4.82, respectively. A 10-day course of therapy using cefaclor (Ceclor) costs $8.26 (*12*). All of these options are acceptable courses of therapy for otitis media in children; clearly, cost is an important consideration in choosing one of them.

*Familiarity with the chosen drug.* A clinician should choose representatives from each of the common families of antibiotics, and should become familiar with these drugs, their antimicrobial spectra, pharmacokinetics, adverse effects, and correct dosages for a variety of disease states. He then should stick with these representatives and come to know them intimately. There are few compelling reasons for the clinician to be equally familiar with oxacillin versus nafcillin or gentamicin versus tobramycin or cephalexin versus cephradine, etc.

*Availability of Therapeutic Drug Monitoring.* Therapeutic drug monitoring is an important clinical tool the impact of which has been felt in clinical medicine over the past five years and whose full flowering is yet to come. Various drugs may now be monitored in the clinical situation. These include many anticonvulsants, such as carbamazepine (Tegretol), ethosuximide (Zarontin), phenobarbital, phenytoin (Dilantin), primidone (Mysoline), and valproic acid (Depakene), as well as theophylline. Antibiotics that commonly are monitored include amikacin, gentamicin, tobramycin, and chloramphenicol.

It is readily apparent why these particular antibiotics have been targeted for therapeutic drug monitoring: their therapeutic index is very narrow or their toxic potential is enormous, or both.

We recently had occasion to treat a young man with chronic granulomatous disease and *Serratia marcescens* osteomyelitis of the finger. The availability of gentamicin concentrations allowed us to increase his gentamicin dose to 8.4 mg/kg/day (7.5 mg/kg/day is the usual maximum daily dose) in order to achieve therapeutic peak and trough concentrations. The narrow therapeutic index of this drug was all too clearly demonstrated several days later by the appearance of proteinuria and cylindruria, heralding the onset of gentamicin nephrotoxicity and necessitating discontinuation of the drug.

Gray baby syndrome resulting from chloramphenicol toxicity is said not to occur when serum chloramphenicol concentrations are <50 mg/L (6). A three-month-old baby with *Hemophilus influenzae* type b meningitis was admitted to our hospital and begun on intravenous ampicillin 400 mg/kg/day and intravenous chloramphenicol 100 mg/kg/day (currently recommended appropriate therapy). Free chloramphenicol peak and trough concentrations on the fifth day of therapy were 53 mg/L and 34 mg/L respectively; both of these values are well above the therapeutic range (10-20 mg/L). Fortunately, no evidence of gray baby syndrome developed and the infant did well, but this example demonstrates graphically the variability in the ability of the liver to conjugate chloramphenicol and points up the necessity for frequent monitoring of chloramphenicol, both in neonates and older children. Chloramphenicol should also be monitored in adults who have any degree of liver impairment. For appropriate conclusions to be drawn from therapeutic drug monitoring, peak and trough values must be collected with meticulous care. If the samples are not drawn at the appropriate time intervals, erroneous conclusions may be reached inadvertently.

Use of therapeutic drug monitoring as a clinical tool should be expanded. Not only will patient care be improved, but there will be a better understanding of the interaction between the patient and the drug.

## Inappropriate Factors Influencing Antibiotic Choice

*Pressure from the patient.* Pressure from the patient to be treated with an antibiotic is a complex and profoundly important problem. In its broadest sense, it is a societal problem. We live in an age of instant gratification. If I see a physician and he doesn't prescribe instant cure I will find another physician who will. Pressure for antibiotic cure is prevalent in internal medicine and even more rampant in pediatric practice. Parents find it very threatening when their child is ill. It robs them of their sleep, disturbs the smooth flow of their lives, and brings them face-to-face with the anxiety, "could my child die?" The pressure on the physician for instant relief of anxiety is phenomenal.

On the other hand, the physician is not entirely without fault in the dynamic interaction that results in inappropriate antibiotic choice. We must assume that he is genuinely motivated to give the best treatment. Unfortunately, this noble motivation is often influenced by a series of widely prevalent misconceptions.

The first such misconception is that fever invariably is caused by infection and that infection responds to antibiotic therapy. This notion is clearly untrue, but nevertheless is commonly heard and commonly acted upon.

The next such misconception says that if a little antibiotic is good, then more is better. Clear data are accumulating that many antibiotic regimens involve excessive amounts and that overkill is unnecessary.

The third misconception, and clearly one of the most dangerous, is the thought that antibiotics as a group are benign, that their use is unlikely to hurt anyone. A recent study of iatrogenic illness at a university hospital found that 36% of 815 consecutive patients on a general medical service had an iatrogenic illness (13). In 9% of the patients admitted, the complication was considered major (threatened life or produced considerable disability). The leading hospital intervention which led to iatrogenic complication was the use of drugs, and the penicillin family of antibiotics accounted for 10% of the major complications. Antibiotics are not harmless substances; the decision to use one and the subsequent choice of one are not trivial decisions.

The last of the most common and most dangerous antibiotic misconceptions centers around the issue of prophylaxis. "If an antibiotic can be used to treat disease, then surely it can also be used to prevent disease." Clearly there are certain circumscribed situations where antibiotic prophylaxis is warranted.

However, the number of situations where the merits of prophylaxis have been studied rigorously and with appropriate scientific design is exceedingly small. In contrast, the number of instances where this axiom is applied with absolutely no scientific basis is immense. Antibiotics are wonderful substances, but unquestionably their misuse has contributed substantially to the emergence of antibiotic resistant strains of bacteria. Finland's data from the Boston City Hospital (*14*) showed that in 1935 most bacteremic infections were caused by Gram-positive cocci; Gram-negative rods were responsible for a mere 12% of bacteremia infections. Within 30 years, after 15-20 years of antibiotic use, 50% of bacteremic infections were caused by Gram-negative organisms, and at present the proportion has reached two-thirds. Examples of bacterial acquisition of antibiotic resistance secondary to antibiotic overuse abound: *Streptococus pneumoniae* resistant to tetracycline, *Neisseria gonorrhoeae* resistant to penicillin, *Staphylococcus aureus* resistant to semi-synthetic penicillin, Shigella resistant first to sulfonamides and then to ampicillin, *Salmonella typhosa* resistant to chloramphenicol, *Hemophilus influenzae* resistant to ampicillin. The list seems endless.

The general public must accept the fact that viral infections must be tolerated by adults and children alike without antibiotic therapy. The physician has a duty to resist pressure from his patient clientele and to educate them toward acceptance of this principle.

*Nonfamiliarity with current antibiotics.* The benefit of continuing medical education is nowhere more obvious than in the area of antibiotic choice. No antibiotic is a good catch-all for most disease. No physician can be content to use his favorite antibiotic for every disease he sees, nor can he be content to use only those antibiotics he learned about in 1940. On the other hand, there is little truth in the notion, "this antibiotic is new, therefore it must be better". An example of this is the group of newer me-too cephamiracles which have nothing compelling to recommend them. In general, more traditional, better studied antibiotics with years of successful use behind them comprise the antibiotic group from which to choose. Nonetheless, physicians must stay current with regard to antibiotic use, indications, dosage, and adverse effects if they are to serve their patients well.

*Pressure from the pharmaceutical representative.* Unfortunately many physicians receive their antibiotic updating from drug company representatives. These representatives are obviously not disinterested parties to the process of antibiotic choice. Unfortunately they are often all too happy to promulgate several of the misconceptions already alluded to, "if it's new, it must be better; if a little is good, then more is better."

As a rule, information from pharmaceutical representatives should be ignored by the clinician, who must be prepared to make an independent assessment of a new antibiotic or to accept the consensus of the infectious disease community. Another excellent source of drug information for the clinician is the *Medical Letter*, a non-profit publication that objectively assesses the relative merits of many drugs.

## Families of Antibiotics and General Indications for Their Use

Some statements can be made regarding the indications for various antibiotics. They cannot be all inclusive, nor can they cover every individual situation that might arise. Antibiotic choice in complex clinical situations may be difficult, and consultation with an infectious-disease service may be necessary.

*Penicillins.* Penicillins are most useful as a group against gram-positive organisms. Usually semi-synthetic penicillinase-resistant penicillins are indicated for infections with *Staphylococcus aureus*. Carbenicillin or ticarcillin are indicated in the treatment of serious *Pseudomonas aeruginosa* infections in combination with an aminoglycoside.

A new oxa-beta penicillin, moxalactam, is currently undergoing clinical trial. Unlike the more traditional penicillins, this drug is not very active against gram-positive organisms but has excellent activity against gram-negative enteric organisms, as well as *Hemophilus influenzae*. It is already apparent that moxalactam will become a respected member of the penicillin family, not only because of its excellent antibacterial spectrum but also because of its ability to penetrate to the cerebrospinal fluid and its relatively few adverse effects.

*Cephalosporins.* Cephalosporins are probably the most inappropriately used antibiotics. In fact, there are no infectious diseases for which the cephalosporins are the drug of first choice. They are indicated for use on patients who have a known allergy to the the drug of choice. Frequently they are used when "broad-spectrum coverage" or "broad-spectrum prophylaxis" is thought to be desirable. "Broad-spectrum coverage" is a phrase that conceals a dearth of rigorous thinking and an abundance of undifferentiated anxiety. "Broad-spectrum prophylaxis" is a contradiction in terms, because prophylaxis is, by definition, narrow antibiotic therapy targeted at a specific organism at the time of suspected exposure.

*The macrolid antibiotics.* At present, erythromycin is the only clinically useful member of the family of macrolid antibiotics. It may be a drug of choice for selected gram-positive infections, including those with *Streptococcus pneumoniae*, many penicillin-resistant strains of *Staphylococcus aureus*, chlamydia infections including neonatal inclusion blenorrhea and the chlamydia pneumonitis syndrome of infancy, Mycoplasma infections, pertussis, campylobacter infections, *Legionella pneumophilia* infection, and diphtheria.

*Aminoglycoside antibiotics.* The aminoglycoside antibiotics (gentamicin, kanamycin, netilmicin, amikacin and tobramycin) are indicated for serious gram-negative enteric infections. Gentamicin acts synergistically with both penicillins and cephalosporins against viridans streptococcus, *Streptococcus faecalis*, and *Staphylococcus aureus*. The combination of gentamicin and either penicillin or ampicillin produces more rapid killing of *Listeria monocytogenes* and group B streptococcus. The combination of gentamicin and carbenicillin or ticarcillin is synergistic for *Pseudomonas aeruginosa* both in vivo and in vitro.

*Clindamycin.* Clindamycin is a drug of choice for serious anaerobic infections. It is active against many anaerobic organisms, including Bacteroides species but is not a good drug for the treatment of clostridial infection. Clindamycin is a good alternative drug against *Staphylococcus aureus*, though its potential for pseudomembranous colitis clearly limits its use. Clindamycin appears to enter bone and abscess cavities well, but does not enter the central nervous system to any significant extent.

*Chloramphenicol.* Chloramphenicol is the drug of choice for infection with *Salmonella typhi* and for brain abscesses. In addition it is a drug of choice for serious anaerobic infections and for Rocky Mountain Spotted Fever, and it is always included in the initial therapy of serious *Hemophilus influenzae* infections.

*Tetracyclines.* A tetracycline antibiotic is the drug of choice for non-gonococcal urethritis, for traveler's diarrhea prophylaxis in some parts of the world, for brucellosis, for *Calymmatobacterium granulomatis* infection, cholera, psittacosis, and Rocky Mountain Spotted Fever. A tetracycline may be a drug of choice also for *Neisseria gonorrhoeae* infection. Tetracyclines should not be administered to pregnant women, infants, or older children under eight years of age.

*Trimethoprim-sulfamethoxazole.* Trimethoprim-sulfamethoxazole is the drug of choice for shigella infection and *Pneumocystis carinii* infection and prophylaxis. It is a third line drug for urinary tract infection and otitis media in children.

*Sulfisoxazole.* Sulfisoxazole is the drug of choice for uncomplicated urinary tract infection.

*Vancomycin.* Vancomycin is an alternative drug for infections with *Staphylococcus aureus* and *S. epidermidis*. It is the drug of choice for methicillin-resistant *S. epidermidis* shunt infections in children.

*Anti-tuberculous drugs.* Isoniazid, rifampin, and ethambutol are all drugs of choice, depending on the specific circumstances, for infection with *Mycobacterium tuberculosis*. Streptomycin, *p*-aminosalicylic acid, cycloserine, and ethionamide are all alternative drugs.

## Conclusion

Appropriate choice of antibiotic is one of the most important decisions a clinician makes. He may be assured of making an appropriate choice if he is familiar with the disease process he is treating, is familiar with a broad range of traditional antibiotics, and engages in clear and rigorous thinking. When he faces a particularly complex or difficult situation, an infectious disease service should be consulted.

## References

1. Finkel, M.J., Magnitude of antibiotic use. *Ann. Int. Med.* **82**, 791-792 (1978).
2. Craig, W.A., Uman, S.J., Shaw, W.R., Ramgopal, V., Eagan, L.L., Leopold, E.T., Hospital use of antimicrobial drugs. *Ann. Int. Med.* **82**, 793-795 (1978).
3. Kass, E.H., Antimicrobial drug usage in general hospitals in Pennsylvania. *Ann. Int. Med.* **82**, 800-801 (1978).
4. Anon, Preventive therapy of tuberculosis infection. *Morbidity and Mortality Weekly Report* **24**, 71 (1975).
5. Shulman, J., Common mistakes in antibiotic usage, In *Practical Aspects of Antibiotic Review,* (C. Kunin, Ed.), Am. Health Consultants, p. 23, 1979.
6. Meissner, H.C., and Smith, A.L., The current status of chloramphenicol. *Pediatrics.* **64**, 348-356 (1979).
7. Appel, G.B., Neu, H.C., Gentamicin in 1978. *Ann. Int. Med.* **89**, 528-538 (1978).
8. Tedesco, F.J., Barton, R.W., Alpers, D.H. Clindamycin-associated colitis. A prospective study. *Ann. Intern. Med.* **81**, 547-548 (1974).
9. Lusk, R.H., Fekety, F.R, Silva, J., et al., Gastrointestinal side effects of clindamycin and ampicillin therapy. *J. Inf. Dis* **135**, S111-S119 (1977).
10. Idsoe, O., Guthe, T., Willcox, R.R., and DeWeck, A.L. Nature and extent of penicillin side reactions with particular reference to fatalities from anaphylactic shock, *Bull. WHO* **38**, 159-188 (1968).

11. Hieber, J.P., Nelson, J.D.: A pharmacological evaluation of penicillin in children with purulent meningitis. *N. Engl. J. Med.* **297**, 410-413 (1977).

12. Anon, Two new oral cephalosporins. *Medical Letter* **21**, 85-87 (1979).

13. Steel, K., Gertman, P.M., Crescenzi, C., Anderson, J. Iatrogenic illness on a general medical service at a university hospital. *N. Engl. J. Med.* **304**, 638-642 (1981).

14. McGowan, J.E., Barnes, M.W., Finland, M. Bacteremia at Boston City Hospital: Occurrence and mortality during 12 selected years (1935-1972) with special reference to hospital-acquired cases. *J. Infect. Dis.* **132**, 316-335 (1975).

# 30

# Interpretation of Antimicrobial Concentrations in Serum

## John P. Anhalt, M.D.

The principal goal of antimicrobial therapy is eradication of the infectious agent with minimal toxicity to the patient. This represents a unique situation for therapeutic monitoring, because the beneficial effects of a drug are not derived from direct actions on the physiology of the patient. In contrast to other medications, the direct effects of antimicrobials on a patient are of concern only from the standpoint of toxicity. Nevertheless, the same principles that apply to measurements of concentrations in blood and to therapeutic monitoring of other drugs apply to antimicrobials. It is in the definition of therapeutic range and the assessment of toxicity that it becomes necessary to consider the complex interaction that exists between the infectious agent, the drug, and the patient.

## General Principles

The determination of the concentration of an antimicrobial in serum or other fluids is justified only when that concentration can be correlated with benchmarks of efficacy or excess and cannot be predicted adequately from dosage. Various methods have been developed to calculate dosages based on desired concentrations in serum and estimated values for absorption, distribution, metabolism, and excretion. The adequacy of these predictions varies with the clinical situation and the acceptability of error. For most antimicrobials, the range between therapeutic and toxic concentrations is large, and the tendency has been to administer doses that assure concentrations in serum that are several-fold the assumed minimum effective value. Assays are not required for these drugs unless there is evidence that the concentration in serum may be markedly different from usual. For example, such factors as severe renal disease, dialysis, and use of oral medication in patients with malabsorption syndromes may indicate the need for assays. The effects of dialysis on elimination of many antimicrobials is sufficiently predictable, however, that assays are not always needed for dosage adjustment (1). Occasionally, assays are indicated for fluids from infection sites where drug penetration is

*Dr. Anhalt is in the Section of Clinical Microbiology, Department of Laboratory Medicine at the Mayo Clinic and Mayo Foundation, Rochester, MN 55901.*

variable or uncertain, such as bile, synovial fluid, or cerebrospinal fluid. Rarely, failure to observe clinical improvement is alone cause to obtain an assay. A relatively small number of antimicrobials—the most common being aminoglycosides, chloramphenicol, and vancomycin—exhibit a narrow range between therapeutic and toxic concentrations, and calculated dosages are often inadequate to assure appropriate values in serum. These calculations are particularly inaccurate for critically ill patients in whom rapid attainment of maximum concentrations is needed to treat a life-threatening infection. In addition, the calculations do not account for the effects of fever on decreasing peak concentrations, the effects of metabolic variation resulting from disease, or the effects of other drugs, which may cause inactivation or change the rate of elimination. Lastly, compliance in taking a prescribed dose is rarely a significant problem with parenteral antimicrobial therapy of hospitalized patients. Medication errors do occur, however, and can result in extremely unusual drug concentrations that necessitate serum assays.

Related to the subject of doing serum assays to avoid excessive drug amounts is the question of whether other, perhaps better, indicators of impending toxicity exist. Generally, alternative indicators of acute toxicity do not exist for antimicrobials. For example, the renal toxicity of aminoglycosides can be demonstrated in the absence of discernible increases in serum creatinine concentration (2), because even with total renal failure, serum creatinine increases at the rate of only 11 mg/L (100 $\mu$mol/L) per day. Serum creatinine may also increase in critically ill patients for a variety of reasons besides drug toxicity. Similarly, clinical indications are inadequate to predict impending cardiovascular collapse from chloramphenicol toxicity (3).

## Therapeutic Range

The desired therapeutic concentration of an antimicrobial is often defined relative to the concentration necessary to inhibit or to kill the infecting organism in an in vitro susceptibility test. When one considers the great differences existing between these tests and the clinical situation, the sometimes poor correlation with clinical outcome is not surprising. Hewitt and McHenry (4) have reviewed studies, for example, showing that 12% of patients with bacteremia survived with inappropriate or no antimicrobial therapy, while 16% of patients receiving presumably appropriate therapy had persistent infections. Undoubtedly, the natural defense mechanisms of the patient greatly influence the outcome of antimicrobial therapy. Also important are the effects of associated therapy, such as surgical drainage of an abscess, and the rate at which an infection resolves. One might assume that the best correlation between concentrations in serum and clinical efficacy would be found in treatment of infections in which host defenses play a relatively minor role or are suppressed. Such is the case in endocarditis and in treatment of immunosuppressed patients; and for these cases, correlations have been demonstrated between the antimicrobial activity in serum and clinical response (5,6). (The antimicrobial activity in serum is determined as the highest dilution of the serum that will completely inhibit or kill the infecting organism.)

Of at least equal importance to attaining a target concentration of an antimicrobial is appropriate drug selection, which also is guided by susceptibility tests. An organism is generally considered susceptible to a particular drug when the minimum concentration that inhibits multiplication of the organism is less, usually by one-half to one-quarter, than the attainable peak concentration of that drug in serum or other fluid with normal doses. This definition, though often clinically useful, must be modified by experience in treating specific infections. For example, infections with staphylococci that produce $\beta$-lactamase cannot be treated adequately with penicillin, even though they will often appear to be inhibited by concentrations of penicillin well below the attainable serum concentrations. Similarly, penicillin or ampicillin may be used to treat some infections from enterococci, but should not be used alone to treat enterococcal endocarditis because they do not effectively kill these organisms. Also, an organism may be considered resistant to an antimicrobial if the infection involves deep tissues, but may be considered sensitive if the infection is in the bladder and the drug is concentrated in urine.

Table 1 shows the interpretive criteria, based on the minimal inhibitory concentration (MIC), for selected antimicrobials. These data are from a proposed standard issued by the National Committee for Clinical Laboratory Standards (7). A more comprehensive listing of susceptibilities and attainable concentrations can be found in the review by Hewitt and McHenry (4).

## Assessment of Toxicity

Just as the determination of minimum effective concentrations is complicated by the interaction of the patient with the organism, determination of toxicity is complicated by the fact that antimicrobials are usually given only during an acute illness. Adverse effects resulting from treatment may be the result of the illness or concurrent therapy instead of antimicrobial. The difficulty in establishing toxic concentrations is illustrated by the case of aminoglycosides, where today, almost two decades after introduction of gentamicin, there is uncertainty still as to what the toxic concentrations are, whether ototoxicity and nephrotoxicity are related truly to dose or to serum concentration, the importance of length of therapy on development of toxicity, and to what extent concurrent therapy with a cephalosporin or a penicillin influences toxicity (4, 8-11). In most cases, the toxic values for antimicrobials have not been precisely defined. Instead, the concentrations attained with doses shown to be effective in clinical trials are considered desirable. It is assumed that concentrations in excess of these are of no greater benefit and may increase the likelihood of adverse effects. Table 2 lists the usual serum concentrations and the toxic concentrations for selected antimicrobials. More extensive data are available in reviews by Hewitt and McHenry (4) and by Gerson and Anhalt (13).

## Specimen Collection

*Type and preservation.* The most appropriate specimen for common antimicrobials is serum. Plasma can be used in some assay procedures; however, anticoagulants may interfere. In one study, for example, the heparin used to anticoagulate plasma bound as much as 32% of a physiological concentration of gentamicin (14). Some assays, such as for sulfonamides, were originally performed on whole blood, but there is little reason to continue this practice. Measurements of urinary concentrations of antimicrobials are rarely indicated, and the results are difficult to interpret.

Data concerning optimum storage conditions for clinical specimens are generally lacking. Because the rate of chemical reactions that would lead to decreases in the apparent concentration in serum are slower at low temperatures, it has been our practice to assay all serum specimens immediately or to store them at -20 °C or lower for no more than two days. However, some drugs and drug combinations are particularly unstable: the combination of an aminoglycoside and a $\beta$-lactam drug, usually carbenicillin or ticarcillin, is particularly unstable, and significant losses may occur rapidly even at -20 °C (15). This reaction can be almost eliminated by addition of a $\beta$-lactamase. The cephalosporins are very unstable in serum, presumably because of the presence of lipoproteins *(16)*. Addition of sodium dodecyl sulfate to a final concentration of 10 g/L at pH 6 or below will stabilize cephalosporins; however, for clinical purposes, they are stable for two days at -20 °C without a stabilizer. There is a need for detailed studies of specimen stability, because some drugs show a paradoxical decrease in stability upon freezing, presumably because of local concentration effects.

*Timing.* It has become customary to monitor aminoglycoside therapy by measurement of "peak" and "trough" concentrations, although the rational basis for this has been questioned *(9)*. The time at which peak values occur is highly variable and varies with the individual, the drug, and the route of administration. For practical purposes, however, we recommend that serum for measurement of peak concentrations should be obtained 1 h after an intramuscular injection or, to allow for distribution, 30 min after an intravenous infusion. For oral medications, the time of maximum concentrations is even more variable, although a serum sample drawn 1 to 2 h after a dose is usually adequate. Most antimicrobials are administered with a dosage interval that exceeds the half-life. Therefore, accumulation is minimal, and serum for peak determinations can be obtained after the first two or three doses. Trough values are more accurately obtained, because they always occur immediately before a subsequent dose. (An exception to this can occur when a slowly activated pro-drug is administered, as in the case of the intravenous preparation of chloramphenicol.) It should be emphasized, however, that determinations of peak and trough values are not justified for all drugs. When the reason for an assay is to avoid acute toxicity or to document attainment of a presumably effective concentration, a peak value is all that is required. When the goal is to avoid accumulation, a trough concentration is more accurate and useful.

## Choice of Methodology

With few exceptions, chloramphenicol being the most notable, the toxicity of antimicrobials is not of rapid onset, and the speed of most assays is adequate for clinical purposes. Similarly, the precision and accuracy of most carefully performed assays are adequate. Reeves and Wise *(12)*, for example, concluded that for aminoglycosides, a 95% confidence limit of ±25 to 30% is adequate, and that for other drugs, such as penicillin, a 95% confidence limit of ±50% would suffice. The most important consideration for clinical assays is specificity, because therapy with multiple antimicrobials is common, and a laboratory cannot rely on having accurate information concerning concurrent therapy. In addition, microbiologically active metabolites of antimicrobials may be present. Of the available assays, the most specific are chromatographic,

immunologic, or enzymatic. Bioassays are the least specific, and because an increasing number of specimens contain multiple antimicrobials, they are inadequate.

## Specific Drug Classes
### Aminoglycosides

The aminoglycosides are a family of antibiotics with a broad spectrum of antimicrobial activity. Streptomycin was the first aminoglycoside to be discovered (1944), followed by neomycin (1949), kanamycin (1957), gentamicin (1963), tobramycin (1967), and amikacin (1972). Sisomicin and netilmicin are in various stages of clinical trials in the United States. Assays for aminoglycosides accounted for 77% of the antimicrobial assays done at the Mayo Clinic in 1980.

*Antimicrobial activity and uses.* The aminoglycosides are bactericidal agents that act by binding to bacterial ribosomes and inhibiting protein synthesis. Their entry into bacteria requires an oxygen-dependent active transport system; thus, they are inactive under anaerobic conditions. They are active against most staphylococci, and in fact, kanamycin was used originally for this purpose before the β-lactamase-resistant penicillins were available *(17)*. Today, they are rarely used alone to treat staphylococcal infections, but may be used in combination with nafcillin or oxacillin. Aminoglycosides are inactive against most streptococci; however, in combination with penicillin or ampicillin, various ones are active against viridans streptococci, enterococci, and *Streptococcus agalactiae* (group B streptococci). The principal use of aminoglycosides is in the treatment of serious infections due to aerobic, Gram-negative bacilli, including *Pseudomonas aeruginosa*. Many of these organisms, particularly *P. aeruginosa*, have developed resistance to streptomycin and kanamycin. Because of this resistance, streptomycin is used now primarily for treatment of enterococcal or viridans streptococcal endocarditis and tuberculosis, and kanamycin is used only rarely. Gentamicin, tobramycin, and amikacin have retained activity against most Gram-negative bacilli and *P. aeruginosa*. However, resistance is variable among clinical isolates, and susceptibility testing is required. Against *P. aeruginosa*, the combination of an aminoglycoside with ticarcillin or carbenicillin is often used because of synergistic activity. Neomycin is no longer administered parenterally because of its great potential for toxicity. It is used orally to reduce bowel flora and is contained in some irrigation fluids used postoperatively. A laboratory may still be called upon to measure neomycin, however, because toxic concentrations in blood can be attained by these routes *(18)*.

*Chemistry and pharmacology.* Aminoglycosides are highly polar and insoluble in lipids. They all contain at least one aminosugar that is linked through a glyco-

**Table 1.** Classification of Microbial Susceptibility

MIC[a], mg/L

| | Susceptible | | Resistant | |
| Antibiotic | Very susceptible | Moderately susceptible | Moderately resistant | Very resistant |
|---|---|---|---|---|
| Gentamicin | ≤0.5 | 1-4 | 8-64 | >64 |
| Tobramycin | ≤0.5 | 1-4 | 8-64 | >64 |
| Amikacin | ≤2 | 4-16 | 32-64 | >64 |
| Kanamycin | ≤2 | 4-16 | 32-64 | >64 |
| Streptomycin | Not used alone against common bacteria | | | |
| Cephalosporins | ≤2 | 4-16 | 32-256 | >256 |
| Penicillin[b] | ≤0.03 | 0.06-16 | 32-128 | >128 |
| Oxacillin or nafcillin | ≤2 | - | - | >2 |
| Chloramphenicol | ≤1.0 | 2-8 | | ≥16 |
| Vancomycin | ≤0.5 | 1-4 | | >4 |

[a]Minimal inhibitory concentrations (MIC values) are from an NCCLS proposed standard for dilution susceptibility tests (7).

[b]Staphylococci with MICs ≥0.06 mg/L may produce β-lactamase. All β-lactamase-producing staphylococci should be considered resistant to penicillin.

**Table 2.** Usual Doses and Desirable Concentrations of Selected Antimicrobials

| Antibiotic | Usual dose[a] | Desirable concn, mg/L[b] | | Toxic range, mg/L |
| | | Peak | Trough | |
|---|---|---|---|---|
| Gentamicin Tobramycin Sisomicin Netilmicin | 1.7 mg/kg every 8 h | 5-8 | 1-2 | >10-12 |
| Kanamycin Amikacin | 5.0 mg/kg every 8 h | 20-25 | 5-10 | >30-35 |
| Streptomycin | 7.5 mg/kg every 12 h | 5-20 | <5 | >40-50 |
| Chloramphenicol | 15 mg/kg every 6 h | 20 | 10 | >50 |
| Vancomycin | 1 g every 12 h | 30-40 | 5-10 | >90[c] |

[a]For adults with normal renal function.

[b]Peak concentrations 1 h after intramuscular dose or 30 min after intravenous dose.

[c]Avoid sustained concentrations greater than 30 mg/L.

sidic bond to other portions of the molecule. At physiologic pH, they exist as polycations. These chemical properties account in part for their similar pharmacokinetic properties (8,9, 19). They are poorly absorbed after oral administration, but repeated oral or rectal administration may give toxic concentrations in patients with poor renal function. Absorption also may occur through denuded skin or by irrigation of surgical wounds. Streptomycin is given intramuscularly; the other agents may be given either intramuscularly or intravenously. Absorption is complete after intramuscular injection, with peak concentrations occurring 0.5 to 3 h after the dose; however, the concentration in serum obtained 1 h after intramuscular injection will usually be at least 70% of the actual peak concentration. Aminoglycosides distribute into the extracellular fluid volume, the apparent volume of distribution (in liters) being numerically 30% of body weight (in kilograms). Infants and young children require larger doses (on the basis of body weight) to attain peak concentrations similar to those of adults (20); however, neonates and pre-term infants require extension of the dosage interval to 12 or 18 h, respectively, to prevent trough concentrations from greatly exceeding 2 mg/L (21). Aminoglycosides do not penetrate into cerebrospinal fluid or the eye sufficiently to produce therapeutic concentrations when administered parenterally. Concentrations in bile, pleural fluid, bronchial secretions, and synovial fluid are 25 to 50% of those in serum. Aminoglycosides are concentrated in renal cortical tissue, the degree of concentration varying with the aminoglycoside. Schentag et al. (19) have speculated that the differences in nephrotoxicity may be related to the differences in affinity for renal cortical tissue. Except for streptomycin, which is about 30 to 35% protein-bound, other aminoglycosides have been reported not to be protein-bound. This conclusion, however, has been disputed. Recent studies with gentamicin showed that protein binding may occur to the extent of 17 to 27% (14).

Aminoglycosides are excreted almost entirely through the kidney by glomerular filtration, and more than 90% of a dose can be recovered from urine eventually. Recovery from urine during the first few days of therapy is lower because of tissue accumulation (19). These drugs are neither metabolized nor excreted appreciably in bile. In patients with normal renal function, the serum half-life is 2 to 3 h. This half-life is prolonged with renal insufficiency, and in anephric patients values from 30 to 110 h have been found (8). After the final dose of drug, a second phase of elimination can be identified, apparently related to slow release of the aminoglycoside from tissues. This phase has been most thoroughly studied for gentamicin and tobramycin, and half-lives of 112 and 146 h, respectively, have been reported (19). Thus, 0.1 to 0.4 mg of these drugs per

liter may persist in serum for several days after therapy is stopped. Aminoglycosides are removed by hemodialysis, and to a lesser extent, by peritoneal dialysis.

Because each aminoglycoside has about the same volume of distribution, similar doses give similar concentrations in serum (Table 2).

*Toxicity and therapeutic monitoring.* Adverse allergic reactions occur in about 1 to 3% of patients. The major adverse reactions are dose-related neuromuscular blockade, nephrotoxicity, and ototoxicity.

Neuromuscular blockade may occur with parenteral administration or when aminoglycosidic solutions are used for peritoneal lavage. Fortunately, it can be reversed by administration of calcium.

Nephrotoxicity from aminoglycosides is characterized by proximal tubular necrosis and results in proteinuria, granular cylinduria, and increasing serum creatinine. Increased excretion of $\beta_2$-microglobulin and various enzymes in urine occurs early. These changes also result in an increasing elimination half-life for the aminoglycoside. Streptomycin causes very little nephrotoxicity. The other aminoglycosides produce clinically evident toxicity in 2 to 10% of patients (8). With very sensitive measures of renal function, Trollfors et al. (2) detected damage in virtually all patients in whom peak concentrations of gentamicin were 4.0 to 6.8 mg/L at least once during 10 to 14 days of therapy. Most nephrotoxicity is reversible with discontinuation of therapy, and experiments in rats have shown that regeneration of tubular epithelium and recovery of renal function may occur even with continuation of therapy (22).

Although ototoxic effects may be detected in 10 to 20% of patients treated with aminoglycosides for long periods, clinically overt ototoxic reactions occur in only 1 to 3% of patients (8). Damage is reversible in about half of these cases. The different aminoglycosides show different potentials for affecting the vestibular and auditory portions of the eighth nerve. Gentamicin, tobramycin, and streptomycin affect the vestibular portion to a greater extent than the auditory portion, whereas kanamycin and amikacin affect the auditory portion preferentially, causing loss of high-tone perception.

The aminoglycoside concentrations related to onset of toxicity are poorly defined, and the work of Trollfors et al. (2) may indicate that nephrotoxicity is a continuum, from subclinical effects with low concentrations to clinically significant effects at higher concentrations. Nevertheless, the authors of several extensive reviews of the literature have concluded that the concentrations listed in Table 2 probably minimize toxicity without sacrificing efficacy (8-10). Because of wide variability from patient to patient, dosage adjustments to achieve these values must be based on measurements of drug concentrations. The frequency of these measurements should vary with the clinical situation. Patients with normal renal function who are receiving minimum doses do not require as close monitoring as critically ill patients receiving maximum doses. Mangione and Schentag *(9)* have recommended that most patients can be monitored by measuring a single peak concentration, to assure that the dose is adequate, and measuring trough concentrations every week to guard against drug accumulation. For high-risk patients, monitoring daily or every other day may be necessary. The importance of measuring to assure efficacy was stressed by Noone et al. *(23)*, who found that because of the great emphasis that had been placed on toxicity, patients were often undertreated. These authors recommended measurement of peak and trough concentrations twice weekly during prolonged therapy or whenever renal function changed. The clinical benefits of adjusting dosages according to concentrations in serum has been shown by Bootman et al. *(24)* in a retrospective study of burn patients with Gram-negative sepsis. The survival of patients whose dosages were adjusted according to serum concentrations was approximately twice the survival rate of a preceeding group whose dosages had not been adjusted in that manner.

## Chloramphenicol

Chloramphenicol was first isolated in 1947 from a strain of *Streptomyces venezuelae* and was marketed shortly thereafter in 1949. The drug rapidly achieved a position of frequent and widespread use because of its broad spectrum of activity. Within a few years, however, reports of serious hematologic and metabolic toxicities surfaced, which led to changes in the recommended dosages and curtailment of use. In fact, the fear of these toxicities may have prevented the appropriate use of chloramphenicol in certain life-threatening illnesses *(25)*. Today, there is a resurgence of interest in this drug, particularly for treatment of meningitis and infections with anaerobic bacteria *(25-27)*.

*Antimicrobial activity and uses.* Chloramphenicol binds reversibly to the 50S subunit of microbial ribosomes and inhibits protein synthesis by interfering with attachment of aminoacyl tRNA as well as competitively inhibiting peptidyltransferase. Protein synthesis in the cytosol of eukaryotic cells is not affected because of differences in the ribosomes and peptidyltransferase; however, protein synthesis and electron transport in the mitochondria of eukaryotic cells are affected, which may explain some of the toxicity of chloramphenicol in humans *(25)*.

Chloramphenicol is primarily a bacteriostatic agent and is active against common aerobic and anaerobic bacteria, including *Bacteroides fragilis* and most *Enterobacteriaceae*, as well as rickettsiae, mycoplasmata, and chlamydia. *Pseudomonas aeruginosa, Serratia marcescens,* and *Providencia* are usually resistant.

Against *Haemophilus influenzae*, a notable exception, chloramphenicol is bactericidal at concentrations easily attainable during therapy. A recent report has also shown bactericidal activity at concentrations of 6.25 to 12.5 mg/L against *Streptococcus pneumoniae* and *Neisseria meningitidis (28)*. Against these pathogens, however, ampicillin was bactericidal at much lower concentrations, and the ratio of the minimal bactericidal concentration to minimal inhibitory concentration of chloramphenicol was several-fold. Chloramphenicol is indicated for therapy of anaerobic infections, particularly those involving *B. fragilis;* typhoid fever and invasive infections due to other *Salmonella* species; brain abscess; and meningitis due to ampicillin-resistant *H. influenzae* type b. Chloramphenicol is used, often in combination with an aminoglycoside, for treatment of meningitis due to sensitive species of *Enterobacteriaceae*. McCracken and Eichenwald *(29)*, however, have recommended against the use of chloramphenicol for neonatal meningitis, which is often caused by such organisms; instead, they recommend using a combination of ampicillin and gentamicin. Unless the gentamicin is instilled directly into the ventricles, results have been poor and are no better than with systemic therapy alone. In contrast, other physicians using systemic chloramphenicol have reported successful treatment of neonatal meningitis due to *Escherichia coli (30)* and have implied that chloramphenicol is appropriate therapy when rapid measurements of the drug can be performed *(31)*. Chloramphenicol is the best alternative therapy for meningococcal, pneumococcal, or *Listeria monocytogenes* meningitis in patients allergic to penicillin *(31)*.

*Chemistry and pharmacology.* Chloramphenicol is well absorbed after oral administration of the free diol, which has a bitter taste and is available only in capsules, or of a suspension of the palmitate ester, which is tasteless. The palmitate ester is hydrolyzed by pancreatic lipases in the duodenum to release free chloramphenicol, which is then absorbed *(26)*. Peak concentrations in serum of about 12 mg/L are reached 1 to 2 h after oral administration of a single 1-g dose to an adult. The concentrations produced by the palmitate are slightly lower and are attained more slowly, particularly in very young infants, who may hydrolyze the ester more slowly.

Chloramphenicol is administered intravenously as the water-soluble sodium 3-monosuccinate ester. Under physiologic conditions, the 3-monosuccinate ester rapidly rearranges to a mixture of the 3-monosuccinate and 1-monosuccinate esters *(32)*. These esters undergo hydrolysis to release active chloramphenicol. The site of hydrolysis has not been identified with certainty; however, it has been shown not to occur in vitro in blood. Some have suggested that hydrolysis may occur in the liver, kidney, and at the site of a localized infection (33, 34). The rate of hydrolysis is rapid, but substantial amounts of the succinate esters can be detected in serum drawn 30 min after an intravenous infusion. According to data given by Glazko (33), the concentration of succinate esters 30 min after an infusion is 30 to 40% of the total nitro compounds. The concentrations attained by the intravenous route are slightly less than those produced by an equivalent oral dose. Intramuscular administration of chloramphenicol or its succinate esters is not recommended. Various studies have shown poor or irregular absorption of chloramphenicol; however, the succinate esters are absorbed slowly but reproducibly to give concentrations about one-half of those attained by the intravenous route. In a recent review, Kucers (31) has suggested using the succinate esters by intramuscular route for H. influenzae meningitis and other infections with organisms that are very sensitive to the drug.

The usual dosage for adults and children older than two weeks is 50 mg/kg of body weight per day, divided into four doses given at 6-h intervals by either intravenous or oral routes. High-dose therapy with up to 100 mg/kg per day may be used for some indications. For newborn infants less than two weeks old, the maximum recommended dosage is 25 mg/kg per day in four equal doses at 6-h intervals. Because of differences in metabolism and excretion in this age group, however, concentrations in serum are very unpredictable, and this reduced dosage may lead to subtherapeutic or even toxic concentrations (25).

Chloramphenicol is distributed into an apparent volume in liters that is slightly less than the body weight in kilograms. Koup et al. (35) found, for example, volumes of distribution of 0.92 L/kg in adults with normal liver function and 0.98 L/kg in patients with serum bilirubin concentrations of >15 mg/L. In infants and children, the apparent volume of distribution has been reported to range from 0.78 L/kg to 2.09 L/kg (mean 1.39 L/kg) (36). Chloramphenicol is about 40 to 50% protein-bound in adults (35). In patients with cirrhosis, binding is decreased, and in premature infants protein binding is only 32%. The decreased protein binding in cirrhotics and premature infants cannot be duplicated by addition of bilirubin to normal serum. Chloramphenicol is not bound to erythrocytes. Chloramphenicol penetrates into most tissues and fluids. Concentrations in the cerebrospinal fluid peak at about 0.5 to 1 h after a dose and are 45 to 67% of the peak concentration in serum; the presence of meningitis does not affect the penetration. Chloramphenicol is concentrated in brain tissue and may exceed serum concentrations several fold. The concentrations in saliva are about 25% of concurrent serum concentrations; however, saliva values cannot be used for therapeutic monitoring because the variation in this ratio is too great (37).

Chloramphenicol is metabolized to several microbiologically inactive products before excretion by the kidneys (33). The principal metabolite is the 3-β-glucuronide, which is formed in the liver. (The possible formation of a small amount of 1-β-glucuronide has not been excluded.) In serum, this metabolite may constitute up to 35% of the total nitro compounds present several hours after a dose. In urine, 80 to 95% of a dose is excreted as nitro compounds, and the glucuronide accounts for the greatest part of these; active chloramphenicol accounts for only 5 to 10% of the dose. Other metabolic products containing the nitrobenzene moiety are formed by reductive dehalogenation of the dichloroacetyl group to give a 2-hydroxyacetamide analogue (glycolic acid analogue) of chloramphenicol or by hydrolysis of the acyl group to give 1-p-nitrophenyl-2-amino-1,3-propanediol. In addition, small amounts of aryl amines, formed by reduction of the nitro group on chloramphenicol or its metabolites, are present. These aryl amines are presumably formed in the intestine by bacterial action on the biliary excretion products and are then reabsorbed. Both the glucuronide and 2-hydroxyacetamide analogue, which can accumulate in renal insufficiency, appear to be nontoxic. When chloramphenicol is given as the succinate ester, either intravenously or intramuscularly, 27 to 32% of the dose has been recovered in urine as unhydrolyzed ester. Excretion of chloramphenicol in bile and feces is minimal. Glazko (33) states that <5% of a dose is recovered as nitro compounds in bile, and the amount of active chloramphenicol may be much lower.

The elimination half-life of chloramphenicol is highly variable between individuals and is particularly variable in young infants and newborns. In adults, the half-life is reported to be 1.5 to 4 h, and renal disease alone does not necessitate changes in dosage. The effects of cirrhosis and hospitalization on half-life were studied by Koup et al. (35), who found that for adult patients with serum bilirubin concentrations of ≤15 mg/L, the clearance was 3.57 ± 1.72 mL/min per kilogram, which corresponds to a range of half-lives from 2 to 5.7 h. In patients with bilirubin concentrations of >15 mg/L, the clearance was 1.99 ± 1.49 mL/min per kilogram, which corresponds to a range of half-lives from 3.3 to 23 h. Variation in the elimination and accumulation of chloramphenicol in neonates is even greater than the extremes described for adults. The poorly predictable behavior of chloramphenicol in neonates is due to several factors. Physiologically, the combination of immature hepatic and renal function results in accumulation, owing to slow conjugation of drug and poor elimination of unconjugated drug. This picture is complicated by the sometimes slow hydrolysis of the succinate esters and the many drugs to which neonates are exposed. [One recent study showed that newborns were exposed to an average of six drugs, in addition to those used in routine neonatal care, before being discharged for the nursery (38).] Recent studies involving highly specific assays have answered some of the questions regarding the disposition of chloramphenicol in children and the factors by which it is affected. Glazer et al. (34) studied two groups of low-birth-weight infants (≤2500 g) divided on the basis of age. In the younger group, who were one to eight days old, the elimination half-life ranged from 10.4 h to greater than 48 h, and in one infant, the serum concentration increased between doses. The group of older infants, who were 11 days to eight weeks old, had elimination half-lives of 5.5 to 15.7 h. After various variables were studied, including the presence of hypotension, concentration of unconjugated bilirubin, estimated gestational age, and postnatal age, the only variable that correlated with the half-lives in the two groups was postnatal age. In a separate study, Friedman et al. (39) divided their study groups on the basis of age, weight, and body surface area. These authors found statistically significant shorter half-life with increased age, weight, or surface area. There was, however, a large overlap between the groups: for example, the range of half-lives for infants less than one month old was 2.49 to 14.8 h and the range for those older than one month was 0.87 to 17.8 h. Excluded from their analysis were six patients in whom the concentration of chloramphenicol either did not decrease or actually increased between doses. It is apparent from these studies that direct measurement of chloramphenicol is the only reliable way to adjust dosages in young children.

*Toxicity and therapeutic monitoring.* Chloramphenicol can cause a variety of gastrointestinal and neurological symptoms, including optic and peripheral neuritis, and hypersensitivity reactions. The major toxic problems associated with chloramphenicol are blood dyscrasias and cardiovascular collapse (grey syndrome). Blood dyscrasias are of two types. The most serious is aplastic anemia, which is often fatal and occurs with a frequency estimated to be 1 in 24 000 to 40 000. This form of anemia is not related to dose and usually follows a latent period of two weeks to one year after treatment (27). There have been claims, however, that it is more common after oral therapy than after parenteral therapy. The apparent absence of aplastic anemia with thiamphenicol, a congener of chloramphenicol lacking the nitro group, has led some investigators to postulate that reduction products of chloramphenicol (e.g., aryl amines) formed by bacteria in the intestine may be responsible for this form of toxicity (27).

The other form of anemia is related to dose and is reversed upon stopping therapy. This dose-related anemia is characterized by maturation arrest in the marrow, cytoplasmic vacuolation of early erythroid and myeloid cells, reticulocytopenia, increases in serum iron and in serum iron-binding capacity, and reduced uptake of $^{59}$Fe by erythrocytes (27). Dose-related anemia occurs most frequently with doses of more than 4 g per day or sustained concentrations in serum exceeding 25 mg/L.

The other form of dose-related toxicity, characterized by cardiovascular collapse, occurs primarily in newborn infants (3, 25) but also may occur in older children and adults (25). Toxicity occurs as a result of accumulation of unconjugated chloramphenicol and is probably caused by inhibition of electron transport within mitochondria (25). The first signs of toxicity are abdominal distension, vomiting, and poor feeding. Symptoms may progress rapidly to hypothermia, respiratory depression, and an ashen-gray cyanosis. Death occurs in about 40% of patients. In infants, this toxicity has been related to total serum chloramphenicol concentrations greater than 50 mg/L (3).

The importance of monitoring neonates to maintain serum concentrations in the therapeutic range of 10 to 20 mg/L is illustrated by data from Lietman (25). In this study of 107 neonates less than two weeks old who received the recommended dose of 25 mg/kg per day, three patients had concentrations exceeding 50 mg/L, 57 had concentrations between 20 and 50 mg/L, and 11 had concentrations less than 10 mg/L. Only 36 of the patients, about one-third, had concentrations in the therapeutic range.

### Vancomycin

Vancomycin is a bactericidal antibiotic, active against a variety of Gram-positive bacteria and some Gram-negative cocci. It was isolated from fermentation of *Streptomyces orientalis* in 1956, and shortly afterward was introduced into clinical practice for the treatment of penicillinase-producing staphylococci. With subsequent development of semisynthetic penicillins and cephalosporins active against penicillinase-producing staphylococci, vancomycin was no longer the drug of choice and was used primarily as alternative therapy when the other drugs could not be used.

*Antimicrobial activity and uses.* Vancomycin inhibits cell wall growth and extension by binding to the peptidoglycan and preventing insertion of new subunits (40). A recent resurgence of interest in vancomycin (41, 42) can partly be traced to the fact that vancomycin is effective against methicillin-resistant staphylococci and corynebacteria, which are resistant to commonly used agents and are a cause of endocarditis and sepsis. Vancomycin has also been useful for prevention and treatment of staphylococcal infections in patients undergoing hemodialysis because a single dose of 1 g will persist at therapeutic concentrations for 10 to 14 days (41, 43). Vancomycin may be used in combination with an aminoglycoside to treat enterococcal endocarditis, but should not be used alone in treatment of this disease because it is not bactericidal for enterococci *(42)*. Vancomycin is the agent of choice for staphylococcal enterocolitis when given orally because it is poorly absorbed and reaches high concentrations in the gastrointestinal tract *(41, 42)*.

***Chemistry and pharmacology.*** Vancomycin has a complex chemical structure and a relative molecular mass of 1449 *(44)*. It is an amphoteric glycopeptide with several aromatic nuclei and is relatively unstable in solution. Dosage forms are available as the hydrochloride.

Therapeutic concentrations of vancomycin are achieved in pleural fluid, pericardial fluid, ascitic fluid, and synovial fluid after intravenous administration *(41, 42)*. Therapeutic concentrations are not attained in cerebrospinal fluid after intravenous administration in the absence of meningeal inflammation; however, successful treatment of staphylococcal meningitis with intravenous therapy has been reported *(41)*. Treatment of systemic infections is by intravenous administration only. Intramuscular administration cannot be used because of pain at the site of injection.

The serum half-life of vancomycin in patients with normal renal function is 6 h; approximately 10% of the drug is bound to protein. The usual dosage schedule is 1 g every 12 h, resulting in peak values of 30-40 mg/L and minimum values of 5-10 mg/L in normal adults. In children, the usual daily dose is 25-40 mg/kg. The principal route of excretion of vancomycin is through the kidney, and 90 to 100% of administered drug activity appears in the urine. In oliguric patients, the half-life is greatly prolonged, to approximately six days, and neither hemodialysis nor peritoneal dialysis reduces concentration in serum greatly *(42, 43)*.

***Toxicity and therapeutic monitoring.*** Toxicity reports of fever, phlebitis, and pain at the injection site have decreased in recent years, perhaps because of better purification of the antibiotic and improved methods of administration. Allergic skin rashes, the most common adverse effect, may occur in 4 to 5% of patients. The most significant dose-related toxicity affects the auditory nerve. This occurs rarely when serum concentrations are kept at 30 mg/L or even lower, but the critical concentration for this toxicity has not been determined. Toxicity may be related to the duration of sustained drug concentrations. No serious toxic effects were observed in two series of patients with normal renal function in whom concentrations as great as 90 mg/L were attained, but ototoxic reactions have occurred at drug concentrations of 80 to 100 mg/L in patients with renal insufficiency *(41)*.

Although vancomycin is a drug with only limited indications, assays for it represented 5% of the total antimicrobial assays done at the Mayo Clinic in 1980, a workload surpassed only by that of gentamicin and tobramycin. This is probably a result of the frequent use of vancomycin in patients with renal insufficiency, in whom therapy must be adjusted according to measured drug levels.

## Summary

This review has focused on the principles of antimicrobial therapeutic monitoring. Many of these principles are the same as for other drugs; however, there are significant differences resulting from interactions that exist between the patient, the infectious agent, and the drug. Three groups of antimicrobials-aminoglycosides, chloramphenicol, and vancomycin-have been considered in detail because of their potential for toxicity and frequency of use. Together, they represented 84% of the antimicrobial assays done at the Mayo Clinic in 1980. Assays of penicillins and cephalosporins, representing 16 different drugs, accounted for 14% of the workload. The remainder of the workload was divided among seven different agents. The reason for assaying these drugs was principally not to prevent toxic concentrations, but to document therapeutic concentrations or penetration into unusual sites (e.g., peritoneal fluid). The relatively large number of assays for penicillins and cephalosporins probably reflects their widespread use rather than a need for patients receiving these drugs to be monitored frequently.

## References

1. Bennett, W.M., Muther, R.S., Parker, R.A., et al., Drug therapy in renal failure: Dosing guidelines for adults. Part I: Antimicrobial agents, analgesics. *Ann. Intern. Med.* **93**, 62-89 (1980).
2. Trollfors, B., Alestig, K., Krantz, I., and Norrby, R., Quantitative nephrotoxicity of gentamicin in nontoxic doses. *J. Infect. Dis.* **141**, 306-309 (1980).
3. McCracken, G.H., Jr., Pharmacological basis for antimicrobial therapy in newborn infants. *Am. J. Dis. Child.* **128**, 407-419 (1974).
4. Hewitt, W.L., and McHenry, M.C., Blood level determinations of antimicrobial drugs. *Med. Clin. North Am.* **62**, 1119-1140 (1978).
5. Schlichter, J.G., MacLean, H., and Milzer, A., Effective penicillin therapy in subacute bacterial endocarditis and other chronic infections. *Am. J. Med. Sci.* **217**, 600-608 (1949).
6. Klastersky, J.D., Daneau, D., Swings, G., and Weerts, D., Antibacterial activity in serum and urine as a therapeutic guide in bacterial infection. *J. Infect. Dis.* **129**, 187-193 (1974).
7. *Standard Methods for Dilution Antimicrobial Susceptibility Tests for Bacteria Which Grow Aerobically*, NCCLS proposed standard PSM-7, National Committee for Clinical Laboratory

Standards, Villanova, PA, 1980.

8. Barza, M., and Scheife, R.T., Antimicrobial spectrum, pharmacology and therapeutic use of antibiotics—part 4: Aminoglycosides. *Am. J. Hosp. Pharm.* **34**, 723-737 (1977). Review.

9. Mangione, A., and Schentag, J.J., Therapeutic monitoring of aminoglycoside antibiotics: An approach. *Ther. Drug Monit.* **2**, 159-167 (1980).

10. Smith, C.R., Maxwell, R.R., Edwards, C.Q., et al., Nephrotoxicity induced by gentamicin and amikacin. *Johns Hopkins Med. J.* **142**, 85-90 (1978).

11. Noone, P., Aminoglycoside and cephalosporin toxicity. *J. Antimicrob. Chemother.* **4**, 465-466 (1978).

12. Reeves, D.S., and Wise, R., Antibiotic assays in clinical microbiology. In *Laboratory Methods in Antimicrobial Chemotherapy*, D.S. Reeves, I. Phillips, J.D. Williams, and R. Wise, Eds., Churchill Livingston, London, 1978, pp 137-143.

13. Gerson, B., and Anhalt, J.P., *High-Pressure Liquid Chromatography and Therapeutic Drug Monitoring*, American Society of Clinical Pathologists, Chicago, IL, 1980, pp 81-162.

14. Myers, D.R., DeFehr, J., Bennett, W.M., et al., Gentamicin binding to serum and plasma proteins. *Clin. Pharmacol. Ther.* **23**, 350-360 (1978).

15. Jones, S.M., Blazevic, D.J., and Balfour, H.H., Jr., Stability of gentamicin in serum. *Antimicrob. Agents Chemother.* **10**, 866-867 (1976).

16. Broughall, J.M., Bywater, M.J., Holt, H.A., and Reeves, D.S., Stabilization of cephalosporins in serum and plasma. *J. Antimicrob. Chemother.* **5**, 471-472 (1979).

17. Neu, H.C., Perspectives on antibiotics. In *Seminars in Infectious Diseases,* **1**, L. Weinstein and B.N. Fields, Eds., Stratton Intercontinental Medical Book Corp., New York, NY, 1978, pp 97-121.

18. Masur, H., Whelton, P.K., and Whelton, A., Neomycin toxicity revisited. *Arch. Surg.* **111**, 822-825 (1976).

19. Schentag, J.J., Lasezkay, G., Plaut, M.E., et al., Comparative tissue accumulation of gentamicin and tobramycin in patients. *J. Antimicrob. Chemother.* **4(Suppl. A)**, 23-30 (1978).

20. Echeverria, P., Siber, G.R., Paisley, J., et al., Age-dependent dose response to gentamicin. *J. Pediatr.* **87**, 805-808 (1975).

21. Szefler, S.J., Wynn, R.J., Clarke, D.F., et al., Relationship of gentamicin serum concentrations to gestational age in preterm and term neonates. *J. Pediatr.* **97**, 312-315 (1980).

22. Luft, F.C., Rankin, L.I., Sloan, R.S., and Yum, M.N., Recovery from aminoglycoside nephrotoxicity with continued drug administration. *Antimicrob. Agents Chemother.* **14**, 284-287 (1978).

23. Noone, P., Parsons, T.M.C., Pattison, J.R., et al., Experience in monitoring gentamicin therapy during treatment of serious Gram-negative sepsis. *Br. Med. J.* **i**, 477-481 (1974).

24. Bootman, J.L., Wertheimer, A.I., Zaske, D., and Rowland, C., Individualizing gentamicin dosage regimens in burn patients with Gram-negative septicemia: A cost—benefit analysis. *J. Pharm. Sci.* **68**, 267-272 (1979).

25. Lietman, P.S., Chloramphenicol and the neonate—1979 view. *Clin. Pharmacol.* **6**, 151-162 (1979).

26. Snyder, M.J., and Woodward, T.E., The clinical use of chloramphenicol. *Med. Clin. North Am.* **54**, 1187-1197 (1970).

27. Polin, H.B., and Plaut, M.E., Chloramphenicol. *N.Y. State J. Med.* **77**, 378-381 (1977). Review.

28. Rahal, J.J., Jr., and Simberkoff, M.S., Bactericidal and bacteriostatic action of chloramphenicol against meningeal pathogens. *Antimicrob. Agents Chemother.* **16**, 13-18 (1979).

29. McCracken, G.H., Jr., and Eichenwald, H.F., Antimicrobial therapy in infants and children. Part II. Therapy of infectious conditions. *J. Pediatr.* **93**, 357-377 (1978).

30. Black, S.B., Levine, P., and Shinefield, H.R., The necessity for monitoring chloramphenicol levels when treating neonatal meningitis. *J. Pediatr.* **92**, 235-236 (1978).

31. Kucers, A., Current position of chloramphenicol chemotherapy. *J. Antimicrob. Chemother.* **6**, 1-9 (1980). Review.

32. Burke, J.T., Wargin, W.A., and Blum, M.R., High-pressure liquid chromatographic assay for chloramphenicol, chloramphenicol-3-monosuccinate, and chloramphenicol-1-monosuccinate. *J. Pharm. Sci.* **69**, 909-911 (1980).

33. Glazko, A.J., Identification of chloramphenicol metabolites and some factors affecting metabolic disposition. In *Antimicrobial Agents and Chemotherapy—1966.* American Society for Microbiology, Washington, D.C., 1967, pp 655-665. Review.

34. Glazer, J.P., Danish, M.A., Plotkin, S.A., and Yaffe, S.J., Disposition of chloramphenicol in low birth weight infants. *Pediatrics* **66**, 573-578 (1980). Review.

35. Koup, J.R., Lau, A.H., Brodsky, B., and Slaughter, R.L., Chloramphenicol pharmacokinetics in hospitalized patients. *Antimicrob. Agents Chemother.* **15**, 651-657 (1979).

36. Sack, C.M., Koup, J.R., and Smith, A.L., Chloramphenicol pharmacokinetics in infants and young children. *Pediatrics* **66**, 579-584 (1980).

37. Koup, J.R., Lau, A.H. Brodsky, B., and Slaughter, R.L., Relationship between serum and saliva chlor-

amphenicol concentrations. *Antimicrob. Agents Chemother.* **15**, 658-661 (1979).

38. Aranda, J.V., Turmen, T., and Cote-Boileau, T., Drug monitoring in the perinatal patient: Uses and abuses. *Ther. Drug Monit.* **2**, 39-49 (1980).

39. Friedman, C.A., Lovejoy, F.C., and Smith, A.L., Chloramphenicol disposition in infants and children. *J. Pediatr.* **95**, 1071-1077 (1979).

40. Jordan, D.C., and Reynolds, P.E., Vancomycin. In *Antibiotics, III: Mechanism of Action of Antimicrobial and Antitumor Agents*, J.W. Corcoran and F.E. Hahn, Eds., Springer-Verlag, New York, NY, 1975, pp 704-718. Review.

41. Cook, F.V. and Farrar, W.E., Jr., Vancomycin revisited. *Ann. Intern. Med.* **88**, 813-818 (1978).

42. Geraci, J.E., Vancomycin. *Mayo Clin. Proc.* **52**, 631-634 (1977).

43. Lindholm, D.D., and Murray, J.S., Persistence of vancomycin in the blood during renal failure and its treatment by hemodialysis. *N. Engl. J. Med.* **274**, 1047-1061 (1966).

44. Sheldrick, G.M., Jones, P.G., Kennard, O., Williams, D.H., and Smith, G.A., Structure of vancomycin and its complex with acetyl-D-alanyl-D-alanine. *Nature* **271**, 223-225 (1978).

## Suggested Reading

1. Reeves, D.S., Phillips, I., Williams, J.D., and Wise, R., Eds., *Laboratory Methods in Antimicrobial Chemotherapy*, Churchill Livingstone, London, 1978.

2. Lorian, V., Ed., *Antibiotics in Laboratory Medicine*, Williams and Wilkins, Baltimore, MD, 1980.

3. Gilman, A.G., Goodman, L.S., and Gilman, A., Eds., *Goodman and Gilman's The Pharmacological Basis of Therapeutics*, 6th ed., Macmillan Publishing Co., Inc., New York, NY, 1980, pp 1080-1248.

4. Aranda, J.V., Turmen, T., and Cote-Boileau, T., Drug monitoring in the perinatal patient: Uses and abuses. *Ther. Drug Monit.* **2**, 39-49 (1980).

5. Eichenwald, H.F., and McCracken, G.H., Jr., Antimicrobial therapy in infants and children. Part I. Review of antimicrobial agents. *J. Pediatr.* **93**, 337-356 (1978).

6. Bennett, W.M., Muther, R.S., Parker, R.A., et al., Drug therapy in renal failure: Dosing guidelines for adults. Part I: Antimicrobial agents, analgesics. *Ann. Intern. Med.* **93**, 62-89 (1980).

# 31

# Therapeutic Drug Monitoring of Aminoglycoside Therapy: Relationship to Efficacy and Toxicity

Deborah H. Schaible, Pharm. D.

## Introduction

The aminoglycoside antibiotics are widely used primarily for the management of serious infections caused by gram-negative organisms. They are bactericidal antibiotics with activity against most aerobic gram-negative bacteria. The most commonly used systemic aminoglycosic antibiotics include amikacin, gentamicin, streptomycin, and tobramycin. Streptomycin is primarily utilized in the management of tuberculosis and will not be further discussed in this paper. The remaining three agents will be discussed with regard to factors influencing therapeutic response, nephrotoxicity, and ototoxicity. The relationship of therapeutic drug monitoring to these issues will be emphasized, and guidelines for monitoring will be presented.

## Factors Influencing Therapeutic Response

The clinical efficacy of aminoglycoside therapy is influenced by factors such as microbiological susceptibility, host defense factors, and drug concentration in the serum and at the site of infection. The antibacterial spectra of amikacin, gentamicin, and tobramycin differ little at clinically achievable concentrations in serum except against *Pseudomonas aeruginosa* and some strains of *Proteus*, *Providentia*, and *Serratia* (1). Widespread use of aminoglycosides has resulted in the emergence of resistant bacterial strains. Gentamicin resistance among some gram-negative strains is due to plasmid-mediated transfer of aminoglycoside-inactivating enzyme activity. Due to structural similarities between gentamicin and tobramycin, gentamicin-inactivating enzymes usually also affect tobramycin. However, some strains of gentamicin-resistant *Pseudomonas* do retain sensitivity to tobramycin (1).

Amikacin has fewer structural sites susceptible to attack by the aminoglycoside-inactivating enzymes. Most of the common aerobic gram-negative bacilli retain susceptibility to amikacin even after development of tobramycin and gentamicin resistance (2).

---

*Dr. Schaible is Clinical Pharmacy Coordinator for Intensive Care Medicine at the Children's Hospital National Medical Center, Washington, D.C.*

---

Susceptibility testing of aerobic gram-negative organisms should be performed against all three aminoglycosides, and amikacin therapy should remain reserved for use against all strains resistant to both tobramycin and gentamicin. Selection of an aminoglycoside for initial management of a patient with suspected gram-negative sepsis should be based upon the evolving susceptibility patterns of gram-negative organisms within a hospital.

The status of the individual patient's immune system may also influence therapeutic outcome. Patients who have poor defense systems due to neutropenia, previous drug administration (antineoplastics, corticosteroids), radiation therapy, or severe systemic illness may require higher aminoglycoside serum concentrations or a combination of synergistic antibiotics for effective antibacterial activity.

Peak concentrations in serum associated with clinical efficacy are in the range of 5-10 mg/L for gentamicin (and tobramycin) and 20-30 mg/L for amikacin. These peak concentrations in serum usually exceed the minimum inhibitory concentration for the susceptible gram-negative bacilli by at least two-fold. Predose (trough) concentrations in serum of less than 2 mg/L for gentamicin/tobramycin and less than 10 mg/L for amikacin also have been recommended. Evidence for a relationship between aminoglycoside toxicity and peak and nadir concentrations in serum has formed the basis for these guidelines (3).

The site of the infection also may influence therapeutic efficacy. Central nervous system, bronchial, and biliary penetration may be unpredictable, and concentrations attained at these sites may be inadequate to eradicate an infection. In general, when aminoglycosides are used in the management of meningitis, pneumonia, or biliary tract infections, peak concentration in serum should be in the high therapeutic range. Peak concentrations in serum of 8 mg/L or higher have been associated with successful treatment of gram-negative pneumonia (4).

## Drug Administration and Monitoring of Drugs in Serum

Aminoglycoside antibiotics are generally administered by either the intramuscular or intravenous routes for systemic infections. They are poorly absorbed after oral administration. Intramuscular and intravenous administration yield similar concentrations in serum in most adult and pediatric patients (3).

Initial dosage selection may be made on the basis of nomograms which take into account such variables as patient age, sex, and lean body weight. One limitation of these nomograms is that they assume average pharmacokinetic parameters which may not apply to all patients. After initial nomogram-based dosage selection, adjustments should be based upon the results of drug concentrations in serum and the use of basic pharmacokinetic principles.

Despite the recognition that knowledge of drug concentrations in serum is essential to monitoring therapy, few physicians have received training in basic clinical pharmacokinetics. As a result, both the ordering and interpretation of aminoglycoside concentrations in serum may be less than optimal. Three retrospective studies have demonstrated that only 14-22% of aminoglycoside concentrations in serum are both obtained and interpreted correctly. This results in a waste of time and funds for both the patient and institution. Improvement in these statistics after establishment of a therapeutic drug monitoring program may be used to justify the cost of such a program (4).

Careful attention should be given to the timing of blood specimen collection for determination of aminoglycoside concentrations in serum. In addition to the aforementioned problems with physician interpretation of test results, problems may be encountered with the relationship between the time and route of drug administration and specimen collection. When administered by intramuscular injection, peak concentrations in serum should be obtained within 1 h. After intravenous administration as a 30-50 min infusion, peak concentrations in serum should be obtained 30 min after the termination of the infusion to allow for drug distribution to occur. Consistent with the pharmacokinetic principle that greater than 90% of the eventual steady-state concentration in serum is attained after four half-lives, concentrations in serum may be obtained after 24-48 h of therapy (5).

Any interpretation of data concerning drug concentration in serum must take into account drug infusion characteristics and their potential influence on drug delivery. Pediatric intravenous infusion systems designed to deliver solutions at slow intravenous infusion rates have been associated with unexpected delays in drug delivery. This is a particular problem when drugs are injected into the intravenous tubing at sites most distal to the needle (6). The timing of drug delivery varies with the physiochemical

properties of the drug, the site of injection into the infusion system, and the rate of flow through the system. Drug delivery cannot always be calculated by dividing the volume to be delivered by the rate of infusion. This problem has been documented for gentamicin and chloramphenicol in systems with flow rates of 29 mL/h (6, 7).

## Nephrotoxicity

The incidence of aminoglycoside-induced nephrotoxocity has been reported to vary from 5 to 40%. Some of this variation in incidence may be attributed to differences between studies in patient population, surveillance techniques, and the definition of nephrotoxicity (8).

This nephrotoxicity has been attributed to specific damage of cells which line the renal proximal tubule. Aminoglycosides have been shown to concentrate in renal cortical tissue to levels which exceed concentrations in serum by several-fold (9). The existence of their accumulation and persistence in renal tissue has been further supported by the recovery of gentamicin from the urine for 10-30 days after discontinuation of therapy (10). An evaluation for accumulation in renal cortical tissue should include trough aminoglycoside concentrations in serum. Rising trough concentrations to greater than 2-2.5 mg/L for gentamicin and greater than 10 mg/L for amikacin have been associated with subsequent nephrotoxic reactions. The dosing interval may also affect the risk for nephrotoxicity. Both animal and human studies have demonstrated increased nephrotoxicity with administration of a daily dose by continuous, as compared to intermittent, infusion (11).

Elevations of creatinine in serum and urea nitrogen in blood remain the most commonly used indicators of renal dysfunction. Nephrotoxicity has been defined as any increase in creatinine in serum by 5.0 mg/L or more during therapy or within one week of the last dose (11). One limitation of this definition is that these changes in serum chemistry values may be relatively late indicators of nephrotoxicity (3). The recent development of more sensitive indicators of nephrotoxicity has enabled its detection five to ten days prior to elevations in serum creatinine (9).

Early changes in renal function associated with aminoglycoside adminstration include impaired urinary concentrating capacity, proximal tubular transport dysfunction, and the presence of increased protein and certain enzymes in the urine. The early impairment in ability to concentrate the urine may at least partially explain why patients with aminoglycoside nephrotoxicity may be in functional "renal failure" while maintaining a normal volume of urine output.

Early aminoglycoside-induced proteinuria involves increased urinary excretion of $\beta_2$-microglobulins. The presence of increased urinary concentrations of this protein has been associated with renal proximal tubular injury, observed by both light and electron microscopy before any observed reduction in glomerular filtration rate (9).

A variety of enzymes may be found in increased concentrations in the urine of aminoglycoside-treated patients. These include renal lysosomal enzymes as well as enzymes from the proximal renal tubules. However, tests for this enzymuria do not accurately predict the later development of frank nephrotoxicity and reduced glomerular filtration rate. This enzymuria may be too sensitive and nonspecific as an indicator of toxicity. Indeed, abnormal enzymuria has been documented during 70% of the courses of aminoglycoside therapy in a population of cystic fibrosis patients who never developed subsequent evidence of nephrotoxicity (12). Abnormal enzymuria has also occurred in febrile and critically ill patients (1).

Predisposing risk factors for the development of nephrotoxicity include increased patient age, prolonged duration of therapy, frequent drug administration, reduced renal mass, and concomitant administration of other nephrotoxic drugs. Age-related differences in susceptibility to aminoglycoside nephrotoxicity have not been carefully defined in humans. However, older animals appear more susceptible to aminoglyoside nephrotoxicity than are younger animals (9).

The selection of a particular aminoglycoside may also influence the risk for nephrotoxicity. Animal studies show gentamicin and amikacin to be more nephrotoxic than tobramycin. This is supported by studies of relative accumulation of these compounds in renal tissue which show less accumulation with tobramycin than with gentamicin. Prospective randomized clinical trials show equal nephrotoxicity for amikacin and gentamicin whereas tobramycin appears to be the least nephrotoxic (3, 11, 13).

## Ototoxicity

The exact incidence of ototoxicity is unknown but has been estimated to be 3 to 24% (1). As with nephrotoxicity, the variable incidence probably relates to differences in both definition and evaluation of ototoxic reactions. When *symptomatic* vestibular toxicity is assessed, a 2% incidence is reported. However, more sensitive audiometric and vestibular testing reveal a greater than 30% incidence of asymptomatic ototoxicity (3).

Aminoglycosides may affect both the auditory and labyrinthian portions of the eighth cranial nerve. Early ototoxicity is characterized by subtle hearing loss, usually bilateral, for high frequency sounds. This may be followed by tinnitus and total deafness. This process may be permanent or may be reversed after discontinuation of therapy.

Assessment for hearing loss should include audiometric testing in addition to clinical evaluation. Audiograms are necessary to detect early changes in high frequency sound conduction that may not be evident on physical examination. Newer testing procedures such as brainstem auditory evoked responses have not yet gained widespread use in the evaluation of aminoglycoside ototoxicity. Adverse vestibular effects include vertigo, abnormalities of gait and problems with ocular movements. In conjunction with the patient history and physical examination, sophisticated electronystagmography may be used to evaluate these ocular effects (14).

Predisposing factors to the development of ototoxicity include renal impairment, a prolonged treatment course, and coadministration of other potentially ototoxic drugs such as furosemide and ethacrynic acid, two loop-inhibiting diuretics. It is imperative that high risk patients be evaluated before, during, and after discontinuation of therapy. Many patients may have a pre-existing hearing loss; one study has shown that 75% of hospitalized patients had abnormal audiograms prior to aminoglycoside therapy (1).

Ototoxicity of aminoglycosides appears to relate to their slow penetration into the perilymph and endolymph fluid of the inner ear with subsequent damage to the cochlear hair cells. Peak concentrations in the inner ear are achieved at 2-4 h after drug administration. Concentrations in the inner ear decline more slowly than concentrations in serum and aminoglycoside half-life in the inner ear fluid has been noted to be 10-12 h. Since aminoglycoside penetration is gradual, the transiently high concentrations in serum obtained shortly after drug administration probably do not reflect concentrations in the inner ear. However, persistently elevated concentrations in serum throughout a dosage interval or a prolonged duration of therapy probably increases the risk of ototoxicity. To minimize the toxic risk, trough concentrations in serum of gentamicin should be maintained below 2.5 mg/L (3, 14).

## Recommendations for Monitoring

Therapeutic drug monitoring of aminoglycoside therapy plays an important role in assuring drug efficacy while attempting to minimize toxicity.

Recommendations for such a monitoring program should include:

1. assessment of patient variables such as site of infection, bacterial agent, pre-existing disease states (renal failure or immunocompromise), and concomitant drug therapy
2. maintenance of peak concentrations in serum in the range of 5-10 mg/L for gentamicin/tobramycin and 20-30 mg/L for amikacin
3. avoidance of trough concentrations higher than 2 mg/L for gentamicin/tobramycin and 10 mg/L for amikacin
4. assessment of renal, auditory, and vestibular function before, during, and after therapy.

## References

1. Meyers, B.R., The aminoglycosides. In *Antimicrobial Therapy*, B.M. Kogan, Ed., W.B. Saunder Co., Philadelphia, PA, 1980.
2. Price, K.E., Defuria, M.D., and Purisano, T.A., Amikacin, an aminoglycoside with marked activity against antibiotic resistant clinical isolates. *J. Infect. Dis.* **134** (Suppl), S249-S261 (1976).
3. Yee, G.C., and Evans, W.E., Reappraisal of guidelines for pharmacokinetic monitoring of aminoglycosides. *Pharmacotherapy* **1**, 55-75 (1981).
4. Bollish, S.J., Kelly, W.N., Miller, D.E., and Timmons, R.G., Establishing an aminoglycoside pharmacokinetic monitoring service in a community hospital. *Am. J. Hosp. Pharm.* **38**, 73-76 (1981).
5. Schentag, J.J., Gentamicin. In *Basic Clinical Pharmacokinetics*, M.E. Winter, Ed., Applied Therapeutics, Inc., San Francisco, CA,
6. Gould, T., and Roberts, R.S., Therapeutic problems arising from the use of the intravenous route for drug administration, *J. Pediatr.* **95**, 465 (1979).
7. Nahata, M.C., Powell, D.A., Glazer, J.P., and Hilty, M.D., Effect of intravenous flow rate and injection site on the in vivo delivery of chloramphenicol succinate and in vivo kinetics. *J. Pediatr.* **79**, 463-466 (1981).
8. Noone, P., Parsons, T.M.C., and Pattison, J.R., et al., Experience in monitoring gentamicin therapy during treatment of serious gram-negative sepsis. *Brit. Med. J.* **1**, 477-481 (1974).
9. Kaloyanides, G.J., and Pastoriza-Munoz, E., Aminoglycoside nephrotoxicity. *Kidney International* **18**, 571-582 (1980).
10. Schentag, J.J., and Jusko, W.J., Renal clearance and tissue accumulation of gentamicin. *Clin. Pharmacol. Ther.* **22**, 364-370 (1977).
11. Smith, C.R., Lipsky, J.J., and Laskin, O.L., et al., Double blind comparison of the nephrotoxicity and auditory toxicity of gentamicin and tobramycin. *N. Engl. J. Med.* **302**, 1106-1109 (1980).
12. Reed, M.D., Vermeulen, M.W., and Stern, R.C., et al., Are measurements of urine enzymes useful during aminoglycoside therapy. *Pediatr. Res.* **15**, 1234-1239 (1981).
13. Schentag, J.J., Plaut, M.E., and Cerra, F.B., Comparative nephrotoxicity of gentamicin and tobramycin: Pharmacokinetic and clinical studies in 201 patients. *Antimicrob. Agents Chemother.* **19**, 859-866 (1981).
14. Lerner, S.A., and Matz, G., Aminoglycoside ototoxicity. *Am. J. Otolaryng.* **1**, 169-179 (1980).

# 32

# Aminoglycosides: Applied Pharmacokinetics

**Darwin Zaske, Pharm.D., F.C.P.**

## Introduction

Because of their unique spectrum of activity with the common pathogens causing hospital acquired infections, aminoglycoside antibiotics are widely used. Unfortunately, the dosages and concentrations in serum that are required for maximum efficacy approximate those associated with toxicity—usually nephrotoxicity and ototoxicity, the incidence of which reportedly range between 3 and 10% for the commonly used aminoglycosides, gentamicin, tobramycin, and amikacin. These antibiotics are used to treat infections that have a very high risk of mortality, but at the same time there must be concern for their potential toxicity. Their concentrations in serum must be measured and their dosages adjustered to ensure maximum safety and efficacy.

Patients with compromised renal function eliminate these antibiotics more slowly. There are nomograms based on serum creatinine or creatinine clearance for adjusting the dosages in such patients *(1)*, but the wide inter-patient variation in these relationships precludes really acceptable precision in making these dosage adjustments. Measuring the highest and lowest concentration in serum has been suggested as a further means of monitoring and adjusting the dosage in patients with severe Gram-negative infections *(2)*. This ultimately leads to a trial-and-error period with various dosages, before the desired serum concentrations are attained—an interval that can well be excessively long and expose patients to a higher risk of treatment failure or toxicity. Further, Anderson et al. *(3)* have demonstrated that the empirical use of maximum peak and minimum values in serum leads to dosage errors and inappropriate use of serum concentration/time data.

A method has been developed and applied in which serum concentration/time data from a patient are used to calculate the drug's kinetic parameters *(4)*. After the clinician has determined the therapeutic endpoint in terms of maximum and minimum concentrations in serum, the optimum dosage regimen may be calculated for the individual patient, based on the drug's kinetic parameters. Use of this method allows

*Dr. Zaske is Associate Professor, College of Pharmacy and Division of Surgical Sciences, School of Medicine, University of Minnesota at St. Paul-Ramsey Medical Center, St. Paul, Minnesota, 55101.*

the clinician to attain the desired serum concentrations rapidly, thus obviating the trial-and-error period. The optimum dosage and concentrations in serum can be calculated and attained within 12 to 24 h after starting the treatment. The improved analyses now available for the aminoglycoside antibiotics have remarkably increased their clinical use. Here, I describe the rationale for these serum assays and specific considerations in providing the drug-monitoring services.

## Drug Administration

Aminoglycoside antibiotics are given several ways. Infusions during 30–60 min are commonly used and may be safer for the patient. This method of administration allows sufficient time for the antibiotic to equilibrate with tissues and induce their lethal effects on the bacteria. After infusion, the drug is eliminated from the body, decreasing the concentrations within the inner ear and the kidney, and thereby reducing the risk of toxicity. Aminoglycosides diffuse into in vivo tissue level models more slowly than do other antibiotics. Models indicate that by maintaining an optimum concentration for 30 to 60 min, higher concentrations of these antibiotics in tissue may be achieved. In addition, the drug equilibrates with tissues during the 30 to 60 min infusion, which simplifies the pharmacokinetic principles of the drug, allowing use of a simple one-compartment model to describe the disposition of the drug after its infusion. In hospitals, the nursing staff should have a consistent policy for administering these drugs, to decrease the likelihood of error as nurses change nursing stations.

Some investigators suggest infusing the drug continuously, but this may be very difficult to do in an intensive-care unit where the patient may be receiving many intravenous medications. A higher incidence of toxicity has also been suggested. In addition, the aminoglycoside antibiotics only need to be in brief contact with the bacteria to exert their killing effect, so once the antibiotic concentration reaches the optimum level, the drug can be eliminated from the body, thus reducing the risk of oto- and nephrotoxicity. For this reason, continuous infusions have not been recommended or widely used for these aminoglycoside antibiotics. In the European literature, bolus injections of aminoglycosides have been suggested, which minimizes nursing time. However, this incurs an increased risk of ototoxicity from the very high transient concentrations that result from these bolus injections.

## Serum Sampling

The time when serum samples are obtained from the patient is extremely important in improving estimates of drug elimination. Ideally, serum should be sampled after the first dose and over two or three biological half-lives of the drug. By using serum samples after the first dose, a predose value is not required, thus reducing the number of serum samples needed for calculating our dosage regimen. This allows an optimal decline in concentration and improves our kinetic estimates. The number of samples necessary precisely to estimate our kinetic parameters can be as few as three or four. If more samples are obtained, the cost to the patient is increased, but estimates of the kinetic parameters are not markedly improved. If fewer than three or four samples are used, our estimate of kinetic parameters has substantially more error. In patients with normal renal function, the sampling intervals should be 15–30 min, 1–2 h, and 2–4 h after the infusion is complete. In patients with abnormal renal function, the drug's half-life (in hours) can be estimated by multiplying the serum creatinine concentration (in mg/dL) by four. The sampling interval should be over two to three half-lives. For example: if a patient has a serum creatinine of 4 mg/dL, the estimated half-life is 16 h. Ideal sampling times are 2, 30, and 60 h post-infusion. The time of the infusion and the time for each sample must be carefully recorded if one is correctly to define the concentration/time relationship in each patient (Figure 1). (See *Patient Case, Step One,* below)

## Serum Assays

Patients with severe Gram-negative sepsis must receive optimum dosages quickly if they are to survive. Noone et al. *(6)* reported improved survival rates when optimum concentrations in serum are attained within the first 72 h of therapy. In patients with optimal concentrations, the survival rate was 84%; in patients with subtherapeutic concentrations, the survival rate was 23%. Patients with Gram-negative sepsis cannot tolerate prolonged periods of bacteremia, especially older patients whose cardiovascular system may fail during acute Gram-negative sepsis. Thus, aminoglycoside samples should be measured within each 12- to 24-h period, so the clinician can promptly individualize his patient's therapeutic regimen.

In major metropolitan areas, there are several practical advantages to centralizing aminoglycoside assays to one hospital, especially in the early phases of implementing these services. The central laboratory receives a larger number of serum samples for assay and thus is more cost-efficient. In addition, results of serum assays are more quickly available to assist the clinician in treating his patient. Thus, centralizing the analytical analysis

reduces costs to the patient and increases the utilization of this data in patient care settings.

Of the several techniques for assaying aminoglycoside antibiotics, the earliest was a microbiological method. This method was neither as sensitive nor as precise as currently available methods, and it required a prolonged interval before zones of inhibition could be read and results reported to the clinician. In addition, its reproducibility has been questioned. The other, more recent techniques include radioimmunoassay, radioenzymatic, "high-performance" liquid-chromatographic, and gas–liquid chromatographic methods. These methods are rapid and have good precision and sensitivity for concentrations that are clinically important, but they are expensive if few patients' samples are run in relation to the number of control samples. Newer assay methods now in development may offer advantages. For clinical purposes, any of the commonly used assay methods can be used to measure serum concentrations and individualize the patient's dosage. Available laboratory personnel, instrumentation, and projected utilization are important factors in determining which assay methodology is selected.

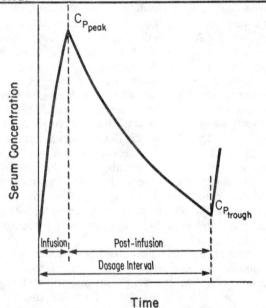

**Fig. 1.**  Drug concentration in serum as a function of time, indicating infusion period and post-infusion period.

To determine the drug's half-life or elimination rate constant, three serum concentration times are needed in the post-infusion interval. The peak concentration ($CP_{peak}$) is the fitted concentration immediately after the infusion.

## Serum Concentration/Time Data

After the concentration in serum has been measured, the concentration/time data should be plotted on semi-log paper. This allows easy assessment of the data, and any errors, including transcription errors may be obvious after visually inspecting the fit of the data. This visual inspection improves confidence of the consultant in making a dosage prediction for an individual patient. In addition, the data plot can also be used to obtain initial estimates of the drug's half-life or elimination rate constant ($k_d$). In this way, institutions without computer facilities can obtain the necessary kinetic parameters without sophisticated computer technology (See *Step Two,* below).

There are several different mathematical methods for fitting the serum concentration/time data.

One, nonlinear regression analysis, requires rather sophisticated computer technology. Although the most nearly accurate, this method depends on access to a large computer, and may be impractical for the clinical setting.

Another is the use of the log of serum concentration vs. time and least squares regression analysis of the log of serum concentration rather than concentration. This method of data fitting is widely available now that inexpensive hand-held calculators are available. When the data fit well, this method provides accurate estimates of the kinetic parameters, but if the data are nonlinear, bias in kinetic parameters may result. The data are weighted for lower concentrations because values for similar concentrations occupy a larger part of the lower end of the log scale. This weighting may influence the fitting of the data and the estimates of the kinetic parameters. However, the error is generally negligible for most patients and does not substantially affect the calculated dosage regimens. Thus, this method provides a very practical clinical approach to fitting serum concentration/time data.

The peak serum concentration immediately after the infusion is obtained from the serum concentration/time data. The exact time of the infusion period must be carefully recorded, as well as the time of serum sampling. The peak value is that found immediately after infusion and should not be extrapolated back to the start of the infusion. (Certain computer programs may inadvertently extrapolate a concentration back to the start of the infusion if the data are not appropriately entered into the program.) This can make a substantial error in calculating a patient's distribution volume, and ultimately will result in a major error in dosage regimen. For example, the relation of concentration vs. time is illustrated for a hypothetical patient in Figure 1. The peak value immediately after the infusion is indicated. If the fitted line were extrapolated to the start of the infusion, the peak concentration would be markedly higher and would incorrectly estimate the "true" peak value, which occurs immediately after the infusion.

## Half-life and Elimination Rate Constant

Methods are now available for using serum concentration/time data to determine each patient's dosage. The necessary pharmacokinetic parameters are the drug's half-life, elimination rate constant, and distribution volume. The half-life and elimination rate constant are obtained from the post-infusion concentration/time data for serum, which describe the rate of drug elimination (Figure 1). The drug's half-life is the time required for the serum concentration to decrease by 50% from the previous value. The elimination rate constant is related to the half-life and can be determined as follows:

$$K_d = \frac{0.693}{T_{\frac{1}{2}}}$$

The elimination rate constant has reciprocal units of time (e.g., $h^{-1}$) (See *Step Three,* below).

There is wide interpatient variation in the drug elimination rate; variation is similar for tobramycin, gentamicin, and amikacin. It is seen even if patients are categorized according to states of renal function (Figure 2). In patients with a normal serum creatinine concentration, gentamicin's half-life can vary from 0.5 to 33 h. In patients with a normal creatinine clearance ($\geq$100 mL/min per 1.73 $m^2$ of body surface), the drug's half-life ranges between 0.5 to 7.5 h. Thus, to obviate excessively long periods during which concentrations are subinhibitory, the dosing interval must be adjusted for

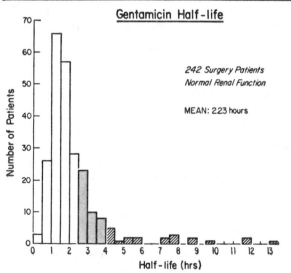

**Figure 2.** Interpatient variation found in gentamicin half-life in 242 surgery patients with normal renal function

The reported range was 2.5-4 h.

the individual patient's rate of elimination. In addition, half-lives in some patients will be long, and so the dosing interval must be prolonged to prevent excessively high minimum-value concentrations, which may increase the risk of toxicity. These data and the patient's clinical condition must be considered by the clinician in selecting an optimal dosage regimen for specific patients.

## Distribution Volume

The "distribution volume" describes a hypothetical or pharmacological space within which a particular drug distributes itself. It is the dose administered divided by the change in serum concentration. For example, if a patient receives 80 mg of gentamicin in a single dose and the change in serum concentration is 8 mg/L, the distribution volume is 80 mg divided by 8 mg/L, or 10 L. Because aminoglycosides are frequently administered over 30-60 min, a substantial amount of drug may be eliminated *during* the infusion period. This is especially important in patients with more rapid rates of drug elimination such as patients showing a drug half-life of 30 min. Thus, equations and mathematical models to calculate the volume of distribution must consider the amount of drug that is eliminated during the infusion. The amount of drug eliminated from the previous dose must also be considered in the mathematical equation. The following equation takes into account the fraction of drug elim-

### Gentamicin Distribution Volume

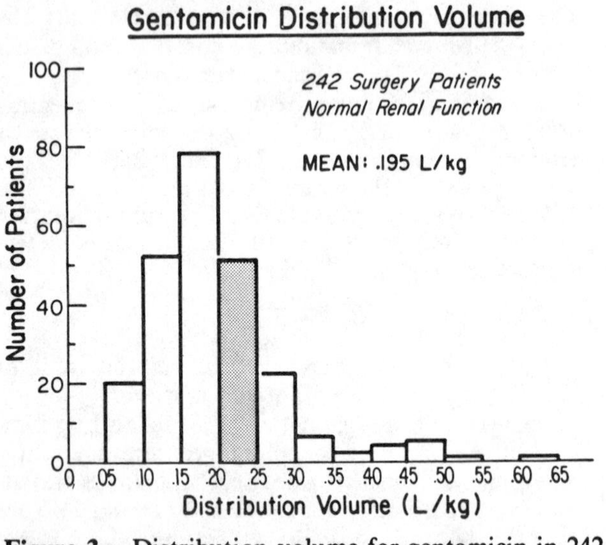

**Figure 3.** Distribution volume for gentamicin in 242 surgery patients

Previously, the distribution volume was thought to be consistent from patient to patient and to approximate the extracellular fluid compartment of 20-25% of body weight. As can be seen, there is considerable variation here.

inated during the infusion period ($t'$) if one knows (a) the peak concentration after infusion ($Cp_{max}$), (b) the concentration before infusion ($Cp_{min}$), (c) the elimination rate constant ($K_d$), and (d) the infusion rate ($K_o$). The infusion rate ($K_o$) is calculated by dividing the dose (mg/kg of body weight) by the infusion period ($t'$); it has units of time and mass (mg/kg per h). The distribution volume has units of volume and mass (L/kg) in this equation:

$$V_d = \frac{K_o}{K_d} \frac{1 - e^{-kdt'}}{Cp_{max} - (Cp_{min} e^{-kdt'})}$$

(See *Step Four*, below).

For the aminoglycoside antibiotics, the distribution volume is similar to the volume of the extracellular fluid compartment, which in healthy adults is between 20 and 25% of body weight. In patients who are dehydrated the drug distribution volume is frequently lower; in patients who have a large extracellular fluid compartment, such as patients in congestive heart failure, the drug distribution volume is frequently larger. Thus, there is a large inter-patient variation in this kinetic parameter for all aminoglycoside antibiotics (Figure 3). This parameter is particularly important because a patient's dose will vary directly with the drug's distribution volume.

## Dosage Interval

A patient's dosage interval (T) is calculated from the desired maximum concentration ($Cp_{max-D}$), the desired minimum concentration, the elimination rate constant ($K_d$), and the infusion period ($t'$). The equation for calculating each patient's dosage interval is:

$$T = \frac{-1}{K_d} ln \frac{Cp_{min-D}}{Cp_{max-D}} + t'$$

These calculated dosing intervals must be rounded to correspond to practical intervals for the nursing staff, which are 4, 6, 12, 24, and 48 h (See *Step Five*, below).

## Dose

Each patient's dose ($K_o$) is calculated to produce a desired change in concentration from the drug's distribution volume ($V_d$), the desired peak concentration ($Cp_{max-D}$), the elimination rate constant ($K_d$), the dosing interval (T), and the infusion period ($t'$). The equation for calculating the dose is:

$$K_o = K_d V_d Cp_{max-D} \frac{1 - e^{-kdT}}{1 - e^{-kdt'}}$$

For adults, the dose must be rounded to the nearest 10 mg increment for gentamicin and tobramycin and to the nearest 25 mg increment for amikacin.

After a patient's dosage is individualized, subsequent maximum and minimum concentrations should be measured during the course of therapy to further titrate to the patient's optimum dosage. In patients with a low or a high volume, these concentrations should be measured in a period of two or three days of treatment. In patients with rapidly changing renal function, maximum and minimum concentrations should be measured daily if necessary. In patients who are clinically stable, maximum and minimum concentrations should be measured after five to seven days of treatment. Further dosage adjustments may be required to maintain therapeutic concentrations.

### Intra-Patient Variation

Patients also demonstrate an intra-patient variation for gentamicin, tobramycin, and amikacin. Because 80-95% of the aminoglycoside is eliminated via the kidney, changing renal function can result in changing elimination. This can be generally assessed by measuring serum creatinine, creatinine clearance, or serum urea nitrogen.

Several other factors have also been identified that are independent of changes in renal function, e.g., a change in the drug's distribution volume that follows rehydration of the dehydrated patient by administering intravenous fluids. Or a drug's distribution volume may change as a result of treatment such as surgical drainage of peritoneal abscess, reversal of congestive heart failure, or decrease in excessive fluid intake. In addition, drug clearance may decrease during the treatment, perhaps as a result of physiological changes occurring during the treatment of Gram-negative sepsis, or as a direct result of a decrease in fever, which will result in decreased cardiac output, decreased renal blood flow, and decreased glomerular filtration rate, and thus a decrease in the drug's elimination rate by the kidney. Also, the drug may accumulate in the tissue in some patients, with a resulting decrease in drug clearance (5). Such patients should have aminoglycosides measured in their serum during the course of treatment.

### Patient Safety

The incidence of both ototoxicity and nephrotoxicity reportedly ranges between 3 and 10%. Other studies evaluating subclinical changes in both kidney function and eighth cranial nerve function suggest that the incidence of toxicity may even exceed 10% in patients treated with aminoglycosides. Some estimates of subclinical oto- and nephrotoxicity are as high as 25% of patients treated with aminoglycosides. The initial 1065 patients treated with individualized dosing of gentamicin in our institution were evaluated for nephrotoxicity and overt signs of clinical ototoxicity. Patients who had a change in serum creatinine greater than 5 mg/L

from baseline were defined as having a substantial change in candidates for drug toxicity. Of these 1065 patients, 16 showed a significant change in serum creatinine concentration during the course of therapy. Eight of the 16 patients had a severe hypotensive episode at onset of sepsis. In these patients, serum creatinine increased rapidly during the early days of therapy, and this was thought to be ascribable to hypotension rather than to therapy with gentamicin. Eight of the initial 1065 patients had a significant increase in serum creatinine that was attributed to gentamicin. The change in serum creatinine was small, which would indicate that their individualized regimens prevented serious changes in kidney function secondary to therapy with aminoglycosides. None of these patients required hemodialysis as a result of renal damage. Individualizing dosages of aminoglycosides seemingly decreases the incidence of nephrotoxicity and perhaps also its severity.

In addition, these same 1065 patients were evaluated for ototoxicity. None exhibited overt signs of either cochlear or vestibular dysfunction. We have done detailed analysis of eighth cranial nerve function, including audiometry and electronystagmography. Our early findings indicate that even subclinical changes in cochlear function and vestibular function can be prevented by individualizing the dosage regimens.

### Efficacy

During the past several years, the major reason for measuring concentrations of gentamicin in serum, and adjusting dosage regimens was to ensure optimal concentrations and improve the efficacy of therapy. Noone et al. (6) reported a response rate of 89% in patients with Gram-negative pneumonias who had therapeutic concentrations of gentamicin in their serum, but the response rate in patients who did not attain therapeutic concentrations was 43%. In a large series of burn patients (7), adjusting gentamicin dosages to ensure therapeutic concentrations increased the patient-survival rate from 33% to 64% for the entire hospital course. Also in burn patients, a complication of *Pseudomonas* sepsis, ecthyma gangrenosum, is reportedly consistently fatal, but substantial number of such patients responded to gentamicin treatment, although they required extremely high dosages to achieve therapeutic concentrations (8). In controlling concentrations in burn patients, dosages frequently were required that exceeded those commonly recommended. In one patient, the required gentamicin dose was 30 mg/kg per day, six times the maximal recommended daily dose (8).

### Cost/Benefit

The additional expense of measuring concentrations in serum is substantial and it should be questioned whether the added costs improve patient care. From a recent study, the costs of providing this service were determined (*9*). These costs were in fact balanced by the benefit realized by the increase in patient survival (*10*). The benefit from improved patient safety was not included in these analyses. Even so, the cost/benefit ratio indicated that society realizes a favorable outcome from these services. The cost/benefit ratio ranged from 1/4.5 to 1/24.0, indicating that society realizes 4.5 to 24 dollars for every dollar that the service cost.

## Team Effort

Individualization of aminoglycoside antibiotics requires a multidisciplinary approach. Frequently, members of this team includes the primary physician, nurse, clinical pharmacist, clinical chemist, clinical microbiologist, medical technologist, pathologist, infectious disease internist, and pediatrician. A marked improvement in patient safety and efficacy is likely when such a functional team approach is used. This requires effective communication among all of the members of this team. Initially, extensive training is required to ensure that the aminoglycoside antibiotic is being administered appropriately, that serum values are being obtained properly, and that the concentration/time data are being interpreted correctly. The application of this method allows the clinician to identify patients who are rapid or slow eliminators of aminoglycosides and to determine each patient's individual dosage regimen. With a successful team approach, patients receiving aminoglycosides in your hospital will likely benefit by improved efficacy and safety from individualized regimens.

## Example of a Patient Case

### Step One

Our patient is a 32-year-old, 130-pound pregnant woman, who was admitted on January 21 with premature contractions. Her leukocyte count is 16,500, and her differential indicates 96% polymorpho-nucleocytes. Her serum urea nitrogen concentration is 6 mg/dL, and her serum creatinine concentration is 5 mg/L. On January 22nd, a premature infant (26-weeks gestational age) is delivered without complications. On January 23rd, the patient's temperature increased to 39.9°C. On physical examination, the patient is found to have abdominal tenderness, and periendometritis or endometritis are suspected. Blood, urine, and endometrial cultures were obtained. Intravenous therapy with antibiotics is initiated: penicillin 5 million units every 6h and gentamicin 65 mg every 8h. The patient received the first dose of gentamicin on January 23rd at 2400 hours.

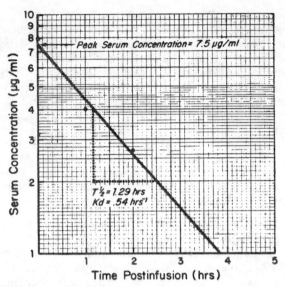

**Figure 4.** Time post gentamicin infusion versus serum concentration in sample patient.

Drug concentrations in serum were measured after the second dose of gentamicin, which was infused from 0800 to 0900h. The time that the specimens were obtained and the concentrations were as follows:

| Time, h | Conc, mg/L |
| --- | --- |
| 0755 | 0.5 |
| 0900 | 7.9 |
| 1000 | 4.0 |
| 1100 | 2.7 |

### Step Two

Plot the serum concentration time data on semi-log paper and determine the line of best fit (*Answer:* see Figure 4).

### Step Three

Determine the drug's half-life, elimination rate constant, and peak serum concentration after infusion from the line of best fit (*Answer:* see Figure 4).

### Step Four

Using the data presented in the case history, determine the patient's distribution volume of gentamicin from the equation. (*Answer:* the distribution volume is 6.95 L or, when standardized to body weight, 0.12 L per kilogram.)

### Step Five

Determine the patient's dosage interval to obtain a peak serum concentration of 8 mg/L and a "trough" of 1 mg/L, for a 60-min infusion. (*Answer:* the calculated dosing interval is 4.87 h. This interval is rounded to a practical increment of 4 or 6 h. A 6-h interval was selected in this patient whose clincial signs were stable.)

### Step Six

Determine the patient's dose to obtain the same peak and trough serum concentrations with use of a 6-h dosing interval. (*Answer*: the calculated dose is 68.9 mg. This would be rounded to 60 or 70 mg, which can be accurately measured by the nursing staff. In this patient 70 mg would be selected. Thus, the patient's dosage regimen would be 70 mg every 6 h.)

### References

1. Hull, H.J., and Sarubbi, F.A., Gentamicin serum concentrations; pharmacokinetic predictions. *Ann. Int. Med.* **85,** 183-189 (1976).

2. Barza, M., Brown, R.N., Shen, D., et al., Predictability of blood levels of gentamicin in man. *J. Infec. Dis.* **132,** 165-174 (1975).

3. Anderson, A.C., Hodges, G.R., and Barnes, W.G. Determination of serum gentamicin sulfate levels. *Arch. Intern. Med.,* **136,** 785-787 (1976).

4. Sawchuk, R.J., Zaske, D.E., Cipolle, R.J., et al., Kinetic model for gentamicin dosing with the use of individual patient parameters. *Clin. Pharmacol. Ther.* **21** 365-371 (1977)

5. Schentag, J.J., Jusko, W.J., Plaut, M.E., et al. Tissue persistence of gentamicin in man. *J. Am. Med. Assoc.* **283,** 327-329 (1977)

6. Noone, P., Parsons, T.M.C., Pattison, J.R. et al., Experience in monitoring gentamicin therapy during treatment of serious gram-negative sepsis. *Br. Med. J. i,* 477-481 (1974).

7. Zaske, D.E., Strate, R.G., Solem, L.F., et al., Improved burn patient survival with individualized gentamicin dosages. *American Burn Association, 11th Annual Meeting, New Orleans, 1979.*

8. Solem, L.D., Zaske, D.E., and Strate, R.G., Ecthyma gangrenosum: survival with individualized antibiotic therapy. *Arch. Surg.* **114,** 580-583 (1979).

9. Bootman, J.L., Zaske, D.E., Wertheimer, A.I., et al., Cost of individualizing aminoglucoside dosage regimens. *Am. J. Hosp. Pharm.* **36,** 368-370 (1979).

10. Bootman, J.L., Wertheimer, A.I., Zaske, D.E. et al., Individualizing gentamicin dosage regimens in burn patients with gram-negative septicemia: A cost benefit analysis. *J. Pharm. Sci.* **267,** 267-272 (1979).

# 33

# Use of Vancomycin in Treatment of *Staphylococcus epidermidis* Endocarditis in an Infant

**Roger L. Boeckx, Ph.D.**
**Deborah H. Schaible, Pharm.D.**

A.H. is a 17-month-old male infant who was admitted for the management of a 20% lower extremity scald burn. During his five-month hospitalization, he developed multiple problems including respiratory failure followed by adult-type respiratory distress syndrome necessitating mechanical ventilation for three months, multiple bouts of bacterial sepsis, and bacterial endocarditis.

The last problem, bacterial endocarditis, was associated with positive cultures for a methicillin-resistant strain of *Staphylococcus epidermidis*. The organism was, however, sensitive to vancomycin, and a six-week course of vancomycin was begun. The patient was begun on a regimen of 150 mg of vancomycin every 6 h (40 mg/kg/day) which resulted in peak and trough concentrations in serum of 38 mg/L and 15 mg/L, respectively. After six days the dosage was adjusted to 150 mg every 8 h (30 mg/kg/day). During the next two weeks, peak vancomycin concentrations in serum ranged between 27 and 39 mg/L and trough concentrations ranged between 8 and 10 mg/L.

After 21 days of vancomycin therapy, the patient developed pneumonia. Cultures from tracheal aspirates and bronchial brush border biopsies were positive for *Pseudomonas aeruginosa*. The organism was sensitive to aminoglycosides, and the patient was begun on gentamicin in addition to the vancomycin. Initial gentamicin therapy was with 37 mg every 12 h (5 mg/kg/day) which produced peak and trough concentrations in serum of 4.5 and 1.1 mg/L, respectively. The gentamicin regimen was changed to provide 37 mg every 8 h resulting in peak and trough concentrations of 7.0 and 1.6 mg/L.

Gentamicin was discontinued after 14 days of therapy. Repeat cultures were negative for *P.*

*Dr. Boeckx is Associate Director of Clinical Chemistry at Children's Hospital National Medical Center and Associate Professor of Child Health and Development at the George Washington University School of Medicine and Health Sciences in Washington, D.C. Dr. Schaible is Clinical Pharmacy Coordinator for Intensive Care Medicine at Children's Hospital National Medical Center in Washington, D.C.*

*aeruginosa.* Vancomycin was discontinued after a total of six weeks of therapy. All subsequent blood cultures were negative for staphylococci; however, the infant remained hospitalized a total of five months for the management of his burns.

This case describes the use of vancomycin in a child with *Staphylococcus epidermidis* endocarditis. Although not a new drug by any means, vancomycin is experiencing a renaissance due to the frequent appearance of *S. epidermidis* infections resistant to other antibiotics. Vancomycin has been shown to be effective in the treatment of a number of staphylococcal infections in children (*1*), specifically skin and soft-tissue infections, osteomyelitis, pneumonia, shunt infections, endocarditis, and septicemia.

Vancomycin is a member of a small group of glycopeptide antibiotics. The group is comprised of compounds such as actinoidin and ristocetin, as well as vancomycin. However, the latter is the only compound in clinical use. Vancomycin was discovered in the early 1950s as part of a search for new antibiotics which were effective against the large number of strains of staphylococci which had become resistant to penicillin, erythromycin, and tetracycline. The compound, later to be named vancomycin, was discovered in the culture medium of a new soil bacterium *Streptomyces orientalis*. This organism had been isolated from soils collected in the jungles of Borneo. Purification of the compound by ion-exchange chromatography and crystallization produced vancomycin hydrochloride of sufficient purity to allow structural determinations.

Early attempts to discern the structure of vancomycin (*2*) revealed the presence of glucose, aspartic acid, *N*-methylleucine, *o*-chlorophenol, and a new sugar which was named vancosamine (*3*). Nuclear magnetic resonance spectrometry eventually allowed the complete structure of the molecule to be described. Williams and Kalman (*4*) showed that the molecule is polycyclic, contains two chlorinated $\beta$-hydroxytyrosines, three phenylglycines, *N*-methylleucine, aspartic acid amide, and glucose in addition to vancosamine. All of the components listed above, except for the carbohydrates, are interconnected in a seven-member peptide chain held in the form of three rings (Figure 1). The molecular weight of vancomycin is 1,448, and the empirical formula is $C_{66}H_{75}N_9O_{24}$.

Vancomycin functions by inhibiting bacterial cell-wall synthesis. The molecule binds tightly to any peptide chain with a D-alanylalanine at the carboxyl terminal. It is postulated that vancomycin binds to the peptide chain of the peptidoglycan precursor and that the stearic hindrance produced by the large vancomycin molecule is sufficient to inhibit substrate binding to peptidoglycan synthetase (6). In addition to its effect on cell-wall synthesis, vancomycin is thought to alter cell-membrane permeability (7) and RNA synthesis (8).

Vancomycin is primarily effective against gram-positive organisms including most strains of *Staphylococcus aureus*, *Staphylococcus epidermidis*, *Streptococcus pneumoniae*, and *Clostridium sp.* However, gram-positive organisms, myobacteria, and fungi are usually resistant.

The preferred method of administration of vancomycin is a slow (30-60 min) intravenous infusion. More rapid administration is associated with an intensely pruritic erythema multiform-like rash (9). Intramuscular administration causes severe pain and orally administered vancomycin is only minimally absorbed. Oral administration is effective only in the treatment of antibiotic-induced diarrhea or enterocolitis caused by *S. aureus* or *C. difficile*.

Vancomycin is predominately excreted by the kidneys via glomerular filtration. Altered renal function has a profound effect on the pharmacokinetics of the drug. In patients with normal renal function, the elimination half-life ranges from 5 to 11 h (10) whereas in the anuric patient the vancomycin elimination half-life may be prolonged to 7.5 days (11). Vancomycin is not removed by hemodialysis, and consequently shunt infections in dialysis patients may be eradicated with once-weekly intravenous vancomycin (11).

Reports of CSF penetration of vancomycin show results which vary with the degree of meningeal inflammation. In one study of 11 adult subjects (12) with noninflamed meninges, no CSF vancomycin could be detected when concentrations in serum ranged from 4.8-10 mg/L. These concentrations are significantly lower than the recommended therapeutic range. In the presence of meningeal inflammation, CSF penetration may be adequate.

One study has shown effective penetration of vancomycin into the ventricular fluid of children with staphylococcal shunt infections. Ventricular vancomycin concentrations in fluid averaged 18% of concomitant concentrations in serum and were associated with sterilization of the CSF (1). These

reports of variable CNS penetration make it imperative to carefully monitor the use of vancomycin in CNS infections. Direct intraventricular injection of vancomycin may be required in some cases in which infection cannot be eradicated (13).

Vancomycin was initially considered to be both a nephrotoxic and ototoxic compound. Since reformulation and purification of the dosage form in the early 1960s, reports of nephrotoxicity and ototoxicity have been rare. Some no longer consider vancomycin to be a significant nephrotoxin when used alone (14). Animal studies have failed to show that vancomycin alone is either ototoxic or nephrotoxic (15-17). However, when vancomycin is used in patients with impaired renal function or in patients receiving other potentially nephrotoxic or ototoxic drugs (such as aminoglycoside antibiotics or loop-inhibiting diuretics such as furosemide or ethacrynic acid), both renal and auditory function should be monitored. Nephrotoxicity has ben reported in animal studies when tobramycin and vancomycin are used concomitantly. This occurs at drug concentrations in serum usually not associated with nephrotoxicity (18).

Current indications for vancomycin therapy in severe staphylococcal infections include infections caused by methicillin-resistant strains, infections in patients who are allergic to penicillins and cephalosporins, infections that fail to respond to other regimens, and a number of special situations such as shunt infections in hemodialysis patients and antibiotic-induced diarrhea (19).

Vancomycin concentrations can be measured in serum and other body fluids. Biological assays using *Bacillus subtilis* as the test organism have been successfully used (18). Recently, a radioimmunoassay

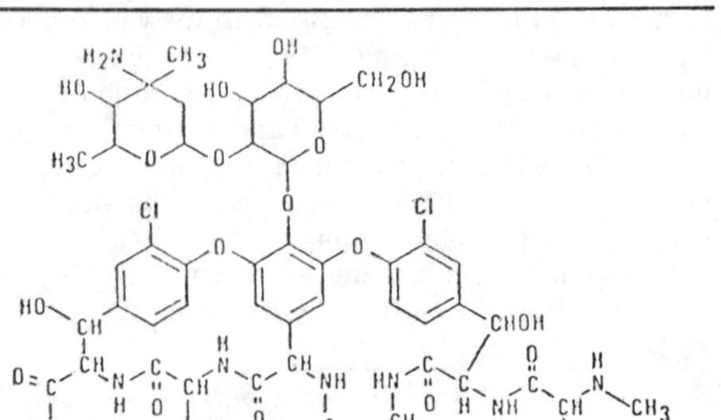

**Fig. 1.** Chemical structure of vancomycin (5)

(20) and a high performance liquid chromatographic assay (9) have been developed. Due to the potential for nephrotoxicity and the altered elimination of the drug in the presence of decreased renal function, vancomycin concentrations in serum should be monitored during therapy. As is the case for the aminoglycosides, the relatively short half-life and the exclusively renal route of elimination make monitoring of both peak and trough concentrations mandatory. Exact guidelines for concentrations in serum associated with optimum therapeutic efficacy remain to be defined. It has been recommended that peak concentrations be maintained between 25 and 40 mg/L, and that trough concentrations should be less than 12 mg/L (21). These concentrations exceed the MIC (minimal inhibitory concentration) and MBC (minimal bacterial concentration) for staphylococci (20).

## Vancomycin Profile

### Chemical Information

| | |
|---|---|
| Trade name: | Vancocin |
| Chemical name: | Vancomycin Hydrochloride |
| pKa: | ? |
| Mol. mass: | 1448 |
| Melting point°C: | ? |
| Water solubility: | Greater than 100 mg/mL |

### Absorption and Distribution

| | |
|---|---|
| Dose absorbed: | Orally administered drug is not absorbed |
| Peak level in plasma, time: | ½-1 h after infusion |
| Protein bound: | 55% |
| Vd: | 0.5-1.25 L/kg |

| Form in urine | % excreted | Active | Detectable in blood |
|---|---|---|---|
| Unchanged drug | Approx 100% | Yes | Yes |

| | Adults | Children |
|---|---|---|
| Half-life: | 5-11 h | 2-10 h |
| Steady state, time: | 20-44 h | 8-40 h |

### Dosage and Blood Levels

| | Adults | Children |
|---|---|---|
| Recommended dose: | 1-2 g/day | 30-40 mg/kg/day |
| Effective levels: | 25-40 mg/L | 25-40 mg/L |
| Toxic levels: | Above 50 mg/L | Above 50 mg/L |

### Monitoring Methods

HPLC (5), Microbiological (18), Radioimmunoassay (19)

## References

1. Schaad, V.B., Nelson, J.D., and McCracken, G.H., Jr., Pharmacology and efficacy of vancomycin for staphylococcal infections in children. *Rev. Infect. Dis.* **3**, S282-S288 (1981).
2. Marshall, F.J., Structure studies on vancomycin. *J. Med. Chem.* **8**, 18-22 (1965).
3. Smith, R.M., Johnson, A.W., and Guthrie, R.D., Vancosamine: A novel branched chain amino sugar from the antibiotic vancomycin. *J. Chem. Soc.* **6**, 361-362 (1972).
4. Williams, D.H., and Kalman, J.R., Structural and mode of action studies on the antibiotic vancomycin. Evidence from 270-MHz proton magnetic resonance. *J. Am. Chem. Soc.* **99**, 2768-2774 (1977).
5. Uhl, J.R., and Anhalt, J.P., High Performance liquid chromatographic assay of vancomycin in serum. *Therapeutic Drug Monitoring* **1**, 75-83 (1979).
6. Watanakunakorn, C., The antibacterial action of vancomycin. *Rev. Infect. Dis.* **3**, S210-S215 (1981).
7. Jordan, D.C., and Malloy, H.D.C., Site of action of vancomycin on *Staphylococcus aureus*. *Antimicrob. Agents Chemother.* **4**, 489-494 (1964).
8. Jordan, D.C., and Inniss, W.E., Selective inhibition of ribonucleic acid synthesis in *Staphylococcus aureus* by vancomycin. *Nature* **184**, 1894-1895 (1959).
9. Schaad, V.B., McCracken, G.H., Jr., and Nelson, J.D., Clinical pharmacology and efficacy of vancomycin in pediatric patients. *J. Pediatr.* **96**, 119-126 (1980).
10. Krogstad, D.J., Moellering, R.C., Jr., and Greenblatt, D.J., Single-dose kinetics of intravenous vancomycin. *J. Clin. Pharmacol.* **20**, 197-201 (1980).
11. Cunha, B.A. Quintiliani, R., Deglia, J.M., Izard, M.W., and Nightingale, C.M., Pharmacokinetics of vancomycin in anuria. *Rev. Infect. Dis.* **3**, S269-S272 (1981).
12. Geraci, J.E., Heilman, F.R., Nichols, D.R., Wellman, W.E., and Ross, G.T., Some laboratory and clinical experiences with a new antibiotic, vancomycin. *Proc. Staff Meet. Mayo Clin.* **31**, 564-582 (1956).
13. Congeni, B.L., Tan, L., Salstrom, S.J., and Weinstein, L., Kinetics of vancomycin after intraventricular and intravenous administration. *Pediatr. Res.* **13**, 459 (1979).
14. Appel, G.B., and Neu, H.C., The nephrotoxicity of antimicrobial agents. *N. Engl. J. Med.* **296**, 722-729 (1977).

15. Brummett, R.E., Effects of antibiotic-diuretic interactions in the guinea pig model of ototoxicity. *Rev. Infect. Dis.* **3**, S216-S223 (1981).

16. Wold, J.S., and Turnipseed, S.A., Toxicology of vancomycin in laboratory animals. *Rev. Infect. Dis.* **3**, S224-229 (1981).

17. Aronoff, G.R., Sloan, R.S., Dinwiddie, C.B., Jr., Glant, M.D., Fineberg, N.S., and Luft, F.C., Effects of vancomycin on renal function in rats. *Antimicrob. Agents Chemother.* **19**, 306-308 (1981).

18. Sabath, L.D., Casey, J.I., Ruch, P.A., Stumpf, L.L., and Finland, M., Rapid microassay of gentamicin, kanamycin, neomycin, streptomycin, and vancomycin in serum or plasma. *J. Lab. Clin. Med.* **78**, 457-463 (1971).

19. Kirby, W.M.M., Vancomycin therapy in severe Staphylococcal infections. *Rev. Infect. Dis.* **3**, S236-S239 (1981).

20. Crossley, K.B., Rotschafer, J.C., Chern, M.M., Mead, K.E., and Zaske, D.E., Comparison of a radioimmunoassay and a microbiological assay for measurement of serum vancomycin concentrations. *Antimicrob. Agents Chemother.* **17**, 654-655 (1980).

21. Cook, F.V., and Farrar, W.E., Vancomycin revisited. *Ann. Int. Med.* **88**, 813-818 (1978).

# 34
# Chloramphenicol: A Case History

Roger Boeckx, Ph.D.

This case is that of a 3-week-old white female, the full-term product of an uncomplicated pregnancy and delivery.

One day before admission the infant vomited after a feeding and had one copious stool. She fed poorly during the rest of the day and slept through her night feeding, which her mother stated to be unusual. All other family members, including a 2-year-old brother, were well.

Early on the day of admission, the child appeared pale, listless, and sweating; she would not feed and appeared limp, and without spontaneous movements. The infant was brought to the Emergency Department. On admission she was described as markedly lethargic with a "septic stare," and difficulty in breathing. Temperature was 37.2° C, pulse rate 180/min, and respirations were shallow. She weighed 3 kg. The child was intubated and arterial blood gases at this time were: $pO_2$ 143 mmHg, $pCO_2$ 43 mmHg, pH 7.12. The infant was given 10 mL albumin solution, 8 mmol bicarbonate and 500 mL of an intravenous solution consisting of 50 g/L glucose and 1/3 strength saline. A spinal tap showed 15,000 leukocytes/mm$^3$ and was described as purulent with 100% polymorphonuclear cells. A Gram stain showed numerous Gram-negative bacilli. Glucose concentration in the cerebrospinal fluid was 200 mg/L; protein was not measured.

The patient was diagnosed as having meningitis complicated by septic shock and was given 200 mg of chloramphenicol and 350 mg of ampicillin and transferred to the Intensive Care Unit.

At this time, laboratory studies showed: hemoglobin, 147 g/L; hematocrit, 41%; leukocytes, 3000/mm$^3$ (4% bands, 6% neutrophils, 67% lymphocytes, 11% monocytes, 12% atypical lymphocytes); serum sodium, 143 mmol/L; potassium, 4.3 mmol/L; chloride, 101 mmol/L; total $CO_2$, 10 mmol/L; urea nitrogen, 90 mg/L; creatinine, 9 mg/L; calcium, 44 mmol/L; prothrombin time, 172% of control; partial thromboplastin time, 210% of control; platelet count, 81,000/mm$^3$; pH, 7.28; $pO_2$, 120 mmHg; $pCO_2$, 50 mmHg. The patient had persistent hypotension and was treated with intravenous dopamine and epinephrine.

The patient's neurological status degenerated rapidly with pupils becoming at first sluggish and then nonreactive to light. Seizures began late in the day, necessitating anticonvulsant therapy with intravenous phenobarbital.

---

*Dr. Boeckx is the Assistant Director of Clinical Chemistry at Childrens Hospital, National Medical Center, Washington, D.C.*

---

An initial loading dose of 30 mg of phenobarbital was given, followed by 15 mg every 12 h for the subsequent 36 h. A maintenance regimen of 5 mg/kg per day given in two doses at 12 h intervals was begun thereafter. Intravenous phenytoin was begun early on the 3rd day of admission, the dosage being 8 mg/kg per day divided in two doses every 12 hours. On day 3, a peak phenobarbital concentration was 27 mg/L, and a peak phenytoin concentration was 8 mg/L. The patient also received furosemide, dexamethasone and mannitol to combat cerebral edema. Chloramphenicol dosage was maintained at 50 mg/kg per day in two doses. The highest value for serum taken 2 hours after a dose was 53 mg/L; the lowest value, that for a sample taken 1 h before the next dose was, 43 mg/L.

Counter-immunoelectrophoresis of urine and serum confirmed the presence of *Hemophilus influenzae*.

Despite continuing aggressive therapy, the infant became unresponsive to pain, showed decerebrate movements, and expired on the third hospital day.

This case illustrates the use of chloramphenicol in an infant with *H. influenza* meningitis. It also serves to illustrate the often fragile nature of the newborn or young infant. The child presented with advanced meningitis and septic shock after showing signs of illness for only one day. Despite aggressive therapy, the shock was irreversible and the child succumbed. In most cases, however, the treatment described would be more successful, and would result in a successful resolution of the illness.

Although chloramphenicol concentrations were considerably above the usually recommended range of 10 to 20 mg/L, the symptoms described are not due to chloramphenicol toxicity. This infant received a regimen that has been shown to be appropriate for her age. It is conceivable that the hypotension might have resulted in a significant decrease in hepatic perfusion with resultant loss of liver metabolism of the drug.

Chloramphenicol is the drug of choice in a case of this type. When faced with a seriously ill infant with meningitis, the antibody chosen must cover a wide range of organisms and must be able to cross the blood brain barrier. As is illustrated by this case, it is sometimes not possible to wait long enough for the organism to be identified and for susceptibility studies to be completed.

## The Pharmacology of Chloramphenicol

Chloramphenicol is a potent antibacterial and antirickettsial agent isolated in 1947 from *Streptomyces venezuelae*. It was first successfully used in the treatment of typhus in 1947 (*1*). Since then it has been shown to be an effective agent in the treatment of infections by a number of other Gram-positive and Gram-negative organisms and rickettsiae. It acts by inhibiting ribosomal protein synthesis by depressing the activity of peptidyl transferase, effectively uncoupling translocation from peptide bond formation.

Chloramphenicol inhibits mycoplasma and the molluscan phase of schistosomiasis, but is inactive against fungi, yeast, viruses, protozoa and most strains of *Pseudomonas*. The fact that many strains of *Hemophilus influenza type b* are killed in the pres-

ence of chloramphenicol concentrations of only 10 mg/L has made chloramphenicol a major drug in the treatment of *H. influenza* meningitis and pneumonia. Its use has increased as the number of ampicillin resistant *H. influenza* isolates has increased.

Certain bacteria are resistant to chloramphenicol owing to their ability to produce a specific acetyltransferase that catalyzes the acetylation of the 3-hydroxyl group of the propanolol side chain. *E. coli* can acquire resistance by transfer of a resistance factor (R factor), a plasmid, during conjugation. Some Gram-

# Chloramphenicol

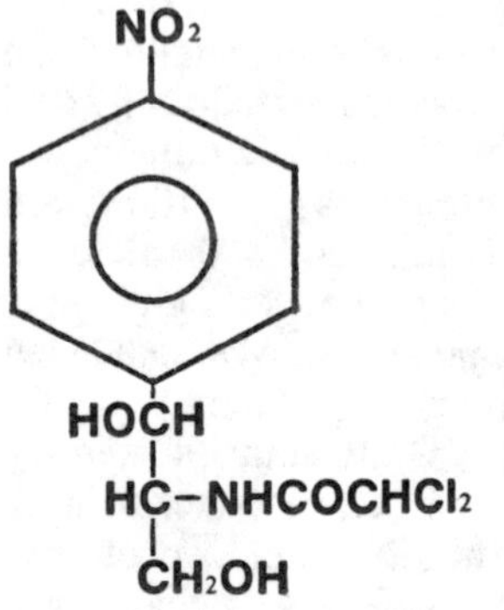

**Trade name:** Chloromycetin
**pKa:** 5.5
**Mol. wt.:** 323.14
**mp,°C:** 150.5 - 151.5
**Water solubility:** 2.5 mg/mL at 25°C
**Chemical name:**

D-threo-*N*-dichloroacetyl-1-*p*-nitrophenyl-2-amino-1,3-propanediol

**Dose absorbed:** 75-90%
**Peak plasma level, time:** 20-40 $\mu$g/mL, 2 h after a 4 g dose (adult)
**Protein bound:** 60% (at peak)
**Vd:** 0.57 L/kg

| Form in urine | % Excreted | Active | Detectable in blood |
|---|---|---|---|
| unchanged drug: | 5-10% | yes | yes |
| monoglucronide: | 70-80% | no | no |
| arylamine: | trace | no | no |
| glycolic acid metabolite: (newborn only) | trace | no | no |

| | Adults | Children |
|---|---|---|
| Half time: | 1.5-3.5 h | 2 h |
| Steady state, time: | 8-18 h | 10 h |

| | Adults | Children | Infants 1st week | Infants 2-4 weeks |
|---|---|---|---|---|
| Recommended dose: | 50-100 mg/kg/d *** | 50-100 mg/kg/d** | 25 mg/kg/d* | 50 mg/kg/d* |
| Effective levels: | 10-20 $\mu$g/mL | 10-20 $\mu$g/mL | 10-20 $\mu$g/mL | 10-20 $\mu$g/mL |
| Toxic levels: | > 25 $\mu$g/mL | > 25 $\mu$g/mL | > 25 $\mu$g/mL | > 25 $\mu$g/mL |

**Monitoring methods:** GLC, HPLC, Radioenzymatic, Bioluminescense

\*dosed at 12 h intervals
\*\* dosed at 6 h intervals
\*\*\* dosed at 4 h intervals

positive organisms, such as *Staphylococcus aureus* have also shown chloramphenicol resistance. There is, however, no trend toward an increasing prevalence of resistance.

The drug diffuses rapidly throughout the body, and detectable concentrations are found in serum 20 min after oral ingestion. Peak values are reached within 2 h. The liver is the major organ of metabolism, and most of the chloramphenicol conjugated there is re-absorbed from the gut and excreted in the urine.

Chloramphenicol is metabolized by the conjugation systems of the endoplasmic reticulum of the liver, which means that it can interfere with the metabolism of other drugs; tolbutamide, phenytoin, and dicumarol for example, can be inhibited by therapeutic doses of chloramphenicol. Since children with meningitis often develop intractable seizures, it is not uncommon for them to receive one or two anticonvulsants while on chloramphenicol therapy.

Although the biological half-life of chloramphenicol in adults is about 2 h (2), the metabolism of the drug in the newborn is significantly different and is dependent upon gestational and postnatal age (3, 4). The immaturity of the enzyme systems responsible for conjugation and excretion of chloramphenicol place the newborn at risk of accumulating active chloramphenicol. Although the recommended dosage regimen now takes into account the relative immaturity of the conjugation system and the rapid maturation of the system in the first six weeks of life, high concentrations of chloramphenicol in serum are still observed in infants receiving this drug.

The toxic effects of excessive chloramphenicol concentrations can be serious and are not necessarily limited to the immediate neonatal period. Anemia, with a normocellular marrow, is occasionally described and occurs when concentrations in plasma are maintained over 25 mg/L. Patients usually recover completely when therapy is stopped. Other toxic effects include nausea, diarrhea, vomiting (with oral administration), digital parasthesias, and optic neuritis, especially in children with cystic fibrosis.

A more serious and life-threatening reaction in the newborn and especially in premature infants was first described in 1959. The "gray baby" syndrome, presumably caused by inhibition of the mitochondrial electron transport chain by high concentrations of chloramphenicol, is the most serious complication of chloramphenicol therapy in this age group. Most cases have been related to excessively high doses of chloramphenicol, generating concentrations in plasma far in excess of 50 mg/L. Symptoms usually appear three to four days after therapy is begun. The syndrome begins with abdominal distension, progressive cyanosis, green stools, vasomotor collapse, and often death, usually within two days. Early recognition and cessation of chloramphenicol administration has resulted in reversal with complete recovery.

While this syndrome has been most frequently associated with excessively high dose therapy in neonates, serious dose independent reactions have been described at chloramphenicol concentrations closer to the therapeutic range.

A very small proportion of patients receiving chloramphenicol (between 1 in 24,000 and 1 in 200,000) develop a serious hypersensitivity manifested primarily by a severe blood dyscrasia. Over 70% of these cases presented with aplastic anemia, and in those cases of complete bone marrow aplasia, the fatality rate was 100%. The outcome is unrelated to dose, length of therapy, or route of administration.

The potential for severe adverse effects and a lack of clear understanding of the pharmacokinetics of chloramphenicol in the newborn makes the use of therapeutic monitoring mandatory when the drug is used in this age group. Ideally the concentration of chloramphenicol in serum should be maintained below 25 mg/L and preferably between 10 and 20 mg/L.

Gas chromatographic (5), high performance liquid chromatographic (HPLC) (6), radioenzymatic (7), and bioluminescent (8) methods have been described. Earlier colorimetric procedures suffered from interference by bilirubin and nonactive metabolites of chloramphenicol. Pickering et al. have recently compared three methods for measuring chloramphenicol in serum (7). Gas chromatographic methods make use of an analog of chloramphenicol as an internal standard and require the use of electron-capture detectors (5, 7). A gas-chromatographic mass/spectrometric procedure is also described (7). Radioenzymatic methods make use of chloramphenicol acetyl transferase, isolated from specific strains of *E. coli,* to transfer radioisotopically labeled acetate from acetyl-CoA to chloramphenicol (7). The acetylated derivative is then extracted and counted. All three methods are specific and give reliable results.

A reversed-phase HPLC method, requiring very small sample sizes has also been described (6), and more recently, a specific "micro-scale" procedure employing bioluminescence has been developed (8).

### References

1. Meissner, H.C., and Smith, A.L., The current status of chloramphenicol. *Pediatrics* **64**, 348-356 (1979).

2.  G. Ireland, Ed., *Drug Monitoring Data Pocket Guide,* American Association for Clinical Chemistry, Washington, D.C., 1980, p. 19.

3.  Lietman, P.S., Chloramphenicol and the neonate — 1979 view. *Clinics in Pharmacol.* **6,** 151-162 (1979).

4.  Glazer, J.P., Danich, M., Yachette, S., et al., Disposition of chloramphenicol in newborn infants. *Pediatr. Res.* **12,** 405 (1978).

5.  Resnick, G.L., Corbin, D., and Sandberg, D.H., Determination of serum chloramphenicol utilizing gas-liquid chromatography and electron capture spectrometry. *Anal. Chem.* **38,** 582-585 (1966).

6.  Petersdorf, S.H., Raisys, V.A., and Opheim, K.E., Micro-scale method for liquid-chromatographic determination of chloramphenicol in serum. *Clin. Chem.* **25,** 1300-1302 (1970).

7.  Pickering, L.K., Hoecker, J.L., Kramer, W.G., et al., Assays for chloramphenicol compared: Radioenzymatic, gas chromatographic with electron capture, and gas chromatographic mass spectrometric. *Clin. Chem.* **25,** 300-305 (1979).

8.  Boeckx, R.L., and Brett, E.M. A micro-method for the measurement of chloramphenicol in serum by bioluminescence. *Clin. Chem.* **26,** 971 (1980).

# 35

# Antibiotics: Methods For Analysis

**Robert J. Cipolle, Pharm.D.**

## Introduction

The health-science community has allocated enormous time, energy, and resources to improving diagnostic techniques and instrumentation, but only minimal emphasis on optimizing drug therapy once the diagnosis has been established. This generalization is particularly true with respect to antimicrobial therapy. Recent advances in anaerobic bacteriology, radiologic investigations, and epidemiology have improved the clinicians' ability to make a diagnosis and determine the causative organism. However, once diagnosis and pathogen have been established, antibiotic therapy is often based on "package-insert" recommendations. Factors known to influence drug disposition, improve efficacy, or minimize toxicity are seldom taken into account.

Over the past decade drug monitoring has repeatedly been demonstrated to improve efficacy and minimize symptoms of toxicity of several antibiotics (1-3). Most work in this area has involved the aminoglycoside antibiotics, including gentamicin, tobramycin, and amikacin. The wide interpatient variation in distribution and elimination of these drugs makes essential the careful monitoring of concentrations in serum, to ensure therapeutic and avoid potentially toxic concentions (4-8). Individualized dosing with aminoglycosides allows control of the concentrations of these antibiotics and improves efficacy and safety (9-11).

These advances in individualizing antibiotic dosage regimens have been made clinically practicable because rapid and accurate antibiotic assays are available. Additionally, this rapidly growing awareness of the utility of antibiotic assays has increased the demand for improvements in assay sensitivity, specificity, and timeliness, as well as reduction in cost. The purpose of this communication is to acquaint the practitioner and laboratorian with the major assay methods now available for antimicrobials as well as the potential advantages and limitations of each.

## Microbiological Assay

Originally, most antibiotic assays were microbiological assays. Several bioassay techniques were developed and used in clinical laboratories, including the agar diffusion, agar or broth dilution, turbidimetric, and urease methods. Agar diffusion is the most widely used technique. The diffusion of antibiotic can be vertical (in tubes) or horizontal (on plates). The latter is more practicable. Its principle is similar to that of the

*Dr. Cipolle is Assistant Professor, College of Pharmacy at the University of Minnesota, and Associate Director of Pharmaceutical Services at St. Paul-Ramsey Medical Center St. Paul, Minnesota 55101.*

disc-diffusion susceptibility test (12). For the bioassay, autoclaved agar is poured into a flat dish, the indicator organism being either incorporated in the agar or poured onto the agar surface. The plates are dried and paper discs (or wells) saturated with test serum or standard antibiotic concentrations are placed on the plates. The diameter of the growth-inhibition zone for each of the standard discs is measured. A regression curve is constructed, to establish the relationship between a measured growth-inhibition zone and the corresponding antibiotic concentration. The size of the growth-inhibition zone surrounding the disc or well that contains the test serum is then compared, with use of the regression curve, and from this the antibiotic concentration of the test serum is calculated.

The several limitations to microbiological methods for antimicrobial agents include the considerable time often required before results are available, and the need for appropriate indicator organisms to constantly be available, making prior notification of the laboratory essential. Bioassay techniques often require 12 to 48 h. If a heavy inoculum of a fast-growing test organism is used, a preliminary reading of the growth inhibition zones can be made after 3 to 5 h (13).

Several antibiotic assays, especially for aminoglycosides, can be considerably affected by the composition of the growth medium, and by ion concentrations, pH, and temperature changes. The antimicrobial activity of aminoglycosides is enhanced in alkaline environments, so careful pH control is required. The degree of ionization of these agents as well as the ionic composition of the media can influence the bacterial uptake and diffusion of aminoglycosides. Optimally, test or control samples should be diluted with normal pooled serum rather than with broth. This may be especially important for antibiotics that are highly bound to serum proteins, because serial dilutions with broth may mask the inhibitory effect of serum proteins and the lysing effect of complement. In the case of patients with serious metabolic diseases, it may be necessary to use the patient's own antibiotic-free serum as a control to establish the standard curve and for any dilutions of specimens obtained after drug administration (14).

Generally, bioassay techniques require relatively large volumes of sample (5mL), thereby limiting their value in neonates, pediatric patients, and other patients from whom such volumes are not appropriate. Large specimen requirements also limit the usefulness of bioassays for pharmacokinetic and metabolic studies that require numerous serial determinations of antibiotic concentration. Microbioassays have been developed that require small volumes of sample material (14), but also require time-consuming dilutions and lack specificity similar to the agar diffusion methods. Additionally, very small zones of growth-inhibition around the test sample discs (or wells) are difficult to interpret, and limit the sensitivity of bioassays. The upper limit of these assays is also restricted to a growth-inhibition zone that is small enough not to overlap the neighboring zones produced by the standard discs. To determine the higher concentrations often present in urine samples, additional, often unforeseen dilutions are required.

Therapy with a combination of antibiotics is often required, especially in hospitalized patients. Serum samples from such patients pose additional problems. Analysis for individual antibiotic concentrations requires additional laboratory technology, equipment, and personnel time. Quantitating a single antibiotic concentration in a specimen from a patient receiving multiple antibiotic therapy can be facilitated by (a) inactivating other antimicrobials (by using beta-lactamase, $p$-aminobenzoic acid) before the analysis, (b) using a strain of test organism that is selectively sensitive to one of the antibiotics in the sample, and (or) (c) separating the drugs (by electrophoresis) in the specimen before microbiological analysis (15).

The importance of monitoring antibiotics in patients who are receiving chemotherapy for cancer is well established. However, several of the commonly used antineoplastic agents reportedly inhibit the activity of some antibiotics. Moreover, many antineoplastic agents have intrinsic antimicrobial activity and therefore can interfere with bioassays in patients who are receiving both types of drugs. Wright and Matsen (16) reported that the presence of 5-fluorouracil resulted in as much as a 100% positive error in cephalothin concentrations when bioassay techniques were used. Similar interference may result in patients' specimens that contain doxorubicin or dactinomycin.

Microbiological techniques have the advantage that a wide variety of antimicrobial assays are available. If single-drug therapy is used virtually any antimicrobial concentration can be quantified by use of bioassay techniques. The equipment and personnel required are readily available in most hospitals and reagent costs for routine determinations are minimal.

### Radioimmunoassay

During the past decade there has been a rapid expansion in the clinical application of radioimmunoassay (RIA) techniques, which incorporate basic principles of immunology, radiochemistry, and engineering. The essence of the radioimmunoassay system is the immune reaction, the binding of antibody to antigen (17). The basic reagents are antibody, labelled antigen, and unlabelled antigen. The labelled antigen is "tagged" with a radionuclide, an atom that spontaneously decays and releases radioactivity (alpha, beta, or gamma radiation, or x-rays).

In the presence of a fixed limited amount of antibody, labelled and unlabelled antigens compete for attachment to antibody sites. The antigen antibody complex is separated from the unbound antigens by use of a second antibody, to the first antibody. This complex precipitates and can be separated by centrifu-

gation. The radioactivity in the bound precipitate is measured. Gamma-emitting isotopes are measured by transferring the sample to be measured into a well drilled in a crystal of sodium iodide. In sodium iodide radioactive energy is converted to light energy pulses, in direct proportion to the amount of radioactivity present. The light energy can then be measured with a spectrometer. When isotopes that emit beta radiation are used, a liquid scintillation counter is required. A liquid medium is used that converts the radioactive energy to light energy. Beta emitters, tritium ($^3$H) and carbon-14 ($^{14}$C), and gamma emitters, iodine-125 ($^{125}$I), are the most common radioisotopes used in commercially prepared RIA systems. Results for the unknown specimen are compared with those in a standard curve constructed by using known concentrations of unlabelled antigen (drug). The standard curve for radioimmunoassays is plotted on logit-log paper and should be linear within the range of measured concentrations. Advantages of RIA techniques over the traditional biological drug assays include greater specificity and sensitivity, small volume of sample material required, assay speed, and potential for automation. The specificity of an RIA depends on the availability of antibodies that will react with a specific antigen (drug), but do not cross react with other substances in the sample material. The specificity of the radioimmunoassay techniques for antibiotics is exemplified by the availability of an antibody produced against tobramycin bovine serum albumin conjugate, which is essentially nonreactive with gentamicin or sisomicin. Despite the close structural similarities of these antibiotics, an assay must be able to distinguish among the several aminoglycoside antibiotics used in clinical practice. It is common for a patient's therapy to be changed from one aminoglycoside antibiotic to another depending on final culture and sensitivity results. It is essential to distinguish between structurally similar antibiotics, to ensure that therapeutic but nontoxic concentrations of the agent as present.

RIA systems are considerably more sensitive than are most biological drug assays. Such techniques have been used to detect biologically potent substances in concentrations as low as picograms per milliliter. In general, commercially available RIAs for aminoglycoside antibiotics provide reliable results in the low range of 0.5 to 1 mg/L. Lower antibiotic concentrations, often required in pharmacokinetic studies, can be quantitated by altering dilutions of reagents and sample in the assay protocol. Another advantage of RIA systems that often is important in pharmacokinetic investigations, is the small sample required. Less than a few hundred microliters of specimen is required, this often facilitates measuring antibiotic concentrations in newborns and other patients from whom sample material is unusually limited. A clinical laboratory that does RIA can make assay results available to the clinician within 2 to 4 h of receipt of the sample, timeliness that is essential for antibiotic assays such as aminoglycosides, because most patients require dosage adjustments early in their course of treatment.

The primary disadvantages of the RIA include the expensive equipment (scintillation counter) required and the need for highly specific antibodies and suitable radiolabelled drug reagents. Extemporaneous preparation of specific antibodies and radiolabelled drug is too expensive and time consuming for most clinical laboratories. Commercially prepared reagents currently are available for several biological and pharmacological substances. Radioimmunoassays have been developed to assist in the diagnosis of many disease states as well as in monitoring drug concentrations, and are now widely used. Walker's excellent review *(18)* of RIA procedures, interpretation, pitfalls, and quality-assurance measures would be useful for analysts who have limited experience with RIA and its contributions to diagnosis and patient management.

### Radioenzymatic Assay

Radioenzymatic assays have been developed for several antibiotics primarily the aminoglycosides. In these techniques an enzyme mediated by *Escherischia coli* R-factor is used that adenylates aminoglycosides. This reaction involves ATP, which is labelled with $^{14}$C. The amount of $^{14}$C incorporated into the aminoglycoside is measured to determine the amount of drug present. Radioenzymatic assay and RIA for the aminoglycoside antibiotics yield similar results *(19,20)*. Tetracycline and chloramphenicol interfere with radioenzymatic assays for aminoglycoside antibiotics and lipemic sera can result in lower gentamicin concentrations when this assay technique is used. Also, enzyme immunoassays for gentamicin have been described in which a peroxidase gentamicin conjugate competes with gentamicin for binding to an antibody absorbed to a polystyrene solid phase *(21)*. This method is generally less sensitive than RIA techniques and variations in the immunological activity of the conjugate have been reported.

### Enzyme-Multiplied Immunoassay Technique (EMIT®)

The EMIT® system combines principles of the immunoassays and enzyme kinetics. This assay depends on photometric determination of the activity of an enzyme that attaches to the drug to be quantitated. The enzyme is inactivated when bound by drug-specific antibody. The enzyme activity is related to the amount of drug present in the sample. Some EMIT assays utilize a "reverse" principle, in which the enzyme is only activated by binding to the drug-specific antibody. With these techniques, the velocity of the enzyme reaction is inversely proportional to the concentration of drug in the sample *(22)*.

The EMIT assays have the advantages that "labelled" and "unlabelled" drug need not be separated, and less-expensive and widely available spectrophotometric instrumentation is used. Additionally, because this system does not require meticulous separation or extraction procedures, EMIT analyses require little technical training and are easily automated. The procedure requires only a few minutes and less than 100 $\mu$L of sample material.

EMIT assays are now available for only two antibiotics, gentamicin and tobramycin, and the assays are rapid and highly specific. However, the accuracy below 1 to 2 mg/L is limited, unless one deviates from the standard automated procedures. This may be a potentially important limitation to the aminoglycoside assays because the desired "trough" concentrations of gentamicin and tobramycin are <2 mg/L. EMIT assays for several other drugs and for use in qualitative urine screens are available, which may increase the utilization of the instrumentation required.

The high specificity, simplicity, and timeliness of EMIT assay systems have led to their increased use by clinical laboratories, emergency hospitals, police, and medical examiners. The recent addition of antibiotic assays to the EMIT system further complement the use of these techniques as a tool for therapeutic drug monitoring.

### Fluorescent Immunoassay

A substrate-labelled fluorescent immunoassy (FIA) is also available for a few antibiotics. This assay is also based on principles of competitive protein binding to quantitatively measure drug concentrations. A conjugate, consisting of drug bound to a fluorogenic enzyme substrate, and free drug compete for antibody binding sites. Hydrolysis of the unbound conjugate produces a fluorescent product, the fluorescence intensity of which is related to the drug concentration in the specimen. As with the enzyme immunoassays, the fluorescent assays do not require handling of radioactive materials, but assays for only a few drugs currently are available.

### Latex Agglutination Inhibition Test

The latex agglutination inhibition card-test has recently become available for gentamicin serum determinations. Gentamicin-sensitized latex particles react with anti-gentamicin antisera. Addition of serum containing gentamicin inhibits the agglutination reaction. The gentamicin concentration is determined by comparing the inhibition caused by 12 different dilutions of test serum with known standard concentrations. Less than 100 $\mu$L of serum is needed, the test requires 20 to 30 min, and results can be read visually under high intensity light. The possible results are limited by the dilution scheme used, and when assessed with control area this assay has a mean coefficient of variation of 14%.

### "High-Pressure" Liquid Chromatography

Possibly the most promising advancement in drug assay methodology has been the application of chromatographic technology. Recently, "high pressure" liquid chromatography (HPLC) has been applied to the quantitation of various drugs, including antimicrobial agents (Table 1). Advantages of chromatographic techniques for assaying antimicrobial agents are high specificity (Table 2) and wide versatility. Throughout the past decade, liquid column-chromatographic technology has been further developed,

**Table 1. Antimicrobials Commonly Used For Which HPLC Assays Have Been Developed[a]**

Aminoglycosides
    Amikacin
    Gentamicin
    Netilmicin
    Tobramycin

Amphotericin B
Ampicillin
Amoxicillin

Cephalosporins
    Cefamandole
    Cefazolin
    Cephalexin
    Cephalothin
    Cephradine
Chloramphenicol
Erythromycin
5-Fluorocytosine
Metronidazole
Nitrofurantoin
Rifampin
Tetracycline
Trimethoprim/sulfamethoxazole

[a] Adapted from Yoshikawa et al. *(25)*

resulting in more efficient columns and therefore in improved separation. The major advantages of HPLC over standard liquid-chromatographic technologies include improved resolution, shorter analysis time, increased sensitivity, more durable columns, smaller sample size required, and possibilities for automation *(23,24)*.

HPLC procedures involve three basic techniques: (a) solvent extraction of the drug from the biological sample, (b) separation by chromatography, and (c) detection and quantitation by spectrometry or fluorometry.

Extracting the antimicrobial from the specimen is a critical step in HPLC procedures. Such procedures should be rapid, uncomplicated, and quantitative. The extraction method used is dictated by the chemical properties of the antibiotic studied. For determination of total antibiotic concentrations, protein-antibiotic complexes must be dissociated; this is done by use of organic solvents, acids, or ultrafiltration. Aminoglycoside antibiotics, which have a low affinity for proteins, are extracted by absorption or ion-exchange chromatographic techniques *(25)*.

Once the antibiotic has been extracted from the biological specimen, it must be separated or isolated from other compounds in the specimen. Several sepa-ration techniques are used in the various antimicrobial assays. In general, a mobile phase containing the antibiotic is applied to a stationary phase, and the antibiotic is separated into the stationary phase. The type of separation technique utilized depends on the properties of the particular antibiotic, including its solubility and ionization characteristics. In the case of liquid-liquid chromatography (partitioning) the stationary phase is polar, the mobile phase is nonpolar. In reverse-phase liquid-liquid chromatography, the polarity of the phases is reversed. The most frequently used column material for the quantitation of antimicrobial agents is a nonpolar stationary phase consisting of octadecylsilane. Ion-pair chromatographic techniques are used for the separation of ionic or ionizable drugs. An organic ion of opposite charge to the antimicrobial is added to the sample, then partition chromatography is used to separate the ion-pair. In several HPLC assays for aminoglycosides reverse-phase ion-pair techniques are used.

Most antimicrobial agents used in clinical practice have high molar absorptivity or fluorescence in the ultraviolet-visible spectrum and thus can be detected and quantitated by spectrometry. The aminoglycoside antibiotics are poorly fluorescent or absorptive, and therefore other detection techniques are required. Fluorescent derivatives of them are made and quantitated fluorometrically *(24)*.

The general lack of interference by other compounds present in the specimen is a major advantage of HPLC assays. Patients quite commonly receive multiple-antibiotic therapy, so assays must be specific. The high specificity of HPLC assays allows for determination of both the parent antibiotic and its metabolites, thus HPLC assays are highly useful in pharmacokinetic and metabolic studies of antimicrobials. The high specificity and the versatility of HPLC assays is a result of the numerous mobile phase compositions that are available and the many separation techniques which can be used.

**Table 2. Procedures Required to Ensure Antibiotic Assay Specificity**

| Assay | Procedure |
|---|---|
| Bioassays | inactivation of other substances with antimicrobial activity |
| Immunoassays (radio, enzymatic) | separation of unlabelled drug by precipitation or adsorption |
| EMIT | selective activation of enzyme (internal) |
| Chemical Assays (GLC, HPLC) | extraction and separation from interfering substances or metabolites |

Major disadvantages of chromatographic procedures include requirements of expensive equipment and highly trained personnel. Initial equipment costs usually range between $10,000 and $30,000. These high equipment costs may be offset if the instrumentation is optimally used for quantitation of drugs and other chemical substances. Yoshikawa et al. (25) reviewed the utilization of HPLC techniques for the quantitation of antimicrobial agents and Maitra et al. (26) reviewed HPLC and other techniques for aminoglycoside assays.

## Comments

An often-neglected aspect of antibiotic assay procedures is sample collection. Samples that are inappropriately collected can be assayed with the most sophisticated technology and still provide no useful information. Probably the most important factor affecting antibiotic assay results is the timing of the sample collection. The most appropriate time to collect the sample or samples varies with the situation. The "peak" concentrations in serum after an intravenous dose is that concentration in a specimen collected just after the injection. The peak concentrations in serum after intramuscular or oral doses can be highly variable and estimating when the peak serum concentration occurs may lead to substantial errors in dosage recommendations. The "trough" or "nadir" concentration, generally most informative, is the lowest concentration achieved in a dosing interval. Regardless of route of administration, the minimum serum concentrations during any dosing interval will be just before the next scheduled dose. In all situations, the exact time the specimen was collected, as well as the time the drug was administered must be recorded.

Timing of specimen collection is also important from the laboratory point of view. Advance notification that an assay is to be requested is always helpful, but sometimes impractical and seldom practiced. Prior notification facilitates timely preparation of the necessary reagents and instrumentation and so minimizes turnaround time. It may also allow the laboratory to "batch" samples, thus reducing costs and personnel time per sample. Batching specimens may not be possible for antibiotic assays if prompt results are required in order to make timely adjustments in therapy. The clinical laboratory must be able to respond to requests for a single drug concentration determination required by the practitioner to maximize a patient's antimicrobial therapy. Another often-neglected aspect of antimicrobial assays is the clinical information required to maximally utilize assay results. It is essential to know whether or not other drugs are present in the specimen. This helps determine the most appropriate assay method, and therefore such information must include antineoplastic agents as well as other antimicrobials the patient may be taking for other infections including (e.g.) tetracycline for acne or isoniazid prophylaxis. Results of antimicrobial assays are most frequently used as a tool to assist in making therapeutic decisions, including dosage adjustments. In these cases, the patient's infectious diagnosis, clinical condition, age, body weight, and estimates of renal and hepatic function must be incorporated with the assay results if the patient's drug therapy is to be optimal.

Antimicrobial assays are indicated in various situations. Most frequently, assay results are used to determine a patient's dosage requirements, thus maximizing safety and efficacy. Compliance with prescribed dosage regimens can most effectively be ensured through periodic analysis of serum or urine concentrations. Medical-legal aspects of serum level monitoring are also influencing the use of antibiotic assays. Aminoglycoside toxicity has repeatedly been associated with elevated peak and trough concentrations, which can be avoided by proper monitoring and controlling serum concentrations. Additionally, antimicrobial assay technology has facilitated the further examination of pharmacokinetic parameters, dose-concentration relationships, and concentration-effect relationships of several antibiotics.

The decision as to which analytical method is preferable for antimicrobial assays depends on several conditions (Table 3). Each institution must determine its needs and project future needs resulting from developing programs in therapeutic drug monitoring. Questions to be addressed include: Will the antibiotic assays be used for monitoring patients in the clinical environment for research purposes, or for both clinical and research purposes? If the determinations will be made from clinical specimens and the results incorporated into a patient's treatment regimen, assay characteristics such as specificity, versatility, turnaround time, and cost are most influential when choosing the optimal assay procedure. If the assay results are to be utilized for research purposes only, assay characteristics including sensitivity, sample size required, and possibilities for batching are most influential. The decision as to which analytical method to be used must also take into account existing instrumentation and expertise. If an institution is presently quantitating digoxin specimens by RIA, it would be advantageous to strongly consider RIA for vancomycin or aminoglycoside assays. Similarly, if lidocaine determinations are currently being performed using an EMIT system, this same instrumentation can be used for gentamicin and tobramycin assays.

Multiple institutions may find it economically advantageous to centralize antimicrobial assays in a single laboratory. Doing so decreases the number of antibiotic assays that must be made available by each institution, thereby increasing the productivity of the centralized instrumentation and laboratory personnel. Substantial cost savings can be realized and shared by all participating institutions, but there may be problems with transportation of unstable samples, slower turnaround time, and communication breakdown.

In all approaches to the utilization of antibiotic assays, a team effort is required. Representatives from several departments throughout an institution must work cooperatively to develop analytical techniques, select appropriate antimicrobial therapy, design opti-

**Table 3. Comparison of Major Antimicrobial Assays**

| Assay | Specificity | Sensitivity | Precision | Rapidity | Versatility |
|---|---|---|---|---|---|
| Microbiological horizontal/vertical, well/disc diffusion | Multiple antibiotic or antineoplastic therapy may require manipulation of specimen to permit analysis of individual antibiotic concentration. | Variable, dependent on technique seldom <1 mg L | Results influenced by composition of medium, test organisms, and variance in technique | Requires several hours, 38 h to 48 h | Potentially highly versatile, especially for single antibiotic specimens. |
| Radioimmunoassay (RIA) (radioenzymatic) | Production of highly specific antibodies permits analysis of a single antibiotic in a specimen containing antimicrobials. | Recommended unmodified procedures permit reliable results as low as 0.5 mg/L. Procedures modifications permit determination of lower concentrations. | Good precision, CV 5-10% | Results routinely available within 2 h. | Antibiotic assay commercially available for gentamicin, sisomicin, vancomycin, kanamycin. Many non-antibioassays available. |
| Enzyme Multiplied Immunoassay Technique (EMIT®) | Highly specific | Antibiotic sensitivity 1-2 mg/L. | Limited below 1-2 μg/mL without deviating from recommended procedures. | Rapid, procedure requires a few minutes. | Limited to gentamicin and tobramycin, however assays for most frequently monitored cardiovascular, anticonvulsant, bronchodilator and toxicologic available. |
| High-pressure liquid chromatography | Very highly specific, metabolites can be analyzed separately from parent compounds. | Highly sensitive, often <0.5 mg/L. | CV generally 5%. | Most HPLC procedures require 30 to 60 min. | Potential application nearly unlimited, assays available for all aminoglycosides, most cephalosporins, chloramphenicol and many other pharmacologic agents. |

| Assay | Equipment Requirements | Reagent costs | Sample size | Major disadvantages | Major advantages |
|---|---|---|---|---|---|
| Microbiological horizontal/vertical, well/disc diffusion | Minimal, available in all microbiology laboratories | Variable, but inexpensive for most assays | Large, generally 1 to 5 mL, micro techniques available which require 1 mL. | Lack of specificity, low precision, slow turnaround time, minimal sensitivity and large sample size may limit use in pharmacokinetic/metabolic studies, trained personnel required. | Widely available, versatile and minimal instrumentation required. |
| Radioimmunoassay (RIA) (radioenzymatic) | Moderately expensive, radiochemical counter spectrometer/scintillation counters. | Inexpensive | Very small, 50 to 200 μL | Separation phase required to ensure specificity, requires handling radioactive materials, highly trained personnel required. | Adequate sensitivity, rapid turnaround, wide application for non-antimicrobial assays. |
| Enzyme Multiplied Immunoassay Technique (EMIT®) | Relatively inexpensive spectrophotometry, instrumentation costs $1000 to $10,000. | Inexpensive | Very small, 100 μL | Limited antibiotic assays available, procedures require adaptation to maximize sensitivity. | Automation possible, inexpensive instrumentation, minimal personnel training required, highly specific. |
| High-pressure liquid chromatography | Expensive, instrumentation costs $8000 to $30,000. | Variable, but inexpensive for most assays | Small, less than 1 mL. | Very highly trained personnel and expensive instrumentation required, limited capacity. | Most useful for metabolic studies, automation possible, extremely specific, highly versatile. |

mal dosage regimens, and monitor drug therapy. Laboratorians, infectious disease specialists, medical staff, pharmacologists, pharmacokineticists, nursing and technical personnel, are all responsible for selected, yet important aspects of antimicrobial therapy.

## References

1. Solem, L.D., Zaske, D.E., and Strate, R.G., Ecthyma gangrenosum, survival with individualized antibiotic therapy. *Arch. Surg.* **114**, 580 (1979).
2. Loebl, B.C., Marvin, J.A., Curreri, P.W., et al., Survival with ecthyma gangrenosum: A previously fatal complication of burns. *J. Trauma* **14**, 370 (1974).
3. Black, S.B., Levine, P., and Shinefield, H.R., The necessity of monitoring chloramphenicol levels when treating neonatal meningitis. *J. Pediatrics* **92**, 235 (1978).
4. Noone, P., Beale, D.E., Pollock, S.S., et al., Monitoring aminoglycoside used in patients with severely impaired renal function. *Br. Med. J.* **ii,** 470 (1978).
5. Barza, M., Brown, R.B., and Shen, D., et al., Predictability of blood levels of gentamicin in man. *J. Infect. Dis.* **132**, 165 (1975).
6. Kaye, D., Levison, M.E., and Labovitz, E.D., The unpredictability of serum concentrations of gentamicin: Pharmacokinetics of gentamicin in patients with normal and abnormal renal function. *J. Infect. Dis.* **130**, 150 (1974).
7. Jackson, G.C., and Riff, L.J., Pseudomonas bacteremia: Pharmacologic and other basis for failure of treatment with gentamicin. *J. Infect. Dis.* **124**, (Suppl), S185 (1971).
8. Anderson, E.T., Young, L.S., and Hewitt, W.L., Simultaneous antibiotic levels in "breakthrough" Gram-negative rod bacteremia. *Am. J. Med.* **61**, 493 (1976).
9. Sawchuk, R.J., and Zaske, D.E., Pharmacokinetics of dosing regimens which utilize multiple intravenous infusion. *J. Pharmacokinet. Biopharmacol.* **4**, 183 (1976).
10. Noone, P., Parsons, T.M.C., and Pattison, J.R., et al., Experience in monitoring gentamicin therapy during treatment of serious gram-negative sepsis. *Br. Med. J.* **1,** 477 (1974).
11. Zaske, D.E., Cipolle, R.J., and Strate, R.G., Gentamicin dosage requirements: Wide interpatient variations in 242 surgery patients with normal renal function. *Surgery* **87**, 164 (1980).
12. Garrod, L.P., Lambery, H.P., and O'Grady, F.,

*Antibiotics and Chemotherapy,* Churchill Livingstone, Edinburgh London and New York, 1973, pp 490-531.
13. Sabath, L.D., Casey, J.J., Ruch, P.A., et al., Rapid microassay of gentamicin, kanamycin, neomycin, streptomycin, and vancomycin in serum or plasma. *J. Lab. Clin. Med.* **78**, 457 (1971).
14. Simon, H.J., and Yin, E.J., Microbioassay of antimicrobial agents. *Appl. Microbio.* **19**, 573 (1970).
15. Carlsom, A., Dornbusch, K., and Hagelberg, A., Use of electrophoresis in the identification and quantification of antibiotics administered in combinations. *Scand. J. Infect. Dis.* **9**, 46 (1977).
16. Wright, D.N., and Matsen, J.M., Bioassay of antibiotics in body fluids from patients receiving cancer chemotherapeutic agents. *Antimicrob. Agents. Chemother.* **17**, 417 (1980).
17. Broughton, A., and Strong, J.E., Radioimmunoassay of antibiotics and chemotherapeutic agents. *Clin. Chem.* **22**, 726 (1976).
18. Walker, W.H.C., An approach to immunoassay. *Clin. Chem.* **23**, 384 (1977).
19. Minshew, B.H., Holmes, R.K., and Bacter, C.R., Comparison of radioimmunoassay with an enzymatic assay for gentamicin. *Antimicrob. Agents. Chemother.* **7**, 107 (1975).
20. Smith, D.E., Van, Otto, B., and Smith, A.L., A rapid chemical assay for gentamicin. *N. Engl. J. Med.* **286**, 583, (1972).
21. Standefer, J.C., and Saunders, G.C., Enzyme immunoassay for gentamicin. *Clin. Chem.* **24**, 1903 (1978).
22. Schobben, F., and Van der Kleijn, E., Drug determinations in body fluids by technique (EMIT®). *Eur. J. Drug. Met. Pharmacokinetics.* **4**, (1977).
23. Koup, J.R., Brodsky, B., Lau, A., and Beam, T.R., High-performance liquid chromatographic assay of chloramphenicol in serum. *Antimicrob. Agents. Chemo.* **14**, 439 (1978).
24. Nilsson- Ehle, I., High-pressure liquid chromatography as a tool for determination of antibiotics in biological fluids. *Acta Pathol. Microbiol. Scand.* Sect B., Suppl. 259, 61 (1977).
25. Yoshikawa, T.T., Maitra, S.K., Schotz, M.C., and Guze, L.B., High-pressure liquid chromatography for quantitation of antimicrobial agents. *Rev. Infect. Dis.* **2**, 169 (1980).
26. Maitra, S.K., Yoshikawa, T.T., Guze, L.B., and Schotz, M.C., Determinations of aminoglycoside antibiotics in biological fluids: A review. *Clin. Chem.* **25**, 1361 (1979).

# IV. Bronchodilatory Drugs

# 36

# Asthma

### F. Estelle R. Simons, M.D.

## Introduction

Asthma is a common disorder affecting at least 5% of the population. It is a major cause of restricted physical activity and absenteeism from school or work. It is also a frequent cause of hospitalization and of visits to a physician. For practical purposes it can be described as obstruction to airflow resulting in symptoms such as wheeze, cough, shortness of breath, and a sensation of "tightness" in the chest. These symptoms are reversible, either spontaneously or after a bronchodilator is given. Asthma can begin at any time in life, even in infancy. Its severity varies greatly from patient to patient, from occasional mild attacks, to frequent severe attacks and/or intractable chronic disease. Severity may also vary in the same patient over a lifetime, or from season to season, or even over a day, or a few hours. Young patients with asthma often have "allergies" and coexisting disorders such as eczema or allergic rhinitis, and usually have a family history of allergic disease.

Symptoms of asthma occur because of narrowing of the lumen, or central air passage, of the air-conducting tubes, the trachea and bronchi. This occurs because of constriction of the muscles in the wall, swelling of the lining or mucosa, and outpouring of mucus into the lumen. Many different stimuli cause this narrowing. These include exercise, exposure to cold air, irritants such as smoke or other atmospheric pollutants or allergens such as pollen, dust, and animal danders, and ingestion of aspirin, or tartrazine (yellow dye `FD&C number 5) (Table 1). Emotional or psychological disturbances do not cause asthma, but may result in exacerbations. In each patient with asthma more than one trigger factor is usually found. Allergens are seldom the sole provoking factors for asthma symptoms. It is not known precisely how the various provoking factors cause the symptoms of asthma. One current theory is that the neurological control of the bronchial smooth muscle is abnormal. Irritant receptors in the airways of asthmatics seem to have lower-than-normal threshold for response to stimulation, resulting in constriction. The stimu-

lating or provoking factors which act in this manner include pollutants, viruses, exposure to cold air, or indirect heat loss from the airway during exercise. A second theory is that some stimuli, including allergens and physical factors such as exercise, trigger chemical mediator release from specialized mast cells in the airways. The mediators released include histamine and other substances such as slow-reacting substance of anaphylaxis (leukotrienes), which cause prolonged contraction of bronchial smooth muscle. Mediators may also cause reflex bronchospasm by stimulation of the irritant receptors. Third, there is the possibility that the smooth muscle in the airways may itself be abnormal in the asthma (1-3).

## Pathology

Deaths from asthma are now quite rare, fortunately, due to improved understanding of the pathophysiology of the disease and due to more effective methods of prevention and management of severe acute attacks. In patients dying from asthma, the lungs are greatly over-distended. Focal areas of atelectasis (collapse) are present. Plugs of mucus containing eosinophils, respiratory columnar epithelial cells, and squamous cells are present in the conducting airways. There is marked swelling of the mucosa, thickening of the basement membrane, hypercellularity of the submucosa and dilatation of capillaries in the submucosa. There is also hypertrophy and hyperplasia of the smooth muscle in the bronchial walls.

## Laboratory Findings in Asthma

1. *Eosinophilia.* The percentage of eosinophils in the blood, normally about 1 to 3% of the total white cell pool, is often elevated in patients with asthma. This can be determined from the differential white

*Dr. Simons is Head of the Section of Allergy and Clinical Immunology and Associate Professor in the Department of Pediatrics, Faculty of Medicine, The University of Manitoba, Winnipeg, Man., Canada.*

### Table 1. Provoking Factors in Asthma

Allergens eg. animal danders, pollens, dust
Infection, especially viral upper respiratory infections
Physical Exertion, especially running
Cold Air, weather changes
Irritants, eg. cigarette smoke, other air pollutants
Drugs such as aspirin
Emotional
Other

blood cell count and the total leukocyte count, but measurement of the total eosinophil count by specialized techniques is preferable. In patients with asthma, the total eosinophil count will decrease temporarily following treatment with $\beta$-adrenergic agonist drugs such as epinephrine, and after corticosteroid treatment. Other causes of moderate eosinophilia ($1000-5000/mm^3$) include parasitic infections, adverse reactions to drugs, and some immunodeficiency diseases (4).

2. *Examination of secretions*. Sputum obtained from an asthmatic may contain eosinophils and granules from disrupted eosinophils. Other characteristic microscopic entities are Curschmann's spirals which are inspissated mucus threads containing fine fibrils, eosinophils, and exfoliated epithelial cells. Charcot-Leyden crystals are thin, colorless, pointed structures 20-40 $\mu$m long, which are hexagonal on cross section. They are sometimes absent in freshly expectorated sputum, then appear after the specimen has been standing for a while (3).

Nasal mucus may also be examined for eosinophils. The optimal method of obtaining nasal secretions for examination consists of having the patient blow into plastic wrap, and then transferring the mucus to a glass slide, air-drying the slide and staining with Hansel's or Wright's stain.

3. *Immunoglobin E (IgE)*. This immunoglobulin is normally present in low concentrations in human serum. Detection of IgE requires specialized tests such as the paper disc radioimmunosorbent test. Normal IgE levels are age-related, peaking at age seven to 10 years. Total serum IgE concentrations are often, but not always, elevated in young patients with asthma, particularly if there is associated eczema.

The presence or absence of IgE specific for an allergen, for example, grass pollen or cat dander, may be detected by the sensitive, time-honored method of skin testing or by analyzing the patient's serum in the radioallergosorbent test (RAST). In the RAST, serum containing an unknown amount of specific IGE is incubated with an allergen such as grass pollen or dog dander that has been coupled to an insoluble matrix. Radiolabeled anti-IgE is added. After various incubation and washing procedures, the anti-IgE-IgE-allergen complex is counted in a gamma spectrometer to determine the amount of specific IgE that was present in the serum. The results of RAST tests correlate well with skin tests and bronchial and nasal challenge tests with specific allergens (5).

4. *Blood gases*. Hypoxemia can be found in asymptomatic asthmatic patients, and in severe acute asthma, hypoxemia is universal. Early in an asthma attack, hypocapnia usually occurs, as well as respiratory alkalosis due to hyperventilation. As airway obstruction progresses, and the asthma attack worsens, arterial $pCO_2$ becomes normal and then increases above the normal range, and respiratory acidosis ensues. If a patient has severe acute asthma, frequent measurement of arterial $pO_2$, $pCO_2$ and pH are required in order to anticipate respiratory failure. This is present if the $pCO_2$ reaches 45 torr, or if arterial oxygen decreases to 50 torr.

5. *Cultures/serology.* Sputum cultures in asthmatics rarely yield pathogenic organisms, unless the patients are hospitalized for severe acute asthma and are receiving ventilatory assistance, in which case nosocomial infections caused by *Pseudomonas* or *Enterobacter* species may be identified. Sputum cultures are often required in older patients with asthma, in order to rule out chronic bronchitis. Viral cultures of the nasopharynx and acute and convalescent titers to common respiratory viruses are sometimes performed in a severe acute asthma episode to document the virus provoking the attack.

6. *Pulmonary function tests.* These provide objective confirmation of reversibility of airflow obstruction and are therefore useful in diagnosis. They are also frequently performed to assess the severity of obstruction to airflow, to evaluate the response to treatment, and to evaluate the response to physical exertion.

7. *Chest radiographs.* Chest radiographs are helpful in acute asthma for ruling out foreign bodies, pneumonia, etc., and for assessment of complications such as pneumothorax (free air in the pleural space), and atelectasis (collapse of lung tissue).

8. *Other.* Examples of additional laboratory tests which may be useful in making the diagnosis of asthma include sweat chloride test for ruling out cystic fibrosis; measurement of immunoglobulins G, A, and M for ruling out hypogammaglobulinemia or agammaglobulinemia; $\alpha$-1 antitrypsin for ruling out $\alpha$-1 antitrypsin deficiency; precipitins for the measurement of IgG precipitating antibody to rule out hypersensitivity pneumonitis; quantitation of urinary 5-hydroxyindoleacetic acid, the chief metabolite of serotonin, to rule out the carcinoid syndrome; and electrocardiograms for identifying cardiac problems.

## Treatment of Chronic Asthma

Although asthma cannot be cured, with optimal treatment most patients should be able to live relatively normal lives (*1-3, 6, 7*). An individualized treatment program is developed for each patient (Table 2) and attention is paid to adequate rest and

### Table 2. Treatment of Asthma: Summary

| Chronic Asthma | Acute Asthma |
|---|---|
| Avoidance of Provoking Factors | Oxygen |
| Drugs: theophylline | Drugs: beta-2 adrenergic agonist |
| cromolyn | |
| beta-2 stimulator | theophylline |
| corticosteroids | corticosteroids |
| Immunotherapy | Intravenous fluids |

nutrition. The basis of treatment is identification and avoidance of triggering factors for the asthma. For example, a patient with asthma who is allergic to cats and only wheezes when exposed to cats will be asymptomatic if he avoids cats. If a patient has allergies to many things, a beneficial effect will often be observed if some or all of these materials are removed from his environment. Pollens and molds are difficult to avoid, but measures such as air-conditioning and electrostatic air filters can reduce the pollen and mold counts in a specific portion of the environment and may result in considerable relief of symptoms when the patient is in that area. Exercise is the only triggering factor for asthma which should not be avoided; indeed, regular exercise is recommended for all patients with asthma although some patients will require medication before exercise to be able to participate.

The role of immunotherapy (allergy shots) in the management of chronic asthma in allergic patients is controversial at present (*1*, *6*). Although it is still widely used, numerous physicians are beginning to believe that the invasiveness, discomfort, expense, and time required for the treatment is not justified in many patients. It is much more difficult to prove the effectiveness of allergy shots in asthma than to prove their effectiveness in some other allergic diseases, because asthma is triggered by so many factors besides allergies.

Medication may be required intermittently or regularly in chronic asthma, depending on the severity and frequency of the patient's symptoms. Four classes of drugs are commonly used in the treatment of chronic asthma; methylxanthines (theophylline), $\beta$-adrenergic stimulators, cromolyn, and corticosteroids (*1-3*, *6*, *7*). The drug or the drug combinations used depends to some extent on the personal preference of the prescribing physician. There is continuing work to develop new drugs including new atropine-like drugs which lack atropinic side effects, clinically useful prostaglandins with bronchodilator effects, drugs which inhibit calcium influx or inhibit microtubular aggregation in mast cells and smooth muscles, and oral cromolyn-like agents.

*Theophylline.* Theophylline causes bronchodilation and inhibition of release of mediators of inflammation. It also improves mucociliary transport, prevents or reverses respiratory muscle fatigue, and stimulates respiration. The beneficial effects of theophylline have been attributed to inhibition of phosphodiesterase, and increased intracellular CAMP. However, phosphodiesterase inhibition probably does not occur with the serum theophylline concentrations generally achieved in vivo. Theophylline may also act as a prostaglandin antagonist, may antagonize adenosine, or may affect intracellular calcium concentrations.

Theophylline is rapidly and completely absorbed when administered as liquid or a plain uncoated tablet. Sustained-release products have variable bioavailability, bust some of these formulations provide constant absorption and eliminate fluctuation in concentrations in serum. In older children and adults requiring long-term around-the-clock treatment with theophylline these products facilitate improved compliance as they need to be given only twice daily.

Theophylline is eliminated from the body by biotransformation in the liver. Age is an important determinant of clearance rates. In children over one year of age, clearance is generally more rapid than in adults and half-life values are shorter. Requirements for theophylline on a milligram-per-kilogram basis are larger in young children than in adults and in teenagers. Factors which decrease clearance include cirrhosis, congestive heart failure, pulmonary edema, drugs such as erythromycin or cimetidine administered concurrently, fever, viral respiratory infections, immunization for influenza, and ingestion of a low-protein, high-carbohydrate diet. Smoking cigarettes, or marijuana, on the other hand, causes clearance rates to increase and increases dose requirements.

The toxic effects of theophylline include hyperactivity, nervousness, insomnia, headaches, seizures, unconsciousness, abdominal pain, nausea, vomiting and hematemesis. Theophylline also causes diuresis, tachycardia and other cardiac arrhythmias, and may cause hypertension or hypotension. If iatrogenic or accidental poisoning does occur, there is no specific antidote. Before 1975, theophylline was used in fairly low doses in order to avoid adverse effects, particularly in children, and in many patients it did not provide optimal bronchodilation. When the ability to measure theophylline concentrations in serum readily became widespread, patients with rapid clearance rates could be identified by their low theophylline concentrations in serum and could be given higher theophylline doses safely. Presently, the most commonly used methods of theophylline measurement are high-performance liquid chromatographic methods and the enzyme immunoassay (EMIT, Syva). Both have the advantages of small sample size, rapidity, and ease of performance. The correlation between the two methods is excellent (*8*). With both assays, there is no interference with other xanthines or uric acid, or commonly used medications. Dry reagent immunoassays with colorimetric indicators are now being evaluated. The therapeutic range over which bronchodilation is maximal and adverse effects uncommon has been defined as 5 to 20 $\mu$g/mL. Monitoring is indicated to aid in finding an optimal dose, to check for compliance with treatment, to ascertain the cause of lack of response to treatment, and to identify toxicity.

Children may outgrow their theophylline doses and should have levels checked yearly, or twice yearly during growth "spurts," or if any factor potentially affecting clearance is identified in the patient.

Theophylline passes freely into body fluids such as breast milk and saliva. Salivary levels are approximately 50% of serum concentrations. Monitoring of salivary theophylline concentrations has been advocated but is not widely practiced because of variations in the saliva/serum ratio, and the difficulty in obtaining saliva samples from a sick or uncooperative patient (9).

2. *Beta-Adrenergic stimulators*. Beta-Adrenergic agonists act by binding reversibly to $\beta$-adrenergic receptors, located in the membrane of smooth muscle cells and mast cells, as well as other cell types. The binding produces conformational changes in the enzyme, leading to the increase of intracellular cAMP, the "second messenger," and inhibition of mast cell mediator generation and smooth muscle contraction. The potency of a $\beta$-2 agonist depends on the proportion of receptors which the drug occupies at a given concentraion and the ability of the drug to trigger the biological effect once the receptor is occupied. Newer $\beta$-2 agonists such as metaproterenol, terbutaline, and salbutamol (albuterol) have greater bronchodilator effects relative to cardiovascular effects. They have increased duration of action compared to the older $\beta$-1 agonists epinephrine and isoproterenol. Also, they are palatable and effective when given orally.

Beta-2 adrenergic agonists administered by pressurized aerosols provide convenient rapid relief of intermittent asthma or prevention of exercise-induced asthma. Patients who have difficulty in mastering the technique of inhalation are helped by the use of a "spacer" placed between the orifice of the metered-dose aerosol and the patient's mouth. In some studies, beta-2 adrenergic agonist subsensitivity has been found after repeated dosing. This subsensitivity may be reversed by corticosteroid treatment. Beta agonists may cause tremor, nervousness, headaches, tachycardia, blood pressure changes, and increase in insulin and decrease in serum glucose and potassium. These adverse effects may be caused by beta-1 agonists but also by beta-2 agonists, particularly if the recommended doses are exceeded. They are less common after inhalation of the drugs than after oral administration. Skeletal muscle tremor is a direct effect of stimulation of beta-2 receptors in the muscles.

3. *Cromolyn*. Cromolyn is not a bronchodilator. Its structure is unlike that of any other antiasthmatic drug. Cromolyn is said to stabilize the mast-cell membrane, preventing release of mediators of allergic disease. It is used prophylactically and is not useful if given after an asthma attack has started, as it does not reverse the effect of mediators already released. Cromolyn must be administered by inhalation, as less than 1% of a dose is absorbed after oral administration. When the patented tubo-inhaler device (Spinhaler) for powder inhalation is used, about 75% of the dose is delivered to the airways but only 10% reaches the peripheral airways. The remainder is deposited in the mouth and pharynx, swallowed, and passed in the stools without biotransformation. Cromolyn may also be given via face mask and compressor or as a metered-dose pressurized aerosol. One of the chief advantages of cromolyn is its lack of toxicity. The most common adverse effects are transient bronchospasm, cough, and dryness in the throat shortly after inhalation. Very rarely, adverse reactions consisting of dermatitis, myositis, or gastroenteritis have been observed. In the long-term management of asthma, cromolyn is effective in about 70% of patients. It tends to be more effective in young, allergic asthmatics than in older patients. Most, although not all, treatment failures occur early, and some are due to a poor technique of administration of the drug.

4. *Corticosteroids*. In chronic asthma, corticosteroids are reserved for use when there is failure of response to bronchodilators and cromolyn. Although the mechanism of their action is not fully understood, it involves formation of specific messenger ribonucleic acid (RNA) and stimulation of intracellular protein receptors. Among other things, corticosteroids have anti-inflammatory actions and facilitate the effect of $\beta$-agonists. If taken by mouth daily for more than a few weeks they cause inhibition of linear growth, excess weight gain, cushingoid appearance, posterior subcapsular cataracts, acne, hypertension, and other serious side effects. Because of these side effects, the lowest doses of corticosteroids which control symptoms in a particular patient are used for as short a time as possible. If long-term corticosteroid treatment is required, side effects can be avoided almost entirely with the use of short-acting compounds such as prednisone, prednisolone, or methylprednisolone given in a single dose every 48 h at 8:00 a.m. Side effects may also be prevented by the use of inhaled corticosteroids with high topical activity such as beclomethasone dipropionate, beclomethasone valerate, triamcinolone acetonide, and flunisolide. These drugs prevent asthma with minimal suppression of the hypothalamic-pituitary-adrenal axis. *Candida albicans* is frequently isolated from the oropharynx of patients receiving aerosolized steroids. Patients receiving corticosteroids by any route chronically require extra corticosteroids by the intravenous or oral route during a severe asthma episode or during stress such as surgery or trauma.

## Management of Acute Asthma in Children

The goals of treatment of acute asthma are to preserve life, and to free the patient from wheeze, cough, and shortness of breath. Initial treatment measures include administration of oxygen and a $\beta$-adrenergic agonist such as injected epinephrine or terbutaline, or metaproterenol or salbutamol (albuterol), nebulized and inhaled by face mask, and careful observation. If a patient requires admission to hospital, he will continue to receive intermittent inhalations of a $\beta$-2 agonist by face mask, with oxygen, and also fluids and medications such as theophylline and corticosteroids given by the intravenous route (10). Theophylline therapy in acute asthma is based on the principle that therapeutic and toxic effects vary directly with the log of drug concentrations in serum. The signs and symptoms associated with theophylline toxicity may also be caused by adrenergic drugs, by the intercurrent viral infections which so frequently provoke severe acute asthma, or by other factors. Consequently, the ability to obtain rapid measurement of concentrations in serum is mandatory for optimal use of the drug. Without these measurements, patients must be underdosed in order to avoid toxicity. Ideally, sufficient drug is given intravenously to maintain concentrations in serum in the middle to upper portions of the therapeutic range, that is, about 15 to $18 \mu g/mL$. For these purposes a loading dose of 6 or 7 mg/kg aminophylline is usually given followed by an initial maintenance dose of 0.65 to 1.0 mg/kg/h administered by constant infusion pump. The loading dose is diluted with intravenous fluid and injected slowly over 15 min. The maintenance dose may be required for several days and should be adjusted as necessary to yield serum theophylline concentrations in the therapeutic range. Corticosteroids such as methylprednisolone or hydrocortisone are life-saving in severe acute asthma. Significant improvement in blood gases occurs within 3 h after starting corticosteroids, although pulmonary function tests may not improve significantly for many hours or even days. Antibiotics formerly were liberally used in asthma treatment. It is now recognized that the infections which provoke acute asthma are usually viral rather than bacterial, and there is seldom an indication for the use of antibiotics.

## Summary

Asthma is a complex disorder with multiple possible provoking factors. Although there is no cure for it at present, the major advances in the pharmacologic management of both chronic and acute asthma in the past decade have radically improved the quality of life for many asthmatic patients.

## References

1. Simons, F.E.R., Asthma in childhood. In *Seminars in Respiratory Medicine* 1, 147-166 (1979).

2. Ellis, E.F., Allergic disorders, In *The Textbook of Pediatrics*, V.C. Vaughan, R.J. McKay and R.E. Behrman, Eds., W.B. Saunders Co., Philadelphia, PA, pp 611-625, 627-635. 11th Edition (1979).

3. Bernstein, I.L., Asthma in adults. In *Allergy Principles and Practice*, E. Middleton, C.E. Reed and E.F. Ellis, Eds., The C.V. Mosby Co., St. Louis, MO, p 743-770 (1978).

4. Ottesen, E.A., and Cohen, S.G., The eosinophilia, and eosinophil-related disorders. *Ibid.*, pp 584-632.

5. Yunginger, J.W., and Gleich, G.J., The impact of the discovery of IgE on the practice of allergy. *Pediatr. Clin. North Am.* 22, 3-15 (1975).

6. Leffert, F., The management of chronic asthma. *J. Pediatr.* 97, 875-885 (1980).

7. Weinberger, M., Hendeles, L., and Ahrens, R., Clinical pharmacology of drugs used for asthma. *Pediatr. Clin. North Am.* 28, 47-75 (1981).

8. Boeckx, R.L., Frith, E.M., and Simons, F.E.R., Comparison of a high performance liquid chromatographic and an enzyme immunoassay technique for quantitation of theophylline in serum. *Ther. Drug Monitor.* 1, 65-73 (1979).

9. Hendeles, L., Burkey, S., Bighley, L., and Richardson, R., Unpredictability of theophylline saliva measurements in chronic obstructive pulmonary disease. *J. Allergy Clin Immunol.* 6, 335-338 (1979).

10. Shapiro, G.G., Simons, F.E., Pierson, W.E., and Bierman, C.W., The management of status asthmaticus in children. In *The Critically Ill Child Diagnosis and Management.* Clement A. Smith, Ed., W.B. Saunders Co., Philadelphia, PA, 1977, pp 178-193. Second Edition.

# 37

# A Case Report on Theophylline in the Newborn

**Mhairi G. MacDonald, MBChB, FRCP(E), FAAP, DCH**

The effectiveness of theophylline in the management of neonatal apnea is well described (1). It decreases both the number and severity of apneic episodes. This case illustrates the importance of monitoring the concentration of theophylline in blood at appropriate intervals, particularly in extremely tiny premature babies during the first few weeks of postnatal life.

## Case Presentation

D.D., a 1050-g premature boy, was born to a 24-year-old mother after a 28-week gestation. Apgar scores were 5 and 7. He exhibited very mild respiratory distress shortly after birth and his chest roentgenogram was consistent with hyaline membrane disease. On the second postnatal day severe apnea with bradycardia developed, which was refractory to standard therapy. The apnea could not be related to infection or onset of other pathological condition. Therapy with theophylline* was initiated, using a loading dose of 6 mg/kg body wt. and a maintenance dose of 2 mg/kg every 8 h. The loading dose effected a serum concentration of about 10 mg/L, and apnea was effectively controlled until day 4, when the infant's heart-rate was noted to be increased to between 180 and 210 beats/min. The serum theophylline concentration at this time was 24 mg/L. The next dose was missed and the maintenance dose was dropped to 2 mg/kg every 12 h. Standing orders were written to withhold theophylline if the infant's pulse rate exceeded 180 beats/min. The serum theophylline concentration at 24 h was 21 mg/L and at 48 h 17 mg/L. Thereafter apnea was well controlled at a concentration in serum of 11 mg/L (range, 2 mg/L).

On the 21st day the infant developed seizure activity. A complete investigation revealed no obvious etiology and the serum theophylline concentration was 9 mg/L on a theophylline dosage of 2 mg/kg every 8 h, orally. Phenobarbital therapy was instituted. Apnea and seizure activity were controlled with phenobarbital and theophylline until day 33, when regular jerking body movements and twitching of the tongue were noted. Two hours later, generalized seizures occurred. It was then discovered that the infant's oral theophylline solution had been incorrectly prepared. As a result, the infant had received 10 times the prescribed maintenance dose for three days; a total of nine to 10 doses. The serum theophylline concentration at the time of generalized seizures was 55 mg/L, with a serum phenobarbital concentration of 18 mg/L. Therapy with theophylline was withdrawn, maintenance phenobarbital was continued, and no additional anticonvulsants were given. The seizures resolved in 6 h and did not recur. Serum theophylline concentrations remained above the therapeutic range for 48 h.

The pulse rate exceeded 180 beats/min only briefly once before the overdose was recognized, with irritability the only manifestation of theophylline toxicity noted before the seizures. The infant appeared normal when he was discharged from the hospital at age two months.

## Discussion

Unusually small premature infants, particularly those weighing less than 1500 g at birth, frequently exhibit irregular respirations. This phenomenon is thought to be related to immaturity of the brainstem center that controls respiration. Apnea of prematurity would appear to be an exaggeration of this normal irregularity, so that breathing ceases altogether for periods longer than 15-20 s. These episodes can endanger the life of the infant when they are associated with slowing of the heart and cyanosis. In these circumstances the baby will often not recover from the apnea unless resuscitated.

Apnea is observed in 25% of neonates who weigh less than 2500 g at birth. The incidence varies with fetal maturity, with a reported incidence of 85% in preterm neonates weighing less than 1000 g at birth. If the apnea does not respond to simple measures such as tactile stimulation, continuous positive airway pressure (CPAP) is initiated and the baby is fully screened for predisposing factors such as hypoglycemia and infection. If severe apnea persists and no other pathological condition is found, the infant is treated with theophylline.

The extremely long biological half-life of theophylline (about 30 h in the premature infant weighing less than 1550 g) is probably responsible for the accumulation and early toxicity seen in this patient. Toxicity at the age of four days manifested itself clinically with onset of tachycardia. However, the subsequent history shows that the clinician cannot rely on the onset of minor side effects to warn him of severe toxicity.

---

*Dr. MacDonald is the Director of Outreach Program, Children's Hospital National Medical Center, Washington, D.C.*

---

*As intravenous Aminophyllin, which contains 80% theophylline.

## THEOPHYLLINE PROFILE

| | |
|---|---|
| **Trade Name:** | Elixophyllin |
| **Generic:** | Theophylline |
| **Chemical Name:** | 1, 3-Dimethylxanthine |
| **Chemical structure:** | |

| | |
|---|---|
| **pK$_a$:** | 8.6 |
| **Rel. Molecular Mass** | 180.17 |
| **Melting point, °C:** | 270-274 |
| **Solubility in water:** | 8.3 g/L |

### ABSORPTION AND DISTRIBUTION

| | |
|---|---|
| **Percentage of oral dose absorbed:** | 95-100% adults   80% newborns |
| **Peak Conc. in Plasma:** | 2-3 h in adults; mean, 2 hrs in newborns, but very variable. |
| **Protein bound:** | Adult 55-60%. Value is probably lower in newborn. |
| **V$_d$:** | Adults: 0.351—0.701 L/kg |
| | Newborn: 0.33—1.03 L/kg |

### URINARY EXCRETION AND METABOLISM

| | % Daily dose excreted | Active | Detectable In Blood |
|---|---|---|---|
| **Unchanged drug** (adult values) | 2-14 | Yes | |
| **1,3-Dimethyl uric acid** (adult values) | 35-44 | No | |
| **1-Methyl uric acid** (adult values) | 13-20 | Yes | Not in newborns |
| **3-Methylxanthine** (adult values) | 29-44 | No | Not in newborns |
| **Caffeine** | Up to 50 in premature infants | Yes | Only in newborns |

| | Adults | Children | Newborns |
|---|---|---|---|
| **Half-life, h:** | 3-8 | 1-8 | 17-45 |
| **Time to steady state, h:** | 16-37 | 6-44 | Very variable. Without loading dose >1 week. |

### DOSAGE AND CONCENTRATIONS IN BLOOD

| | | | |
|---|---|---|---|
| **Recommended dosage** (mg/kg body wt per day) | 13 | 24 | Loading dose* 5.5-6 mg/kg i.v. Maintenance dose: 2 mg/kg each 12 h, i.v. |
| **Effective conc., mg/L:** | 10-20 | 10-20 | 6-15 |
| **Toxic conc., mg/L:** | >20 | >20 | >15-20 |

* Usually given as Aminophyllin

Seizure activity is a recognized manifestation of severe theophylline toxicity in adults and has also been reported previously in the neonate (2). At 33 days of age this baby had seizure activity owing to theophylline overdose, despite the fact that a standing order had been written that included instructions to withhold theophylline if the infant's pulse rate exceeded 180 beats/min. The clinical picture was further confused by the fact that the infant was known to have a seizure disorder unrelated to drug toxicity. Had data on drug concentration in serum not been available, the theophylline toxicity might not have been recognized, and the dose of phenobarbital might have been increased inappropriately, or other unnecessary anticonvulsants added to the therapeutic regimen.

## References

1. Aranda, J.V., and Turmen, P., Methylxanthines in apnea of prematurity. *Clin. Perinatol.* **6,** 87-108 (1979).

2. Gal, P., Roop, C., Robinson, H., and Erkan, N.V., Theophylline-induced seizures in accidentally overdosed neonates. *Pediatrics* **65,** 547-549 (1980).

## Suggested Reading

Lucey, J.F., Shannon, D.C., and Soyka, L.F., Eds. *Apnea of Prematurity: Report of the 71st Ross Conference on Pediatric Research.* Ross Laboratories, Columbus, OH, 1977.

# 38

# A Case History:
# Theophylline and Caffeine in Premature Neonates

### James Standefer, Ph.D.

Theophylline is widely used as a respiratory stimulant and its therapeutic use in treating neonatal apnea has been accepted (*1, 2*). The primary pathway for biotransformation of theophylline in neonates is different from that in adults which involves demethylation and oxidation to produce 1-methyluric acid, 1,3-dimethyluric acid, and 3-methylxanthine (*3*). In contrast to adults, biotransformation of theophylline in neonates involves primarily *N*-methylation to produce caffeine (*4*). That is, metabolism of 1,3-dimethylxanthine (theophylline) in neonates produces 1,3,7-trimethylxanthine (caffeine). A significant amount of caffeine can accumulate in neonates who receive theophylline for treatment of apnea, and the combined therapeutic effects of both methylxanthines should be considered when the therapeutic efficacy of a particular theophylline dose is considered (*4*). While the levels of theophylline in serum in neonates are generally related to dose, the concentration in serum of its metabolic product, caffeine, is not as closely related to theophylline dose (Figure 1). At theophylline dose levels of less than 5 mg/kg/day, the caffeine in serum may be greater than theophylline while at higher theophylline doses, the caffeine is usually lower than theophylline.

To illustrate the conversion of theophylline to caffeine in neonates in a clinical setting, a case history is presented which involves a 30-week gestational age male infant who was delivered by caesarean section. This infant developed respiratory distress shortly after delivery. He was treated with oxygen, prophylactic antibiotics, and theophylline. During the following weeks he experienced intermittent, acute hypoxic episodes which were relieved by a combination of increased oxygen pressure, terbutaline, and muscle relaxants. The infant remained on chronic oxygen therapy for eight months during which there were several unsuccessful attempts to remove him from a high oxygen atmosphere. Also during this eight month treatment period he was on continuous theophylline therapy with doses ranging from an initial dose of 4

mg/kg/day to a discharge dose of 13 mg/kg/day. Because of multiple intermittent episodes of unexplained fever, unusual irritability with nausea and vomiting plus difficult fluid balance, the theophylline dose appropriate to the expected therapeutic range was difficult to maintain. An additional complicating factor in premature neonates such as this patient is the longer half-life of theophylline, 30 ± 6.5 h (*2*), compared to children, 3.5 ± 1.1 (*5*) and adults, 8 ± 2 (*5*). This longer half-life translates to a longer time to achieve equilibrium and consequently a longer interval between dose adjustments.

Concentrations of theophylline and caffeine in serum were monitored at regular intervals during the treatment period and are shown in Figure 2. All samples were collected immediately prior to the next dose and thus the plotted values reflect "trough" values and are within the mid-portion of the expected therapeutic range for neonates of 5 to 20 mg/L.

During the initial three months of theophylline therapy, the caffeine concentration in serum follows the theophylline concentration in serum in a parallel fashion. After this initial 12-week period caffeine

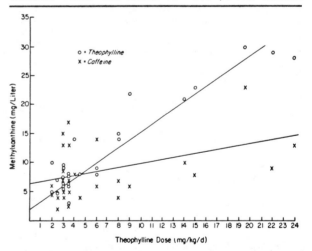

**Figure 1.** Concentration of theophylline and caffeine in serum from premature neonates on various levels of chronic theophylline therapy. The regression statistics for theophylline are $y = 1.3x + 2.0$, $r^2 = 0.90$ and for caffeine $y = 1.9x - 2.4$, $r^2 = 0.15$.

*Dr. Standefer is Director, Clinical Chemistry, University of New Mexico Hospital, Albuquerque, NM 87106.*

appeared only during the twentieth week and was not detected thereafter. One explanation for finding little or no caffeine in serum after several weeks of theophylline therapy is a decreasing rate of conversion of theophylline to caffeine to be expected when the $N$-methylation pathways in the infant's liver decrease relative to the demethylation and oxidation pathways that are important in adult liver.

Two samples collected during the twentieth week of therapy contain caffeine while samples collected two weeks before and several weeks after contain no caffeine. While there is no obvious explanation for this brief appearance of caffeine, it is tempting to speculate that concentrations in serum induced by a higher dose (20 mg/kg/day) during weeks 14 through 18 may have induced a temporary return to the $N$-methylation pathway during this transitional stage of the metabolic pathways. Obviously more data are required to support such speculation and perhaps the 12 to 20 week postnatal period should be studied more carefully for evidence of transitional metabolic pathways in the liver.

The clinical condition of the infant did not significantly change during this interval; however, his theophylline dose was changed from an intravenous dose of 15 mg/kg/day to an oral dose of 11 mg/kg/day in response to a concentration in serum of 21 mg/L (eighteenth week of therapy, Figure 2). Similar changes from intravenous to oral medication had occurred several times during his therapy with no change in the caffeine concentration in serum.

This case exemplifies theophylline metabolism in an infant during chronic therapy. Theophylline is converted to caffeine in neonates and it may accumulate to clinically significant levels. This conversion may be attenuated after several weeks of therapy, perhaps due to the appearance of other metabolic pathways in the developing liver. Our experience indicates that caffeine may be found occasionally in clinically significant concentrations in the serum of older infants (up to two years old). Thus, if the caffeine concentration is lower due to a transition of metabolic pathways, the transition interval must vary considerably depending on individual differences among patients and their disease states.

The clinical efficacy of using only caffeine in the management of neonatal apnea has been evaluated and shown to be effective (6). A significant decrease in the mean number of apneic episodes was noted (13.6 vs. 2.1) after initiation of caffeine therapy in a group of 18 low-birth-weight infants.

While the expected therapeutic range for caffeine is not established, caffeine is effective at concentrations in serum similar to those of theophylline and the interim therapeutic range may be taken as 5 to 20 mg/L in neonates (*1 and unpublished observations*). With regard to the relative toxicity of caffeine and theophylline, the LD$_{50}$ for caffeine in neonatal rats is approximately 35% higher than the LD$_{50}$ for theophylline (7). Additionally, a follow-up study of sequelae associated with caffeine treatment in preterm apneic infants showed no difference in growth and neurologic development between control and caffeine-treated infants (8).

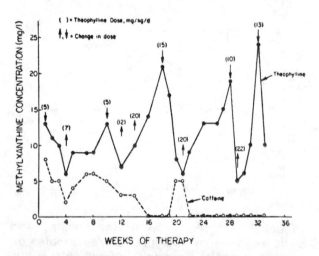

**Figure 2.** Theophylline and caffeine concentrations in one patient receiving chronic theophylline therapy: Theophylline ●——●, Caffeine ○----○.

### Caffeine Profile

| | |
|---|---|
| Generic name: | Caffeine |
| Chemical name: | 1,3,7-Trimethylxanthine |
| Mol. wt.: | 194.20 |
| Melting point: | 236° C |
| Solubility in H$_2$O: | 17 g/L (increased as citrate) |
| pKa: | 14 |
| Protein binding: | 20% (estimated) |
| Volume of distribution: | 0.5 L/kg |
| Urinary excretion (48 h): | 1-Methyluric acid (26%) and 1-methylxanthine (16%) |
| Recommended dose (neonates): | 10 mg/kg (loading) 5-20 mg/kg/day (maintenance) |
| Time to peak levels (oral dose): | 1 h |
| Half-life: | Neonates 40-230 h Adults, 3.1 h |
| Effective levels, mg/L: | Neonates 5-20 |
| Toxic levels, mg/L: | Greater than 20 |

In conclusion, caffeine accumulates to clinically significant levels in neonates receiving theophylline and, because caffeine is an equally potent drug for treatment of apnea, its concentration in serum should be monitored.

## References

1. Shannon, D.C., Gotay, F., et al., Prevention of apnea and bradycardia in low-birthweight infants. *Pediatrics* **55**, 589 (1975).

2. Aranda, J.V., Sitar, D.S., et al., Pharmacokinetic aspects of theophylline in premature newborns. *New Engl. J. Med.* **295**, 413 (1976).

3. Cornish, H.H., and Christman, A.A., A study of the metabolism of theobromine, theophylline, and caffeine in man. *J. Biol Chem.* **228**, 315 (1957).

4. Bory, C., Baltassat, P., Porthault, M., et al., Metabolism of theophylline to caffeine in premature newborn infants. *J. Pediatr.* **94**, 988 (1979).

5. Hendeles, L., Weinberger, M., and Johnson, G., Theophylline. In *Applied Pharmacokinetics*, W.E. Evans, J.J Schentag, and W.J. Jusko, Eds. Applied Therapeutics, San Francisco, CA, 1980, p 95.

6. Aranda, J.V., Gorman, W., et al., Efficacy of caffeine in treatment of apnea in the low-birth-weight infant. *J. Pediatr.* **90**, 467 (1977).

7. Warsyzawski, D., Gorodischer, R., and Kaplanski, J., Comparative toxicity of caffeine and aminophylline (theophylline ethylenediamine) in young and adult rats. *Biol Neonate* **34**, 68 (1978).

8. Gunn, T., Metrakos, K., et al., Sequelae of caffeine treatment in preterm infants with apnea. *J. Pediatr.* **94**, 106 (1979).

# V. Psychoactive Drugs

# 39

# Guidelines for Therapeutic Monitoring of Tricyclic Antidepressant Plasma Levels

**Paul J. Orsulak, Ph.D.**
**Joseph J. Schildkraut, M.D.**

*Reprinted from Therapeutic Drug Monitoring, Vol. 1, pages 199-208, 1979.*

**Summary:**

A brief review of the literature surrounding the relationship between plasma levels of tricyclic antidepressants currently available in the United States and clinical efficacy is presented. While therapeutic ranges for plasma levels of some tricyclic antidepressants are reasonably well established, the relationships between plasma levels of others and clinical efficacy require further clarification. Conditions under which plasma level measurements are clinically useful and factors that alter steady-state plasma levels are discussed.

Individual variability in the response to drugs is a crucial but often neglected fact of pharmacotherapeutics, and the importance of individualizing the dosage of potent drugs in order to maximize therapeutic effectiveness and safety is generally accepted (1-3). The correlation between plasma levels of some tricyclic antidepressants and therapeutic effects suggests that measurement of tricyclic antidepressant plasma levels may provide valuable information for improved clinical management of depressed patients (4). Individual differences in drug metabolism (5,6), wide interpatient variability of plasma tricyclic antidepressant concentrations in patients on fixed doses (7-9), and the fre-

*Dr. Orsulak is Assistant Professor of Psychiatry, Harvard Medical School, and Technical Director or the Psychiatric Chemistry Laboratory, New England Deaconess Hospital, Boston, MA. Dr. Schildkraut is Professor of Psychiatry, Harvard Medical School, Boston, MA.*

quently encountered noncompliance with prescribed dose schedules (10,11) make the measurement of plasma levels a useful way of determining if a patient is receiving an adequate trial of a particular tricyclic antidepressant.

There is growing awareness among psychopharmacologists and clinical chemists that the determination of plasma levels of tricyclic antidepressant medication may be important in determining clinical efficacy, monitoring compliance, and managing side effects. However, the complexity of therapeutic monitoring of the tricyclic antidepressant plasma levels is often overlooked. At present, only the parent compounds and the demethylated metabolites of some tricyclic antidepressants are measured. Many other tricyclic metabolites are also psychoactive (12,13) and may also have to be measured to insure maximum utility of the biochemical data and to prevent toxicity.

Comprehensive reviews of the literature surrounding plasma levels of tricyclic antidepressants and clinical efficacy have recently appeared (14,15) and several reviews dealing with the clinical use of tricyclic antidepressants have also been published during the past year (16-18). The purpose of this paper is not to duplicate these efforts, but rather to outline and present the salient points of the relationship between tricyclic antidepressant plasma levels and clinical efficacy for the tricyclic antidepressants that are currently available in the United States. These include imipramine, desipramine, amitriptyline, nortriptyline, protriptyline, and doxepin. The authors hope that the material presented will serve as a guideline for the practicing clinician who is attempting to utilize therapeutic monitoring of these drugs as part of his effort to improve the clinical management of depressed patients.

## Relationships Between Plasma Concentrations and Antidepressant Response

### Imipramine

Both imipramine and its monodemethylated metabolite, desipramine, are usually found in plasma from depressed patients being treated with imipramine. Several investigators have now examined the relationship between plasma levels of imipramine plus desipramine and clinical response (13,19,20). These studies have found that antidepressant response rate to imipramine therapy is quite low for patients with plasma levels below 150 ng/ml. Clinical response then increases with increasing plasma levels up to 250 ng/ml and appears to plateau at this level. Depressed patients who do not respond at a plasma level as high as 250 ng/ml are not likely to respond at higher levels, and increasing their plasma levels only serves to increase side effects (20).

Of the several types of nonschizophrenic depressive disorders studied so far, only the unipolar delusional patients failed to demonstrate an association between blood levels and clinical response in these studies (13, 20).

Other studies have demonstrated the importance of measuring both imipramine and its demethylated metabolite, desipramine, individually in plasma (6, 19). These studies indicate that the concentrations of imipramine and desipramine must be greater than 45 ng/ml and 75 ng/ml, respectively, for maximum therapeutic effect to be achieved in patients treated with imipramine. A more recent study (21) reported that the ratio of imipramine to desipramine was significantly higher among patients who responded to imipramine treatment than it was among patients who failed to respond to imipramine. Since the range in these two groups overlapped (0.8-1.8 in responders versus 0.4-1.9 in nonresponders), and because this relationship may not exist in all patients, clinical utility of this ratio may be limited.

### Nortriptyline

The recommended therapeutic plasma levels of nortriptyline are between 50 and 150 ng/ml based on several Scandinavian and American studies (22-27). However, in contrast to imipramine, the relationship between plasma levels and clinical response to nortriptyline is curvilinear, i.e., patients with plasma levels either below 50 ng/ml or above 150 ng/ml tend to respond less favorably to treatment with this drug than do patients with plasma levels within this range. Levels above this range have also been associated with an increased incidence of side effects in addition to the decreased antidepressant response (26).

### Amitriptyline

Amitriptyline and its monodemethylated metabolite, nortriptyline, are both usually found in plasma from patients treated with amitriptyline. A number of recent studies have found a relationship between clinical response and total plasma levels of amitriptyline plus nortriptyline. Unlike imipramine and nortriptyline, however, the exact therapeutic range and the nature of the relationship between blood levels and clinical efficacy in various groups of depressed patients is not well understood and a relationship has not been observed in all studies.

Several studies have reported a positive correlation between clinical efficacy and plasma concentrations of amitriptyline plus nortriptyline. These studies suggest that antidepressant response rate is more favorable in patients who achieve plasma levels greater than 120 ng/ml and then increases with increasing total plasma levels (of amitriptyline plus nortriptyline) up to around 250 ng/ml (28-30).

Other studies have found a curvilinear relationship between the plasma levels of amitriptyline plus nortriptyline and therapeutic effect. These studies reported that the lower limit of the "therapeutic window" is approximately 80 ng/ml and that the upper limit of the "window" is approximately 220 ng/ml (25,31,32).

In contrast to the studies that reported a relationship between plasma levels and clinical efficacy, two studies (33,34) failed to find any relationship between clinical response and the plasma levels of amitriptyline, nortriptyline, or amitriptyline plus nortriptyline in patients treated with amitriptyline. One of these studies (33) has been criticized, however, because it may not have included patients for whom tricyclic antidepressants were appropriate, and for problems related to collection, storage, and transport of specimens since it was a multicenter study (35). The other study (34) found only a weak association between plasma levels of amitriptyline and clinical improvement in the more severely depressed patients, suggesting that factors other than plasma level alone may play a role in predicting response to antidepressant therapy with amitriptyline. This provocative finding, when taken with those outlined above, clearly indicates that further studies on the relationship between therapeutic outcome and plasma levels of amitriptyline and its metabolites are required.

### Protriptyline

Currently available data suggest that the relationship between plasma levels of protriptyline and therapeutic response may also be curvilinear. In one study

(36), patients with plasma levels within the range from 165 to 260 ng/ml showed better response to protriptyline than patients who had plasma levels outside this range. In another study (37), in which the maximum plasma level of protriptyline achieved was 167 ng/ml, patients with plasma levels above 70 ng/ml had better clinical outcomes than did those patients with plasma levels below 70 ng/ml. While these two studies suggest that plasma concentrations of protriptyline between 70 and 260 ng/ml may be therapeutic and that poor antidepressant response results when plasma levels are outside this range, the optimal therapeutic range for protriptyline remains to be clarified.

### Doxepin

As with protriptyline, there have been few studies relating plasma levels of doxepin and its demethylated metabolite, desmethyldoxepin, to clinical response in patients treated with this drug. One study (38) reported that plasma levels of doxepin plus desmethyldoxepin must exceed 110 ng/ml for most patients to have a good antidepressant response to this drug, while case reports indicate that patients respond more favorably to therapy with doxepin at plasma levels of doxepin plus desmethyldoxepin between 150 and 250 ng/ml (39,40). A therapeutic range for doxepin alone of 75 to 200 ng/ml has been proposed (41), but the demethylated metabolite was not mentioned.

Although these reports suggest that the therapeutic range for doxepin (plus desmethyldoxepin) lies between 110 ng/ml and 250 ng/ml, definite statements cannot be made on the basis of the presently available data.

### Desipramine

Desipramine is the major psychoactive metabolite of imipramine and is itself an effective antidepressant; however, very few studies to date have attempted to relate plasma levels of desipramine to therapeutic efficacy. A therapeutic range of 150 to 300 ng/ml for patients being treated with desipramine has been proposed (41) and the limited data available tend to support this range. Two small studies from the same group of investigators found a positive correlation between plasma levels of desipramine (29 to 318 ng/ml) and clinical response in patients treated with this drug (42). These investigators also found, in another study (43), that two subjects with plasma levels of 167 and 290 ng/ml responded more favorably than did one subject with a plasma level of 43 ng/ml and two subjects with plasma levels over 440 ng/ml. A recent case report (44) also found that a depressed patient who failed to respond to desipramine therapy at conventional doses but low plasma levels (10 ng/ml)

responded when high doses of desipramine were administered and the blood level rose to 145 ng/ml.

Clearly, the relationship between the plasma levels of desipramine and its antidepressant efficacy remains to be clarified by future studies.

### Discussion

Although many of the studies outlined in the previous sections are confounded by differences in the methodology, statistical treatment of the data, and patient populations that were used, it appears from the available evidence that plasma measurements of at least some of the tricyclic antidepressants can provide valuable additional information for the treatment and management of psychiatric patients.

Recent studies have shown that therapeutic monitoring of tricyclic antidepressant plasma levels can be useful in managing the treatment of elderly patients. One study (45) demonstrated that older patients treated with a given dose of tricyclic antidepressant often develop higher steady-state plasma levels than do younger individuals. Another study (46) showed that geriatric patients can attain extremely high plasma levels of tricyclic antidepressants when treated with only modest doses, while conventional doses can lead to toxic levels in such patients.

Recent reports on the cardiac side effects of tricyclic antidepressants (47-49) have focused attention on the need to avoid toxic plasma levels of these drugs in patients with cardiac disease, and there is general agreement that plasma level measurements can be useful in determining the optimal dose to be given to such patients (11).

Race can also play a significant role in determining the steady-state plasma tricyclic antidepressant levels in patients taking these drugs. Ziegler and Biggs (50) showed that blacks achieved higher steady-state plasma levels of nortriptyline than did white patients receiving similar doses.

The presence of other medications and drug-drug interactions may also significantly alter steady-state plasma levels of tricyclic antidepressants (13,51). For example, hydrocortisone, neuroleptics, and methylphenidate are known to inhibit the metabolism of tricyclic antidepressants by the liver, thus producing higher plasma levels (52), while barbiturates, chloral hydrate, and glutethimide appear to stimulate liver microsomal activity, thus lowering tricyclic antidepressant levels in plasma (53). Benzodiazepines appear to have no effect on the rate of tricyclic antidepressant metabolism (54).

Cigarette smoking also lowers steady-state plasma levels of tricyclic antidepressants, presumably by induction of liver metabolizing enzymes (13,40).

Although therapeutic monitoring of tricyclic antidepressant plasma levels can improve the treatment and management of depressed patients, clinically applicable methods for selection of those patients who actually need, or are likely to respond to, a particular antidepressant are required. The notion that differences in the underlying biochemical pathophysiology of the various subtypes of depressions may lead to differences in the clinical effects of tricyclic antidepressant drugs is exemplified by studies showing that pretreatment levels of urinary 3-methoxy-4-hydroxyphenylglycol (MHPG) may provide a biochemical criterion for predicting differential responses to treatment with various tricyclic antidepressant drugs (55-59).

Even though further studies of the relationship between plasma levels of tricyclic antidepressants and their therapeutic efficacy are required, it is clear that plasma level determinations can help the clinician to arrive more quickly at the optimal dosage of some tricyclic antidepressant drugs and that therapeutic monitoring of plasma levels can eliminate some of the uncertainty associated with the use of these drugs in clinical practice.

Great strides have been taken in recent years in the analysis of the tricyclic antidepressants by gas chromatography, gas chromatography-mass spectrometry, and high pressure liquid chromatography, and the major responsibility for routine analyses of these drugs is shifting from the research laboratory to the clinical laboratory. However, not all laboratories engaged in the analysis of tricyclic antidepressants are in a position to provide the necessary supporting information required to deal with psychiatric patients being treated with these drugs. A program of continuing education, quality control, and appropriate reference methodology remains to be established in this area of clinical chemistry to insure the quality of laboratory results and to provide the fundamental data and clinical expertise needed to apply therapeutic monitoring effectively to the utilization of tricyclic antidepressants.

Finally, the clinician who uses therapeutic monitoring of tricyclic antidepressants should remember that plasma levels should be used only in conjunction with a thorough clinical evaluation and should never be a substitute for careful medical observation and judgment.

## Acknowledgment

This work was supported in part by an Alcohol, Drug Abuse and Mental Health Administration grant from the National Institute of Mental Health (MH 15413).

## References

1. Koch-Weser J: Serum drug concentrations as therapeutic guides. *N Engl J Men* 287:227-231, 1972
2. Koch-Wesser J: The serum level approach to individualization of drug dosage. *Eur J Clin Pharmacol* 9:1-8, 1975
3. Pippenger CE: Therapeutic drug monitoring: An overview. *Ther Drug Monitoring* 1:3-9, 1979
4. Glassman AH, Perel JM: Tricyclic blood levels clinical outcome: a review of the art. In: *Psychopharmacology: A Generation of Progress,* ed. by MA Lipton, A DiMascio and KF Killam, New York, Raven Press, 1978, pp 917-922
5. Asberg M: Treatment of depression with tricyclic drugs—Pharmacokinetic and pharmacodynamic aspects. *Pharmakopsych Neuro-Psychopharmakol* 9:18-26, 1979
6. Gram LF, Reisby N, Ibsen I, Nagy A, Dencker SJ, Bech P, Petersen GO, Christiansen J: Plasma levels and antidepressant effect of imipramine. *Clin Pharmacol Ther* 19:318-324, 1976
7. Boethius G, Sjoqvist F: Doses and dosage intervals of drugs—Clinical practice and pharmacokinetic principles. *Clin Pharmacol Ther* 24:255-263, 1978
8. Braithwaite R, Montgomery S, Dawling S: Nortriptyline in depressed patients with high plasma levels. II. *Clin Pharmacol Ther* 23:303-308, 1978
9. Ziegler VE, Wylie LT, Biggs JT: Intrapatient variability of serial steady-state plasma tricyclic antidepressant concentrations. *J Pharm Sci* 67:554-555, 1978
10. Biggs JT, Chang SS, Sherman WR, Holland WH: Measurement of tricyclic antidepressant levels in an outpatient clinic. *J Nerv Ment Dis* 162:46-51,1976
11. Asberg M, Sjoqvist F: On the role of plasma level monitoring of tricyclic antidepressants in clinical practice. *Commun Psychopharmacol* 2:381-391, 1978
12. Calil HM, Potter WZ, Rapaport J, Zavadil AP, Sutfin T, Goodwin FK. Hydroxylated metabolites of imipramine and desipramine in man. *Society of Biological Psychiatry, 34th Annual Scientific Program,* May 10-13, 1979
13. Perel JM, Stiller RL, Glassman AH: Studies on plasma level/effect relationships in imipramine therapy. *Commun Psychopharmacol* 2:429-439, 1978
14. Risch SC, Leighton LY, Janowsky DS: Plasma levels of tricyclic antidepressants and clinical efficacy: Review of the literature — Part I. *J Clin Psychiatry* 40:4-16, 1979

15. Risch SC, Huey LY, Janowsky DS: Plasma levels of tricyclic antidepressants and clinical efficacy: Review of the literature — Part II. *J Clin Psychiatry* 40:58-69, 1979

16. Hollister LE: Tricyclic antidepressants (first of two parts). *N Engl J Med* 299:1106-1109, 1978

17. Hollister LE: Tricyclic antidepressants (second of two parts). *N Engl J Med* 299:1168-1172, 1978

18. Rosenbaum AH, Maruta T, Richelson E: Drugs that alter mood. I. Tricyclic agents and monoamine oxidase inhibitors. *Mayo Clin Proc* 54:335-344, 1979

19. Reisby N, Gram LF, Bech P, Petersen GO, Ortman J, Ibsen I, Dencker SJ, Jacobsen O, Krautwald O, Sondergaard I, Christiansen J: Imipramine: Clinical effects and pharmacokinetic variability. *Psychopharmacology* 54:263-272, 1977

20. Glassman AH, Perel JM, Shostak M, Kantor SJ, Fleiss JL: Clinical implications of imipramine plasma levels for depressive illness. *Arch Gen Psychiatry* 34:197-204, 1977

21. Muscettola G, Goodwin FK, Potter WZ, Claeys MM, Markey SP: Imipramine and desipramine in plasma and spinal fluid. *Arch Gen Psychiatry* 35:621-625, 1978

22. Asberg M, Cronholm B, Sjoqvist F, Tuck D: Relationship between plasma level and therapeutic effect of nortriptyline. *Br Med J* 3:331-334, 1971

23. Kragh-Sorensen P, Hansen CE, Baastrup PC, Hvidberg EF: Self-inhibiting action of nortriptyline's antidepressive effect at high plasma levels. *Psychopharmacologia (Berl)* 45:305-312, 1976

24. Kragh-Sorensen P, Hansen CE, Baastrup PC, Hvidberg EF: Relationship between antidepressant effect and plasma level of nortriptyline. Clinical studies. *Pharmakopsych Neuro-Psychopharmakol* 9:27-32, 1976

25. Ziegler VE, Clayton PJ, Biggs FT: A comparison study of amitriptyline and nortriptyline with plasma levels. *Arch Gen Psychiatry* 34:607-612, 1977

26. Kragh-Sorensen P: Correlation between plasma levels of nortriptyline and clinical effects. *Commun Psychopharmacol* 2:451-456, 1978

27. Sorensen B, Kragh-Sorensen P, Larsen N-E, Hvidberg EF: The practical significance of nortriptyline plasma control. *Psychopharmacology* 59:35-39,1978

28. Braithwaite RA, Goulding R, Theano G, Bailey J, Coppen A: Plasma concentration of amitriptyline and clinical response. *Lancet* 1:1297-1299, 1972

29. Kupfer DJ, Hanin I, Spiker DG, Grau T, Coble R: Amitriptyline plasma levels and clinical response in primary depression. *Clin Pharmacol Ther* 22:904-911, 1977

30. Kupfer DJ, Hanin I, Spiker D, Neil J, Coble P, Grau T, Nevar C: Amitriptyline plasma levels and clinical response in primary depression. II. *Commun Psychopharmacol* 2:441-450, 1978

31. Vandel S, Vandel B, Sandoz M, Allers G, Bechtel P, Volmat R: Clinical response and plasma concentration of amitriptyline and its metabolite nortriptyline. *Eur J Clin Pharmacol* 14:185-190, 1978

32. Montgomery SA, McAuley R, Montgomery DB, Braithwaite RA, Dawling S: Dosage adjustment from simple nortriptyline spot level predictor tests in depressed patients. *Clin Pharmacolinetics* 4:129-136, 1979

33. Coppen A, Ghose K, Montgomery S, Rama Rao VA, Bailey J, Christiansen J, Mikkleson PI, vanPraag HM, van de Poel F, Minsker EJ, Kozulja VG, Matussek N, Kungkunz G, Jorgensen A: Amitriptyline plasma concentration and clinical effect. *Lancet* 1:63-66, 1978

34. Robinson DS, Cooper TB, Ravaris CL, Ives JO, Nies A Bartlett D, Lamborn KR: Plasma tricyclic drug levels in amitriptyline-treated depressed patients. *Psychopharmacology* 62:223-231, 1979

35. Potter WZ, Goodwin FK: Antidepressant drug levels and clinical response (Letter). *Lancet* 1:1049-1050, 1978

36. Whyte SF, MacDonald AJ, Naylor GJ, Moody JP: Plasma concentrations of protriptyline and clinical effects in depressed woman. *Br J Psychiatry* 128:384-390, 1976

37. Biggs JT, Ziegler VE: Protriptyline plasma levels and antidepressant response. *Clin Pharmacol Ther* 22:269-273, 1977

38. Freidel RO, Raskind MA: Relationship of blood levels of Sinequan to clinical effects in the treatment of depression in aged patients. In: *Sinequan (Doxepin HCl): A Monograph of Recent Clinical Studies,* ed. by J Mendels and J Amsterdam, New York, Excerpta Medica, 1975, pp 51-53

39. Green DO: Clinical importance of doxepin antidepressant plasma levels. *J. Clin Psychiatry* 5:481-482, 1978

40. Jobson K, Burnett G, Linniola M: Weight loss and a concomitant change in plasma tricyclic levels. *Am J Psychiatry* 135:237-238, 1978

41. Biggs JT: Clinical pharmacology and toxicology antidepressants. *Hosp Pract* 13:79-84, 1978

42. Khalid R, Amin MM, Ban TA: Desipramine plasma levels and therapeutic response. *Psychopharmacol Bull* 14:43-44, 1978

43. Amin MM, Cooper R, Khalid R, Lehmann HE: A comparison of desipramine and amitriptyline

plasma levels and therapeutic response. *Psycho-pharmacol Bull* 14:45-46, 1978

44. Amsterdam J, Brunswick DJ, Mendels J: High dose desipramine, plasma drug levels and clinical response. *J Clin Psychiatry* 40:141-143, 1979

45. Nies A, Robinson DS, Friedman MJ, Green R, Cooper T, Ravaris CL, Ives JO: Relationship between age and tricyclic antidepressant plasma levels. *Am J Psychiatry* 134:790-793, 1977

46. Applebaum PS, Vasile RG, Orsulak PJ, Schildkrut JJ: Clinical utility of tricyclic antidepressant blood levels: A case report. *Am J Psychiatry* 136:339-341, 1979

47. Bigger JT, Kantor SJ, Glassman AH, Perel JM: Cardiovascular effects of tricyclic antidepressant drugs. In: *Psychopharmacology: A Generation of Progress,* ed. by MA Lipton, A DiMascio, and KF Killam, New York, Raven Press, 1978, pp 1033-1046

48. Kantor SJ, Glassman AH, Bigger JT, Perel JM, Giardina DV: The cardiac effects of therapeutic plasma concentrations of imipramine. *Am J Psychiatry* 135:534-538, 1978

49. Glassman AH, Bigger JT, Giardina EV, Kantor SJ, Perel JM, Davies M: Clinical characteristics of imipramine-induced orthostatic hypotension. *Lancet* 1:468-472, 1979

50. Ziegler VE, Biggs BT: Tricyclic plasma levels: Effects of age, race, sex, and smoking. *JAMA* 438:2167-2169, 1977

51. Hollister LE: Interaction of psychotherapeutic drugs with other drugs and disease states. In: *Psychopharmacology: A Generation of Progress,* ed. by MA Lipton, A DiMascio, and KF Killam, New York, Raven Press, 1978, pp 987-992

52. Gram LF, Overo KF: Drug interaction: Inhibitory effect of neuroleptics on metabolism of tricyclic antidepressants in man. *Br Med J* 1:463-465, 1972

53. Alexanderson B, Evans DAP, Sjoqvist F: Steady-state plasma levels of nortriptyline in twins: Influence of genetic factors and drug therapy. *Br Med J* 4:764-768, 1969

54. Silverman G, Braithwaite RA: Benzodiazepines and tricyclic antidepressant plasma levels. *Br Med J* 3:18-20, 1973

55. Fawcett J, Maas JW, Dekirmenjian H: Depression and MHPG excretion. *Arch Gen Psychiatry* 26:246-251, 1972

56. Maas JW, Fawcett J, Dekirmenjian H: Catecholamine metabolism, depressive illness and drug response. *Arch Gen Psychiatry* 26:252-262, 1972

57. Schildkraut JJ: Norepinephrine metabolites as biochemical criteria for classifying depressive disorders and predicting responses to treatment: Preliminary findings. *Am J Psychiatry* 130:695-699, 1973

58. Beckmann H, Goodwin FK: Antidepressant response to tricyclics and urinary MHPG in unipolar patients. *Arch Gen Psychiatry* 32:17-21, 1975

59. Modai I, Apter A, Golomb M, Wijsenbeek H: Response to amitriptyline and urinary MHPG in bipolar depressive patients. *Neuropsychobiology* 5:181-184, 1979

# 40

# Clinical Pharmacology of Tricyclic Antidepressants: A Brief Review

**Paul J. Orsulak, Ph.D.**

The value of measurements of their concentration in plasma as an adjunct to the use of some therapeutic drugs has been firmly established and the capability of measuring therapeutic concentrations of drugs has changed both clinical chemistry and pathology. Many drugs, including anticonvulsants, antibiotics, and antiarrhythmic drugs, are being measured, and there is growing awareness that the determination of tricyclic antidepressant drugs in plasma can be important in the treatment and management of psychiatric patients to determine efficacy, to monitor compliance, and to control side effects.

The correlation between concentrations of some tricyclic antidepressants in plasma and their therapeutic effect has been well documented, and such measurements can provide valuable information for improved clinical management of depressed patients. Individual variability in response to drugs makes it necessary to individualize dosage, to maximize therapeutic effectiveness and safety (1, 2). Large differences in drug metabolism (3, 4) and frequently encountered noncompliance with prescribed dose schedules (5) make such measurements a useful way of determining whether a patient is receiving an adequate therapeutic trial of a tricyclic antidepressant.

Over the past 10 years, there has been a technological revolution in the practice of medicine, and utilization of the laboratory by physicians has increased. The increasing interest in monitoring the tricyclic antidepressants (and other therapeutic drugs) in plasma is related to the availability of new and (or) more reliable techniques for their analysis. Gas chromatography and high-pressure liquid chromatography are currently being used to analyze for these drugs, and advances in the development of immunoassay methods for the tricyclic antidepressants appear promising. However, not all laboratories engaged in the analyses for tricyclic antidepressants understand the various aspects of therapy with these drugs or are in a position to provide the necessary supporting information needed to deal with psychiatric patients.

---

*Dr. Orsulak is Assistant Professor of Psychiatry, Harvard Medical School, and Technical Director of the Psychiatric Chemistry Laboratory, New England Deaconess Hospital, both in Boston, MA.*

Comprehensive reviews of the literature surrounding the correlation between plasma levels of tricyclic antidepressants and clinical efficacy have appeared recently (6, 7) and several reviews dealing with the clinical use of tricyclic antidepressants have been published (8-10). Guidelines for therapeutic monitoring of tricyclic antidepressants have also been published (11) and appeared earlier in this series (12). The methodology for analyzing these drugs has also been reviewed recently (13). The purpose of this paper is not to provide a comprehensive review of these areas again, but rather to outline and present salient aspects of the chemistry, pharmacology, and therapeutic use of tricyclic antidepressants as background material for laboratory scientists engaged in the analysis of these drugs. I hope that the material presented will serve as a ready reference and provide some of the fundamental information that the laboratory needs to improve its clinical expertise and apply therapeutic monitoring of tricyclic antidepressant drugs effectively.

## Clinical Indications

Tricyclic antidepressants are approved for use primarily in treating depressive disorders (9, 14). This indication is quite broad, even though evidence from clinical studies suggests that the drugs are specifically useful in the autonomous or endogenous depressions. These are depressions characterized by a lack of responsiveness to environmental events or interpersonal interactions, along with such symptoms as loss of appetite, anergia, anhedonia, psychic retardation, decreased productivity, and disturbances of major body rhythms, including sleep, sexual drive, and motor activity.

Tricyclic antidepressants are also approved for use in treating childhood enuresis, and are quite effective for this purpose (9). However, drug therapy is not the preferred approach to this problem, because beneficial effects last only as long as active drug is being given. There are no data on the relationship between tricyclic antidepressant concentrations in plasma and clinical effectiveness for treating this disorder.

Tricyclic antidepressants are used to treat chronically painful states that cannot be definitely diagnosed as part of another disorder. Tricyclic antidepressants are also being used to treat anorexia nervosa, a disorder related to depression, to treat patients with migraine and obsessive compulsive phobic states, and to treat children with school phobias, hyperkinesis, and minimal brain damage *(9, 15)*. Again, there are no data on the relationship between concentrations in plasma and clinical efficacy for these disorders.

Even when tricyclic antidepressants are used to treat depressed patients, special caution is generally advised when certain patients are treated. Patients with histories of schizophrenic disorders and manic episodes require close observation during treatment, because these drugs have the potential for precipitating psychosis or mania although these drugs are indicated for treatment of acute depressive episodes in these patients *(16)*. Tricyclics should not be administered to patients during the acute recovery period after myocardial infarction, nor should they usually be given to patients taking monoamine oxidase inhibitor antidepressants. They should also be avoided in pregnant and lactating women because safe use of the drugs in these patients has not been established and reports have documented that these drugs pass through breast milk to nursing infants *(15, 17)*.

## Mode of Action

Although research thus far has not provided conclusive evidence, it is thought that the principal action of the tricyclic antidepressants is to increase the functional availability of the neurotransmitters norepinephrine and serotonin at nerve endings in the brain by blocking re-uptake of these two neurotransmitters into the presynaptic nerve terminal. The effect of this inhibition is to increase the amount of neurotransmitter at the post-synaptic receptor site. As summarized in Table 1, the different tricyclic antidepressants available in the United States exhibit different degrees of inhibition of the re-

uptake of norepinephrine and serotonin *(18, 19)*. The tertiary amine tricyclic antidepressants, amitriptyline and imipramine, more potently inhibit re-uptake of serotonin into the nerve endings, whereas the secondary amine tricyclic antidepressants, nortriptyline and desipramine, more potently inhibit re-uptake of norepinephrine *(20)*. Desipramine has little effect on the re-uptake of serotonin, whereas amitriptyline primarily inhibits re-uptake of this neurotransmitter. The uptake inhibition properties of protriptyline and doxepin are less well known. Although the exact relationship between the ability of these drugs to inhibit the re-uptake of biogenic amines and their antidepressant effects is not known, this effect has contributed significantly to the "biogenic amine hypothesis" of depression *(21)*.

In addition to their ability to inhibit the re-uptake of neurotransmitters, the tricyclic antidepressants exhibit various degrees of sedative action. Tertiary amines — such as doxepin, amitriptyline, and imipramine — are most sedative and the secondary amine tricyclics are somewhat less sedating. Protriptyline is virtually devoid of this action. This difference in drugs often is pertinent when a choice must be made by the clinician, to avoid side effects, but apparently it is unrelated to their antidepressant efficacy.

Tricyclic antidepressants also exhibit both peripheral and central anticholinergic (i.e., atropinic) action. The anticholinergic action leads to the most common and unwanted side effects of these drugs, which are described below in the section on side effects. Amitriptyline is the strongest anticholinergic agent and, as shown in Table 1, desipramine is the weakest, with the others exhibiting varying degrees of anticholinergic effects in between these two extremes. Like the sedative side effects, the differences sometimes affect the choice

### Table 1. Pharmacological Properties of Tricyclic Antidepressant Drugs

| Drug | Effect on biogenic amine reuptake | | Anticholinergic effect | Sedation |
|---|---|---|---|---|
| | Norepinephrine | Serotonin | | |
| Amitriptyline | 0 | + + + + | + + + | + + + |
| Imipramine | + + | + + + | + + | + + |
| Nortriptyline | + + | + + | + + | + + |
| Desipramine | + + + + | 0 | + | + |
| Protriptyline | ? | ? | + + | 0 |
| Doxepin | ? | ? | + + + | + + + |

0 = least potent to + + + + = most potent

of antidepressant used to treat a particular patient.

More recent studies of the mechanism of action of the tricyclic antidepressants have demonstrated that these compounds, along with electroconvulsive therapy, cause a decrease in the ability of norepinephrine to stimulate cyclic AMP formation in the brain (22). The time course of this apparent desensitization of norepinephrine receptors was on the order of two to three weeks, i.e., a period of time compatible with that usually required for clinical response to these drugs. The exact mechanism whereby tricyclic antidepressants cause this change in sensitivity to norepinephrine is not known, but based on these data, a modification of the biogenic amine hypothesis suggests that at least some forms of depression are due to increased sensitivity of the noradrenergic cyclic AMP-generating system in the brain, whereas mania is a result of decreased sensitivity of this receptor system.

Recent findings suggest that one aspect of the relationship between tricyclic antidepressants and their ability to block the uptake of different central nervous system neurotransmitters may provide a clinically applicable method for selecting those patients who actually need or are likely to respond to a particular antidepressant. Studies have shown that pretreatment concentrations of the norepinephrine metabolite, 3-methoxy-4-hydroxyphenylglycol (MHPG), in urine may provide a chemical criterion for predicting differential responses to treatment with various tricyclic antidepressant drugs. In three studies (23-25), depressed patients with low urinary MHPG excretion before treatment responded more favorably to treatment with imipramine or desipramine than did patients who excreted higher levels of MHPG in their urine; in contrast, depressed patients with higher levels of urinary MHPG before treatment responded more favorably to treatment with amitriptyline than did patients with lower levels (26, 27).

## Dosage

The tricyclic antidepressants are administered orally. Generally, these medications are begun at fairly low doses and the dose is increased gradually over several days to reach therapeutically effective doses. Table 2 lists the approximate dose ranges for average adults and elderly patients. Because recent studies indicate that there is pronounced variation in individual rates of metabolism, absorption, and distribution of tricyclic antidepressants, these doses are estimates (9, 10). In middle-aged, physically healthy patients of average weight (60 to 90 kg), the typical starting dose of a tricyclic antidepressant is about 50 to 75 mg/day. The dose is then increased by about 25 mg/day every two or three days until an average dose of 150 mg/day (for

imipramine, amitriptyline, or desipramine) is reached by the end of the first week. Adverse effects, such as dry mouth, hypotension (light-headedness), difficulty in urinating, or drowsiness, often limit the increase in dosage of these medications (10). Based on clinical effect and the concentration attained in plasma, the dose of tricyclic antidepressant is then increased up to the maximum indicated for each drug. Elderly patients generally require much less tricyclic antidepressant; thus the usual dose range in these patients is considerably lower than it is for younger patients.

In patients who eventually respond to tricyclic antidepressants, improvement in sleep, appetite, and even mood can occur within 7 to 10 days, although generally the full effect of medication does not come until the end of the second or third week and occasionally later. If clinical response is slight by this time, further increase in dosage may be warranted. In cases where concentrations in plasma are within appropriate therapeutic ranges, indicating an adequate trial, but where clinical response is minimal, lithium is sometimes co-administered with the antidepressant (10).

Once a patient responds to a tricyclic antidepressant, the dosage may be reduced gradually to a maintenance range. However, concentrations in plasma should remain within the therapeutic range. Patients may be treated with maintenance doses for an additional two to three months and, depending upon the treatment course, the number of previous episodes, and the severity of the depression being treated, the dosage may then be gradually tapered off over one to two additional months.

**Table 2.  Dosage Ranges for Tricyclic Antidepressant Drugs**

|  | Average dose, mg/day | |
| Drug | Adult patient | Elderly patient |
| --- | --- | --- |
| Imipramine | 75 - 300 | 20 - 100 |
| Desipramine | 150 - 300 | 20 - 100 |
| Amitriptyline | 150 - 300 | 20 - 100 |
| Nortriptyline | 50 - 150 | 10 - 75 |
| Protriptyline | 30 - 60 | 10 - 30 |
| Doxepin | 200 - 400 | 30 - 200 |

From:  Rosenbaum, A.H., Maruta, T., and Richelson, E., Drugs that alter mood. I. Tricyclic agents and monoamine oxidase inhibitors. *Mayo Clin. Proc.* **54,** 335-344 (1979).

**Table 3.   Tricyclic Antidepressant Drug Preparations**

| Generic name | Trade name | Source |
|---|---|---|
| **Amitriptyline** | Amitril | Warner/Chilcott |
| | Amitriptyline HCl | Purepac Pharmaceutical Co. |
| | Elavil | Merck Sharp & Dohme |
| | Endep | Roche Laboratories |
| | Etrafon | Schering Corp. |
| | Limbitrol | Roche Labs. |
| | SK-Amitriptyline | Smith Kline & French Labs. |
| | Triavil | Merck Sharp & Dohme |
| **Nortriptyline** | Aventyl HCl | Eli Lilly and Co. |
| | Pamelor | Sandoz Pharmaceuticals |
| **Imipramine** | Antipres | Lemmon Pharmacal Co. |
| | Imavate | A.H. Robins Co. |
| | Imipramine HCl | Philips Roxane Labs., Inc. |
| | Imipramine HCl | Purepac Pharmaceutical Co. |
| | Janimine Filmtab | Abbott Labs. |
| | Presamine | USV Pharmaceutical Corp. |
| | SK-Pramine | Smith Kline & French Labs |
| | Tofranil | Geigy Pharmaceuticals |
| **Desipramine** | Norpramin | Merrell-National Labs. |
| | Pertofrane | USV Pharmaceutical Corp. |
| **Doxepin** | Adapin | Pennwalt Pharmaceutical Div. |
| | Sinequan | Pfizer Laboratories Div. |
| **Protriptyline** | Vivactyl | Merck Sharp & Dohme |

Table 3 lists the tricyclic antidepressants that currently are available in the United States, by generic name, trade name, and supplier. All of these preparations are available for oral administration, supplied in amounts ranging from 10 to 150 mg per tablet or capsule. Elavil (Merck) is available in liquid form for intramuscular injection, but this form is rarely used to treat depression. Etrafon (Schering) and Triavil (Merck) contain the antipsychotic, perphenazine, while Limbitrol (Roche) contains chlordiazepoxide (Librium).

## Metabolism and Pharmacokinetics

The pharmacokinetics of tricyclic antidepressants have been studied extensively in man, but data are generally available only for adult patients. Data for pediatric patients are, in contrast, scarce, even though these drugs are widely used to treat childhood enuresis and depression.

Tricyclic antidepressants are metabolized by two major routes: N-demethylation of the side chain and ring hydroxylation of the nucleus of the molecule. Monodemethylation of the tertiary amines, amitriptyline and imipramine, results in formation of the active demethylated metabolites, nortriptyline and desipramine, so that when tertiary amines are used to treat depressed patients, both the parent tricyclic antidepressant and the major (demethylated) metabolite are present in the plasma. Further demethylation results in the formation of inactive metabolites.

Imipramine and its principal active metabolite, desipramine, are both metabolized further by hydroxylation. Desipramine is oxidized to 2-hydroxydesipramine while the parent imipramine is converted to 2-hydroxyimipramine. These compounds are then either excreted in this form or conjugated to form glucuronides. Other minor metabolic pathways include N-oxidation of imipramine, dealkylation of the molecule by removal of the entire side chain resulting in the formation of iminodibenzyl, and further demethylation of desipramine to yield didesmethylimipramine.

Amitriptyline is also metabolized by N-demethylation to an active metabolite, nortriptyline, but this process is slower than for imipramine. In addition, amitriptyline is metabolized to desmethylnortriptyline, which is inactive. All of these compounds can be hydroxylated in the 10-position of the aliphatic ring (rather than by hydroxylation of the aromatic ring, as with imipramine). This hydroxylation is stereospecific and gives rise to cis and trans isomers in a constant ratio. The 10-hydroxy metabolites are either excreted in this form or conjugated with glucuronide acid before excretion.

It has long been assumed that the hydroxylated metabolites of tricyclic antidepressants are pharmacologically inactive. However, recent studies (28, 29) have shown that the hydroxylated metabolites of imipramine and desipramine have strong cardiovascular activity and can inhibit biogenic amine uptake. In addition, studies have shown that the concentration of hydroxylated metabolites in plasma can be as high as the concentration of imipramine (30).

The metabolic breakdown of tricyclic antidepressants can be significantly decreased by concurrent administration of neuroleptics, i.e., antipsychotic medications. These drugs appear to inhibit the metabolism of the demethylated derivatives, desipramine and nortriptyline, often resulting in increased concentrations in blood despite stable oral doses. Oral contraceptives may also significantly impair the metabolic breakdown of amitriptyline; in contrast, barbiturates, chloral hydrate, and glutethimide appear to stimulate the metabolism of these compounds.

Steady-state concentrations in plasma observed in the course of treatment with tricyclic antidepressants are poorly related to the dose administered orally and values in patients given similar doses of tricyclic antidepressants can vary from 10- to 30-fold (3, 4). This wide variation is probably related to the first-pass metabolism of these drugs in the intestine and liver.

Tricyclic antidepressant drugs have relatively low and variable bioavailability (Table 4) when taken by mouth, owing to extensive first-pass metabolism in the liver. Protein binding of them in plasma has been shown to range from about 70% to nearly 96% for these drugs, and this may partly account for the very large apparent volumes of distribution (15).

Tricyclic antidepressants, including imipramine, desipramine, amitriptyline, nortriptyline, doxepin, and protriptyline, are virtually completely absorbed in the gastrointestinal tract (15). Concentrations in plasma are generally greatest 4 to 8 h after administration of a single oral dose and values ranging from 10 to 100 $\mu g/L$ have been observed after oral administration of a single 50- to 75-mg dose of imipramine or desipramine and single doses of 25 to 50 mg of amitriptyline or nortriptyline. After imipramine administration, desipramine concentrations become measurable in plasma within 2 to 3 h and may exceed those of the parent compound after about 12 h.

Tricyclic antidepressants are filtered through the glomerulus, then passively reabsorbed in the distal tubule. Acidification of the urine may increase total drug excretion by 10 to 40% in patients treated with imipramine. This increase is ascribable to a 50- to 100-fold increase in the amont of unconjugated derivatives, mainly imipramine and desipramine (31).

Studies using radioactively labelled tricyclic antidepressants have shown that 60 to 85% of administered dose is recovered in the urine within 6 to 8 days (15).

Maximal urinary excretion is reached 3 to 6 h after administration, but the amount excreted during the first 24 h is highly variable.

For imipramine and amitriptyline, less than 5% of the administered dose can be recovered in the urine as the parent compound or the demethylated active metabolite. About 45 to 60% of administered imipramine appears in the urine as glucuronide conjugates of the hydroxylated metabolites, about 15 to 30% as free 2-hydroxy metabolites. Similar ratios are observed for amitriptyline and nortriptyline. The remainder of the drug (about 20%) is excreted as nonextractable, more polar metabolites.

Pharmacokinetic information on other tricyclic antidepressant drugs, including protriptyline and doxepin, fairly limited, but the data available suggest that they behave like amitriptyline and nortriptyline. Of note, however, is the extremely long half-life of protriptyline (54 to 198 h) and its unique metabolic breakdown, which may lead to the formation of a stable epoxide, as shown by studies in the rat *(32)*.

### Side Effects

In addition to their ability to inhibit the "biogenic amine pump," tricyclic antidepressant drugs exhibit varying degrees of peripheral and central anticholinergic (i.e., atropine-like) action. Although the side effects resulting from this action are usually not serious, they can be extremely uncomfortable and in rare cases they can be dangerous. Although there is little current evidence to indicate a relationship between concentrations of particular tricyclic antidepressants in plasma and the occurrence or severity of particular side effects, measurements in plasma can be particularly useful in assisting the physician to determine a proper course of action when significant side effects are present.

The principal anticholinergic side effects of tricyclic antidepressants are dry mouth, urinary retention, blurred vision, postural hypotension (light-headedness), and constipation. Central nervous system side effects may also include confusion, agitation or increased irritability, and speech difficulties, but these usually occur in association with toxic concentrations of tricyclic antidepressants.

Several methods can be used to help alleviate the anticholinergic side effects: decreasing the dosage, giving the entire dose at bedtime rather than administering the drug on a divided-dose schedule, or changing to another tricyclic antidepressant that has less anticholinergic effect (see Table 1). Administration of a cholinergic agent such as physostigmine is generally reserved for treating severe toxic reactions.

Tricyclic antidepressants also exhibit various antihistaminic effects, including sedation. Patients develop a tolerance to this effect and reasonable accommodation is possible if dosage is increased slowly and alcoholic beverages are avoided.

Patients taking tricyclic antidepressants often gain weight, which may also be mediated by the antihistaminic effect of these drugs. Patients do not develop tolerance to this reaction and need to watch their caloric intake closely to avoid gaining weight excessively. Such weight gains can cause altered drug concentrations in plasma and lead to loss of antidepressant effect, because heavier individuals sometimes require larger doses of tricyclic antidepressant to maintain clinical effect.

Among the more serious adverse effects of tricyclic antidepressants are direct effects on the heart. Cardiovascular effects include electrocardiographic abnormalities, arrhythmias, palpitations, tachycardia, and orthostatic hypotension. The EKG abnormalities in-

**Table 4. Pharmacokinetic Properties of Tricyclic Antidepressant Drugs**

| Drug | Plasma half-life, h | Peak time, oral dose, h | Bioavailability, % | Protein binding, % | Vol of distribution, L/kg | Time to steady state, days |
|------|---------------------|-------------------------|---------------------|---------------------|----------------------------|-----------------------------|
| Amitriptyline | 17 - 40 | 2 - 8 | 56 - 70 | 82 - 96 | n/a | 4 - 10 |
| Nortriptyline | 15 - 93 | 2 - 8 | 46 - 79 | 93 - 95 | 20 - 57 | 4 - 19 |
| Imipramine | 6 - 24 | 1 - 6 | 29 - 77 | 76 - 96 | 10 - 40 | 2 - 5 |
| Desipramine | 12 - 76 | 2 - 8 | ~90 | 73 - 92 | 22 - 60 | 2 - 11 |
| Protriptyline | 54 - 198 | 6 - 12 | ~85 | ~92 | 15 - 31 | 10+ |
| Doxepin | 8 - 36 | 2 - 6 | ~27 | ? | 9 - 33 | 2 - 8 |

clude T-wave changes, QRS changes, and intraventricular conduction delays *(10)*. Recent studies have correlated plasma levels of tricyclic antidepressant with EKG findings and indicate that conduction defects, at least, do not occur when concentrations of the drug in plasma are within the therapeutic range, but only after values exceed therapeutic ranges *(10)*.

Additional side effects of tricyclic antidepressants that occur relatively rarely include allergic reactions, altered serum enzyme activities, hematologic abnormalities, and central nervous system effects including tremors, tardive dyskinesias, and seizures *(10)*.

At toxic concentrations ($>1000 \mu g/L$), patients can exhibit respiratory depression, hypoxia, coma, convulsions, cardiac arrhythmias, and respiratory arrest *(10)*. However, some patients tolerate extremely high plasma concentrations of tricyclic antidepressants without adverse effects; thus therapeutic monitoring currently must be used in conjunction with a thorough clinical evaluation.

## Drug Interactions

The presence of other medications — and medical or neurological disorders — needs to be considered carefully and understood when interpreting values for tricyclic antidepressants in plasma. These interactions can significantly alter steady-state concentrations *(10, 33)*. For example, hydrocortisone and other corticosteroids, neuroleptics (antipsychotics), and methylphenidate are known to inhibit hepatic metabolism of tricyclic antidepressants, thus producing higher concentrations in plasma. In contrast, barbiturates, chloral hydrate, and glutethimide appear to stimulate liver microsomal activity, thus lowering tricyclic antidepressant concentrations. Benzodiazepines (e.g., Valium, Librium, and other tranquilizers) appear to have no effect on the rate of tricyclic antidepressant metabolism. The cardiotoxic effects of tricyclic antidepressants are potentiated by quinidine and procainamide, probably through increased concentrations of the tricyclic antidepressant drugs and their metabolites in plasma.

Virtually all centrally acting drugs used in the treatment of hypertension, such as clonidine (Catapres), alphamethyldopa (Aldomet), propranolol (Inderal), and metoprolol (Lopresor), interfere with the action of tricyclic antidepressants and generally have to be replaced with peripherally acting agents when hypertensive patients are being treated for depression. Co-administration of tricyclic antidepressants and guanethidine decreases both the antidepressant effect of the tricyclic agents and the hypertensive effects of guanethidine.

Alcohol also increases the metabolism of tricyclic antidepressants, resulting in decreased effect, while sedatives have an additive effect with tricyclic antidepressants. There is increased risk of troublesome atropine-like side effects, particularly in the elderly, if tricyclic antidepressants are administered with anticholinergic agents, anti-parkinsonian drugs, or some antihistamines (e.g., diphenhydramine). Tricyclic antidepressants are not usually administered concurrently with monoamine oxidase inhibitor antidepressants and, if given inadvertently, this mixture can result in agitation, tremor, hyperpyrexia, convulsions, and coma.

Antidepressants also increase the central nervous system depressant effects of sedatives, including barbiturates, chloral hydrate, glutethimide, oxazepam (Serax) and flurazepam (Dalmane).

## Guidelines for Therapeutic Monitoring

Although many of the studies of the relationship between concentrations of tricyclic antidepressants in plasma and clinical outcome are confounded by differences in methodology, statistical treatment of data, and patient populations studied, it appears from the available evidence that plasma measurements of tricyclic antidepressants can provide valuable information for the treatment and management of psychiatric patients *(11, 34, 35)*.

Such measurements can aid the physician in determining a proper course of action when drug toxicity is readily confused with the underlying disorder or when large individual differences in drug metabolism, such as those seen in elderly patients, lead to poor correlation between administered dose and plasma concentrations *(36)*. They are also useful when the pharmacokinetic consequences of drug interaction (e.g., co-administration of antipsychotic medications and hypertensive medications or more than one tricyclic antidepressant) are unknown, or when compliance is poor, or for a drug like nortriptyline that exhibits a "therapeutic window" where efficacy may be lost at higher concentrations in the absence of toxicity and where the relative amounts of the parent drug and metabolites can influence the clinical response.

Therapeutic drug monitoring is also advised for patient populations such as rapid or slow metabolizers, or in those patients for whom there is clear need to keep dosage and concentration at the minimum effective level, such as in the elderly, children, pregnant women, nursing mothers, or patients with cardiovascular, hepatic, or renal disease (who may exhibit altered protein binding or renal clearance).

Therapeutic monitoring of tricyclic antidepressants is also essential when treating non-responsive patients (assuming a correct diagnosis) before switching medication or altering the dose of an appropriate medication. It is particularly indicated when alterations in medication result in doses that exceed the recommended limits for a particular drug.

Recent studies (37,38) have also demonstrated that it may be possible to predict the optimal dose of tricyclic antidepressant for a particular patient on the basis of determinations in plasma after an oral "test dose" of drug, but this technique is not used routinely at present.

Valid measurements of tricyclic antidepressants require attention to several factors that alter their concentrations in plasma, including such things as the age, sex, and race of the patient, and sample-collection techniques. These factors and potential sources of error have been reviewed in detail recently (11, 39).

## Methods of Analysis

In the decade since the initial studies demonstrating the clinical applicability of monitoring tricyclic antidepressants, more than 100 methods for the analysis of tricyclic antidepressants have been described (13). The low concentrations of these drugs found in plasma presented formidable technical difficulties during the early years, and many attempts were made to develop suitable methods involving spectrophotometry, spectrofluorometry, thin-layer chromatography, or isotope derivative analysis. Contemporary methods of analysis for tricyclic antidepressant drugs include gas chromatography with a nitrogen-specific detector, and high-pressure liquid chromatography. Mass-fragmentographic methods are generally considered to be the most reliable and specific, but these techniques require access to expensive mass spectrometry equipment. Attempts to develop immunoassay techniques that would be clinically convenient and relatively inexpensive appear promising, but specific antibodies have yet to be developed for all of the tricyclic antidepressants.

In choosing a method for therapeutic monitoring of tricyclic antidepressants, several issues need to be considered. The method chosen must be specific, i.e., capable of measuring the antidepressant drug (and active metabolite) individually without interference from other metabolites or other drugs that may be administered concurrently. It must also be sensitive enough to measure concentrations as low as 5 to 10 $\mu$g/L in 1- to 2-mL plasma samples. The assay should have a routine intra-assay and inter-assay precision (CV) of 10% or less over the therapeutic range, and be rapid enough to provide results within 24 h after specimens are received in the laboratory.

Because both gas-chromatographic and liquid-chromatographic techniques can meet most of these criteria (13), the choice of a particular method can be based on other factors, including availability or cost of equipment, the skill and experience of the laboratory staff, and the particular requirements of each laboratory. Both gas-chromatographic and liquid-chromatographic techniques are quite suitable for the analysis of the tricyclic antidepressants and their demethylated metabolites, but high-performance liquid-chromatographic techniques may prove more suitable for the analysis of the hydroxylated metabolites if these are also being measured. Chromatographic techniques, including gas chromatography and (or) high-pressure liquid chromatography, will probably be required in most laboratories because of the number of new antidepressants that are currently being investigated (13). Immunoassay techniques may prove to be quite convenient and cost effective, but the need to measure new antidepressant drugs and their metabolites as they are developed may preclude the immediate application of immunoassay techniques to all antidepressants on the market. Thus, laboratories engaged in therapeutic monitoring of antidepressant medications may find themselves in the position of having to utilize at least two different techniques to provide the full range of analyses with maximum cost effectiveness.

## Comment

The value of therapeutic drug monitoring as an adjunct to treatment of depressed patients with tricyclic antidepressants is becoming more firmly established, and the major responsibility for therapeutic monitoring of these drugs has shifted from the research laboratory to the clinical laboratory. Recent advances in development of methods of analyzing for tricyclic antidepressants have resulted in a dramatic increase in the number of laboratories performing these determinations. However, not all laboratories engaged in the analysis of these drugs are in a position to provide the necessary supportive information required to deal with psychiatric patients being treated with these drugs. Although the role of the clinical laboratory in assisting the physician in treating patients is a controversial area, it has been recommended that all laboratories engaged in therapeutic drug monitoring be in a position to provide fundamental data and supporting information to the physician requesting it.

This is particularly true for the tricyclic antidepressant drugs. The therapeutic ranges for some tricyclic antidepressant drugs are reasonably well established, but the relationship between concentration in plasma and clinical efficacy requires further clarification for some others. In addition, a wide range of new antidepressants are currently being tested in the United States, so the clinical laboratory will probably be faced with new questions from physicians and psychiatrists treating depressed patients. Sources of error in collection and analysis of specimens are wide and varied and not generally well known and understood. Accurate information is required concerning procedures needed to ensure proper collection of specimens and precise determinations.

During the coming years, a number of factors will impact on therapeutic monitoring of antidepressant medications. Clinically applicable methods for selection of those patients who actually need or are likely to respond to particular antidepressants have been introduced (i.e., the determination of urinary MHPG) and will be refined. Novel, perhaps more rapidly acting, antidepressants are likely to be developed and the clinical methods used for selecting patients to be treated with the antidepressants and methods for assessing treatment outcome will become more standardized.

Ongoing studies are focusing on individual pharmacokinetic and pharmacodynamic properties of the currently available tricyclic antidepressants in an attempt to identify the most significant correlations with clinical effect. Studies thus far suggest that the strongest correlation will be found between values for total tricyclic antidepressant in plasma (parent and all active metabolites) and therapeutic outcome. These studies are also beginning to suggest that factors other than concentration in plasma alone, such as the subtype of depressive disorder being treated, may play a role in determining the response to antidepressant therapy. Such distinctions will significantly enhance the reliability of treatment with these agents.

These changes, when coupled with appropriate levels of therapeutic drug monitoring and continuing education of both physicians and laboratory personnel, will ultimately ensure more accurate and effective treatment of patients with depressions.

## Acknowledgement

This work was supported in part by an Alcohol, Drug Abuse and Mental Health Administration grant from the National Institute of Mental Health (MH 15413).

## References

1. Koch-Weser, J., Serum drug concentrations as therapeutic guides. *N. Engl. J. Med.* **287,** 227-231 (1972).
2. Koch-Weser, J., The serum level approach to individualization of drug dosage. *Eur. J. Clin. Pharmacol.* **9,** 1-8 (1975).
3. Asberg, M., Treatment of depression with tricyclic drugs - pharmacokinetic and pharmacodynamic aspects. *Pharmakopsych. Neuropsychopharmacol.* **9,** 18-26 (1976).
4. Gram, L.F., Reisby, N., Ibsen, L., et al., Plasma levels and antidepressant effect of imipramine. *Clin. Pharmacol. Therap.* **19,** 318-324 (1976).
5. Biggs, J.T., Chang, S.S., Sherman, W.R., and Holland, W.H., Measurement of tricyclic antidepressant levels in an outpatient clinic. *J. Nerv. Ment. Dis.* **162,** 46-51 (1976).
6. Risch, S.C., Huey, L.Y., and Janowsky, D.S., Plasma levels of tricyclic antidepressants and clinical efficacy: Review of the literature — Part I. *J. Clin. Psychiatry* **40,** 4-16, (1979).
7. Risch, S.C., Huey, L.Y., and Janowsky, D.S., Plasma levels of tricyclic antidepressant and clinical efficacy: Review of the literature — Part II. *J. Clin. Psychiatry* **40,** 58-69 (1979).
8. Hollister, L.E., Tricyclic antidepressants (first of two parts). *N. Engl. J. Med.* **299,** 1106-1109 (1978).
9. Hollister, L.E., Tricyclic antidepressants (second of two parts). *N. Engl. J. Med.* **299,** 1168-1172 (1978).
10. Rosenbaum, A.H., Maruta, T., and Richelson, E., Drugs that alter mood. I. Tricyclic agents and monoamine oxidase inhibitors. *Mayo Clin. Proc.* **54,** 335-344 (1979).
11. Orsulak, P.J., and Schildkraut, J.J., Guidelines for therapeutic monitoring of tricyclic antidepressant plasma levels. *Ther. Drug Monitoring* **1,** 199-208 (1979).
12. Orsulak, P.J., and Schildkraut, J.J., Guidelines for therapeutic monitoring of tricyclic antidepressant plasma levels. *Therapeutic Drug Monitoring Continuing Education and Quality Control Program,* Am. Assoc. Clin. Chem., November 1979.
13. Scoggins, B.A., Maguire, K.P., Norman, T.R., and Burrows, G.D., Measurements of tricyclic antidepressants. Part I. A review of methodology. *Clin. Chem.* **26,** 5-17 (1980); Part II. Applications of methodology. *Clin. Chem.* **26,** 805-815 (1980).
14. Byck, R., Drugs and the treatment of psychiatric disorders. In *The Pharmacological Basis of Therapeutics,* 5th ed., L.S. Goodman and A. Gilman, Eds., MacMillan, New York, NY, 1975, pp 153-200.
15. Morselli, P., Antidepressant drugs. In *Drug Disposition During Development,* P. Morselli, Ed., Spectrum Press, New York, NY, 1978, pp 439-449.
16. Shader, R.I., Ed., *Manual of Psychiatric Therapeutics,* Little, Brown and Co., Boston, MA, 1975.

17. Sovner, R., and Orsulak, P.J., Excretion of imipramine and desipramine in human breast milk. *Am. J. Psychiatry* **136**, 451- 452 (1979).

18. Maas, J.W., Biogenic amines and depression: Biochemical and pharmacological separation of two types of depression. *Arch. Gen. Psychiatry* **32**, 1357-1361 (1975).

19. Maas, J.W., Clinical implications of pharmacological differences among antidepressants. In *Psychopharmacology: A Generation of Progress,* M.A. Lipton, A. DiMascio, and K.F. Killam, Eds., Raven Press, New York, NY, 1978, pp 955-960.

20. Maas, J.W., Clinical and biological heterogeneity of depressive disorders. *Ann. Intern. Med.* **88**, 556-563 (1978).

21. Schildkraut, J.J., Current status of the catecholamine hypothesis of affective disorders. In *Psychopharmacology: A Generation of Progress,* M.A.Lipton, A. DiMascio, and K.F. Killam, Eds., Raven Press, New York, NY 1978, pp 1223-1234.

22. Sulser, F., Vetulani, J., and Mobley, P.L., Mode of action of antidepressant drugs. *Biochem. Pharmacol.* **27**, 257-261 (1978).

23. Fawcett, J., Maas, J.W., and Dekirmenjian, H., Depression and MHPG excretion. *Arch. Gen. Psychiatry* **26**, 246-251 (1972).

24. Maas, J.W., Fawcett, J., and Dekirmanjian, H., Catecholamine metabolism depressive illness and drug response. *Arch. Gen. Psychiatry* **26**, 252-262 (1972).

25. Rosenbaum, A.H., Schatzberg, A.F., Maruta, T., Orsulak, P.J., Cole, J.O., Grab, E.L., and Schildkraut, J.J., MHPG as a predictor of antidepressant response to imipramine and maprotiline. *Am. J. Psychiatry* **137**, 1090-1092 (1980).

26. Schildkraut, J.J., Norepinephrine metabolites as biochemical criteria for classifying depressive disorders and predicting responses to treatment: Preliminary findings. *Am. J. Psychiatry* **130**, 695-699 (1973).

27. Beckmann, H., and Goodwin, F.K., Antidepressant response to tricyclics and urinary MHPG in unipolar patients. *Arch. Gen. Psychiatry* **32**, 17-21 (1975).

28. Potter, W.Z., Calil, H.M., Zavadil, A.P., and Goodwin, F.K., Steady-state concentrations of hydroxylated metabolites of tricyclic antidepressants in patients: Relationship to clinical effect. *Psychopharmacol. Bull.* **16**, 32-34 (1980).

29. Potter, W.Z., Calil, H.M., Manian, A.A., et al., Hydroxylated metabolites of tricyclic antidepressants: Preclinical assessment of activity. *Biol. Psychiatry* **14**, 601-613 (1979).

30. Perel, J.M., Stiller, R.L., and Glassman, A.H., Studies on plasma level/effect relationships in imipramine therapy. *Commun. Psychopharmacol.* **2**, 429-439 (1978).

31. Gram, L.F., Kofod, B., Christiansen, J., and Rafaelson, O.J., Imipramine metabolism, pH dependent distribution and urinary excretion. *Clin. Pharmacol. Therap.* **12**, 239-244 (1971).

32. Hucker, H.B., Balleto, A.J., Demetriades, J., et al., Epoxide metabolites of protriptyline in rat urine. *Drug Metabolism Disposition* **3**, 80-83 (1975).

33. Avery, G.S., and Heel, R.C., Guide to the clinically more important drug interactions. Appendix C in *Drug Treatment: Principles and Practice of Clinical Pharmacology and Therapeutics,* 2nd ed., G.S. Avery, Ed., Adis Press, Sydney, Australia, 1980, pp 1252-1272.

34. Shader, R.I., and Greenblatt, D.J., Clinical indications for plasma level monitoring of psychotropic drugs. *Am. J. Psychiatry* **136**, 1590-1591 (1979).

35. Baldessarini, R.J., Status of psychotropic drug blood level assay and other biochemical measurements in clinical practice. *Am. J. Psychiatry* **136**, 1177-1180 (1979).

36. Appelbaum, P.S., Vasile, R.G., Orsulak, P.J., and Schildkraut, J.J., Clinical utility of tricyclic antidepressant blood levels: A case report. *Am. J. Psychiatry* **136**, 339-341 (1979).

37. Usdin, E., Ed., Symposium on plasma monitoring of tricyclic antidepressants. *Commun. Psychopharmacol.* **2**, 371-456 (1978).

38. Cooper, T.B., and Simpson, G.M., Prediction of individual dosages of nortriptyline. *Am. J. Psychiatry* **135**, 333-335 (1978).

39. Orsulak, P.J., and Gerson, B., Therapeutic monitoring of tricyclic antidepressants: Quality control considerations. *Ther. Drug Monitoring:* in press (1980).

# 41

# Monitoring Imipramine Concentrations In the Plasma of Elderly Patients: A Case Study

Paul J. Orsulak, Ph.D.
Paul S. Appelbaum, M.D.

This case illustrates the value of monitoring the concentrations of tricyclic antidepressants of elderly patients during therapy. Both imipramine and its monodemethylated metabolite, desipramine, are usually found in plasma from depressed patients who are being treated with imipramine. The antidepressant response rate to imipramine therapy is quite low for patients whose plasma concentrations of imipramine plus desipramine are less than 150 $\mu$g/L. Clinical response increases with concentrations up to 250 $\mu$g/L, but then appears to level off. Depressed patients who do not respond to concentrations in plasma as great as 250 $\mu$g/L are unlikely to respond to higher concentrations; further increasing the concentration only serves to increase side effects.

## Case Study

Ms. A, a 68-year-old woman with a history of recurrent unipolar depressions since her teens, has had more than 13 hospitalizations at several institutions during the past 15 years. During that period, she received several courses of electroconvulsive therapy with modest response and was also treated with phenothiazines and lithium, without success. Tricyclic antidepressant therapy was first initiated in 1969, when Ms. A was 59 years old, and she exhibited some clinical response to a combination of amitriptyline (75 mg/day) and the antipsychotic, perphenazine (6 mg/day). Her recovery was complete when the amitriptyline dosage was increased to 200 mg/day. However, from 1970 to 1975, she had many recurrent episodes of depression, some of which were treated with amitriptyline. Clinical benefit during this period was greatest when the patient received perphenazine (12 mg/day) in addition to amitriptyline (125 mg/day).

In June 1976, the patient stopped taking amitriptyline and her depression recurred. On rehospitalization, she was treated with amitriptyline (100 mg/day) without perphenazine and began to improve, but soon became disoriented with severe memory deficit, incon-

Dr. Orsulak is Assistant Professor of Psychiatry, Harvard Medical School, and Technical Director of the Psychiatric Chemistry Laboratory, New England Deaconess Hospital, both in Boston, Massachusetts.

Dr. Appelbaum is a Clinical Fellow in Psychiatry, Harvard Medical School, Boston, Massachusetts.

tinence, somnolence, and, ultimately, coma. Amitriptyline was discontinued and extensive neurological examination, including lumbar puncture, brain scan, and electroencephalogram revealed no cause for these symptoms. Eight days after amitriptyline was discontinued, the syndrome resolved. The patient's depression persisted despite treatment with acetophenazine (60 mg/day), but she responded when imipramine (50 mg/day) was added to the antipsychotic medication.

During a subsequent depressive episode in 1977, Ms. A again improved on imipramine (75 mg/day) when it was combined with acetophenazine (40 mg/day), but she experienced what appeared to be intermittent relapses when the imipramine dose was increased to 100 mg/day.

Ms. A had been successfully maintained on imipramine (75 mg/day) until a sudden decompensation led to rehospitalization in February 1978. As in previous depressive episodes, she was agitated and diaphoretic. She would not cooperate with formal mental status testing. Results of physical examination, liver function tests, and the remainder of her routine clinical chemistry tests were all within normal limits. Her weight was approximately 49 kg.

At the time of this admission, the dose of imipramine was increased to 100 mg/day and acetophenazine (20 mg/day) was added. The patient failed to respond to this regimen after two weeks, which prompted the measurement of tricyclic antidepressants in her plasma. Given the relatively low dose of imipramine being used, the physician expected to find low plasma concentrations but was surprised to discover that the patient's value for total plasma tricyclic antidepressants was 805 $\mu$g/L (imipramine = 193 $\mu$g/L, desipramine = 612 $\mu$g/L), well above the usual therapeutic range. Imipramine was stopped on March 8, but therapy with acetophenazine was continued. Plasma tricyclic antidepressants were again measured on March 9 and found to total 696 $\mu$g/L (imipramine = 174 $\mu$g/L, desipramine = 522 $\mu$g/L). Physical examination at this point failed to reveal evidence of atropinic (i.e., anticholinergic) toxicity. There was no facial flushing, dry mouth, or difficulty with urination; pulse rate was 120/min, the skin was diaphoretic, and the pupils were reactive to light and were not dilated. Three days after therapy with imipramine was discontinued, Ms. A became less agitated, cooperated with nursing staff for the first time, and began to converse socially and to play the piano. Mental status examination revealed a clear sensorium, marked improvement of depressive mood, and no evidence of psychosis. The next day, treatment with imipramine was resumed at a dose of 25 mg/day and, on March 20, the patient was stable and recompensated. Plasma tricyclic antidepressants concentration totaled 252 $\mu$g/L (imipramine = 51 $\mu$g/L, desipramine = 201 $\mu$g/L) and Ms. A was then discharged.

She was readmitted to the hospital on March 31 because her depressive syndrome had re-emerged. Her plasma tricyclic antidepressant value had declined to 143 $\mu$g/L (imipramine = 23 $\mu$g/L, desipramine = 120 $\mu$g/L), which is below the therapeutic range. Poor medication compliance may have caused this decrease. The following day, the dose of imipramine was increased to 25 mg and 50 mg on alternate days. Three weeks later, on April 20, the patient remained unimproved and acetophenazine dosage was increased from 20 mg/day to 40 mg/day. One week later, the patient recompensated, becoming pleasant and talkative. On May 2, her plasma drug concentration was 307 $\mu$g/L (imipramine = 85 $\mu$g/L, desipramine = 222 $\mu$g/L). Ms. A was discharged on May 12 and, upon re-examination three months later, remained in remission while continuing to receive imipramine (25 mg/day alternating with 50 mg/day) and acetophenazine (40 mg/day).

Two years later, Ms. A remains stable on this dose regimen of imipramine and acetophenazine. This is the longest period that she has remained out of the hospital in the past 15 years.

## Discussion

In the case presented here, accepted clinical practice would have called for an increase in the dosage of imipramine in the face of the failure to respond to a modest dose (100 mg/day) even though this dose is near the maximum dose recommended in elderly patients. However, when plasma tricyclic antidepressants were measured, it became clear that the value was approaching the toxic range and that a decrease in dosage, rather than an increase, was indicated. In the absence of this determination, neither clinical psychiatric evaluation nor physical examination would have led to the proper psychopharmacologic response.

The tricyclic antidepressant, imipramine (a dibenzazepine derivative), and other related compounds—including desipramine, amitriptyline, nortriptyline, protriptyline, and doxepin — are the drugs most commonly prescribed in the treatment of depression.

The principal pharmacological action of the tricyclic antidepressants is inhibition of the "biogenic amine pump." Inhibition of the reuptake of biogenic amine neurotransmitters (norepinephrine and serotonin) into the presynaptic nerve endings from which they were released is thought to be of importance in the antidepressant action of these drugs. The effect of this inhibition is an increase in the amount of neurotransmitter available at the postsynaptic receptor site. In addition to their ability to inhibit the "amine pump," the tricyclic antidepressants exhibit peripheral and central anticholinergic action and a sedative effect.

## Fig. 1. Principal Pathways of Imipramine Metabolism

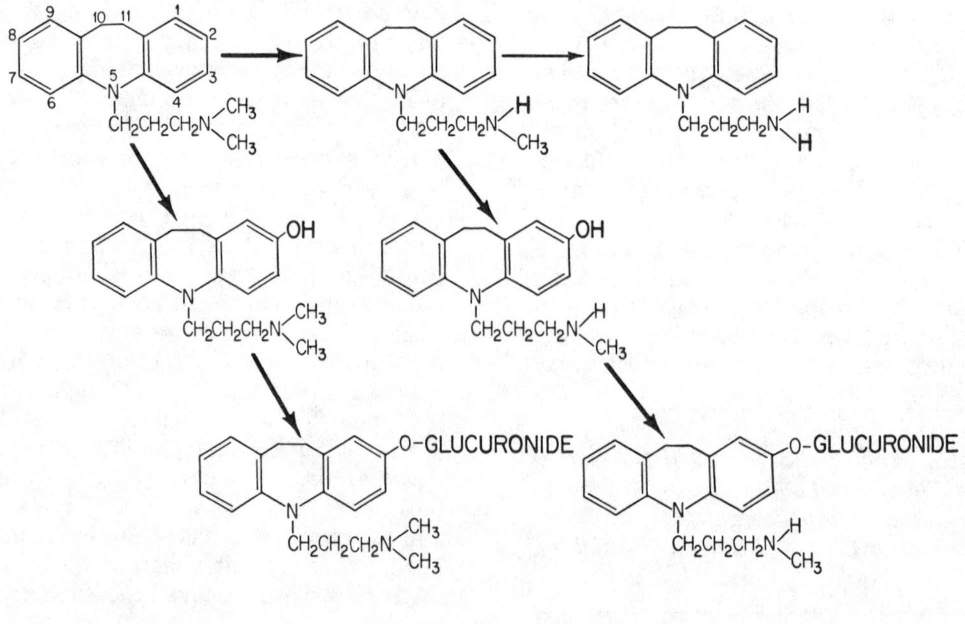

The anticholinergic properties of the tricyclic antidepressants result in the most common side effects, including postural hypotension, dry mouth, and urinary retention.

Imipramine is readily metabolized by N-demethylation to the active antidepressant, desipramine, and by aromatic ring hydroxylation. As with the other metabolic pathways, it has long been assumed that the hydroxylated metabolites of imipramine and desipramine are inactive. However, recent studies have shown that the hydroxylated metabolites have strong cardiovascular actions and can inhibit biogenic amine uptake. In addition, their concentrations in plasma can be as high as the concentration of imipramine.

The tricyclic antidepressants, including imipramine, are administered orally. Generally, these medications are begun at fairly low doses and the dose is increased gradually over several days until therapeutically effective concentrations are achieved. In middle-aged, physically healthy patients of average weight (60 to 90 kg), the typical starting dosage of imipramine is 75 mg/day, which is then increased by 25 mg/day every two or three days until an average dose of 150 mg/day is reached. Adverse effects, such as hypotension (lightheadedness), difficulty urinating, or drowsiness, often limit the increase in dosage of these medications. Based on clinical effect and concentrations measured in plasma, the dose of imipramine can then be increased up to 250 to 300 mg/day. Elderly patients, as illustrated in this case, often require less tricyclic antidepressant medication and the usual dose range for imipramine is 20 to 100 mg/day, although doses as high as 150 mg/day can be used if blood pressure and cardiac rhythms are checked regularly.

Monitoring the concentration of tricyclic antidepressants in plasma can be extremely useful in managing the treatment of elderly patients, because older patients treated with a given dose of tricyclic antidepressant often develop higher steady-state concentrations in plasma than do younger individuals. Ms. A appeared to exhibit a decreased tolerance for tricyclic antidepressants as she aged, a finding which emphasizes the need for caution in prescribing tricyclic antidepressants for geriatric patients and for monitoring concentrations in plasma in such patients.

An additional factor that may have contributed to the attainment of toxic concentrations of tricyclic antidepressants is the concurrent administration of the antipsychotic, acetophenazine. Phenothiazines inhibit the metabolism of tricyclic antidepressants, and especially the metabolism of demethylated derivatives such as desipramine, and so antidepressant concentrations in blood can increase even on a constant dosage. In the case described here, every determination showed much higher concentrations of the demethylated derivative, desipramine, than imipramine, which is consistent with the finding that phenothiazines inhibit the metabolism of demethylated tricyclic antidepressant drugs.

Several factors in Ms. A's case point to the value of monitoring tricyclic antidepressant concentrations in plasma. This can be most useful when drug toxicity is readily confused with the underlying disorder; when large individual differences in drug metabolism, such as those seen in elderly patients, lead to poor correlation between administered dose and plasma concentration; when the pharmacokinetic consequences of drug interaction (e.g., co-administration of antipsychotic medication and tricyclic antidepressant medication) are unknown; or, when non-compliance is suspected. Such clinical laboratory determinations can facilitate arriving at the optimal dosage of some tricyclic antidepressants and can provide valuable information for the treatment of nonresponsive patients before the dosage of medication is changed or therapy with other drugs is substituted. The availability of these monitoring procedures promises to increase the precision and reliability of pharmacological treatment of depressed patients.

## Bibliography

Appelbaum, P.S., Vasile, R.G., Orsulak, P.J. and Schildkraut, J.J., Clinical utility of tricyclic antidepressant blood levels: a case report. *American Journal of Psychiatry* **136**, 339-341 (1979).

Glassman, A.H. and Perel, J.M., Tricyclic blood levels and clinical outcome: a review of the art. In *Psychopharmacology: A Generation of Progress*, M.A. Lipton, A. DiMascio, and K.F. Killam, Eds., Raven Press, New York, N.Y., 1978, pp. 917-922.

Glassman, A.H., Perel, J.M., Shostak, M., Kantor, S.J. and Fleiss, J.L., Clinical implications of imipramine plasma levels for depressive illness. *Arch Gen Psychiat* **34** 197-204 (1977).

Nies, A., Robinson, D.S., Friedman, M.J., Green, R., Cooper, T., Ravaris, C.L. and Ives, J.O., Relationship between age and tricyclic antidepressant plasma levels. *Am J Psychiat* **134** 790-793, 1977.

Orsulak, P.J. and Schildkraut, J.J., Guidelines for therapeutic monitoring of tricyclic antidepressant plasma levels. *Therap Drug Monitoring* **1** 199-208 (1979).

Shader, R.I. and Greenblatt, D.J., Clinical indications for plasma level monitoring of psychotropic drugs. *Am J Psychiat* **136** 1590-1591 (1979).

Shader, R.I., ed.: *Manual of Psychiatric Therapeutics,* Little Brown and Co., Boston (1975).

# Imipramine and Desipramine Profile

| Generic Name: | **imipramine** | **desipramine** |
|---|---|---|
| Chemical name: | (N, N-dimethylaminopropyl) - iminodibenzyl hydrochloride | (N-methylaminopropyl) - iminodibenzyl hydrochloride |
| | | |
| Molecular weight: | 280.40 free base/ 316.87 (HCl) | 266.37 free base/ 302.84 (HCl) |
| Melting point (hydrochloride): | 174-175 °C | 208-218 °C |
| Solubility in water (hydrochloride): | freely soluble | freely soluble |
| $pK_a$: | 9.5 | 9.5 |
| | | |
| Dose absorption (oral) — | | |
|    time to peak plasma concentration, h: | 1-6 | —— |
|    percentage of oral dose absorbed: | 29-77% | —— |
|    percentage of protein bound: | 80-95% | —— |
| | | |
| Volume of distribution, L/kg body wt.: | 10-20 | —— |
| | | |
| Urinary excretion, % daily dose — | | |
|    imipramine, unchanged: | 1-4% | —— |
|    desipramine: | 1-4% | —— |
|    2-hydroxyimipramine | | |
|    2-hydroxydesipramine | 15-36% | —— |
|    2-hydroxyimipramine glucuronide } | | |
|    2-hydroxydesipramine glucuronide } | 45-60% | —— |

## Clinical Pharmacology

| | |
|---|---|
| Recommended dose, mg/day, average adult: | 75-300 |
| Recommended dose, mg/day, elderly adult: | 20-100 |
| Half-life, hours: | 9-24 |
| Time to steady state, days: | 2-5 |
| Therapeutic range, $\mu$g/L (IMI + DMI): | 150-250 |
| Toxic conc., $\mu$g/L (IMI + DMI): | 500-1000 |

# 42

# Clinical Utility of Measuring Amitriptyline in Plasma: A Case Study

**Paul J. Orsulak, Ph.D.**
**Russell G. Vasile, M.D.**

Individual variability of response to tricyclic antidepressants and individual differences in the metabolism of these drugs are both well documented. Measuring concentrations of tricyclic antidepressants in plasma helps determine whether a patient is receiving an adequate dosage of a particular drug, especially when drug toxicity may be confused with the signs and symptoms of the depressive disorder being treated, when the pharmacokinetic interactions of co-administered drugs are unknown, or in elderly patients where age may be a factor in deciding what is an adequate dosage of a tricyclic antidepressant.

Although the exact therapeutic range and the nature of the relationship between drug concentrations in blood and clinical efficacy in various groups of depressed patients being treated with amitriptyline are not well understood, the following case illustrates the utility of measuring amitriptyline in the plasma. In this patient, small changes in dose led to extremely large changes in the concentrations of this antidepressant in plasma.

## Case Study

The patient, a 65-year-old married white woman, presented with a history of three months of a depressive syndrome manifested by anergia, anhedonia, psychic retardation, decreased productivity, mild diurnal variation (feeling worse in the morning), and feelings of helplessness, hopelessness, and worthlessness. In addition, she had lost 9 lbs. during the last two months and had diminished appetite. There was no evidence of thought disorder and no evidence of recent history of mania or hypomania. The patient's syndrome had an autonomous or endogenous quality (i.e., it was not responsive to environmental events or interpersonal interactions) and had proven resistant to treatment both with amitriptyline and imipramine in doses as high as 350 mg/day in successive trials extending over a six-

Dr. Orsulak is Assistant Professor of Psychiatry, Harvard Medical School and Technical Director, Psychiatric Chemistry Laboratory, Department of Pathology, New England Deaconess Hospital, Boston, MA.

Dr. Vasile is Instructor in Psychiatry, Harvard Medical School and Staff Psychiatrist, Massachusetts Mental Health Center, Boston, MA.

week period. In fact, the patient noted that on high doses of the medication she "felt worse," and she described feelings of dizziness and depersonalization (a sense of feeling unreal, distant, or "in a fog").

After this initial assessment, amitriptyline (75 mg/day) and perphenazine (12 mg/day) were prescribed. Additionally, she participated in supportive psychotherapy and received diazepam (15 mg/day). After three weeks of this combined therapy, she experienced distinct improvement, although mild morning dysphoria persisted. The patient continued on this program of treatment relatively uneventfully for nearly a year, when she noted again that she was "not 100% right," although there were no striking symptoms. She felt that her level of energy and ambition was not fully normal and indicated that she was feeling demoralized. At this point, her physician decided to evaluate her medication program.

The patient's dose of amitriptyline was increased to 100 mg/day, perphenazine (12 mg/day) was continued, and diazepam dosage was reduced to 10 mg/day. Shortly after this alteration in medication, amitriptyline plus nortriptyline was measured in the plasma and found to be 212 μg/L (amitriptyline, 120 μg/L; nortriptyline, 92 μg/L). Even though this value was within the "therapeutic range" for this drug, given the patient's mild but persistent dysphoria, the amitriptyline dosage was increased further, from 100 mg/day to 125 mg/day. Diazepam was discontinued at this time.

To the physician's surprise, the patient did not improve with this increase in amitriptyline, but rather became more depressed during the next two months. She described increasing feelings of agitation, depersonalization, fatigue, and a vague sense of apprehension. The patient did not, however, report experiencing any anticholinergic side effects of amitriptyline such as dry mouth, constipation, postural hypotension, or other overt symptoms that would suggest toxicity. The concentration of amitriptyline plus nortriptyline was now 373 μg/L (amitriptyline, 175 μg/L; nortriptyline, 198 μg/L). Because of this unexpectedly high value, the patient's antidepressant dosage was reduced gradually over a period of 10 days, to 75 mg of amitriptyline per day, whereupon there was a striking clinical improvement: she became clear-headed again, was able to play competitive bridge, and felt less sedated, more optimistic, and physically more comfortable.

# AMITRIPTYLINE AND NORTRIPTYLINE

| | amitriptyline | nortriptyline |
|---|---|---|
| **Generic name:** | amitriptyline | nortriptyline |
| **Chemical name:** | ($N,N$-dimethylaminopropyl-idene) dihydrodibenzocyclo-heptene | ($N$-methylaminopropyl-idene) dihydrodibenzo-cycloheptene |
| **Molecular mass (free base/hydrochloride):** | 277.39/313.86 | 263.37/299.84 |
| **Melting point (hydrochloride):** | 196-197 °C | 213-215 °C |
| **Solubility in water (hydrochloride):** | freely soluble | freely soluble |
| **pK$_a$:** | 9.4 | 9.0 |
| **Dose absorption (oral)—** | | |
| time to peak plasma concentration, h: | 4-8 | — |
| percentage of oral dose absorbed: | 56-70 | — |
| percentage of protein bound: | 82-96 | — |
| **Volume of distribution, L/kg body weight:** | n/a | — |
| **Urinary excretion, % daily dose—** | | |
| amitriptyline, unchanged: | 2-5 | — |
| nortriptyline: | 2-5 | — |
| 10-hydroxyamitriptyline / 10-hydroxynortriptyline | 15-30 | — |
| 10-hydroxyamitriptyline glucuronide / 10-hydroxynortriptyline glucuronide | 40-60 | — |

## Clinical Pharmacology

| | |
|---|---|
| **Recommended dose, mg/d, average adult:** | 150-300 |
| **Recommended dose, mg/d, elderly adult:** | 20-100 |
| **Half-life, hours:** | 17-40 |
| **Time to steady state, days:** | 4-10 |
| **Therapeutic range, $\mu$g/L (ng/mL) (AMI+NOR):** | 120-250 |
| **Toxic level, $\mu$g/L (ng/mL) (AMI + NOR):** | 500-1000 |

Upon re-examination three months later, the patient is continuing in supportive psychotherapy monthly and remains improved, even though her amitriptyline dose has been reduced to 50 mg/day (with perhenazine, 8 mg/day). Her total plasma tricyclic antidepressant concentration is 170 $\mu$g/L (amitriptyline, 102 $\mu$g/L; nortriptyline, 68 $\mu$g/L).

## Discussion

This patient failed to respond to high doses of the tricyclic antidepressant drugs, amitriptyline and imipramine. Consequently, her physician initiated therapy at a relatively low dose of amitriptyline (100 mg/day) and obtained modest clinical improvement. At this dose, values for plasma amitriptyline plus nortriptyline fell within the reported therapeutic range. In an attempt to achieve further clinical improvement, the amitriptyline dosage was increased to 125 mg/day, which increased the concentration of amitriptyline plus nortriptyline in plasma to 373 $\mu$g/L, a value nearly twice that obtained with a 100 mg/day dosage of amitriptyline. This increased dose and the striking increase in concentrations in plasma were accompanied by clinical deterioration rather than further improvement as might have been expected. The availability of data on drug concentration in plasma at this time led the treating physician to suspect the existence of a "therapeutic window" for this patient. In the absence of such data, accepted clinical practice would have called for further increases in the dose of amitriptyline in the face of continued clinical deterioration and probably would have led to toxic side-effects in this patient.

Amitriptyline and its monodemethylated metabolite, nortriptyline, are both usually found in plasma obtained from depressed patients being treated with amitriptyline. Unlike other antidepressant drugs, however, the therapeutic range for amitriptyline and the relationship between circulating concentrations and clinical efficacy is not well understood. Several studies have reported a positive correlation between clinical effect and concentrations of amitriptyline plus nortriptyline in plasma. These studies suggest that antidepressant response rate is more favorable in patients for whom these values exceed 120 $\mu$g/L, and increases with increasing concentrations of amitriptyline plus nortriptyline up to 250 $\mu$g/L. In other studies a curvilinear relationship was found, indicating that there is a "therapeutic window" of about 80 to 220 $\mu$g/L for this drug. In contrast, other investigators found no relation betweeen clinical response and the concentrations of either amitriptyline, nortriptyline, or amitriptyline plus nortriptyline in plasma. Considered together, these studies suggest that factors other than concentrations in plasma alone - such as the subtype of

depressive disorder being treated - may play a role in predicting response to antidepressant therapy with amitriptyline.

Tricyclic antidepressants, including amitriptyline, are generally administered orally. Drug therapy is generally begun at a fairly low dose (25 to 50 mg/day), and the dose is then gradually increased during several days to one that is therapeutically effective. In middle-aged, physically healthy patients of average weight (60 to 90 kg), the usual therapeutic dose of amitriptyline is between 150 and 300 mg/day, but the patient's tolerance of the medication often becomes a limiting factor.

One of the principal pharmacological actions of the tricyclic antidepressants is thought to be inhibition of the "biogenic amine pumps": inhibition of the re-uptake of the neurotransmitters norepinephrine and serotonin into the presynaptic nerve endings from which they were released. The effect of this inhibition is to increase the amount of neurotransmitter available at the post-synaptic receptor site.

In addition to their ability to inhibit the amine pump, many tricyclic antidepressants exhibit varying degrees of peripheral and central anticholinergic (i.e., atropine-like) action and sedation. The principal anticholinergic side-effects include dry mouth, urinary retention, and postural hypotension. Side-effects may also include confusion, agitation, or increased irritability, but these usually occur only in association with toxic concentrations of medication. Amitriptyline is the most potent anticholinergic agent among the tricyclic antidepressants, although it is not nearly as potent as atropine in this respect. These adverse effects often limit increases in dosage of tricyclic antidepressants and, in particular, of amitriptyline.

Several aspects of the present case point to the value of monitoring amitriptyline in plasma, even though the exact therapeutic range for this drug has not been firmly established. Individual differences in drug metabolism can lead to poor correlation between administered dose and concentration of the tricyclic antidepressant drugs in plasma. In this case, increasing the dose of amitriptyline from 100 to 125 mg/day resulted in an increase in the value for amitriptyline plus nortriptyline in plasma from 212 to 373 $\mu$g/L, almost double as a result of a 25% increase in dose.

Such monitoring also is extremely useful in managing the treatment of elderly patients, because they often show higher steady-state concentrations in plasma than do younger individuals on similar doses. This patient required a relatively low dose (50 to 75 mg/day) of amitriptyline to maintain clinical effect, which is consistent with the doses recommended for elderly patients.

Monitoring can also be extremely useful for drugs

with a "therapeutic window," the term for a situation where efficacy may be lost at higher concentrations in plasma, even in the absence of toxicity. Although the existence of a therapeutic window has not been firmly established for amitriptyline, the data in this case suggest that such a window might exist for some patients.

An additional factor that may have contributed to the unexpectedly high concentration of amitriptyline in this patient is the concurrent administration of the antipsychotic drug perphenazine. Phenothiazines inhibit the metabolism of tricyclic antidepressants, thereby increasing their concentrations in blood, even on low oral doses.

Although doses of tricyclic antidepressant drugs have usually been determined empirically, effective doses may range from as little as 25 mg/day to more than 300 mg/day, depending on the age of the patient, concurrent drug administration, and many other factors. Monitoring can assist the clinician in arriving more quickly at optimum doses of the particular antidepressant chosen, can provide valuable information for treating a nonresponsive patient, and can increase the precision and reliability of pharmacological treatment of depressed patients even when the exact therapeutic range is not well established.

## References

Asberg, M., Treatment of depression with tricyclic drugs -- pharmacokinetic and pharmacodynamic aspects. *Pharmakopsych. Neuro-Psychopharmakol.* **9,** 18-26 (1976).

Boethius, G., and Sjoqvist, F., Doses and dosage intervals of drugs -- clinical practice and pharmacokinetic principles. *Clin. Pharmacol. Ther.* **24,** 255-263 (1978).

Hollister, L.E., Monitoring tricyclic antidepressant plasma concentrations. *J. Am. Med. Assoc.* **241,** 2530-2533 (1979).

Orsulak, P.J., and Schildkraut, J.J., Guidelines for therapeutic monitoring of tricyclic antidepressant plasma levels. *Therap. Drug Monitoring* **1,** 199-208 (1979).

Shader, R.I., and Greenblatt, D.J., Clinical indications for plasma level monitoring of psychotropic drugs. *Am. J. Psychiat.* **136,** 1590-1591 (1979).

# 43

# New Antidepressant Drugs: A Brief Review

Paul J. Orsulak, Ph.D.

The introduction of psychotropic agents in the 1950s dramatically altered treatment of patients with psychiatric illnesses. Despite the major achievements of the tricyclic antidepressants and the monoamine oxidase inhibitor antidepressants, treatment with these agents is still far from perfect. Tricyclic antidepressants and monoamine oxidase inhibitors are effective antidepressants, but in many cases they are prescribed somewhat uneasily, because of their potentially serious side effects. However, promising new classes of antidepressants are beginning to open a new era in the treatment of depression. These agents, which often have a more rapid onset of action, may be biologically more specific, may have fewer side effects, and may be effective in patients with refractory depressions. However, they pose significant new problems for those engaged in therapeutic monitoring of these drugs because methodology is poorly developed, and information on both basic pharmacology and the relationship between serum conentrations and clinical effectiveness is limited.

From the mid-1950s until 1980, only six tricyclic antidepressants were on the market in the United States. These included imipramine and its demethylated metabolite desipramine, amitriptyline and its demethylated metabolite nortriptyline, doxepin, and protriptyline. Doxepin also has a demethylated metabolite, desmethyldoxepin, which has never been marketed as an antidepressant. Recently, however, a number of new compounds have found their way onto the U.S. market (Table 1). These include a new tricyclic antidepressant, trimipramine, marketed as Surmontil® by Ives Laboratories; and the tetracyclic antidepressant maprotiline, marketed by Ciba-Geigy as Ludiomil®, and amoxapine, marketed as Asendin® by Lederele Laboratories. A benzodiazepine, alprazolam (Xanax®) which has antidepressant properties, was released at the end of 1981, and the triazolpyridine compound trazodone or Desyrel® appeared early in 1982.

During the past decade, research on antidepressant pharmacotherapy has been active throughout the world, and as many as 40 or 50 new compounds are in various stages of development or clinical evaluation. During the past several years, a number of these agents in addition to the ones listed above have been given significant attention. In addition to maprotiline and amoxapine, other tetracyclic compounds including mianserin and oxaprotiline, an analog of maprotiline, are being tested. Bicyclic drugs with antidepressant properties such as zimelidine and fluoxetine, the

*Dr. Orsulak is Assistant Professor of Psychiatry, Harvard Medical School, and Technical Director of the Psychiatric Chemistry Laboratory, New England Deaconess Hospital, both in Boston, MA.*

## Table 1. New Antidepressant Drug Preparations

| Generic name and structure | Trade name | Source |
|---|---|---|
| Trimipramine | Surmontil | Ives Laboratories |
| Maprotiline | Ludiomil | Geigy Pharmaceuticals |
| Amoxapine | Asendin | Lederle Laboratories |
| Trazodone | Desyrel | Mead Johnson |
| Alprazolam | Xanax | Upjohn |

tetrahydroisoquiniline compound nomifensine, and the chloropropiophenone bupropion, as well as many other compounds, are actively undergoing evaluation at the present time.

Comprehensive reviews of the literature surrounding correlations between concentrations of the traditional tricyclic antidepressants in plasma and clinical efficacy have appeared and several reviews dealing with the clinical use of tricyclic antidepressants have also been published (see References). However, little organized information is available on the basic pharmacology, therapeutic monitoring, or analyses of these new antidepressants. The purpose of this paper will be to provide a review of the basic pharmacology of the new compounds that have appeared on the market, including trimipramine, maprotiline, trazodone, and alprazolam. This paper will also summarize the available information pertinent to therapeutic monitoring of these drugs and review some of the problems that the laboratory engaged in therapeutic monitoring of antidepressants will face because of their availability, and it will provide a brief discussion of some of those compounds which are currently under active investigation and may appear as antidepressants in the near future.

## Need For New Antidepressants

Despite the effectiveness of the traditional tricyclic antidepressant drugs, their spectrum of limitations and problems, including significant side effects, their potentially lethal nature when used for suicide attempts, and their generally slow onset of action have provided the impetus for continued research aimed at finding new antidepressant agents. The limitations and problems of the tricyclic antidepressants need to be kept in mind when evaluating the comparative advantages and disadvantages or clinical information on the new compounds.

The traditional tricyclic antidepressants have been shown to be "effective" in only between 60 and 80% of unselected inpatients or outpatients with depressive disorders, and often patients improve but do not completely recover; that is, symptoms may be reduced significantly but patients still exhibit many of the symptoms of depression. Clinical response, when it occurs, is often delayed and gradual. Occasionally patients may feel markedly better after a few days but gradual progressive improvements in the first one to four weeks is more common. Early, rapid, and complete improvement is not usually achieved with the traditional tricyclic antidepressants.

The common and troublesome side effects of the tricyclic antidepressants result from their anticholin-

ergic activity. Although these side effects are usually not serious, they can be extremely uncomfortable and in rare cases can be dangerous. Principal anticholinergic side effects include dry mouth, constipation, urinary retention, memory difficulties, and delirium. The tricyclic antidepressants often produce oversedation, with this effect occurring most commonly when patients are treated with amitriptyline or doxepin. Postural hypotension is a common problem limiting rapid dosage increase, particularly in elderly patients, but it also may be troublesome in younger patients. Tremor and unpleasant stimulation are more common with desipramine (and the monoamine oxidase inhibitors), but they sometimes occur with other tricyclic antidepressants as well. Tachycardia and quinidine-like electrocardiographic changes occur with tricyclic antidepressants at usual doses, progressing to heart block in rare patients.

Overdosage of antidepressants results in severe arrhythmia, and current drugs must be used with extreme caution in patients with heart disease. Treatment with tricyclic antidepressants can also result in diaphoresis, skin rashes, and sexual dysfunctions in both men and women. Convulsions, although rare, also occur. The tricyclic antidepressants also can precipitate manic excitement or hypomania in both bipolar depressed patients and some patients with unipolar depressions, and can exacerbate schizophrenic episodes.

In some patients, initial favorable response disappears without obvious cause, and is often resistant to further manipulation of dosage. Tricyclic antidepressants block the action of many antihypertensive drugs, and are subject to significant drug interactions. These drugs also tend to cause persistent weight gain at normal doses, and virtually all of them can be lethal at 20 to 50 times the usual daily therapeutic dose.

Many of the new compounds being developed and particularly those described below offer promise of effectiveness without some of the side effects or limitations that confront the clinician utilizing tricyclic antidepressants. Some of them exhibit virtually no unpleasant anticholinergic side effects or worrisome cardiovascular toxicity (trazodone and alprazolam), while the tetracyclic antidepressants maprotiline and amoxapine may have a more rapid onset of action than the tricyclic drugs. Studies have demonstrated particular efficacy in certain subtypes of depressive disorders. For example, nomifensine and bupropion may be especially useful in psychomotor retarded depressions. Long-term studies also indicate sustained efficacy with trazodone, indicating that it may be safe for extended treatment.

## Trimipramine

The tricyclic antidepressant trimipramine (Surmontil®) was introduced into the United States by Ives Laboratories at the end of 1980. While the drug is new to the U.S. market, it has been in use in Europe for more than 20 years. Trimipramine appears to be as effective as the older tricyclic antidepressants. Based on limited data, this drug appears to be well tolerated in the elderly, and there are reports that it has a special place in treating patients with mixed anxiety and depression and patients with agitated depressions. It is relatively sedative, like the other tricyclic antidepressants, making it useful in depressed patients with sleep disturbances.

Its principal mechanism of action (Table 2) appears to be blockade of uptake of both norepinephrine and serotonin at presynaptic nerve terminals. In these respects, its activity resembles the other antidepressants, including imipramine, desipramine, and nortriptyline. Like the other tricyclic antidepressants, it exhibits significant anticholinergic side effects, though these are less severe than with amitriptyline, and it does affect cardiac function like the other tricyclic drugs as well. The dosage regimen for trimipramine is similar to that of imipramine or amitriptyline, as shown in Table 3.

At the present time, studies are being performed to examine the relationship between concentration of this new tricyclic antidepressant in plasma and clinical response, but at the present time no data is available relating clinical efficacy to concentration. Drug concentration in plasma in patients being treated with trimipramine resemble those for imipramine and fall between 150 and 300 $\mu$g/L (ng/mL) if patients are

being treated with usual doses. As with the other tricyclic antidepressants, there is probably little correlation between dose and concentrations of this drug in plasma and there is probably significant interindividual variability in the response to this drug and its metabolism. Since trimipramine is a tertiary amine, its metabolism also resembles that of other tricyclic antidepressants. Principal metabolites include the didemethylated iminodibenzyl derivative and conjugated, presumably hydroxylated, compounds. The pharmacological activity of these drug metabolites has not been studied.

## Maprotiline

Maprotiline (Ludiomil®) is one of the two tetracyclic antidepressants introduced at the beginning of 1981. It appears to be as effective as the traditional tricyclic antidepressants in treating depressions.

In clinical trials at relatively low doses (150 mg/day), maprotiline is at least equally effective to similar doses of imipramine or amitriptyline. A number of studies have shown maprotiline to be "faster acting," with the drug being superior to both imipramine or amitriptyline at either three days, one week, or two weeks after initiation of therapy.

This drug primarily blocks reuptake of the biogenic amine norepinephrine in the central nervous system. Maprotiline has virtually no effect on serotonin reuptake, a property which makes it most like desipramine when comparing it to the tricyclic antidepressants.

Like the tricyclic antidepressants, maprotiline exhibits both anticholinergic (or atropine-like) side effects and cardiovascular toxicity, although both of these effects may be less severe than they are for the traditional tricyclic antidepressants (Table 2). It can also precipitate mania or excited states and has been reported to cause more skin rashes. The dosage range for maprotiline in also similar to the tricyclic antidepressants in both adults and elderly patients (Table 3).

Maprotiline has a half-life of approximately 27 to 58 h, which is substantially longer than some of the tricyclic antidepressants. Therefore, a longer period of time (approximately two weeks) is required to reach steady state. While the therapeutic range for this drug has not been clearly established, there is evidence that better clinical improvement occurs at 180 to 400 $\mu$g/L with better responses occurring at the higher drug concentrations in plasma. However, other studies have suggested the possibility of a bimodal relationship between drug concentrations in plasma and clinical response to this antidepressant. In a collaborative study, patients with low pretreatment

### Table 2. Pharmacological Properties of Antidepressant Drugs

| Drug | Effect on biogenic amine reuptake | | Anticholinergic Activity | Cardiovascular Toxocity |
|---|---|---|---|---|
| | Norepinephrine | Serotonin | | |
| **Tricyclics** | | | | |
| Amitriptyline | 0 | +++ | +++ | +++ |
| Imipramine | ++ | ++ | ++ | +++ |
| Nortriptyline | ++ | + | ++ | ++ |
| Desipramine | +++ | 0 | + | ++ |
| Protriptyline | + | + | ++ | +++ |
| Doxepin | + | + | +++ | |
| Trimipramine | ++ | ++ | ++ | +++ |
| **Tetracyclics** | | | | |
| Maprotiline | +++ | 0 | ++ | ++ |
| Amoxapine | ++ | + | ++ | ++ |
| (8-Hydroxy-amoxapine) | (++) | (++) | (?) | (?) |
| **Other Classes** | | | | |
| Trazodone | 0 | +++ | 0 | 0 |
| Alprazolam | 0 | 0 | 0 | 0 |

0 = least potent to ++++ = most potent

24-h levels of the urinary norepinephrine metabolite 3-methoxy-4-hydroxyphenylglycol (MHPG) responded rapidly to maprotiline at lower doses, and at significantly lower blood concentrations, while patients with high pretreatment urinary MHPG levels required significantly higher doses and achieved significantly higher blood concentrations. In the low MHPG group, responders received slightly less than 150 mg/day, and achieved a mean blood level of 138 $\mu$g/L. The high MHPG responders required nearly twice as much medication (258 mg/day) and achieved mean blood levels of 407 $\mu$g/L, more than twice as high. Patients with intermediate MHPG levels did not respond well to this medication in this study.

In summary, maprotiline is an effective, useful antidepressant which may act more rapidly than traditional tricyclic antidepressants such as imipramine or desipramine, and has as its major advantage a slightly reduced side-effect profile.

## Amoxapine

Amoxapine (Asendin®) belongs to a new subclass of tricyclic antidepressant drugs and is referred to as a tetracyclic antidepressant. It is an antidepressant of the dibenzoxazepine class, chemically distinct from other tricyclic antidepressants in that the tricyclic nucleus of amoxapine contains both a nitrogen and an oxygen atom. In addition, its side chain consists of a piperazinyl ring rather than a straight side chain.

Like the tricyclic antidepressants, the principal pharmacologic action of amoxapine is blockade of norepinephrine and serotonin reuptake at presynaptic nerve terminals. Table 2 shows that amoxapine's action is directed primarily toward the blockade of norepinephrine reuptake with less effect on the blockade of serotonin reuptake. The amoxapine metabolite 8-hydroxyamoxapine shows activity comparable to that of the parent compound, with respect to blockade of norepinephrine reuptake, but its effect on blocking serotonin reuptake is greater than that of the parent. Amoxapine is also a weak dopamine blocking agent, a property that distinguishes it from the other tricyclic antidepressants or maprotiline.

The effectiveness of amoxapine has been documented in a large series of controlled clinical trials in which the depressed patients were selected randomly for treatment with either amoxapine, amitriptyline, or imipramine. In general, these studies showed that amoxapine was superior to placebo in treating depressions, but that it was approximately equivalent to imipramine or amitriptyline. These studies also indicated, however, that the onset of

therapeutic action was evident as early as one week after initiating treatment, and that the response to amoxapine could be observed in some patients as early as the third day of treatment. As mentioned previously, the slow onset of therapeutic action of traditional tricyclic antidepressants has been a major disadvantage.

Amoxapine is well tolerated by most patients and severe complications or adverse reactions are similar to other tricyclic antidepressants. Side effects most often recorded include anticholinergic activity, neurological and behavioral changes, and sedative effects. Amoxapine exhibits cardiovascular toxicity approximately equivalent to the tricyclic antidepressants, particularly in high doses and can induce tachycardia, changes in conduction time, and arrhythmias. Overdosage of amoxapine in man is characterized primarily, however, by central nervous system overactivity and convulsions, rather than by cardiac arrhythmias.

Dosage of amoxapine ranges from 150 to 300 mg/day in adults and 50 to 150 mg in elderly patients (Table 3). In hospitalized patients, who are refractory to antidepressant therapy, and who have had no history of convulsive siezures, dosage can be raised cautiously up to 600 mg/day in divided doses. Dosage in elderly patients can also be increased to 300 mg/day in divided doses if required under similar circumstances.

Amoxapine is rapidly absorbed, like other antidepressants, and concentrations in serum reach peak approximately 90 min after oral dose. Amoxapine, the parent compound, has a half-life of approximately 8 h. However, its major metabolite, 8-hydroxyamoxapine (which is also an active inhibitor

### Table 3. Dosage Range of Antidepressant Drugs

| Drugs | Average dose, mg/day | |
|---|---|---|
| | Adult patient | Elderly patient |
| **Tricyclics** | | |
| Amitriptyline | 150-130 | 20-100 |
| Nortriptyline | 50-150 | 10- 75 |
| Imipramine | 75-300 | 20-100 |
| Desipramine | 150-300 | 20-100 |
| Protriptyline | 30- 60 | 10- 30 |
| Doxepin | 200-400 | 30-200 |
| Trimipramine | 150-200 | 50-100 |
| **Tetracyclics** | | |
| Maprotiline | 75-300 | 50- 75 |
| Amoxapine | 200-600 | 150-300 |
| **Other Classes** | | |
| Trazodone | 50-600 | 50-600 |
| Alprazolam | 0.5-4.0 | 0.25-4.0 |

of norepinephrine and serotonin reuptake), is cleared more slowly and has a half-life of 30 h. Another metabolite of amoxapine, 7-hydroxyamoxapine, appears in the blood at lower concentrations and is cleared more rapidly, with a half-life of approximately 6.5 h.

Pharmacokinetic data for amoxapine and its metabolites indicate that steady-state serum concentrations of amoxapine are achieved at the end of two days, and that the 8-hydroxyamoxapine concentration reaches steady state after approximately one week. Because both amoxapine and its 8-hydroxy metabolite exhibit pharmacological activity as inhibitors of norepinephrine and serotonin reuptake, they may both participate in its antidepressant effect. Therapeutic monitoring of this drug therefore requires measurements of both the parent compound and the hydroxylated metabolites.

Studies relating clinical efficacy to concentrations of amoxapine and its metabolites in plasma are limited. Data reported thus far, however, indicate that plasma levels of amoxapine plus 8-hydroxyamoxapine (the major metabolite) are usually within the range of 200 to 500 $\mu$g/L in patients showing good therapeutic response. More important, however, is the fact that the 8-hydroxyamoxapine/amoxapine ratio is near 3:1 or 4:1 at steady state. The relatively high concentration of the hydroxylated metabolite points to the importance of monitoring its concentration as well as that of the parent drug.

Amoxapine can be measured by both gas chromatographic and high-performance liquid chromatographic techniques that are used for the other tricyclic and tetracyclic antidepressants. However, extraction techniques specific for the hydroxylated compounds need to be utilized if the metabolites are to be measured as well. Hydroxylated compounds cannot be measured effectively by gas-liquid chromatography without derivatization, but can be measured using reverse-phase high-performance liquid chromatography. To date, however, no procedures have been published for HPLC separation of the 7- and 8-hydroxy metabolites of amoxapine, although these compounds can be separated by gas-liquid chromatography as trifluoroacetic anhydride derivatives by using electron capture detection.

Amoxapine itself is a metabolite of a potent antipsychotic, loxapine, and while the parent compound and 8-hydroxy metabolite have not been reported to have antipsychotic or neuroleptic activity, the 7-hydroxy metabolite may exhibit neuroleptic properties. While data concerning the relationship of 7-hydroxyamoxapine to either its antidepressant effect or its potential neuroleptic side effects are incomplete, it may be necessary to measure 7-hydroxyamoxapine as well.

## Trazodone

Trazodone (Desyrel®) is the first of a new class of triazolopyridine compounds to be introduced as an antidepressant. This drug appears to have little or no effect on dopamine and norepinephrine reuptake in the central nervous system. Its principal action is blockade of serotonin reuptake. It also exhibits some peripheral $\alpha$-adrenergic blocking activity.

The effectiveness of trazodone in the treatment of endogenous depression and related anxiety was first reported in 1967. Since that time, numerous other studies conducted primarily in Europe and Canada have confirmed the antidepressant properties of this compound. Over the past 13 years, its therapeutic use has been investigated internationally in more than 200 open and controlled clinical trials involving more than 10,000 patients.

Clinical trials comparing trazodone with imipramine, desipramine, chlorimipramine, and amitriptyline have shown that it is as effective therapeutically as the reference drugs. In addition, it is generally well tolerated, apparently has a rapid onset of action, and has virtually no anticholinergic side effects. It also exhibits extremely low cardiovascular toxicity, but as one would expect from its serotoninergic activity, the compound is quite sedating.

The average daily dose for outpatients is between 200 and 300 mg/day, and for inpatients the dosage can range as high as 600 mg/day. However, it is important to note that trazodone has a relatively wide dosage range. Some patients do well on 50 mg/day whereas others require as much as 600 to 800 mg/day to achieve optimal therapeutic effect. The drug is usually administered in divided doses with the single largest dose being given at bedtime.

Like many of the new antidepressants being investigated, concentrations in plasma of trazodone have not yet been established, and in fact, very few procedures for the determination of trazodone in plasma or serum have appeared.

The wide dosage ranges of this drug clearly suggest wide interindividual variability in its metabolism, and point to the importance of individualizing the dosage of this drug in order to maximize the therapeutic effectiveness.

In summary, trazodone appears to be equally effective as an antidepressant when compared to the tricyclic antidepressants for treatment of depressive disorders. It is free of major anticholinergic side effects, but is significantly sedative. It is better tolerated by patients than is imipramine, and possibly may be used safely for long-term maintenance therapy.

## Alprazolam

A recent review on the antidepressant activity of benzodiazepines stated that there is limited evidence to indicate that drugs of this class may have specific antidepressant effects in some patients. Alprazolam (Xanax®) is a new triazolobenzodiazepine which was found to be effective as an antidepressant in patients with unipolar depressions accompanied by symptoms of anxiety, agitation, or insomnia. It was, however, found to be ineffective as an antidepressant in patients with psychomotor retarded or bipolar depressive disorders.

Alprazolam has been compared with both diazepam and placebo in several double-blind control studies involving anxious patients and with placebo alone in four studies. In all studies involving more than 2000 patients, alprazolam was consistently superior to placebo and in three of the studies alprazolam was significantly better than diazepam in relieving anxiety while exhibiting fewer side effects than this reference compound. Because alprazolam was consistently more effective than diazepam in anxious patients diagnosed as having "mixed anxiety depression," alprazolam was then compared to imipramine and placebo in five studies involving almost 1000 depressed outpatients. Alprazolam was superior to placebo and had fewer side effects than imipramine. In two of the five studies imipramine was found not to be more effective than placebo, while alprazolam was more effective than placebo for these patients.

Alprazolam resembles diazepam in animal tests, being generally more potent than diazepam as an anti-anxiety agent. It is also a muscle relaxant but is no more potent than diazepam in this respect, and it does induce sleep, but at higher doses. Alprazolam is also an anticonvulsant and can cause physical dependence of the barbiturate type, but shows only limited cross-dependence with phenobarbital. To achieve physical dependence very high and very frequent dosages are required. Alprazolam is not active in any of the standard pharmacological tests for antidepressants or antipsychotics. It also has no anticholinergic properties and no apparent cardiovascular toxicity.

Alprazolam is better tolerated by patients than imipramine and has a much more rapid onset of action. The dosage range is 0.5 to 4 mg per day, given in single or divided oral doses. At a dose of 0.3 mg/day (equivalent to 5 mg of diazepam) alprazolam is an effective antianxiety drug, and at 0.5 mg/day (equivalent to 25 mg of imipramine) alprazolam is an effective antidepressant for moderate depressions.

Side effects from alprazolam are relatively low in frequency. Drowsiness, hypotension, and increased salivation are the most prevalent side effects.

Additional advantages of alprazolam are its lack of anticholinergic effects and the minimal danger of cardiovascular toxicity or mortality upon overdose.

## Other Antidepressants

In addition to the antidepressants discussed above, a number of other compounds are currently undergoing active investigation, and promise to create a new era of greater specificity in drug management for depression.

Oxaprotiline is a hydroxy analog of maprotiline. It is from five to 50 times more potent than its parent compound in animal models, and in clinical studies was found to be about twice as potent as maprotiline. It is a norepinephrine reuptake inhibitor and like the parent compound possesses anticholinergic side effects, although these are less severe than those observed with maprotiline. Preliminary studies with this compound indicate that its therapeutic concentrations in plasma are relatively low, and fall between 5 and 50 $\mu g/L$. These drug concentrations in plasma are achieved at doses of from 50 to 100 mg/day.

Mianserin is another tetracyclic compound that has been extensively studied in Europe. Mianserin does not exhibit blockade of biogenic amines, including norepinephrine or serotonin. Mianserin is an $\alpha_2$-receptor blocking agent in the central nervous system. Thus it effectively acts as a noradrenergic compound by down-regulating noradrenergic receptors. It is a potent central nervous system histamine-$H_2$ receptor

### Table 4. Pharmacokinetic Properties of Antidepressants

| Drug | Half-life in plasma, h | Peak time, oral dose, h | Time to steady state, days |
|---|---|---|---|
| **Tricyclics** | | | |
| Amitriptyline | 17-40 | 2- 8 | 4-10 |
| Nortriptyline | 15-93 | 2- 8 | 4-19 |
| Imipramine | 6-24 | 1- 6 | 2- 5 |
| Desipramine | 12-76 | 2- 8 | 2-11 |
| Protriptyline | 54-198 | 6-12 | 10+ |
| Doxepin | 8-36 | 2- 6 | 2- 8 |
| Trimipramine | 9 | ? | ~2 |
| **Tetracyclics** | | | |
| Maprotiline | 27-58 | 9-16 | 7-14 |
| Amoxapine | ~8 | ~1.5 | ~2 |
| 8-Hydroxy-amoxapine | ~30 | ~2.1 | ~5 |
| **Other Classes** | | | |
| Trazodone | ~13 | 1.5-2 | ~3 |
| Alprazolam | ~12 | ~1 | ~3 |

blocker, which probably accounts for its main side effects of drowsiness, lethargy, and weight gain. However, it has very few anticholinergic or cardiovascular side effects.

Nomifensine, a drug which has been approved for use in Europe for several years, is a tetrahydroisoquinoline compound that exhibits both norepinephrine and dopamine reuptake blocking activity. It has no effect on serotonin reuptake and is not a monoamine oxidase inhibitor. Clinical studies indicate that it may be useful in psychomotor retarded depressions because it possesses central nervous system activating properties and is not sedative. It has some anticholinergic side effects, but these are much less pronounced that those produced by the tricyclic antidepressants, and it does not appear to be cardiotoxic.

Bupropion belongs to another new family of antidepressants, the chloropropiophenones. It is thought to be a dopaminergic compound (i.e., blocks dopamine reuptake) and appears to have little or no effect on norepinephrine or serotonin reuptake. It also does not inhibit monoamine oxidase. It has virtually no anticholinergic side effects and, like nomifensine, produces central nervous system activation.

In addition to these compounds, another class of drugs comprised of bicyclic antidepressants are also being investigated. These drugs, including zimelidine and fluoxetine, are all highly specific serotonin reuptake inhibitors. They appear to have no effect on dopamine or norepinephrine reuptake and are virtually devoid of anticholinergic side effect. Common side effects of these drugs include nausea, weight loss, diarrhea, and central nervous system activation.

## Comment

A number of new antidepressants have become available in the United States in recent months. Among them are two tetracyclic antidepressants, amoxapine and maprotiline; one new tricyclic antidepressant, trimipramine; and two relatively unique compounds, the triazolopyridine derivative trazodone and the triazolobenzodiazepine alprazolam. Numerous additional compounds are also undergoing investigation at this time, and it clear that the range of chemical structures and pharmacological properties of drugs available for treatment of depressions is expanding rapidly.

While data from all of the studies surrounding the clinical efficacy and utility of these antidepressants will improve our ability to treat these disorders and help to clarify the biological mechanism underlying depressions, this data will also force the psychiatrist and primary care physician to learn how to use a much wider and more divergent range of drugs. Incorporated into the research in this field is an emphasis on development of greater diagnostic specificity correlated with diagnostic criteria used to differentiate subtypes of patients with affective disorders. Proper identification of individual patients or patient groups will be required to achieve the greatest possible effectiveness from this new array of antidepressants.

According to some authors, we will shortly have antidepressants which not only act more rapidly and lack serious side effects, but which may be safe for patients with cardiac disorders or even when taken with suicidal intent.

While more than 100 methods for the analysis of tricyclic antidepressants have been described in recent years, the introduction of these new antidepressants has not been paralleled by technical advances in their analysis. Contemporary methods for the analysis of tricyclic antidepressant drugs including gas chromatography with nitrogen detectors, high-pressure liquid chromatography, and mass fragmentography can probably be applied to the analysis of most of these new compounds. However, few techniques have been published or evaluated for these purposes to date, and we are likely to see in the near future problems similar to those faced by laboratories five years ago when they began to perform analyses of the tricyclic antidepressants. Laboratories engaged in therapeutic monitoring of antidepressant drugs will be faced with a plethora of methods from which to choose and will probably have to utilize a number of techniques to provide the full range of analyses requested.

Laboratories that are just beginning to understand the complexities of monitoring tricyclic antidepressants and that are just beginning to develop the basic pharmacological background and information required to deal with psychiatric patients being treated with antidepressant drugs will now be faced with a whole range of new compounds, for which fundamental data, laboratory procedures, and appropriate reference methodology remain to be established. Laboratory scientists engaged in monitoring these new compounds will have to expand their clinical expertise rapidly and significantly to apply therapeutic monitoring effectively to the utilization of these drugs.

## Selected References

1. Asendin (amoxapine), Professional monograph, Lederle Laboratories, Pearl River, New York, NY, 1981.
2. Ayd, F., Amoxapine: A new tricyclic antidepressant, *Int. Drug Therapy Newsletter* 15, 33-40, 1980.

3. Ayd, F., Trazodone: A unique broad spectrum antidepressant. *Int. Drug Therapy Newsletter* **14**, 33-40 (1979).

4. Boutelle, W.E., Clinical response and blood levels in the treatment of depression with a new antidepressant drug, amoxapine. *Neuropharmacology* **19**, 1229-1231, 1980.

5. Feighner, J.P., Clinical efficacy of the newer antidepressants. *J. Clin. Psychopharm.* **1** (Suppl.), 235-265 (1981).

6. Feighner, J.P., Pharmacology: New antidepressants. *Psychiatric Annals* **10**, 338-394 (1980).

7. Orsulak, P.J., Clinical pharmacology of tricyclic antidepressants: A brief review. This volume, pp 229-238.

8. Orsulak, P.J., and Schildkraut, J.J., Guidelines for therapeutic monitoring of tricyclic antidepressant plasma levels. *Ther. Drug Monitoring* **1**, 199-208 (1979).

9. Pinder, R., Brogden, R., Speight, T., and Avery, G., Maprotiline: A review of its pharmacological properties and therapeutic efficacy in mental depressive states. *Drugs* **13**, 321-387 (1977).

10. Rosenbaum, A.H., Schatzberg, A., Maruta, T., Orsulak, P.J., Cole, J.O., Grab, E.C., and Schildkraut, J.J., MHG as predictor of response to imipramine and maprotiline. *Am. J. Psychiatry* **137**, 1090-1092 (1980).

11. Schatzberg, A., and Cole, J., Benzodiazepines in depressive disorders. *Arch. Gen. Psychiatry* **35**, 1359-1365 (1978).

12. Settle, E., Ayd, F., Trimipramine: Twenty years' worldwide clinical experience. *J. Clin Psychiatry* **41**, 266-274 (1980).

13. Sulser, F., Pharmacology: Current antidepressants. *Psychiatric Annals* **10**, 381-387 (1980).

# 44

# Therapeutic Monitoring of Maprotiline: A Case Study of High-Dose Therapy

**Paul J. Orsulak, Ph.D.**
**Sten Lofgren, M.D.**
**Sandra Lipchus, M.S.**

The value of therapeutic monitoring of tricyclic and tetracyclic antidepressant drugs is becoming more firmly established. The determination of these drugs in plasma can be important in the treatment and management of psychiatric patients to determine efficacy, to monitor compliance, and to control side effects (1). While the correlations between concentrations of some tricyclic antidepressants in plasma and their therapeutic effect have been well documented, therapeutic ranges for all of the tricyclic antidepressants and the newer tetracyclic antidepressants, including maprotiline, have yet to be well documented. However, individual variability in response to drugs, large differences in drug metabolism, and frequently encountered noncompliance with prescribed medication schedules make drug measurements in plasma a useful way of determining whether a patient is receiving an adequate therapeutic trial of an antidepressant.

The following case illustrates the value of monitoring the tetracyclic antidepressant maprotiline and utilizing information on the concentrations of this drug in plasma to tailor drug management to the specific needs of the patient. This case illustrates the value of plasma level measurements even when the therapeutic range for the drug is not firmly established, and emphasizes the strategy of considering each patient individually when interpreting plasma level measurements.

## Case Study

Mr. A, a 53-year-old high level business executive, had experienced his second psychiatric episode and was hospitalized following a serious suicide attempt.

---

*Dr. Orsulak is Assistant Professor of Psychiatry, Harvard Medical School, and Technical Director, Psychiatric Chemistry Laboratory, New England Deaconess Hospital, Boston, MA. Dr. Lofgren is Clinical Instructor in Psychiatry, Harvard Medical School, and a member of the psychiatric staff, McLean Hospital, Belmont, MA. Ms. Lipchus is senior chemist, Psychiatric Chemistry Laboratory, New England Deaconess Hospital, Boston, MA.*

---

The patient described himself as always having been something of a loner, and expressed a sense of feeling awkward in social settings. Following graduation from a prominent college, the patient joined his father's firm. When the patient was 29 years old, his father died and he experienced his first depressive episode. He credits extensive psychotherapy following this episode with enabling him to rise within his company to a senior executive position. At this point in his career he was responsible for several thousand employees and an annual budget in the hundreds of millions of dollars. During the past several years, however, the patient identified episodes of depressive symptoms. He was passed over for promotions and his symptoms gradually increased until, in the fall of 1980, he found it difficult to work and began to be more depressed on a regular basis. By the end of 1980 he was experiencing significant depressive symptoms, including loss of energy, anhedonia, inability to concentrate, inability to sleep, and loss of appetite. He had lost more than 10 pounds. He attempted suicide for the second time, and was admitted to an outpatient psychiatric hospital.

He was initially treated with amoxapine, and was later switched to a monoamine oxidase inhibitor, followed by a combination of imipramine and lithium, all of which had no effect. Blood level measurements indicated that imipramine concentrations during the third drug trial were adequate, but the patient refused to continue medication for any reasonable period of time and was transferred to an inpatient psychiatric hospital.

At the time of this admission to the hospital, laboratory examination, including urinalysis, hematology, and an SMA-12 screen were all within normal limits. A CT scan was performed and read as being normal.

Treatment was instituted with maprotiline on March 20 at 150 mg/day. The drug concentration in plasma approximately 10 days later was 85 µg/L (ng/mL), below the therapeutic range, and the dose of maprotiline was increased to 200 mg/day. After starting on maprotiline, the patient experienced a number of side effects, including urinary retention, which was treated with bethanechol, 75 mg/day, and a rapid heart rate, with some decreased exercise tolerance. At the suggestion of his internist, the cardiac syptoms were treated by the addition of Nadolol, 40 mg/day. Heart rate and exercise tolerance returned to normal.

After approximately four weeks of treatment with maprotiline at 300 mg/day, definite but partial symptomatic relief was noted, with improvement in mood and concentration abilities. The patient was now able to discuss his financial state and described that on review he was quite well situated financially, quite unlike what he had believed when depressed. In spite of the apparent symptomatic improvement, however, a dexamethasone suppression test remained abnormal, suggesting poor prognostic outcome, and the patient still experienced feelings of sadness, loneliness, guilt, and anger, as well as residual difficulties with concentration. On May 19, the concentration of maprotiline in plasma was 207 µg/L. Although the patient was responding at this point, he was seen by a senior consultant. Because the concentration of maprotiline in plasma was in the lower end of the therapeutic range, the consultant decided to increase the dose of maprotiline to increase the concentrations in plasma for this patient.

However, the pharmacy adamantly refused to supply doses of maprotiline higher than 300 mg/day, since this was the upper limit recommended in the package insert. The consultant indicated, however, that plasma level measurements would be continued, and the patient's medication was increased to 400 mg/day. The patient tolerated this dose well and on June 7, approximately two weeks later, the pervasive sadness and anger he had felt for the past month lifted. The concentration of maprotiline in plasma was 282 µg/L on June 23. The patient was discharged on June 30 with clear-cut clinical improvement, and planned to return to his previous employment to resume new duties.

## Discussion

Although the importance of monitoring tricyclic and tetracyclic antidepressants is becoming more apparent, the complexity of therapeutic monitoring is still often overlooked. Therapeutic ranges have not, as some may believe, been firmly established for all of the antidepressants that are currently on the market in the United State.

Therapeutic ranges for the tetracyclic antidepressants, including maprotiline, are just beginning to emerge, but initial reports suggest that the therapeutic range for maprotiline lies between 180 and 400 µg/L (2,4). There are also data to suggest that

maprotiline may have more than one therapeutic range, depending on the subtype of depressed patient being treated (5).

A recent study (5) has reported that pretreatment levels of the norepinephrine metabolite 3-methoxy-4-hydroxyphenylglycol (MHPG) in urine may serve as possible predictors of response to antidepressant drugs, including imipramine and maprotiline. These data are complex, but can be summarized as follows: Patients in this study with relatively low levels of urinary MHPG prior to treatment responded better to treatment with maprotiline or impramine than did patients with higher levels of urinary MHPG. In addition, many of those patients who responded to maprotiline responded after only two weeks of treatment. Findings from this study also suggest that patients with low pretreatment MHPG levels may not only respond better to maprotiline, but may also respond more rapidly and at lower doses and consequently lower blood levels than do patients with high MHPG levels. In this study, patients with low pretreatment urinary MHPG levels were treated with a mean of 138 mg/day of maprotiline. In contrast, the mean dose of maprotiline in the high MHPG responders to this drug was 258 mg/day. Maprotiline concentrations in plasma in these low and high MHPG groups were approximately 185 and 407 µg/L, respectively, near the extremes of the therapeutic range. Therefore, patients with relatively low pretreatment urinary MHPG levels required only half as much medication and achieved half the concentration of maprotiline in plasma that was found in patients who responded to this medication but had pretreatment levels of MHPG in the upper range.

Both tricyclic and tetracyclic antidepressants, including maprotiline, are administered orally. Generally, these medications are begun at fairly low doses and the dose in increased gradually over a number of days to therapeutically effective levels. In middle-aged, physically healthy patients of average weight (60 to 90 kg) the typical starting dose of maprotiline is 75 mg/day, which is then increased by 25 mg/day increments every two or three days until an average dose of 150 to 250 mg/day is reached (6, 7). Adverse effects, such as hypotension, lightheadedness, difficulty urinating, drowsiness, dry mouth, and constipation often limit the increase in dosage of these medications. Based on clinical effect and plasma levels obtained, the dose of maprotiline can then be increased up to 300 mg/day (6, 7). As illustrated in the cited case, however, doses above 300 µg/day are sometimes required to achieve maximal clinical response. In such cases, therapeutic monitoring is essential to ensure that the patient does not attain toxic levels of the medication.

Monitoring the level of antidepressants in plasma is often used when managing the treatment of elderly patients (8), since older patients treated with a given dose of drug often develop higher steady-state drug levels in plasma than do younger individuals. Since this patient was 53 years old, experience would have suggested that he might require lower doses of maprotiline than would younger individuals. In fact, he required significantly higher doses to achieve maximal clinical effect, even though concentrations in plasma barely reached the upper end of the therapeutic range.

The availability of data on drug concentrations in plasma also enabled both the clinician treating the patient and the consultant to determine a proper course of action when side effects were experienced very early in the treatment plan. Medication was not discontinued at the onset of side effects. Rather, the side effects were treated with additional medications and the treatment protocol with maprotiline was continued to obtain maximal clinical efficacy. Also of note is the fact that the side effects which occurred early were not exacerbated by substantial increases in dose and drug concentration of maprotiline.

## Chemical Profile

| | |
|---|---|
| Generic name | Maprotiline |
| Chemical name | N-methyl-9, 10-ethanoan-thracene-9(10H)propanamine |
| Molecular weight (free base/ hydrochloride) | 277.41 / 313.88 |
| Melting point (hydrochloride) | 238-246°C |
| Solubility in water (hydrochloride) | Freely soluble |
| $pK_a$ | 10.5 |
| Dose absorption (oral) | |
|   Time to peak concentration in plasma (h) | 9-16 |
|   Percentage of oral dose absorbed | 100 |
|   Percentage of protein bound | ~88 |
| Volume of distribution, L/kg body weight | ~23 |
| Urinary excretion—% daily dose | |
|   Maprotiline, unchanged | 2 |
|   Acid metabolites | 13 |
|   Basic metabolites, other | 8 |
|   Neutral (alcohol) metabolites | 2 |
|   Conjugated (phenolic) metabolites | 75 |

### Clinical Pharmacology

| | |
|---|---|
| Recommended dose, mg/day, average adult | 75-300 |
| Recommended dose, mg/day, elderly adult | 50-75 |
| Half-life | 27-58 |
| Time to steady state, days | 7-14 |
| Therapeutic range, μg/L (ng/mL) | 180-400 |
| Toxic level, μg/L (ng/mL) | >800 |

## References

1. Orsulak, P.J., and Schildkraut, J.J., Guidelines for therapeutic monitoring of tricyclic antidepressant plasma levels. *Ther. Drug Monitoring* **1**, 199-208 (1979).

2. Fischbach, R., Maprotiline in adult depressed patients: A study of the relation between clinical efficacy and serum concentrations after repeated intravenous and peroral administration. *Drug Res.* **29**, 352-355 (1979).

3. Pinder, R., Brogden, R., Speight, T., and Avery, G., Maprotiline: A review of its pharmacological properties and therapeutic efficacy in mental depressive states. *Drugs* **13**, 321-387 (1977).

4. Miller, P.I., Beaumont, G., Seldrup, J., John, V., Luscombe, D.K., and Jones, R., Efficacy, side-effects, plasma and blood levels of maprotiline (Ludiomil). *J. Int. Med. Res.* **5**, (Suppl.), 101-111 (1977).

5. Schatzberg, A., MHPG for discriminating among subtypes of unipolar depressions and predicting response to maprotiline. *Int. Drug Therapy Newsletter* **15**, 29-31 (1980).

6. Rieger, W., Rickels, K., Norstad, N., Johnson, J., Maprotiline (Ludiomil) and imipramine in depressed in-patients: A controlled study. *J. Int. Med. Res.* **3**, 413-416 (1975).

7. Loque, J., Sachais, B., and Feighner, J., Comparisons of maprotiline analog with imipramine in severe depression: A multicenter controlled trial. *J. Clin. Pharmacol.* **19**, 64-74 (1979).

8. Orsulak, P.J., and Appelbaum, P.S., Monitoring imipramine concentrations in the plasma of elderly patients: A case study. This volume, pp 239-242.

# 45

# Urinary MHPG Levels as Predictors of Response to the Antidepressant Maprotiline

Paul J. Orsulak, Ph.D.
Alan F. Schatzberg, M.D.
Edwin L. Grab, M.S.
Joseph J. Schildkraut, M.D.

Certain pharmacological agents, including antidepressant drugs, which produce alterations in mood and affective state in human subjects also produce significant effects on the disposition and metabolism of catecholamines and indoleamines in the brain. This observation served as the intitial stimulus for research on the possible role of alterations in biogenic amine metabolism in the pathophysiology of the affective disorders (depressions and manias). Moreover, based on these early observations, the possibility was suggested more than 15 years ago (1) that different subgroups of patients with depressive disorders might be characterized by differences in the metabolism of norepinephrine and the physiology of noradrenergic neuronal systems. Further studies from a number of laboratories have now indicated also that pretreatment levels of the norepinephrine metabolite 3-methoxy-4-hydroxyphenylglycol (MHPG) can aid in discriminating among subtypes of depressive disorders (2-5), and aid in predicting response to some antidepressant drugs. When taken together these findings support the role of MHPG as one useful measure in the diagnosis and management of patients with affective disorders. This paper will summarize the results of a study which examined the relationship between pretreatment levels of urinary MHPG and response to the tetracyclic antidepressant maprotiline in order to illustrate the potential clinical use of MHPG levels to predict the likelihood of patients responding favorably or unfavorably to this drug.

_Dr. Orsulak and Dr. Schatzberg are Assistant Professors, Mr. Grab is Lecturer, and Dr. Schildkraut is Professor, Department of Psychiatry, Harvard Medical School, Boston, MA._

_This work was supported in part by grant MH15413 from NIMH and grant RR585 from Division of Research Resources, NIH._

## Physiological Role of Urinary MHPG

During the 1960's, findings from a number of studies suggested that MHPG or its sulfate conjugate was a major metabolite of norepinephrine in the human brain, as it was in the brains of a number of other species. Moreover, it appeared that much of the norepinephrine originating in the brain was excreted in the urine as MHPG. In contrast, relatively little urinary norepinephrine, normetanephrine, epinephrine, metanephrine, or vanillylmandelic acid appeared to derive from the central nervous system, and most of these appeared to originate from the peripheral sympathetic nervous system of the adrenal glands (6).

However, urinary MHPG may derive in part from the peripheral sympathetic nervous system as well as from the brain, and the exact fraction of urinary MHPG which does originate in the brain remains uncertain. For example, on the basis of a recent study in human subjects measuring venous-arterial differences in the concentration of MHPG, Maas et al. (7) estimated that the average contribution by brain to the total body production of MHPG exceeded 60%. However, the findings of this study have been questioned by another investigation (8) which suggested that only about 20% of urinary MHPG comes from norepinephrine in the brain. Hovever, these investigators did note that even if the majority of urinary MHPG were derived from peripheral sources, as suggested by their study, urinary MHPG could still be a biochemical measure of clinical value in subclassifying affective disorders or in predicting therapeutic response to specific forms of treatment.

Although one might intuitively expect levels of MHPG in the cerebrospinal fluid to provide a better index of norepinephrine metabolism in the brain than does urinary MHPG, this does not appear to be the case (5).

Numerous studies have now indicated that pretreatment levels of urinary MHPG may predict responses to certain tricyclic or tetracyclic antidepressant drugs. Depressed patients with "low" pretreatment urinary MHPG levels respond more favorably to treatment with imipramine (2, 9-14), desipramine (2), nortriptyline (15), or maprotiline (13, 16) than do depressed patients with high pretreatment urinary MHPG levels. In contrast, other studies (9, 11, 17, 18) have found that depressed patients with "high" pretreatment levels of urinary MHPG respond more favorably to treatment with amitriptyline than do patients with lower MHPG levels prior to treatment, but this has not been observed in all studies (19-21).

## Methods

This study included 28 depressed patients (13 men and 15 women), who were treated with maprotiline at Mclean Hospital in Belmont, MA, or at the Mayo Clinic. All patients in this study met the Research Diagnostic Criteria for major depressive disorders (22), and all but one of the patients met criteria for endogenous depressive syndrome (23). All of the patients included in the study were free of significant organic, neurological, or medical illness, and all of the patients in the study had a Hamilton Depression Rating Scale (HDRS) (24) score of at least 19 prior to drug treatment, and most had considerably higher scores (range 19-43; mean=31).

During the pretreatment base-line period, 24-h urine specimens were collected for analysis of MHPG, which was determined by modifications of a gas chromatographic method using electron capture detection (25). Prior to the drug treatment, all patients received a physical examination and routine diagnostic laboratory tests were performed. During the base-line period 18 of the patients were hospital inpatients while 10 were outpatients. Base-line HDRS scores were obtained during the urine collection period and on the first day of drug treatment just prior to the first dose of maprotiline. Informed consent was obtained from all patients participating in this study.

Upon completion of the base-line data collection, patients began a four-week trial of maprotiline and received 150 mg/day during the first two weeks. After two weeks of treatment the dosage could be increased to a maximum of 300 mg/day at 50 mg/day every three days. At the two- and four-week points of the study, patients were considered to have been treated with adequate dosage if they had received at least 150 mg/day for the two and four weeks, respectively, unless they showed favorable clinical response at lower doses. Patients who remained in the study but who did not meet these dosage criteria were designated as "inadequate dosage patients." Patients who dropped out were designated as dropouts. To obtain maximal information from the study and to avoid biases, response to treatment was analyzed using data from all patients and excluding dropouts and those with inadequate dosage.

Criterion for clinical response at two weeks was a 40% reduction in HDRS score from base-line, while the criterion after four weeks of treatment was a 60% reduction in HDRS score.

## Results

Since both the range of MHPG levels and the mean excretion of the subjects in this study were similar to those found in previous studies (26) we designated low and high urinary MHPG levels as those $\leq 1950 \, \mu g/day$ and $>1950 \, \mu g/day$, respectively. Patients with low and high urinary MHPG levels were well matched with respect to age ($43 \pm 4$ and $44 \pm 3$ years, respectively).

Table 1 summarizes the results of the study after two weeks of treatment with maprotiline, while Table 2 summarizes the findings after four weeks of treatment with this drug. As shown in Table 1, favorable clinical response after two weeks of treatment occurred with significantly higher frequency in patients with low pretreatment urinary MHPG levels than it did in patients with high pretreatment urinary MHPG levels. Nine of twelve patients with low MHPG levels responded to maprotiline while only three of sixteen patients with high MHPG levels responded to this drug. Similar results were obtained when data were analyzed excluding dropouts or those who had received inadequate dosage, and similar findings were also observed when data was analyzed separately for male and female patients.

As noted in the section on Methods, criterion for response at four weeks required a percentage

## Table 1. Base-line Urinary MHPG and Response to Maprotiline After Two Weeks

|  | Responders | Nonresponders |
|---|---|---|
| Low MHPG ($\leq 1950 \, \mu g/day$) | 9 | 3 |
| High MHPG ($>1950 \, \mu g/day$) | 3 | 13 |

Chi square = 6.71; p < 0.01
Response = % HDRS reduction from baseline $\geq 40\%$

## Table 2. Base-line Urinary MHPG and Response to Maprotiline After Four Weeks

|  | Responders | Nonresponders |
|---|---|---|
| Low MHPG ($\leq 1950 \, \mu g/day$) | 8 | 4 |
| High MHPG ($>1950 \, \mu g/day$) | 3 | 13 |

Chi square = 4.74; p < 0.05
Response = % HDRS reduction from base-line $\geq 60\%$

reduction in HDRS scores from base-line ≥60%. Table 2 shows that patients with low pretreatment urinary MHPG levels also responded more favorably after four weeks to treatment with maprotiline than did patients with higher pretreatment MHPG levels. However, the apparent difference in clinical response in patients with low versus high pretreatment MHPG levels was less pronounced at four weeks than it was at two weeks. This may be explained in part by a high rate of attrition among patients with high MHPG, since only eight of the original sixteen patients with high MHPG were able to complete four weeks of treatment with adequate doses of maprotiline.

The incidence of discontinuing maprotiline therapy and the side effects that prevented continuation of medication further suggest that patients with low MHPG levels tolerate treatment and respond more favorably than patients with high MHPG levels. Of the patients with low MHPG, only two dropped out of the study (both due to allergic reactions) and only one could not tolerate adequate dosage. In contrast, of the patients with high MHPG levels, eight dropped out because of poor clinical response, uncomfortable side effects, or inability to tolerate adequate doses.

Steady-state concentrations of maprotiline in plasma were obtained on some of the patients in this study between weeks 4 and 6. Table 3 shows that patients with high MHPG levels who responded favorably to treatment required higher doses of maprotiline and achieved higher blood levels than did patients with low MHPG who responded to this drug. Although blood levels of maprotiline were determined in only three low MHPG responders, the range in this group was 165 to 203 µg/L. In contrast, four of the five high MHPG responders on whom blood levels were determined had levels greater than 300 µg/L. One high MHPG patient who showed a favorable response to treatment with

maprotiline had a blood level less than 300µg/L between weeks 4 and 6 of this study, but he was the only patient who did meet the criteria for an endogenous depressive syndrome. This observation was consistent with findings of Gram et al. (27) who reported that blood levels of imipramine did not correlate well with clinical response in patients with nonendogenous depressions.

## Discussion

The data provided by this study, while not conclusive, support previous findings that patients with low MHPG levels prior to treatment would respond favorably to the noradrenergic uptake inhibitors like maprotiline. In this study, antidepressant responses occurred more rapidly and at lower doses in patients with low pretreatment MHPG levels than in patients with high MHPG levels. However, antidepressant responses were observed in some patients with high MHPG levels, although their responses occurred later and only after relatively higher doses (and higher concentrations in plasma) of maprotiline were achieved. In addition, patients with low pretreatment urinary MHPG levels respond to relatively lower doses of maprotiline, whereas patients with higher MHPG levels who respond to maprotiline require higher doses and longer periods of drug administration for clinical effect to be observed.

The complex effects on noradrenergic, dopaminergic, and other neurotransmitter systems— including alterations in various indices of presynaptic and postsynaptic receptor functions that are observed after chronic administration of antidepressant drugs (28)—suggest that additional specific empirical trials will be required to assess the value of urinary MHPG levels or any other biochemical measure as clinically useful predictors or response to specific antidepressant drugs. For example, it has recently been reported that patients with normal or high urinary MHPG levels who exhibit dexamethasone suppression respond favorably to treatment with the experimental antidepressant mianserin, whereas patients with low urinary MHPG levels whose cortisol secretion is not suppressed by dexamethasone do not respond to mianserin (29). As a practical clinical matter, however, these findings suggest that measurement of pretreatment urinary MHPG levels may aid in the identification of patients who are likely to respond to treatment with maprotiline.

## Table 3. Maprotiline Doses and Plasma Concentrations at Conclusion (Weeks 4-6) of Study

| Group (N) | Dose mg/day | Drug Conc. in plasma; ug/L |
|---|---|---|
| Low MHPG responder (N=8) | 138 ± 20 | 185 ± 11 |
| High MHPG responder (N=6) | 258 ± 20* | 407 ± 94 |
| Low MHPG nonresponder (N=2) | 274 ± 173 | 200 ± 50 |
| High MHPG nonresponder (N=5) | 170 ± 38 | 181 ± 50 |

*Significantly different from low MHPG responders (p < 0.01).

## References

1. Schildkraut, J.J., The catecholamine hypothesis of affective disorders. *Am. J. Psychiatry* **122**, 509-522 (1965).
2. Maas, J.W., Fawcett, J.A., and Dekirmenjian, H., Catecholamine metabolism, depressive illness and drug response. *Arch. Gen. Psychiatry* **26**, 252-262 (1972).
3. DeLeon-Jones, F.D., Maas, J.W., Dekirmenjian, H., and Sanchez, J., Diagnostic subgroups of affective disorders and their urinary excretion of catecholamine metabolites. *Am. J. Psychiatry* **132**, 1141-1148 (1975).
4. Goodwin, F.K., Post, R.M. Studies of amine metabolites in affective illness and in schizophrenia: A comparative analysis. In *Biology of the Major Psychoses,* D.X. Freedman, Ed., Raven Press, New York, NY, pp 299-332.
5. Schildkraut, J.J., The current status of the catecholamine hypothesis of affective disorders. In *Psychopharmacology: A Generation of Progress,* M. Lipton, A. DiMascio, K.F. Killam, Eds. Raven Press, New York, N.Y., 1978, pp 1223-1234.
6. Maas, J.W., and Landis, D.H., The metabolism of circulating norepinephrine by human subjects. *J. Pharmacol. Exper. Ther.* **177**, 600-612 (1971).
7. Maas, J.W., Hattox, S.E., Greene, N.M., and Landis, D.H., 3-Methoxy-4-hydroxyphenethyleneglycol production by human brain *in vivo. Science* **205**, 1025-1027 (1979).
8. Blombery, P.A., Kopin, J.J., Gordon, E.K., Markey, S.P., and Ebert, M.H., Conversion of MHPG to vanillylmandelic acid. *Arch. Gen. Psychiatry* **37**, 1095-1098 (1980).
9. Beckmann, H., and Goodwin, F.K., Antidepressant response to tricyclics and urinary MHPG in unipolar patients. *Arch. Gen. Psychiatry* **32**, 17-21 (1975).
10. Steinbook, R.M., Jacobson, A.F., Weiss, B.L., and Goldstein, B.J., Amoxapine, imipramine and placebo: A double blind study with pretherapy urinary 3-methoxy-4-hydroxyphenylglycol levels. *Current Ther. Res.* **26**, 490-496 (1979).
11. Cobbin, D.M., Requin-Blow, B., Williams, L.R., and William, W.O., Urinary MHPG levels and tricyclic antidepressant drug-selection. *Arch. Gen. Psychiatry* **36**, 1111-1115 (1979).
12. Maas, J., Bowden, C., Mendels, J., and Koscis, J.H., Neurotransmitter metabolites and the therapeutic response to antidepressant drugs. Presented at the 12th Congress of the College Internationale Neuropsychopharmacologicum. Goteborg, Sweden, June 22-26, 1980.
13. Rosenbaum, A.H., Schatzberg, A., Maruta, T., Orsulak, P.J., Cole, J.O., Grab, E.L., and Schildkraut, J.J. MHPG as a predictor of antidepressant response to imipramine and maprotiline. *Am. J. Psychiatry* **137**, 1090-1092 (1980).
14. Schatzberg, A.F., Orsulak, P.J., Rosenbaum, A.H., Maruta, T., Kruger, E., Cole, J.O., and Schildkraut, J.J., Toward a biochemical classification of depressive disorders IV. Pretreatment urinary MHPG levels as predictors of antidepressant response to imipramine. *Commun. Psychopharm.* **4**, 441-445 (1980-81).
15. Hollister, L.E., Davis, K.L., and Berger, P.A., Subtypes of depression based on excretion of MHPG and response to nortriptyline. *Arch. Gen. Psychiatry* **37**, 1107-1110 (1980).
16. Schatzberg, A.F., Rosenbaum, A.H., Orsulak, P.J., Rohde, W.A., Maruta, T., Kruger, E.R., Cole, J.O. and Schildkraut, J.J. Toward a biochemical classification of depressive disorders IV. Pretreatment urinary MHPG levels as predictors of response to treatment with maprotiline. *Psychopharm.* **75**, 34-38 (1981).
17. Schildkraut, J.J, Norepinephrine metabolites as biochemical criteria for classifying depressive disorders and predicting responses to treatment. Preliminary findings. *Am. J. Psychiatry* **130**, 696-699 (1973).
18. Modai, I., Apter, A., Golomb, M., and Wijsenbeek, H. Response to amitriptyline and urinary MHPG in bipolar depressive patients. *Neuropsychobiology* **5**, 181-184 (1979).
19. Sacchetti, E., Allaria, E., Negri, F., Biondi, P.A., Smeraldi, E., and Cazzullo, C.L., 3-Methoxy-4-hydroxyphenylglycol and primary depression: Clinical and pharmacological considerations. *Biol. Psychiatry* **14**, 473-484 (1979).
20. Coppen, A., Ramo Rao, V.A., Ruthven, C.R.J., Goodwin, B.L., and Sandler, M., Urinary 4-hydroxy-3-methoxyphenylglycol is not a predictor for clinical response to amitriptyline in depressive illness. *Psychopharm.* **64**, 95-97 (1979).
21. Spiker, D.G., Edwards, D., Hanin, I., Neil, J.F., and Kupfer, D.J., Urinary MHPG and clinical response to amitriptyline in depressed patients. *Am. J. Psychiatry* **137**, 1183-1187 (1980).
22. Spitzer, R.L., Endicott, J., and Robins, E. *Research Diagnostic Criteria (RDC) for a Selected Group of Functional Disorders,* 3rd ed.
23. Schildkraut, J.J., Klein, D.F., The classification and treatment of depressive disorders. In *Manual of Psychiatric Therapeutics. Practical Psychiatry and Psychopharmacology,* R.I. Shader, Ed., Little, Brown, Boston, MA, 1975, pp 39-61.

24. Hamilton, M., A rating scale for depression. *J. Neurol. Neurosurg. Psychiatry* **23**, 56-62 (1960).
25. Dekirmenjian, H., and Maas, J.W., An improved procedure of 3-methoxy-4-hydroxy-phenylethyleneglycol determination by gas liquid chromatography. *Anal. Biochem.* **35**, 113-122 (1970).
26. Schildkraut, J.J., Orsulak, P.J., Schatzberg, A.F., Gudeman, J.E., Cole, J.O., Rohde, W.A., and LaBrie, R.A., Toward a biochemical classification of depressive disorders I. Differences in urinary MHPG and other catecholamine metabolites in clinically defined subtypes of depressions. *Arch.* *Gen. Psychiatry* **35**, 1427-1433 (1978).
27. Gram, L.F., Bech, P., Reisby, N., Nagy, A., and Christiansen, J. Factors influencing pharmacokinetics and clinical effects of tricyclic antidepressants. In *Depressive Disorders,* S. Garattini, Ed., Symposia Medica Hoechst 13, Schattauer Verlag, Stuttgart, Germany, 1978, pp 337-346.
28. Sulser, F., Vetulani, J., and Mobley, P.K., Mode of action of antidepressant drugs. *Biochem. Pharmacol.* **27**, 257-261 (1978).
29. Cairncross, K.D., Cobbin, D.M., Pohlen, G.J., Letter to editor. *Brit. Med. J.* **283**, 991 (1981).

# 46

# Lithium: A Case History

**Juan Ramon de la Fuente, M.D.**

## Introduction

Although lithium is almost universally accepted as the drug of choice for the treatment of patients with **bipolar affective disorders (manic-depressive illness)**, as yet no single mechanism explains its therapeutic effects. There is also substantial evidence for its effectiveness as a drug for prophylaxis of recurrent depressions (unipolar affective disorders) and its use is currently being investigated in other medical and psychiatric disorders. Clearly, the full extent of its indications remains to be determined *(1)*.

Because lithium ion can be measured so readily and accurately, and because there is a therapeutic range below which there is no effectiveness and above which there may be considerable toxicity, it is currently the only psychotropic drug that is monitored routinely in standard clinical practice. Despite many studies, the optimal concentration in plasma is uncertain. For treatment of acute mania, concentrations between 0.8 and 1.4 mmol/L have been considered desirable. Generally accepted concentrations for prophylactic purposes range between 0.6 and 1.2 mmol/L. However, lithium has a narrow therapeutic range and acute toxicity *can* appear at concentrations of about 1.5 mmol/L, while symptoms of chronic toxicity may appear at lower concentrations *(2)*.

This report illustrates the correlations between clinical improvement and lithium concentrations in plasma within the therapeutic range, as well as the appearance of signs and symptoms of toxicity when lithium concentrations exceed the therapeutic range.

## Case Report

A 68-year-old white male was admitted to the hospital for evaluation of ascites and peripheral edema, which was found to be secondary to alcoholic liver disease. Shortly after admission the patient developed a manic episode and was transferred to the psychiatric ward. He exhibited most of the typical signs and symptoms of mania: his mood was euphoric but he was easily irritated, his speech was very rapid, and the pace of his psychomotor activity was grossly accelerated. Although garrulous, with stream-of-consciousness

*Dr. de la Fuente is a Fellow in Psychiatry, Mayo Clinic and Instructor in Psychiatry, Mayo Medical School, Rochester, MN.*

speech, his words remained sufficiently relevant to be followed. He was easily distracted, felt "on top of the world" and talked tangentially about some grandiose financial plans. He was suspicious and unwilling to stay in the ward, but finally accepted it if the stay was to be brief. His cognitive functions were difficult to assess, but memory and orientation appeared to be unaffected.

The patient had a history of multiple psychiatric problems for at least 20 years. He had been hospitalized elsewhere on at least 10 different occasions for situations that, according to his relatives, appeared to be quite similar to his present illness. He had been treated with electro-convulsive therapy several times, which had helped substantially, although its effects had not lasted long. Between his manic episodes there had been at least three discernible depressive episodes, but he was never hospitalized for this reason. Otherwise, he had been a very successful businessman and a good father and husband. He had begun to abuse alcohol for the past five years to "sleep better and be a bit more relaxed." He had suffered from insomnia for at least four decades and was described as always being very active, quickly changing from one to another of multiple enterprises. In spite of his wealth, he had long shown a tendency to neglect himself, being almost always ungroomed, unwashed, and untidily dressed. Atypically, we could elicit no family history of affective disorders.

Treatment was started with haloperidol, 2 mg orally three times a day, and lithium carbonate, 300 mg three times a day. Improvement was gradual but steady, and three days later his plasma lithium concentration was 1 mmol/L. During subsequent days, his haloperidol dosage was decreased, but lithium dosage was kept the same. During the following week, plasma lithium concentrations, determined on two different occasions, were 1.1 and 0.9 mmol/L. Haloperidol was discontinued and the patient was kept only on lithium for his third and last week of hospitalization; his plasma lithium concentration was 0.8 mmol/L early in the week, 1.1 mmol/L the day before dismissal. Most manic symptoms had disappeared, although the patient still was experiencing some insomnia.

A week after the patient was dismissed his local physician saw him and—because of borderline hypertension, overweight, and mild hyperglycemia—suggested that he start a 1200-calorie per day diet, containing 90 mmol of sodium.

Three days later the patient was brought to the emergency room in a state of somnolence. His daughter, who brought him, reported noting increasing unsteadiness in his gait during the last 24 h, and that he had had several falling episodes that morning, due to loss of balance, although he had not hit his head or lost consciousness.

On examination, he was grossly ataxic, tremulous, and with generalized weakness. Values for serum sodium, potassium, creatinine, and glucose were within normal limits. Plasma lithium concentration was 1.9 mmol/L. The patient was re-admitted and treated that night with saline diuresis. Plasma lithium concentration the next day was 1.4 mmol/L. The patient was less somnolent but remained ataxic and somewhat dysarthric. Results of an electrocardiogram were normal.

The symptoms of lithium toxicity cleared during the subsequent 48 h, therapy with lithium was re-begun (300 mg three times a day) and the patient was discharged again, at which time his plasma lithium concentration was 0.9 mmol/L. He was given specific instructions to avoid low-sodium diets or the use of diuretics without prior consultation with a psychiatrist. Obviously, the patient was not believed to have an overriding need for antihypertensive treatment at that time.

## Discussion

This case illustrates several important points about the usefulness, safety, and toxicity of therapy with lithium carbonate.

Perhaps the most important one is that it is an effective anti-manic drug at a dosage that is largely determined by its concentration in plasma. Because its effects begin relatively slowly, severely manic patients may require concurrent use of antipsychotic drugs for a few days; conversely, supplemental antidepressants during severe depressive episodes may also be necessary. For lesser degrees of mania, lithium alone usually suffices.

A second major point illustrated in this case report is the need for clinicians to be aware that changes in water and sodium flux may produce changes in lithium concentration. Thus, rigid dieting or fasting, salt restriction, diuretics—in fact, any medical illness that changes water or salt balances—should alert physicians to carefully monitor lithium treatment (3). This may include dose reduction or complete withdrawal.

In cases of toxicity, plasma lithium concentrations may not necessarily reflect the severity of overdose. Values may be quite high early on with mild or moderate symptoms of intoxication, and may be low later on, with severe toxic symptoms. The early signs of toxicity, such as nausea, vomiting, and diarrhea, may be quickly superseded by neurological signs such as lethargy,

weakness, and decreasing levels of consciousness.

In cases of moderate overdose, saline cathartics usually suffice, although treatment with cation-exchange resins theoretically should be useful. Whatever the therapeutic measures, lithium ion should be measured frequently enough to assure that the drug is being eliminated. With adequate management, permanent neurological damage as a consequence of lithium intoxication is much less likely.

Concomitant use of lithium and diuretics has been controversial, but despite the almost universal warnings against such use, diuretic-induced lithium retention has been well documented only with regard to the thiazides. Some preliminary reports suggest that the potassium-sparing group can also cause lithium retention while the loop diuretics do not. At any rate, by appropriate downward adjustment of lithium dosage, the associated use of a thiazide is relatively safe, if the medical condition of the patient remains stable. On the other hand, if a consistent plasma lithium concentration is established while the patient is receiving a diuretic, discontinuing the diuretic without also adjusting the lithium dose could result in its concentration declining below the therapeutic range (4).

Lithium ion is distributed in the total body water, shifting slowly into cells. It is not bound to plasma proteins. It penetrates the brain slowly, but in some areas of the brain concentrations seem higher than

## Lithium Carbonate Profile

| Trades names: | Lithotabs, Lithonate, Eskalith |
| --- | --- |
| pKa: | n/a |
| Rel. Mol. mass: | 73.89 |
| Melting point, °C: | 618 |
| Water Solubility: | 12.8 mg/mL |

| Dose absorbed: | 97% |
| --- | --- |
| Peak plasma level, time: | 1-3 h |
| Protein bound: | 0 |
| $V_d$: | 0.4-1.4 L/kg |

| FORM IN URINE | % excreted | Active | Detectable in blood |
| --- | --- | --- | --- |
| unchanged drug: | 50 | yes | yes |

| | Adults | Children |
| --- | --- | --- |
| Half-life (h): | 8-35* | n/a |
| Steady state, time (d): | 2-7 | n/a |

| | Adults | Children |
| --- | --- | --- |
| Recommended dose (mg/kg/d): | 10-20 | n/a |
| Effective concn (mmol/L): | 0.8-1.4** | n/a |
| Toxic concn (mmol/L): | 2.0 | n/a |

| Monitoring Methods: | flame emission, atomic absorption |
| --- | --- |

*variable with renal function
**monitor trough at 12 h post-dose

those in plasma. Virtually all lithium is excreted unchanged by the kidney and its clearance in steady state is about one-fifth that of creatinine. It is also excreted in saliva and the ratio between the concentrations in saliva and plasma is relatively constant. Thus, saliva may be an appropriate sample for monitoring lithium treatment.

Lithium is rapidly absorbed after an oral dose. Concentrations in the blood are maximum within 1 to 3 h; its elimination half-life is roughly equivalent to its plasma half-life (about 24 h). Steady-state concentrations in plasma can be expected in about five days, although this time is somewhat modified by the amount of fluid brought to the kidney and its sodium content. Lithium carbonate has no active metabolites (see reference 2 for details of clinical pharmacology).

While its relatively long half-life in plasma would seem to make single daily dosage possible, single doses are usually not well tolerated. Three or four equal doses are usually prescribed during the day, and concentrations in plasma are customarily measured about 12 h after the last dose, at a point where absorption and accumulation of lithium from the preceding day's doses has ceased. Initially, lithium was used without measuring it in plasma, but the simple techniques required for such measurements and their unequivocal value in assuring that treatment is adequate support the measurement of plasma concentrations. Additionally, the plasma lithium value provides some assurance to the physician that he is not inducing toxicity. All these factors strongly suggest that therapeutic monitoring of plasma lithium levels is helpful in the clinical management of these patients.

## References

1. Rosenbaum, A.H., Maruta, T., and Richelson, E., 1. Drugs that alter mood. II. Lithium. *Mayo Clin. Proc.* **54**, 401-407 (1979).
2. Hollister, L.E., Lithium and manic depressive disorders. In *Monographs in Clinical Pharmacology*, **1**, *Clinical Pharmacology of Psychotherapeutic Drugs*, D.L. Azarnoff, Ed., Churchill Livingstone, New York, NY 1978, pp 192-226.
3. Lipton, M.A., and Jobson, K.O., Psychopharmacology. In *Psychiatry in General Medical Practice*, G. Usdin and J.M. Lewis, Eds., McGraw-Hill, New York, NY, 1979, pp 561-620.
4. Jefferson, J.W., and Greist, J.H., Lithium and the kidney. In *Psychopharmacology Update: New and Neglected Areas*, J.M. Davis and D. Greenbalt, Eds., Grune and Stratton, New York, NY, 1979, pp 81-104.

# VI. Antineoplastic Drugs

# 47

# Chemotherapy: A Brief Review

James Standefer, Ph.D.

## Introduction

Chemotherapy is a blend of the art and science of using cytotoxic drugs to treat malignant disease. Because there is no "magic bullet" drug that seeks out and with surgical precision destroys only malignant tissue while sparing adjacent normal cells, the physician must exercise skill and judgment in applying the therapy of cytotoxic drugs. In this process, he relies on the laboratory to provide information about whether the cytotoxic drug has been applied excessively. In response to this need, drug-assay laboratories are providing more assays directed toward therapeutic monitoring of cytotoxic drugs.

Although the therapeutic indices for some drugs may be large enough to permit some trial and error while adjusting the concentrations of drug in the blood, this is not generally the case for cytotoxic drugs. For example, the short term side effects of excess phenytoin may be only lethargy and nystagmus, but excess methotrexate can be more directly life-threatening. By definition a cytotoxic drug kills cells - all cells. For this reason, the efficacy of cytotoxic drug therapy depends (a) on adjusting the drug concentration in cells such that normal cells may get sick but don't die, and (b) on the greater susceptibility of fast-growing malignant cells to the drug's cytotoxic effects. In other words, the central aim of chemotherapy is to apply a drug that kills cells in such a way that few normal cells will succumb, but all cancer cells will be killed. This obviously difficult task is only rarely completely successful. More often, successful treatment is measured in terms of months of disease-free existence or in the degree of disease regression, but not in terms of complete remission.

This somewhat pessimistic view of the efficacy of chemotherapy should not dampen the enthusiasm of researchers and clinical laboratorians. There have been some notable success stories in chemotherapy, including the successful treatment of certain leukemias to achieve near-total cure rates. In the 40 to 50 years

that chemotherapy has been applied to malignant disease, treatment of certain cancers have improved significantly, particularly when chemotherapy has been coupled with ablative surgery.

To understand more about chemotherapy, we will look briefly at three types of chemotherapeutic agents: the alkylating agents, the antimetabolites, and the antibiotics. This will be followed by a brief discussion of the laboratory's general task of monitoring drug toxicity with indirect hematologic tests and the more specific task of providing data on cytotoxic drug concentrations in blood.

## History

One of the early instances of chemotherapy, reported in 1931, was the use of mustard gas (dichlorodiethylsulfide) in the topical treatment of a neurogenic sarcoma. Fortunately, this treatment was successful as measured by tumor regression. This rather limited approach was followed in the 1940's by a series of initial in vitro investigations and later clinical trials of other alkylating agents, including chlorambucil and busulfan. These agents proved successful and are still widely used.

A second chemotherapeutic approach in which antimetabolites were used to treat malignant disease was initiated in the late 1940's and applied more vigorously in the 1950's. The folic acid antagonist, methotrexate, and the pyrimidine analog, 5-fluorouracil, emerged as clinically useful antimetabolite drugs. Some of the initial applications of these drugs led to improved cure rates and increased survival for patients with acute lymphocytic leukemia and certain lymphomas.

A third general group of chemotherapeutic agents, the antibiotics, was developed during the 1950's and was shown to be effective in treating certain cancers. Of this group, actinomycin D and streptozocin have enjoyed considerable success against Wilm's tumor and Hodgkin's disease, respectively.

Later, development of other chemotherapeutic agents such as the vinca alkaloids, vincristine and vinblastine, is particularly interesting. These drugs were shown to promote the accumulation of methotrexate inside the cell. Presumably, this promotion of accumulation occurs because of the demonstrated a-

*Dr. Standefer is the Director of the Clinical Laboratory at Bernalillo County Medical Center in Albuquerque, New Mexico.*

bility of these alkaloids to disrupt cellular microtubular structure and function. This would allow more methotrexate to penetrate the cell and to accumulate at its site of action. However, it is not clear whether this combination of drugs leads to increased effectiveness and, indeed, their combination may lead to increased toxicity.

## Cell Cycle

The effectiveness of any chemotherapeutic agent is closely related to its action on the cell at some particular stage of the cell cycle (Figure 1).

During cell division, cells pass through several metabolic stages or phases. These have been generally characterized by the synthetic events that occur within the cell, especially within the nucleus. In the $G_1$ phase, there is a rapid turnover of ribonucleic acid with an increase in synthesis of proteins and other molecules. The $G_1$ phase is followed by the S phase, during which DNA is synthesized. A cell that enters the S phase is generally committed to the remaining phases of the cell reproduction cycle. Following the rather concise period of DNA replication during the S phase, the cell synthesizes cellular proteins and generally regroups its metabolic machinery. This occurs during the $G_2$ phase. The cell then enters the mitotic or M phase, during which very little metabolic activity is apparent while the cell divides. However, microtubule and mitotic spindle formulations are important for cell division and may be inhibited by cytotoxic drugs such as the vinca alkaloids.

Cytotoxic drugs may be effective in any one or all of these cell-division phases. For instance, methotrexate is *phase specific* and kills proliferating cells during the S phase of the cell cycle, while alkylating agents such as carmustine are effective by killing cells throughout the cell cycle, i.e., they are *cycle specific*. Except for cyclophosphamide, which is most effective in the S phase of the cell cycle, alkylating agents generally are cycle specific in that they kill proliferating cells at any stage of the cell cycle. Therefore, those cells that happen to be in the resting phase during the drug treatment would be less affected. This suggests that the effectiveness of a cytotoxic drug is directly related to (a) the differences in proliferation rate between normal and malignant cells and (b) the number of malignant cells that happen to be proliferating at the time of treatment. These relationships appear to especially hold for cycle-specific alkylating agents. For example, proliferating leukemia cells are quite sensitive to busulfan and presumably only a relatively small proportion of those cells that happen to be in the resting phase will survive the treatment. This contrasts with a

### Figure 1. The cell cycle

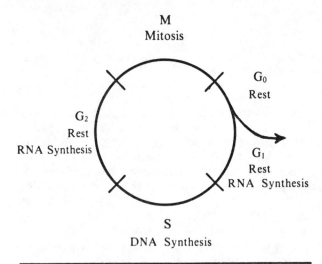

much higher survival of normal hematopoietic cells because a greater proportion of normal cells would be in the resting state.

## Pharmacology

How useful cytotoxic drugs are in treatment of malignant disease depends directly on the pharmacokinetic nuances of each drug. It has been well stated in earlier discussions on therapeutic drug monitoring that in order to achieve the desired therapeutic result an appropriate amount of drug must reach the tissue and remain there for a sufficient time. This obvious process is partially controlled by the pharmacology of the drug, i.e., route of administration, amount absorbed, concentration at the active site, rate of metabolism, and rate of excretion. We will now consider some of these pharmacokinetic parameters for one or two examples of each type of chemotherapeutic agent.

## Alkylating Agents

Alkylating agents have been useful as chemotherapeutic agents because they form covalent alkyl linkages with molecules that have electron-rich centers, such as amines, sulfides, and cyclic ring nitrogens. In particular, the nitrogen atom in the 7 position on the guanine of DNA is susceptible to this alkylation. A wide variety of alkylating agents participate in this reaction, which leads to a distortion of DNA and subsequent interruption of accurate replication. Some examples that are commonly applied therapeutically

(Table 1) include the nitrogen and sulfur mustards, alkyl halides, and a platinum-containing compound.

Cyclophosphamide is an interesting example of a chemotherapeutic agent that must be metabolized to an active form before it will promote alkylation and cell killing. Cyclophosphamide is oxidized by hepatic mixed-function oxidases to 4-hydroxcyclophospha-mide and aldophosphamide. These two metabolites are active alkylating agents and have a serum half-life that is shorter than their parent, cyclophosphamide.

Most alkylating agents are well absorbed from the gastrointestinal tract and are distributed to the extra-vascular space within minutes of absorption. This accounts for their relatively short plasma half-lives and is consistent with renal excretion of a high per-centage of the dose within 24 hours. Generally, most aklylating agents are excreted as inactive metabolites. Cyclophosphamide is an exception: about 40% of it is excreted in its active form and, if renal function is compromised, the drug dose must be reduced appro-priately.

## Table 1. Examples of Chemotherapeutic Agents

| Example | Commonly used abbreviation or synonym |
|---|---|
| *Alkylating Agents* | |
| Semustine | Methyl-CCNU |
| Carmustine | BCNU |
| Cyclophosphamide | -- |
| Cis-platinum | DDP |
| *Antimetabolites* | |
| Fluorouracil | 5-FU |
| Methotrexate | MTX |
| Cytarabine | ara-C |
| *Antibiotics* | |
| Actinomycin D | -- |
| Doxorubicin | Adriamycin |
| Streptozocin | -- |

## Antimetabolites

The antimetabolite drugs, including methotrexate and fluorouracil, are generally phase specific, with a pronounced cell-killing effect manifested in the S phase of the cell cycle. These drugs, as their name implies, are effective because they inhibit the produc-tion of metabolites that are essential for DNA produc-tion. For example, methotrexate directly inhibits tetrahydrofolate dehydrogenase (EC 1.5.1.3), which is the enzyme responsible for converting 7,8-dihydrofol-ate to 5,6,7,8-tetrahydrofolate (THF). THF is a precursor to 5,10-methylene tetrahydrofolate which supplies a methyl group for the conversion of deoxy-uridine to thymidine. Thus, methotrexate indirectly inhibits DNA synthesis by limiting the availability of thymidine, a metabolite that is specific to DNA.

Another antimetabolite drug, fluorouracil, more directly interrupts DNA synthesis by inhibition of thymidylate synthase (EC 2.1.1.45), the enzyme that catalyzes methylation of deoxyuridine to produce thymidine. Additional mechanisms by which fluoro-uracil disrupts cellular metabolism include (a) being incorporated into RNA to produce subsequent con-fusion in the cells synthetic machinery, and (b) in-hibiting cellular utilization of uracil by directly inhibit-ing uracil.

Mercaptopurine is another effective anti-metabo-lite. It is converted in vivo to 6-thioinosinic acid which is incorporated into nucleic acids and also interferes with the de novo synthesis of purines.

As discussed above, the action of alkylating agents is rapid and direct, in that they enter the cells quickly and directly distort DNA replication. By contrast, antimetabolites act more indirectly because they are more effective during those cell-cycle phases in which precursors to DNA synthesis are produced. In fact, one common treatment protocol for relief from cyto-toxic effects of methotrexate therapy ("rescue") relies on this competitive effect. The cytotoxic effects of methotrexate are nullified by supplying leucovorum, a folic acid analog. This effectively bypasses the methotrexate blockade of DNA synthesis and relieves the cytotoxic effects.

Antimetabolites generally are not well absorbed from the gastrointestinal tract and are usually best administered intravenously or intramuscularly. How-ever, some antimetabolites such as methotrexate are well absorbed after oral administration when given in low doses.

The biological half-life of the antimetabolites in plasma varies widely but generally is less than 1 to 3 hours because these drugs are rapidly distributed to tissues. While the extent of antimetabolite metabo-lism varies, a significant percentage of the total dose may be excreted considerably unchanged in the urine during the first 24 hours after the dose.

## Antibiotics

Actinomycin and adriamycin are examples of anti-biotics that are effective cytotoxic drugs. They are phase-specific except that they may affect any phase of the cell cycle in which DNA or RNA is replicated. Those antibiotics which are effective anti-tumor agents are cytotoxic because they associate closely or

**Table 2. Examples of Therapy with Chemotherapeutic Agents**

| Agent | Tumor type | Signs and Symptoms of Toxicity |
|---|---|---|
| Cyclophosphamide | chronic lymphatic and myelocytic leukemia, solid tumors | temporary alopecia, some myelosuppression |
| Carmustine | Hodgkin's disease, multiple myeloma, gliomas | myelosuppression, nausea, vomiting, pigmentation |
| Methotrexate | acute leukemia, choriocarcinoma, osteosarcoma | myelosuppression, stomatitis, renal toxicity |
| Fluorouracil | Breast carcinoma, G.I. adenocarcinoma | alopecia, pigmentation, neurotoxicity |
| **Actinomycin D** | choriocarcinoma, Wilm's tumor, Hodgkin's disease | myelosuppression, alopecia, nausea, vomiting |
| Adriamycin | Hodgkin's disease, lymphomas | cardiotoxicity, alopecia, stomatitis |
| Vinblastine | Hodgkin's disease, testicular tumors | leukopenia, constipation, neurotoxicity |

intercalate with the guanine residues of DNA and disrupt DNA-dependent synthesis of RNA. These drugs are even more effective in disrupting DNA-dependent replication of new complementary DNA. Thus, they are effective in the $G_1$ and $G_2$ and S phases of the cell cycle.

Certain antibiotics have been effective in chemotherapy for a wide variety of solid tumors, such as small-cell carcinoma of lung, choriocarcinoma, and Hodgkin's disease, as well as in some forms of acute leukemia. Generally, these antibiotics are not well absorbed from the gastrointestinal tract and are most effective when given parenterally. These drugs are rapidly cleared from blood to the extravascular compartment with biological half-lives ranging from 2 to 35 min.

## Toxicity

Table 2 lists examples of the three general types of chemotherapeutic agents and some of their toxic effects. The toxicity of chemotherapeutic drugs varies widely but is generally dose-related. Most commonly, nausea and vomiting will occur regardless of the route of administration. More serious cytotoxic effects that may occur include alopecia (loss of hair), myelosuppression (loss of leukocytes and platelets), stomatitis (oral mucosal ulceration), hepatotoxicity (fibrosis and cirrhosis), and nephrotoxicity (renal failure). It should be obvious that this toxicity is the result of the killing of some normal cells during the drug treatment interval that is required to kill cancer cells. Generally, the cytotoxic drug will be most effective when its con-

centration is adjusted to the highest level consistent with survival of normal cells. Thus, a certain degree of toxicity must be anticipated when cytotoxic drugs are applied therapeutically.

## The Clinical Laboratory

The clinical laboratory can provide vital support to chemotherapeutic trials. A primary concern of the physician who directs the patient's chemotherapy is to adjust the drug dosage such that malignant cells are killed with a minimum of trauma to normal cells. The physician needs some objective means of assuring appropriate dosage adjustment, and the clinical laboratory can provide this objective measurement of cytotoxicity in two ways. First, because hematopoietic cells are very sensitive to cytotoxic drugs, a measure of the number of leukocytes and platelets in blood is often a useful index used in monitoring the killing of normal cells. Although this approach to monitoring the degree of cytotoxicity is relatively simple and is readily available in the clinical laboratory, there is a disadvantage. Neither the leukocyte count nor the platelet count decreases with mild cytotoxicity; only when drug exposure produces significant cell-killing will leukopenia and thrombocytopenia be observed. Thus, while decreases in leukocytes and platelets are indicative of effective cytotoxic drug treatment, a more sensitive measure of cytotoxicity would be clinically useful.

A second laboratory approach to monitoring cytotoxic effects of therapeutic drugs is less direct than cell counts, but may prove to be a more sensitive measure of cytotoxicity. This approach is therapeutic drug

**Table 3.** Laboratory Data Collected During Multiple Methotrexate Treatments of a Patient

| Parameter | Treatment number | | | | | |
|---|---|---|---|---|---|---|
| | __20__ | __21__ | __22__ | __23__ | __24__ | __25__ |
| Serum Creatinine, mg/L | 8 | 9 | 11 | 8 | 8 | 23 |
| Creatinine Clearance (mg/min) | 45 | 50 | 42 | 37 | 40 | __a__ |
| Methotrexate concn. in blood, (mol/L) $\times 10^{-7}$ | | | | | | |
| 24 h | 56 | 108 | 74 | 84 | 113 | 5160 |
| 48 h | 5.1 | 5.4 | 6.0 | 7.1 | 8.9 | 1739 |
| 72 h | 1.8 | 1.7 | 1.5 | 1.8 | 3.1 | 372 |
| Leukocyte count, in 1000's/mm³ | 6.8 | 7.2 | 5.7 | 10.0 | 6.6 | 1.2 |
| Platelet count $\times 10^{-6}$ per mm³ | 2.4 | 2.8 | 2.3 | 2.7 | 2.6 | .03 |

__a__ Not measured, owing to acute renal failure.

monitoring of chemotherapeutics and can be applied if the laboratory can measure the concentration and their active metabolites in blood.

It is important to note that a significant number of chemotherapeutic agents are unique in that 1) they are not active until they are metabolized to their active forms, 2) they react irreversibly at the site of action. These rather unique properties may distort the usual pharmacokinetic considerations related to therapeutic drug monitoring and for this reason, therapeutic monitoring has not become a routine procedure for most chemotherapeutic agents. However, drugs such as methotrexate, cis-platinium, fluorouracil, adriamycin and hexamethylmelamine can be measured in serum following therapeutic doses. Some laboratories which support larger cancer treatment centers are being asked to provide assays for these drugs. A general approach by such laboratories is to establish some serum drug concentration as a "cut-off" value, above which excessive cytotoxicity is known to occur. This provides a rationale for assaying the drug concentration in blood, i.e., to determine whether this critical "upper limit" concentration has been exceeded. Additionally, it is important for the clinician to know the length of time during which the drug has exceeded this critical cytotoxic concentration. This can be determined by assaying serum samples drawn at various times after the drug has been administered. By determining what an appropriate drug concentration is for each post-dose interval, excessive cytotoxicity can be more easily assessed. Table 3 gives an example of this type of protocol in which serial blood samples were collected. These data are from a patient who received multiple high doses of methotrexate, with leucovorin rescue. The data suggest that in treatments 23 and 24 the drug concentration in the blood samples drawn at 24 h and 48 h is increasing. This in turn suggests an increasing inability to eliminate methotrexate and a concomitant potential for excessive cytotoxicity, even though the serum creatinine concentration, creatinine clearance, and the hematological studies do not indicate imminent renal failure. In this particular case, the patient did develop renal failure during the subsequent methotrexate treatment, and hemoperfusion with massive leucovorum doses were required to obviate severe cytotoxicity.

Chemotherapy has proven to be a valuable and effective treatment of certain malignant diseases, but as yet, no single cytotoxic drug or combination of cytotoxic drugs has proven 100% effective against a variety of cancers. This lack of 100% reliability should not inhibit aggressive approaches to new modes of chemotherapy, especially when this therapy is used in conjunction with other treatments such as radiation and surgery. The laboratory must also take an aggressive stance because a considerable amount of information about chemotherapeutic agents must be gathered. More information about the pharmacokinetics of most cytotoxic drugs is required and the therapeutic drug monitoring laboratory has both the opportunity and the obligation to join in the effort of providing this information. In this way the TDM laboratory can contribute significantly to the effort of achieving its primary objective of improving patient care.

## References

Cridland, M.D., *Fundamentals of Cancer Chemotherapy,* University Park Press, Baltimore, Md., 1978.

Silver, R.T., Lauper, R.D., and Jarowski, C.I., *A Synopsis of Cancer Chemotherapy,* The Yorke Medical Group, DUN-Donnelley Publishing Corp., New York, N.Y., 1977.

Brule, C., Eckhardt, S.J., Hall, T.C., and Winkler, A., *Drug Therapy of Cancer,* World Health Organization, Geneva, 1973.

# 48

# Clinical Pharmacology of High-Dose Methotrexate Therapy and Pediatric Case History

**Michael A. Pesce, Ph.D.**

Therapy with high doses of methotrexate has been used to treat osteogenic sarcoma, acute lymphatic leukemia, cancer of the head and neck, and other malignancies. Methotrexate acts as an antitumor agent by blocking the metabolism of folic acid: because it is tightly bound to the enzyme dihydrofolate reductase (EC 1.5.1.3), it prevents formation of reduced folates. As a result, purines and thymidylate cannot be formed, and DNA synthesis and cell proliferation is prevented, both in normal and tumor cells. To "rescue" normal cells from the toxic effects of methotrexate, leucovorin (5-formyl tetrahydrofolate) is administrated several hours after methotrexate infusion. Leucovorin acts by replenishing the reduced folate pool by a pathway independent of the enzyme dihydrofolate reductase, and it selectively allows resumption of normal cell division without the recovery of certain tumor cells (1).

Prolonged high-dose methotrexate therapy has been associated with myelosuppression, renal failure, vomiting, dermatitis, alopecia, and hepatotoxicity. High-dose methotrexate therapy has also been suspected to contribute to fatal outcomes. In a survey of cancer treatment centers in the United States, fatalities reportedly occurred in 29 of 498 patients who were receiving high-dose methotrexate with leucovorin rescue (2). Because methotrexate in serum would identify those patients with concentrations such that they are at high risk of developing symptoms of toxicity, methotrexate concentrations in the serum of patients receiving high-dose therapy should be $<1 \mu$mol/L 48 h after the infusion of methotrexate if toxicity is to be avoided. The following case history illustrates the appropriate monitoring.

## Case History

A.M., a 9½-year-old American Indian boy, presented with osteogenic sarcoma. When he was 9 years

Dr. Pesce is the Director of the Special Chemistry Laboratory at Columbia Presbyterian Medical Center and Assistant Professor of Clinical Pathology at Columbia University, College of Physicians and Surgeons.

old he noted pain in his right knee, which gradually worsened until he limped. On admission his temperature was 37 °C, blood pressure 100/80 mmHg, height 137 cm, weight 35 kg, pulse 108/min, respiration 20/min. He was walking on crutches, with no weight bearing on the right leg. Roentgenograms and bone scans were consistent with a diagnosis of osteogenic sarcoma. He was to be treated with chemotherapy, to shrink the tumor before its surgical removal was possible.

Routine chemical studies indicated normal values for sodium, potassium, chloride, serum urea nitrogen, **creatinine, bilirubin, aspartate aminotransferase** (EC 2.6.1.1), alanine aminotransferase (EC 2.6.1.2), lactate dehydrogenase (EC 1.1.1.27), total protein and albumin. His alkaline phosphatase (EC 3.1.3.1) activity was threefold normal. Results of hematological studies, including complete blood count and platelet count, were normal.

Before methotrexate treatment was started the patient was hydrated and the urine made alkaline by intravenous infusion of a 50 g/L dextrose solution containing 42 mmol of bicarbonate per liter, at a rate of 150 mL per hour until the urinary pH exceeded 6.5. Methotrexate therapy was then started. He was given 7.2 g of methotrexate in 900 mL of 50 g/L dextrose solution containing 36 mmol of sodium bicarbonate per liter, intravenously, at a rate of 150 mL per hour for 6 h. One hour after the infusion was started 2 mg of vincristine was given intravenously. Leucovorin rescue was started 2 h after the methotrexate infusion was finished; it was administered intravenously every 3 h for a total of eight doses. Then leucovorin was given orally at 6 h intervals in eight 15 mg doses. Methotrexate and creatinine concentrations were monitored to detect renal failure and toxicity. Before the start of infusion the creatinine value was 6 mg/L; at 24 h it again was 6 mg/L and by 48 h it was 7 mg/L. Methotrexate concentrations, monitored at the end of infusion and at 18, 30, 56, and 68 hours after the infusion, were 340, 13, 1.5, 0.3, and 0.05 μmol/L, respectively. The patient exhibited no symptoms of toxicity because of rapid clearance of the drug which is reflected by the serum methotrexate levels. He was discharged three days after starting therapy and was given 15 mg leucovorin tablets, to be taken every 6 h for one day. He was re-admitted for two more treatments with methotrexate. During neither did he show signs of toxicity. Eighteen days after the first treatment with methotrexate the tumor was surgically removed.

## Discussion

The major route of elimination of methotrexate is by the kidneys. Within 24 h after infusion about 90% of methotrexate is excreted unchanged in the urine. Recently, a metabolite of methotrexate, 7-hydroxymethotrexate, has been detected in the urine of patients who are receiving high-dose therapy, in amounts ranging from 1 to 10% of the total excreted drug (3,4). Substantial amounts of 7-hydroxymethotrexate have also been detected in the serum of patients receiving high-dose therapy (5). Methotrexate is metabolized to 7-hydroxymethotrexate probably in the liver by the enzyme aldehyde oxidase (EC 1.2.3.1). 7-Hydroxymethotrexate neither significantly inhibits the enzyme dihydrofolate reductase nor has any other antifolate activity. Methotrexate is not metabolized to 7-hydroxymethotrexate in patients who are receiving low dose therapy, because the oxidase has a low affinity for the drug. Methotrexate is sparingly soluble in water at pH <7.0 (see page 283) and 7-hydroxymethotrexate is three to fivefold less soluble in water than methotrexate. Methotrexate and 7-hydroxymethotrexate will precipitate out in renal tubules at acid pH, causing renal failure and delayed excretion of methotrexate which is the situation responsible for the resulting toxicity. To minimize the possibility of methotrexate toxicity, the clinician must see that the patient is sufficiently hydrated with an alkaline urine before methotrexate infusion is started.

Serum creatinine values used as a guide in predicting renal failure are determined before and 24 and 48 h after infusion of methotrexate. In theory, if the serum creatinine value is as much as 50% larger than the pre-methotrexate value, renal failure and drug toxicity are more likely. However, in a recent survey (6), the serum creatinine concentration had increased by 50% in only four of seven patients who developed toxicity. Therefore serum creatinine values may not be a good indicator of renal failure and measurement of serum methotrexate is the only reliable way to assess drug toxicity.

Patient A.M. received 7.2 g of methotrexate intravenously during 6 h. Vincristine was given 2 h after the start of therapy, to increase the cellular uptake of methotrexate. Serum methotrexate concentrations exceeding 10 $\mu$mol/L at 24 h or 1 $\mu$mol/L at 48 h after infusion usually indicate delayed excretion of methotrexate, with impending toxicity. A.M. did not develop toxicity because his methotrexate concentrations at 30 and 56 h after infusion were satisfactory. His serum creatinine values did not increase during the course of therapy, which is in harmony with the lack of toxicity.

Of those patients with osteogenic sarcoma who are receiving high doses of methotrexate, concentrations of drug in serum are lower in children than in adults at the end of the 6 h infusion, but 48 h after the infusion, they were the same (7). Methotrexate has a bi-phasic half life, the first phase in children is more rapid than in adults. The first half life of methotrexate in children is 1.2 h, as compared to 2.2 h in adults. Urinary excretion of methotrexate by children is greater than in adults at the end of the 6 h infusion. In the 6 to 24 h period, the amount excreted in the urine by adults exceeded that by children. Thereafter, the amount excreted was the same in both. Evidently there is an age-related difference in the concentration and urinary elimination of methotrexate. However, the type of carcinoma may influence the pharmacokinetics. In children and adults with acute lymphatic leukemia, the pharmacokinetics of methotrexate were similar (8).

There are interactions between methotrexate and other drugs in serum. Salicylates, barbiturates, sulfonamides, phenytoin, or p-aminobenzoic acid diminish renal tubular transport of methotrexate and enhance toxicity. These drugs should not be given in conjunction with methotrexate therapy.

Methotrexate in serum has been measured by microbiological, fluorometric (9), liquid-chromatographic (5), radioimmunoassay (10, 11), competitive protein binding (12), enzyme inhibition (13), and enzyme-multiplied immunoassay techniques. The last two techniques are well suited for rapid monitoring of methotrexate. With the enzyme multiplied assay, serum or plasma is mixed with a reagent consisting of antibodies to methotrexate, $NAD^+$ and glucose 6-phosphate. The methotrexate in the sample binds to the antibody. This solution is added to a reagent containing methotrexate bound to the enzyme glucose-6-phosphate dehydrogenase (EC 1.1.1.49). The enzyme labeled drug combines with any remaining unfilled antibodies sites. The residual enzyme activity is determined by measuring an increase in absorbance of NADH at 340 nm and is related to the concentration of methotrexate in the sample. With the enzyme inhibition system, dihydrofolic acid is reduced to tetrahydrofolic acid and NADPH is oxidized to $NADP^+$ by the enzyme dihydrofolate reductase. Methotrexate in the sample binds the active sites on the dihydrofolate reductase molecule and inhibits the oxidation of NADPH to NADP$^+$. The change in concentration of NADPH, recorded at 340 nm, is related to the concentration of methotrexate in the sample. Methotrexate values as measured in 45 patients by both the enzyme-multiplied and enzyme inhibition systems showed good correlation (14).

The enzyme-multiplied and enzyme inhibition systems are readily adaptable to many of the automated instruments in the laboratory. If a centrifugal analyzer is used to measure methotrexate, as little as 3 $\mu$L of sample can be used, and results obtained in an hour (14). Either serum or plasma samples can be used to measure methotrexate, and the blood can be obtained by skin-puncture.

The toxic effects of methotrexate make it essential that methotrexate results be available within a few hours after the blood is sampled. If the results indicate toxicity, then the patient's urinary flow and pH should be increased, and additional leucovorin given, to prevent the potentially fatal effects of methotrexate.

## References

1. Frei, E., Jaffe, N., Tattersall, M.H.N., Pitman, S. and Parker, L. New approaches to cancer chemotherapy with methotrexate. *N. Engl. J. Med.* **292**, 846-851 (1975).

2. Von Hoff, D.D., Penta, J.S., Helman, L.J. and Slavik, M. Incidence of drug-related deaths secondary to high-dose methotrexate and citrovorum factor administration. *Cancer Treat. Rep.* **61**, 745-748 (1977).

3. Jacobs, S.A., Stroller, R.G., Chabner, B.A. and Johns, D.G. 7-Hydroxymethotrexate as a urinary metabolite in human subjects and rhesus monkeys receiving high dose methotrexate. *J. Clin. Invest.* **57**, 534-538 (1976).

4. Jacobs, S.A., Stoller, R.G., Chabner, B.A. and Johns, D.G. Dose-dependent metabolism of methotrexate in man and rhesus monkeys. *Cancer Treat. Rep.* **61**, 651-656 (1977).

5. Watson, T., Cohen, J.L. and Chan, K.K. High pressure liquid chromatographic determination of methotrexate and its major metabolite, 7-hydroxymethotrexate, in human plasma. *Cancer Treat. Rep.* **62**, 381-387 (1978).

6. Stoller, R.G., Hande, K.R., Jacobs, S.A., Rosenburg, S.A. and Chabner, B.A. Use of plasma pharmacokinetics to predict and prevent methotrexate toxicity. *N. Engl. J. Med.* **297**, 630-634 (1977).

7. Wang, Y.M., Sutow, W.W., Romsdahl, M.M. and Perez, C. Age-related pharmacokinetics of high-dose methotrexate in patients with osteosarcoma. *Cancer Treat. Rep.* **63**, 405-410 (1979).

8. Bratlid, D. and Moe, P.J. Pharmacokinetics of high-dose methotrexate treatment in children. *Europ. J. Clin. Pharmacol.* **14**, 143-147 (1978).

9. Kinkade, J.M., Jr., Vogler, W.R., and Dayton, P.G. Plasma levels of methotrexate in cancer patients as studied by an improved spectrophotofluorometric method. *Biochem. Med.* **10**, 337-350 (1974).

10. Paxton, J.W. and Roswell, F.J. A rapid, sensitive and specific radioimmunoassay for methotrexate. *Clin. Chim. Acta* **80**, 563-572 (1977).

11. Raso, V. and Schreiber, R. A rapid and specific radioimmunoassay for methotrexate. *Cancer Research* **35**, 1407-1410 (1975).

12. Myers, C.E., Lippman, M.E., Eliot, H.M. and Chabner, B.A. Competitive protein binding assay for methotrexate. *Proc. Natl. Acad. Sci. U. S.* **72**, 3683-3686 (1975).

13. Falk, L. C., Clark, D.R. Kalman, S. M. and Long T.F. Enzymatic assay for methotrexate in serum and cerebrospinal fluid. *Clin. Chem.* **22**, 785-788 (1976).

14. Pesce, M.A. and Bodourian, S.H. Unpublished observations.

# 49
# Methotrexate Concentrations in Renal Failure: An Adult Case Study

**James Standefer, Ph.D.**

Methotrexate is an analog of folic acid that serves as an effective antitumor agent because of its competitive inhibition of dihydrofolate reductase (see Figure 1). This enzyme catalyzes a critical step in the series of reactions that provide methyl groups for synthesis of thymidylic acid. This nucleotide precursor is required for DNA synthesis and, therefore, is particularly important for cellular reproduction. The cytotoxicity of methotrexate is thought to be related primarily to its inhibition of thymidylic acid production.

A common protocol for using methotrexate as a therapeutic anti-tumor agent calls for massive doses of the drug, followed by a "rescue" from the cytotoxic effects by administration of 5-formyl-tetrahydrofolic acid (citrovorum factor, leucovorum, folinic acid). Citrovorum factor may be converted to tetrahydrofolic acid and thus provides an essential product of the reaction blocked by methotrexate (Figure 1). Such "high-dose" protocols require the lab to monitor serum methotrexate concentrations, because assaying methotrexate in serum at various times after drug administration is helpful in assessing potential drug cytotoxicity. To avoid excessive cytotoxicity, serum drug values should be less than $1 \times 10^{-5}$, $1 \times 10^{-6}$, and $4 \times 10^{-7}$ mol/L at 24, 48, and 72 h after administration, respectively. The exact maximum allowable methotrexate concentration in serum varies with the dosing protocol; these figures apply generally to the treatment protocol described below.

## Case Study

A 65-year-old woman had radical vulvectomy and a deep pelvic node dissection for removal of a squamous-cell carcinoma of the vulva. Six months after surgery a recurrence of the carcinoma was noted. The patient was selected for a high-dose methotrexate treatment protocol, which called for an initial methotrexate intravenous infusion of 0.5 g/m$^2$ over 6 h and monitoring of serial serum samples for methotrexate assay drawn at 8, 24, 48, and 72 h after the drug infu-

*Dr. Standefer is the Director of the Clinical Laboratory at Bernalillo County Medical Center in Albuquerque, New Mexico.*

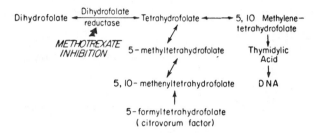

**Fig. 1.** DNA synthesis is limited by methotrexate inhibition of dihydrofolate reductase; citrovorum factor rescues the cell by providing tetrahydrofolate

sion. Rescue from the cytotoxic effects of methotrexate was provided at 24 h post-dose by intravenous infusion of citrovorum factor (10 mg/m$^2$), followed by oral doses of 10 mg/m$^2$ given at 6-h intervals for 48 h. The patient successfully completed several methotrexate treatments, her drug dosage increasing by 0.5 g/m$^2$ at each treatment for a maximum dose of 8 g/m$^2$. Regardless of the dose, serum drug values always were less than $1.0 \times 10^{-6}$ at 48 h (Figure 2).

After one year of drug treatment the patient was admitted for her next scheduled methotrexate treatment with no obviously abnormal physical signs. She had normal values for hematological and clinical chemical studies, including normal platelet and leukocyte counts, a blood urea nitrogen of 130 mg/L, and a serum creatinine of 9 mg/L. Her creatinine clearance was 44 mL/min. A 6-h methotrexate infusion (8 g/m$^2$) was tolerated well by the patient.

Before the infusion, and during the subsequent 24 h, sufficient sodium bicarbonate was included in her intravenous fluids to raise the urine pH above 7.0 and thus avoid crystallization of methotrexate in the renal tubules. This pH also enhanced the urinary excretion of methotrexate, an acid drug.

After methotrexate infusion was completed, citrovorum factor was infused to begin the rescue from the drug's cytotoxic effects. At this time (24 h after the methotrexate dose) the urinary output fell to 40% of fluid intake and the urine had a specific gravity of 1.011. Serum creatinine increased to 23 mg/L. The concentration of methotrexate in the serum drawn at 24 h post-infusion was $5.1 \times 10^{-4}$ mol/L. The serum drug concentration subsequently decreased to $1.7 \times$

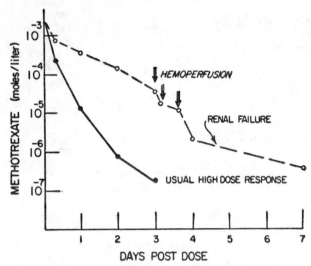

**Fig. 2.** Comparison of serial methotrexate concentrations after high-dose perfusion in one patient before and during renal failure.

$10^{-4}$ mol/L at 48 h.

Because this latter methotrexate value is about 1000-fold higher than that expected to produce severe cytotoxicity, the dose of citrovorum factor was increased 10-fold. As an additional measure to limit the cytotoxicity of methotrexate, the patient's blood was perfused through a charcoal column designed to remove excess methotrexate. Charcoal hemoperfusion requires an arteriovenous shunt, usually placed in the femoral area. However, because of extensive scarring from the radical vulvectomy, the femoral area was not accessible and a Ramirez shut was placed. After 2 h of hemoperfusion (72 h post-medication) the methotrexate concentration was $3.7 \times 10^{-5}$ mol/L. A second charcoal hemoperfusion lowered the serum methotrexate to $2.6 \times 10^{-5}$ mol/L.

The lack of a consistent, substantial drop in the serum methotrexate concentration after hemoperfusion suggested that a considerable amount of the drug was being sequestered in a "pool," which was being slowly cleared by the hemoperfusion procedure. This postulated large extravascular pool of the drug was consistent with the development of bilateral pneumonia during the 24-h to 48-h post-infusion period. A subsequent 8-h hemoperfusion (now at 96 h post-dose) through an amberlite resin column lowered the serum methotrexate to $4.4 \times 10^{-6}$ mol/L (Figure 2).

During the immediate post-hemoperfusion period, the urine output increased, and the patient stabilized with respect to fluid and electrolyte balance. Blood urea nitrogen values returned to less than 200 mg/L and serum creatinine values to less than 10 mg/L.

Although no further hemoperfusion was performed, because of problems in maintaining a patent arteriovenous shunt, the patient's pneumonia responded to rigorous treatment, and subsequent methotrexate determinations showed progressively lower serum drug values. At 14 days post-dose the drug concentration had fallen to $3.5 \times 10^{-7}$ mol/L, well below the expected cytotoxic concentration.

This case illustrates the direct relationship between adequate renal function and therapeutic methotrexate concentrations in the blood. The concentration of methotrexate at 48 h post-infusion was much higher during renal failure than in the same patient during previous treatment protocols. This higher value correlated directly with an increase in serum creatinine and the development of oliguria. Charcoal and resin hemoperfusion significantly lowered blood concentrations of methotrexate and, with increased doses of citrovorum factor, significantly improved the clinical prognosis. The patient was discharged two weeks after admission with no apparent abnormalities from the unusually intensive exposure to methotrexate.

## Characterization of Methotrexate

### Mechanism of Drug Action

Methotrexate is a potent competitive inhibitor of dihydrofolate reductase, an enzyme that is responsible for promoting the conversion of dihydrofolate to tetrahydrofolate (Figure 1). Thus, methotrexate is a potent inhibitor of cell reproduction and is used as an antitumor agent. Large doses (up to 18 g/m$^2$) are given by intravenous infusion because the intestinal absorption is severely limited for doses exceeding 30 mg/m$^2$. This cytotoxic drug is particularly potent against rapidly multiplying cells such as those found in bone marrow, gastrointestinal epithelium, and tumors.

### Drug Interactions

Because methotrexate is bound to proteins, primarily albumin, free methotrexate in serum may be increased in the presence of other drugs that bind strongly to albumin (e.g., salicylates).

The cytotoxic effects of methotrexate may be diminished by drugs that arrest the cell-reproduction cycle in G-phase (e.g. asparaginase, EC 3.5.1.1) and thus limit the inhibition by methotrexate, which is primarily manifested in the S-phase of the cell cycle.

By altering the intestinal flora that metabolize methotrexate, antibiotics may influence the amount of methotrexate reabsorbed in the enterohepatic circulation.

## Clinical Side Effects

The exact clinical side effects observed with methotrexate therapy are related to the dose size and its duration. Low doses (less than 30 mg/m$^2$) have been associated with cirrhosis, intestinal pneumonitis, and osteoporosis. High doses (up to 18 g/m$^2$) may cause vomiting, renal dysfunction, nephrotoxicity, and seizures. Intrathecal methotrexate therapy may result in neurotoxicity manifested by headache, fever, cerebrospinal fluid pleocytosis, and motor dysfunctions after chronic intrathecal therapy.

## Specimen

Blood samples for methotrexate assay should be centrifuged to remove cells as soon as practical, and may be stored at 4 °C for at least 24 h. No significant change occurs in serum methotrexate values in samples stored for two months at −20 °C. The pH of a collected urine specimen should be adjusted to below 5 to limit degradation of methotrexate, which may occur at higher pH values.

## Sampling Interval

For low-dose protocols, a blood sample should be drawn immediately before and 0.5 h (intravenous dose) or 2 h (oral dose) after dosing. For high-dose protocols, blood samples should be drawn at 24, 48, and 72 h after methotrexate infusion.

## Assay Methods

Several approaches to assay of serum methotrexate have been developed. Radioimmunoassay and the kinetic enzymatic methods have been most widely adopted, although the "high-performance" liquid chromatographic technique appears to be a reasonable approach. The radioimmunoassay method may not be entirely specific for methotrexate, because some methotrexate analogs and metabolites can cross react with antisera directed against methotrexate. The kinetic enzymatic assay provides accurate results, but requires isolation and purification of an enzyme; this somewhat complicated procedure may be beyond the scope of most busy clinical laboratories. High-performance liquid chromatography requires extraction and isolation of the drug from serum before adequate sensitivity is obtained. This extraction is complicated by the amphoteric and somewhat hydrophilic character of methotrexate. The following references are representative of the methods currently available for methotrexate assay:

### METHOTREXATE PROFILE

Trade name: Amethopterin

Chemical name: L-(+)-N-p-2. 4-diamino-6-pteridinyl methylamino benzoyl glutamic acid

Chemical structure:

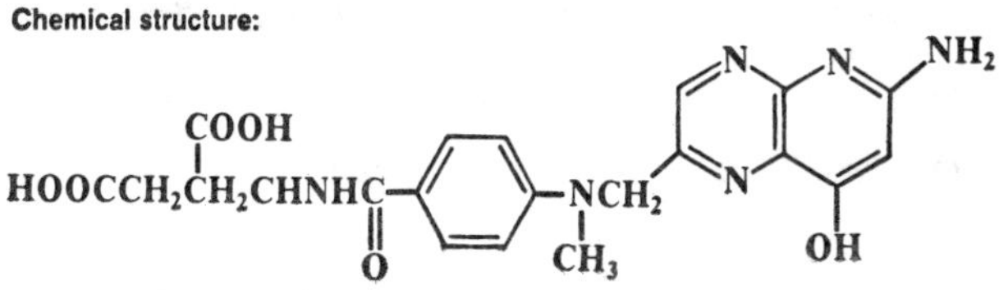

| | |
|---|---|
| Molecular weight: | 454.46 |
| Melting point, °C: | 184-204 |
| Solubility in water, mg/mL: | 8.9, pH 7.0 |
| pK$_a$: | 4.3, 5.5 |

Dose absorption –

| | Oral | IV |
|---|---|---|
| time to peak plasma conc., h: | 1-2 | 0.5-1.0 |
| percentage dose absorbed: | dose related | |

Protein binding –
percentage bound: 50-70

Tissue distribution, V$_d$, L/kg: 0.75

| Urinary excretion, % daily dose – | | Active | Detectable in Blood |
|---|---|---|---|
| as unchanged drug: | 40-50 (low dose) 50-90 (high dose) | yes | yes |
| as 7-hydroxymethotrexate: | 1-20 | no | yes |

| | Adults | Children |
|---|---|---|
| Recommended dose, mg/kg/d: | variable | variable |
| Half-life, h: | triphasic: 0.75, 3.5, 27 | low dose - 1.2 high dose - 10.4 |
| Time to steady state, h: | not applicable | not applicable |
| Effective levels, μg/mL: | 4.5, 24 h 0.45, 48 h | 4.5, 24 h 0.45, 48 h |
| Toxic levels, μg/mL: | > 10$^{-5}$M, 24 h > 10$^{-6}$M, 48 h > 10$^{-7}$M, 72 h | > 10$^{-5}$M, 24 h > 10$^{-6}$M, 48 h > 10$^{-7}$M, 72 h |

Methods available for monitoring: EMIT; RIA

*Radioimmunoassay:* Raso, V., and Schreiber, R., A rapid specific radioimmunoassay for methotrexate. *Cancer Res.* **35,** 1407 (1975).

*"High-performance" liquid chromatography:* Watson, E., Cohen, J., and Chan, K., High pressure liquid chromatographic determination of methotrexate and its major metabolite, 7-hydroxymethotrexate, in human plasma. *Cancer Treatment Rep.* **62,** 381 (1978).

*Kinetic enzymatic:* Wang, Y., Lantin, E., and Sutow, W., Methotrexate in blood, urine, and cerebrospinal fluid of children receiving high doses by infusion. *Clin. Chem.* **22,** 1053 (1976).

*Fluorimetric:* Kinkade, J., Vogler, W., and Dayton, P., Plasma level of methotrexate in cancer patients as studied by an improved spectrophotofluorometric method. *Biochem. Med.* **10,** 337 (1974).

*Biological:* Fountain, J., Hutchinson, D., Waring, G., and Burchenal, J., Persistence of amethopterin in normal mouse tissues. *Proc. Soc. Exp. Biol. Med.* **83,** 369 (1953).

## Bibliography

1. Bleyer, W.A., Methotrexate: Clinical pharmacology, current status and therapeutic guidelines. *Cancer Treatment Rev.* **4,** 87 (1977).

2. Wang, Y., Lantin, E., Sutow, W., Methotrexate in blood, urine, and cerebrospinal fluid of children receiving high doses by infusion. *Clin. Chem.* **22,** 1053 (1976).

3. Djerassi, I., High dose methotrexate (NSC-740) and citrovorum factor (NSC-3590) rescue: Background and rationale. *Cancer Chemother. Rep. Parts* **3, 6,** 3 (1975).

# 50

# Methotrexate: Case History

**C.P. Collier, Ph.D.**
**S.M. MacLeod, Ph.D.**
**S.J. Soldin, Ph.D.**

## Case History

Investigation of a 15-year-old Caucasian girl, who was experiencing pain in her left knee after a seemingly innocent fall, revealed an osteogenic sarcoma of the left distal femur. No metastases were detected and an above-the-knee amputation was performed one month later. Chemotherapy with doxorubicin and high-dose methotrexate commenced 10 days after the amputation.

In our chemotherapy protocol for osteogenic sarcoma, high-dose methotrexate (HD-MTX) therapy with leucovorin (LEU) rescue is administered on days 1 and 28, while doxorubicin (DXR) is administered on days 8, 9 and 10. Repetition of this regimen for six courses constitutes the first part of the chemotherapy program. The DXR is given in doses of 30 mg/$m^2$/day up to a total cumulative dose of 550 mg/$m^2$. Above this recommended limit the frequency of irreversible cardiac toxicity is markedly increased. After adequate hydration, including $NaHCO_3$ to alkalinize the urine above pH 7.0, MTX is administered in a 6-h infusion. The first dose of MTX is approximately 150 mg/kg, while all subsequent doses are approximately 250 mg/kg. LEU rescue is started 2 h after the end of the infusion. The dose is calculated according to surface area and is administered intravenously every 3 h for a total of 24 doses (the last 12 doses may be given orally). Chemotherapy is generally completed with an intensive course of six weekly doses of HD-MTX (250 mg/kg) with LEU rescue. Blood counts must be adequate, blood chemistries normal, and urine pH greater than 7.0 before a course of chemotherapy is started. All drugs except digoxin are held during MTX infusion. Dimenhydrinate may be given for vomiting and codeine for pain and diarrhea.

The patient started with DXR 10 days after surgery and underwent 11 of the 12 courses of chemotherapy, at which time several metastatic lesions were discovered in her lungs. All further interventions were discontinued.

During the chemotherapy courses, various chemical

*The authors are affiliated with the Departments of Clinical Biochemistry and Pharmacology, University of Toronto, and the Research Institute, Hospital for Sick Children, Toronto, Canada.*

parameters were followed, usually at preinfusion, 24-h and 48-h postinfusion times (all times are related to the start of the MTX infusion). Preinfusion BUN concentrations were always within the reference range of 80-200 mg/L. However, postinfusion concentrations were consistently lower, probably due to the forced diuresis. No pattern was observed for the uric acid concentrations which were maintained within the reference range of 20-60 mg/L. Any increases in excretion of uric acid due to diuresis may have been balanced against a possible increase in uric acid formation due to cell lysis and/or a decrease in renal tubular secretion due to competition for the carrier by MTX itself. Creatinine was maintained below 12 mg/L and although several postinfusion values did show an increase, the increments were never >50% of the preinfusion concentrations. For the first six courses of therapy, alkaline phosphatase either remained the same or decreased after the infusion. However, the activities were lower (20-40 U/L) than the reference range of 45-120 U/L. During the last five courses, the measured activities were slightly higher (33-59 U/L) and tended to increase after the infusions, a trend which may be associated with relapse of the disease. Aspartate aminotransferase increased significantly above the upper limit of 25 U/L after each of the first six courses of chemotherapy, with peak activities of 26, 86, 96, 72, 286, and 120 U/L, respectively. The increases during the last five courses were much less, again possibly reflecting the course of the disease.

The serum profile of MTX and its metabolite 7-hydroxy-methotrexate (70H-MTX) obtained during and after the second course of MTX (250 mg/kg) is presented in Figure 1. An HPLC-UV spectrophotometric assay for the simultaneous determination of both compounds was used for the quantitation (1). Administered MTX, which is supplied by Lederle (Cyanamid Canada Inc., Montreal, Quebec, Canada), was found to be pure and free of 70H-MTX after injection onto our HPLC system. 70H-MTX was detected at a concentration of 2.77 $\mu$mol/L in the 15-min sample after the beginning of the infusion. This is the earliest detection time reported to date.

The variability in the patient's 24-h and 48-h MTX and 70H-MTX concentrations in serum is demonstrated in Figure 2. Except for one course (discussed below), 24-h MTX serum concentrations were below the two-standard-deviation upper limit of 5.87 μmol/L [X (1 SD)=2.30 (1.79) μmol/L] observed in our laboratory over the past year after MTX infusions when the above protocol was followed. All 48-h MTX serum concentrations were also within the two-standard-deviation upper limit of 0.59 μmol/L [X (1 SD)=0.27 (0.16) μmol/L]. 70H-MTX levels appear to be more variable as seen in Figure 2. Our mean (1 SD) 70H-MTX serum concentrations for 24 h and 48 h are 35.37 (20.28) μmol/L and 8.92 (6.20) μmol/L, respectively.

The patient's 70H-MTX to MTX ratios at 24 h and 48 h are also presented in Figure 2. At 24 h her ratios were all within the one-standard-deviation range determined for our laboratory over the past year of 10-28 [X (1 SD) = 19 (9)]. However, at 48 h the ratios were widely distributed across and beyond our one-standard-deviation range of 14-64 [X (1 SD) = 39 (25)].

During the third course of chemotherapy, the patient was inadvertently given DXR a few hours prior to her HD-MTX therapy. Fortunately, no obvious clinical or biochemical adverse affects were observed. At 24 h postinfusion, both the MTX and 70H-MTX serum concentrations were above the two-standard-deviation upper limits. By 48 h postinfusion, the patient's ability to handle MTX had recovered and the MTX level was within the expected range, while

the 70H-MTX level was still slightly above the two-standard-deviation limit.

## MTX Pharmacology

When MTX binds competitively to the enzyme dihydrofolate reductase (DHFR) it blocks the production of reduced folates, and this deficiency results ultimately in the inhibition of DNA, RNA, and protein synthesis (2-4). Thus, the normal tissues which are most affected by MTX are those with a rapid cellular turnover and a high growth fraction, including the gastrointestinal tract, bone marrow, and skin. Renal and liver toxicities are additional complications which may occur. The severity of toxicity is directly proportional to the duration of MTX exposure above certain critical concentrations and this varies for each individual tissue. After HD-MTX

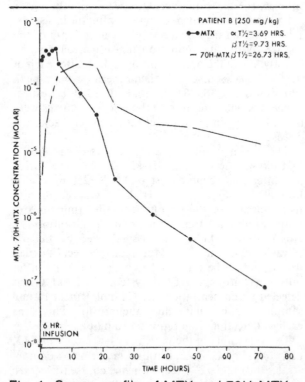

Fig. 1. Serum profile of MTX and 70H-MTX

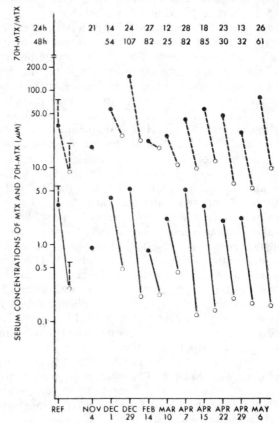

Fig. 2. Serum concentrations of MTX (———) and 70H-MTX ( - - - - ) at 24 h (●) and 48 h (o) after the start of the HD-MTX infusions

The HPLC reference ranges (REF) (+2 SD) from our laboratory are presented for comparison (the actual values are reported in the text). 70H-MTX ratios at 24 h and 48 h are also listed. The last course of chemotherapy is not presented in this graph as the analysis was not performed by HPLC but by EMIT®.

therapy these limits are likely to be exceeded, thus necessitating the use of the rescue agent leucovorin (LEU) to offset the increased frequency of toxic side reactions. As a reduced folate derivative, LEU replenishes the cellular pool of reduced folates, bypassing the MTX block distally, and thus rescuing the cells. Since serum concentrations below 1 $\mu$mol/L at 48 h posttherapy are generally associated with low incidences of toxicity (5), serum MTX monitoring can specify when LEU rescue can safely be discontinued and also identify patients with elevated antifolate levels in whom the standard LEU dosage may prove to be inadequate.

Renal dysfunction due to HD-MTX delays the clearance of the drug, which increases the likelihood of other toxicities occurring. Since precipitation of the drug within the renal tubules is the probable mechanism of the nephrotoxicity (6), it has been suggested that 70H-MTX, which is four times less soluble in urine than MTX, might be an important factor contributing to the nephropathy following HD-MTX therapy. In recent years, most of the nephrotoxicity associated with HD-MTX therapy has been averted by alkalinization of the urine and maintenance of a high urinary output (7). Alkalinization of the urine increases the solubility of MTX and 70H-MTX, as well as ionizing the drug within the renal tubules, thereby retarding its reabsorption and promoting its net renal clearance (2).

## Discussion

Early accounts of HD-MTX therapy reported that 28% of patients may develop prolonged myelosuppression (8), while as many as 6% (29/498) may die of complications associated directly with their drug therapy (9). Nephrotoxicity occurred frequently (17%), with the delayed MTX clearance resulting in failure of the leucovorin rescue and enhanced myelosuppression (8). Currently, renal damage is generally successfully averted through alkalinization of the urine and maintenance of a high urine flow. However, when it does occur, myelosuppression at least may be prevented by extended and more vigorous therapy with LEU (5). Thus, the monitoring of patients for the early detection of impending toxicity is essential (5, 10).

Renal function is commonly monitored through creatinine levels in plasma and/or creatinine clearance. However, the value of these measurements for the early detection of nephrotoxicity has been questioned (3, 5). Monitoring of MTX serum concentrations for the determination of adequate drug clearance has resulted in the definition of safety limits such as <1 $\mu$mol/L at 48 h postinfusion (4). Our patient had levels of <0.05 $\mu$mol/L at 48 h after every infusion,

including the one in which DXR was coadministered. Confirmation of a safe MTX concentration at 48 h following an elevated concentration at 24 h aided the clinicians in their decision regarding extended LEU rescue. 70H-MTX, however, was slightly beyond the acceptable limits at both 24 h and 48 h after this particular course of chemotherapy. The significance of 70H-MTX concentrations in serum is currently being evaluated, especially with respect to correlation with nephro-toxicity.

## References

1. Collier, C.P., MacLeod, S.M., and Soldin, S.J., Analysis of methotrexate and 7-hydroxymethotrexate by high performance liquid chromatography and preliminary clinical studies. *Ther. Drug Monit.*, 1982.
2. Bleyer, W.A., The clinical pharmacology of methotrexate. *Cancer* **41**, 36-51 (1978).
3. Chabner, B.A., Donehower, R.C., and Schilsky, R.L., Clinical pharmacology of methotrexate. *Cancer Treat. Rep.* **65**, 51-54 (1981).
4. White, J.C., Recent concepts on the mechanism of action of methotrexate. *Cancer Treat. Rep.* **65**, 3-12 (1981).
5. Stroller, R.G., Hande, K.R., Jacobs, S.A., Rosenberg, S.A. and Chabner, B.A., Use of plasma pharmacokinetics to predict and prevent methotrexate toxicity. *New Engl. J. Med.* **297**, 630-634 (1977).
6. Jacobs, S.A., Stroller, R.G., Chabner, B.A., and Johns, D.G., 7-Hydroxymethotrexate as a urinary metabolite in human subjects and Rhesus monkeys receiving high dose methotrexate. *J. Clin. Invest.* **57**, 534-538 (1976).
7. Sand, T.E., and Jacobsen, S., Effect of urine pH and flow on renal clearance of methotrexate. *Eur. J. Clin. Pharmacol.* **19**, 453-456 (1981).
8. Frei, E. III, Blum, R.H., Pitman, S.W., Kirkwood, J.M., Henderson, I.C., Skarin, A.T., Mayer, R.J., Bast, R.C., Gornick, M.B., Parker, L.M., and Canellos, G.P., High dose methotrexate with leucovorin rescue: Rationale and spectrum of antitumor activity. *Am. J. Med.* **68**, 370-376 (1980).
9. Van Hoff, D.D., Penta, J.S., and Helman, L.J., Incidence of drug-related deaths secondary to high-dose methotrexate and citrovorum factor administration. *Cancer Treat. Rep.* **61**, 745-748 (1977).
10. Evans, W.E., Pratt, C.B., Tayler, H., Barker, L.F., and Cran, W.R., Pharmacokinetic monitoring of high-dose methotrexate: Early recognition of high-risk patients. *Cancer Chemother. Pharmacol.* **3**, 161-166 (1979).

# VII. Other Drugs

# 51

# Antihypertensive Agents:
# The Role of Therapeutic Drug Monitoring

**Thomas P. Moyer, Ph.D.**

## Introduction

Hypertension, defined as a diastolic blood pressure exceeding 90 mmHg, under standard conditions on more than one occasion, has been identified in more than 10% of the adult American population. Primary (essential) hypertension represents the most common form of the disease, estimated to be the case in eight of every 10 hypertensive adults. Two major studies *(1,2)* have demonstrated that control of hypertension is associated with reduced incidence of cardiovascular disease. Putting these two factors together should lead one to the conclusion that effective control of hypertension would play an important role in improved health care in America.

Blood pressure is under control of numerous physiological factors. A partial listing would include: 1) the hormones aldosterone, angiotensin, and renin; 2) ionic homeostasis, recognized as the role of sodium, potassium, chloride, and plasma water; 3) the sympathetic nervous system, principally via the adrenergic amines; as well as more subtle humor factors such as 4) baroreceptors, autoregulators, and the central nervous system.

Aldosterone is a steroid synthesized in the adrenal cortex, often referred to as a "mineralocorticoid". Release of aldosterone is under control of the renin-angiotensin system in a manner that causes aldosterone excretion to be inversely proportional to extracellular fluid volume and total body sodium (Fig. 1). Aldosterone controls reabsorption of sodium and potassium in the distal tubule of the kidney; increased aldosterone causing increased reabsorption of sodium and exchange of sodium for potassium, thus enhanced potassium excretion. When serum sodium concentration is low or serum potassium is high, release of aldosterone stimulates the kidney to retain sodium and excrete potassium (the influence of potassium on aldosterone release is a direct effect, not mediated through the renin-angiotensin system). Aldosterone is also under limited control by corticotropin (ACTH) secreted by the pituitary, which in turn is under control by the central nervous system (CNS) via the hypothalamic

hormone corticoliberin (CRF).

Renin is a polypeptide synthesized and released by the juxtaglomerular cells of the kidney. A decrease in pressure within the afferent arterioles of the kidney, mechanically detected as the degree of stretch of blood vessel walls, will cause stimulation of glomerular cells (this function also occurs in the myocardium), which respond by releasing renin into the efferent arteriole. The mechanism is often referred to as the "baroreceptor" response to changes in blood pressure. Renin catalyzes the conversion of angiotensinogen to angiotensin I. As this compound passes through the lungs it is converted to the active agent, angiotensin II (Fig. 1). This octapeptide increases blood pressure in several ways. It has a direct effect upon smooth muscle angiotensin receptors which activate the sympathetic nervous system, resulting in constriction of peripheral arterioles. This results in an immediate increase in blood pressure. A second, long-term effect is stimulation of aldosterone synthesis and release from the adrenal cortex. As would be expected, these combined responses result in rhythmic increase in blood pressure; as pressure falls, the baroreceptor system stimulates release of renin to catalyze the conversion of angiotensinogen through several steps to angiotensin II. The immediate effect is a quick constriction of the peripheral vascular system followed by a slower response of aldosterone release, which results in reabsorption of sodium in exchange for potassium, with subsequent volume expansion and increased pressure.

Corticotropin is a polypeptide, synthesized in the pituitary gland and released from it under control of several factors. Direct feed-back inhibition by the concentration of free cortisol in the blood and central nervous system stimulation via hypothalamic release of corticoliberin are the major control mechanisms. Unfortunately, the role the corticotropin in primary hypertension is not well defined; it may well be a minor factor. "Elevated" ACTH concentrations in blood in primary hypertension are generally not demonstrable.

Hypertension is associated not only with the concentration of sodium in blood, but has also been related to the concentration of sodium in the arterial wall. Several workers *(3,4)* related the effect of thiazide diuretics not only to enhanced excretion of sodium, but also to a redistribution of sodium in the arterial wall, which resulted in decreased vascular resistance. These

---

*Dr. Moyer is Consultant in Laboratory Medicine, Mayo Clinic, and Assistant Professor of Laboratory Medicine, Mayo Medical School, Rochester, Minnesota.*

observations have been used to explain a phenomenon commonly observed in the use of thiazide diuretics: initial decrease in total fluid volume followed by a rebound to normal fluid volume several weeks after initiation of thiazide therapy. With decreased vascular resistance, fluid volume may return to normal, but decreased blood pressure is maintained.

## Review of the Common Drugs

### Diuretics

***Thiazides.*** The benzothiadiazides and their related sulfonamides are well-absorbed drugs which inhibit the reabsorption of sodium and chloride in the distal convoluted tubule and the ascending limb of the loop of Henle (Fig. 1). Most recently, several authors have demonstrated that they also have their effect by decreasing the sodium concentration in the arterial wall, which allows the vessel to be more elastic and hence less resistant to blood flow *(3)*. Table 1 lists the commonly used thiazide and sulfonamide diuretics, common dosage, time of peak concentrations in plasma, and half-life. While plasma concentrations are measurable *(5,6)*, a therapeutic concentration has not been established nor has a need for monitoring been indicated. Owing to the variable bioavailability of the various preparations available, Beerman et al. *(6)* and Shah and Needham *(7)* have suggested that there may be greater efficacy in monitoring concentrations of thiazide diuretics in urine, with the only demonstrable need for doing so being to ensure compliance or demonstrate inadvertent or intentional abuse. Screening methods are available *(8)*.

The major clinical complication of diuretic use (except in the case of potassium-sparing diuretics discussed below) is hypokalemia. Sodium is exchanged for hydrogen and potassium in the distal tubule of the kidney (Fig. *1*). If diuretics are used, urinary sodium excretion will be greater than normal. In the distal tubule, a free, uncontrolled exchange occurs and if the excretion of urinary sodium is higher than normal, a greater degree of potassium exchange occurs, resulting in depletion of total body potassium (including plasma) and retention of extracellular sodium. Thus, frequent monitoring of plasma potassium is common when diuretics are used. The maintenance of a plasma potassium concentration >3.5 mmol/L, associated with controlled hypertension, is the best index of adequate therapy. In certain cases of resistant hypertension, when diuretic dosage must be increased, potassium supplementation may be necessary. To avoid the use of potassium supplementation, clinicians place most patients on a sodium-restricted diet, which results in lower urinary sodium excretion, less exchange, and normokalemia without

supplementation.

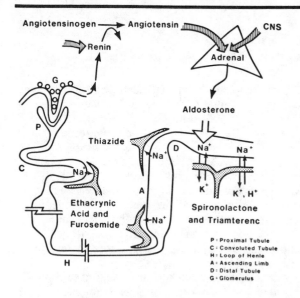

**Fig. 1.** Schematic representation of the renal tubular anatomy, depicting sites of action of antihypertensive agents

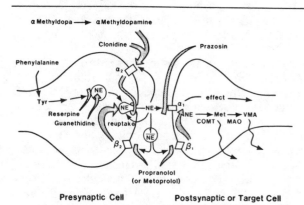

**Fig. 2.** Schematic representation of the adrenergic neuron (site undefined), depicting the sites of action of antihypertensive agents

***Furosemide and ethacrynic acid.*** . These loop-of-Henle diuretics inhibit reabsorption of sodium in the convoluted tubule and in the ascending limb of Henle (Fig. 1). Both of these drugs can produce hypokalemia. Their biological half-lives are much shorter than is true of thiazides (Table 1). Furosemide is used for the control of hypertension associated with chronic renal disease. Guidance for therapeutic monitoring purposes is the same as indicated above for thiazides. Analytical methods are available *(9)*.

***Spironolactone and triamterene.*** The potassium-sparing diuretics are spironolactone, which specifically competes for mineralocorticoid-receptor binding sites in the distal tubule of the kidney, and triamterene, which actively inhibits exchange of sodium for potassium in the renal tubule, but not by competing for aldosterone binding sites. Their action is such that the free exchange of sodium for potassium in the distal tubule, which leads to hypokalemia in thiazide blockade of sodium reabsorption, does not occur, resulting in maintenance of the normokalemic state while sodium reabsorption is blocked. The natriuresis provoked by these diuretics is small, because they act late in the sequence of sodium reabsorption. Usually these drugs are used in conjunction with another diuretic (thiazide) to enhance natriuresis. Overdosage with potassium-sparing diuretics usually results in hyperkalemia, thus serum potassium is the important analyte to consider when monitoring therapy with these drugs. There is no demonstrable case for monitoring concentrations of these drugs in the blood.

## β -Blockers

***Propranolol*** (Inderal, Ayerst) was introduced in 1976 in the United States for control of hypertension. Since then, it has become one of the leading agents used to reduce blood pressure. Although classified as a "β-blocker" (it will block the action of a receptor protein which, when stimulated, causes the release of norepinephrine from postsynaptic nerve cells), it has more than one mechanism of action. Blockade of the β-receptor results in diminished release of norepinephrine or decreased sensitivity to its release. Propranolol, as a β-blocker, diminishes release of norepinephrine from the presynaptic nerve cell (Fig. 2). The reader should be cautioned from drawing the conclusion that decreased norepinephrine release results in decreased vascular muscle tone, resulting in decreased blood pressure. Things are not quite that simple. Michelakis and McAllister *(10)* and Buhler et al. *(11)* proposed that propranolol's mechanism of action was not via relief of vascular tension, but rather by suppressing release of renin. This work has been confirmed by Hollifield et al. *(12)* and by Nies and Shand *(13)*, who suggested that β-blockade was significant when propranolol concentration in blood was 100 μg/L six hours after the dose.

There appears to be considerable interindividual variability in the concentration in blood required for maintainance of adequate antihypertensive activity. Factors influencing this variability include: 1) the high rate of "first-pass" metabolism of propranolol. Propranolol in low orally administered doses is quickly and almost completely metabolized. One of its active metabolites, 4-hydroxypropranolol, has been identified as a possible reason for the interindividual variability. When the dose of propranolol is increased, metabolism and uptake is quickly saturated, and substantial concentrations of propranolol can be measured in the blood. Propranolol in a dosage of 30 mg/day will in a normal adult result in negligible propranolol concentrations in blood, but 4-hydroxypropranolol is present (20 μg/L). At 80 mg/day, the propranolol concentrations becomes significant (100 μg/L in a average individual, 6 h after dose) while 4-hydroxypropranolol concentration does not change (10-20 μg/L). Recently, Walle et al. *(14)* confirmed this inverse relationship between propranolol and 4-hydroxypropranolol blood concentration and daily dosage. They also identified another important metabolite to be considered, 4-hydroxypropranolol glucuronide. 2) Total binding of propranolol by serum proteins in the normal subject amounts to 90-95%. A substantial portion of the population taking propranolol for hypertension control will have some compromised renal or hepatic function, resulting in some interindividual variability in the percentage of the drug that is bound to protein. This, coupled with the observation that a change in percent protein saturation of binding capacity from 90 to 95% results in a twofold decrease in free drug concentration could also explain the interindividual variability observed in the dosing of propranolol. 3) Variability can also be attributed to the interplay of the influence of β-blockade and suppression of renin release in the control of hypertension by propranolol.

While numerous authors have demonstrated a direct relation between drug concentration in blood and β-blockade *(10-13)*, it is difficult to define a therapeutic range for control of hypertension. Some hypertensives

### Table 1. Commonly Used Diuretics

| Diuretic | Usual daily dose, mg | Average half-life, h | Duration of effect, h |
|---|---|---|---|
| Chlorothiazide | 500-2000 | 4 | 6-12 |
| Hydrochlorothiazide | 25-100 | 4 | 6-12 |
| Benzthiazide | 25-50 | 6 | 6-18 |
| Hydroflumethiazide | 25-50 | 10 | 12-24 |
| Bendroflumethiazide | 2-5 | 10 | 18-24 |
| Cyclothiazide | 1-6 | 12 | 18-24 |
| Polythiazide | 4-8 | 18 | 24-36 |
| Ethacrynic acid | 100 | 2 | 6-8 |
| Furosemide | 60 | 6 | 6-10 |
| Spironolactone | 100 | 4 | 6-8 |
| Triamterene | 200 | 6 | 7-10 |
| Chlorthalidone | 25-100 | 48 | 48-72 |

will require circulating concentrations as high as 300 $\mu$g/L for adequate control, others only 100 $\mu$g/L (concentration 6 h after the dose). In either case, it should be noted that propranolol is a relatively safe drug, that there is much interindividual variation in concentrations achieved, and that propranolol is readily metabolized in the liver. Dosage schedules should not be designed with the aim of attaining a specific concentration in the blood; rather, decisions as to dosage should be made on clinical grounds. The principal value of therapeutic drug monitoring lies in identifying the optimum concentration in blood once control has been achieved. Once this target value had been identified for a particular patient, it serves as a reference point for future treatment. Should the patient return at a later date with increased blood pressure, one can quickly establish whether the current drug concentration is near the "target" value established previously (i.e., this is a check of patient compliance). If blood pressure has increased significantly and the plasma propranolol concentration is at the "target" concentration, the existence of a new clinical condition not obvious at the previous workup should be suspected.

**Metoprolol** (Lopresor, Geigy) was introduced for use in the United States in 1978. It has antihypertensive properties similar to propranolol, with certain additional advantages, and its side effects are either not as significant or differ from those of propranolol. To discuss metoprolol, the subclasses of $\beta$-adrenoceptors must be mentioned. $\beta_1$-Adrenergic receptors are associated with cardiac and lipolytic functions; $\beta_2$-adrenoceptors are defined as associated with bronchodilatory and vasodilatory activity. Both propranolol and metoprolol have $\beta_1$ blocking activity, but propranolol also possesses some $\beta_2$ blocking activity. Metoprolol in low doses does not. Thus the unwanted side effects often experienced with propranolol—bronchoconstriction and vasoconstriction—are not a problem when metopolol is used, and thus metoprolol has become popular for use in patients with acute or chronic obstructive pulmonary disease, and in treating hypertension.

The metabolism of metoprolol is like that of propranolol in certain respects. It undergoes significant first-pass metabolism when taken orally. Unlike propranolol, however, only 10-15% of metoprolol is protein bound. It has a biological half-life in the blood of normal adults of 4-5 h, and its metabolites are less active than the parent drug — they play no significant role except in cases of renal impairment. While there is a correlation between decrease of heart rate and blood concentration, studies have failed to demonstrate a correlation between drug concentration and the associated antihypertensive effect of metoprolol (15). The

average normal adult taking 200 mg of metoprolol per day will have a drug concentration of 50-100 $\mu$g/L two h after an oral dose.

## $\alpha$-Agonists

Receptor proteins that cause decreased release of norepinephrine when stimulated are defined as $\alpha$-adrenoceptors. These receptors can be located either presynaptically or postsynaptically and are classified by well-defined criteria outlined in the excellent review article by Weinshilboum (16). The three most commonly used $\alpha$-agonists, $\alpha$-methyldopa, clonidine, and prazosin, are reviewed here.

***Clonidine*** (Catapres, Boehringer Ingelheim) is an $\alpha$-adrenoceptor agonistic, which decreases the release of norepinephrine from presynaptic nerve cells in the central nervous system and in the peripheral arteriolar adrenergic system. The decreased blood pressure produced by clonidine is associated with a decrease in heart rate. The effect is maximum at concentrations of 0.5-2 $\mu$g/L of plasma (17,18). Concentrations greater than 2 $\mu$g/L induce sleep, an effect that decreases during chronic therapy.

The action of clonidine has been related to decreased renin release (19), an effect mediated by an adrenergic mechanism, as substantiated when clonidine failed to alter renin release after denervation of the kidney. Direct injection of clonidine into the central nervous system resulted in a decrease in renin secretion (20).

Clonidine is rapidly and completely absorbed, reaching peak plasma concentrations in 1-2 h. It is concentrated in most tissues, the highest concentrations being found in spleen and submaxillary glands. The concentration in brain tissue is about twice that in plasma (21). Clonidine is 50% protein bound and has a half-life in plasma of 20 h in humans. It is readily metabolized by the liver, the principal metabolites being $p$-hydroxyclonidine (an active metabolite), $p$-hydroxyclonidine glucuronide, and 2,6-(diphenyl)guanidine.

Methods for therapeutic drug monitoring are available (22), although few applications have been documented.

***$\alpha$-Methyldopa*** (Aldomet, Merck Sharpe and Dohme) for many years was thought to be a "false neurotransmitter", causing a decrease in blood pressure by blocking the amine receptor on the postsynaptic side of the neuron. In 1973, Van Zweiten (23) discovered that decarboxylation of $\alpha$-methyldopa was necessary for the hypotensive effect of the drug, that the metabolites $\alpha$-methyldopamine and $\alpha$-methylnorepinephrine were the active components, that their site of action was in the central nervous system, and that they acted not as postsynaptic $\alpha$-agonists, but instead as presynaptic α-agonists (Fig. 2). Quite recently, O'Dea and Mirkin *(24)* demonstrated a correlation between the increased concentration of α-methyldopamine in the blood of patients with renal failure and an exaggerated hypotensive action associated with α-methyldopa. That these findings would be observed was predicted earlier by Freed et al. *(25)*. Concentration of α-methyldopamine in the blood of normal individuals are <20 μg/L; renally impaired patients display concentrations of 0.2 to 0.4 mg/L. O'Dea and Mirkin *(24)* also observed a good correlation between concentration of the sulfate esters of both α-methyldopa and α-methyldopamine in blood, but these compounds are not neuroactive.

There is no correlation between the magnitude of the decline in blood pressure and the concentration in plasma of α-methyldopa (0.2 to 4 mg/L) or its sulfate esters *(26)*. In contrast, Freed et al. *(25)* demonstrated a good correlation between concentrations of α-methyldopamine in cerebrospinal fluid and depressed neurotransmitter (norepinephrine) release, and this observation was associated with the subsequent hypotensive action expected of α-methyldopa.

The biological half-life of α-methyldopa is 2 h, but the antihypertensive effect of the drug may be observed for up to 24 h after a single dose, which also suggests that its action is mediated through one or more active metabolites. One must conclude that measuring circulating concentrations of α-methyldopa is of no value in therapeutic monitoring . Analysis for α-methyldopamine, the active metabolite, in blood in possible *(24)*, but a direct correlation of such measurement with hypotensive action has yet to be demonstrated. The pharmacokinetics of α-methyldopamine are complex, so therapeutic monitoring will require significant consultative support for it to prove useful.

*Prazosin* (Minipress, Pfizer), an aminoquinazoline, is an α-adrenergic blocking drug that acts principally on the peripheral arterial smooth muscle, resulting in decreased total peripheral resistance (Fig. 2). The capacity of prazosin to block postsynaptic α-adrenoceptors selectively means that during therapy with the drug, released norepinephrine can combine with presynaptic α-receptors and inhibit further release of norepinephrine. This may explain the relative lack of tachycardia or increased renin release observed when prazosin is used *(16)*.

Prazosin was introduced in Europe in 1974 and became available in the United States in 1976. It is readily absorbed, is 90-95% protein bound with a biological half-life in blood of 3-5 h. It undergoes significant "first-pass" hepatic metabolism. Peak concentrations in blood of 20 μg/L are reached in 1-2 h *(32)*.

The principal side-effects of prazosin, as would be anticipated for any α-blocking drug, are postural dizziness (but not hypotension), headache, drowsiness, and weakness. These symptoms are generally not as severe as with other antihypertensive drugs such as α-methyldopa. While methods for therapeutic monitoring are available *(32)*, the role of therapeutic monitoring has not yet been defined. Perhaps as use of this drug becomes more common, the role of monitoring therapy by measuring blood concentrations will become important.

## Neuron Blocking Agents

*Guanethidine* (Ismelin, Ciba) is a drug that is commonly used in conjunction with other hypertensive agents because its effects alone, although adequate to control hypertension, are usually accompanied by excessive side effects. When used in conjunction with a diuretic, it has been demonstrated to be an effective antihypertensive agent at doses low enough to produce few side effects. Guanethidine is poorly absorbed: only about 10 to 30% of the dose finally reaches the blood. That which is absorbed is about 50% metabolized upon the first pass through the liver, and the metabolites are generally inactive. Guanethidine is concentrated in tissues and excreted via a multicompartment mechanism; its biological half-life is five days. Infusion of 10 mg of guanethidine per kilogram body weight results in initial concentrations of 30 mg/L of plasma. Two hours after infusion, this concentration is 0.5 mg/L, and the trough concentration is 5 μg/L *(27)*. Concentration in plasma and adrenergic blockade correlate well *(27,28)*. Trough blood concentrations >8 mg/L were associated with a high degree of sympathetic blockade and side effects. Concentrations >15 μg/L resulted in complete blockade, and all patients displayed undesirable side effects (postural hypotension, diarrhea, fatigue, and nasal stuffiness). Guanethidine acts by displacing norepinephrine from the storage vesicles (Fig. 2) in the peripheral adrenergic neuron. This action appears to be selective for norepinephrine storage vesicles of the sympathetic nervous system; the effect was not observed in the adrenal medulla. Drugs that block uptake of norepinephrine, such as tricyclic antidepressants, inhibit the effect of guanethidine by blocking its uptake.

*Reserpine* (many suppliers) was the first antihypertensive drug introduced into clinical medicine. It was first reported to have antihypertensive activity nearly 50 years ago *(29)*. Reserpine acts by blocking amine uptake into the amine storage vesicle in brain, heart, adrenals, spleen, platelets, and mast cells in a manner that is generally irreversible. Once reserpine binds to the membrane of the vesicle, no more catecholamine can be stored. This has been demonstrated by decreases in tissue catecholamine concentration *(28)*. The drug does not display normal pharmacokinetics. Its apparent half-life in plasma is short (30 min) but its therapeutic effect may last for days. For this reason, therapeutic monitoring of reserpine has not been common, although methods *(30)* are available, and peak concentrations between 0.4-3.5 $\mu$g/L of plasma have been observed. Because the drug is membrane bound, and is active in this form, studies to define a therapeutic effect have not been successful *(31)*.

## Vasodilators

*Hydralazine* (many suppliers), a vasodilatory drug, acts directly on the arterial smooth muscle, resulting in dilation of blood vessels. Hydralazine causes an increased heart rate and cardiac output, stimulates renin release, and is associated with sodium retention and volume expansion. Thus, therapy with hydralazine is usually accompanied by a diuretic and a drug that slows heart rate, most commonly propranolol. The mechanism of action of hydralazine is not well understood. It appears that hydralazine is concentrated in blood vessel walls and in some way inhibits metalloenzymes by selectively binding the metal needed for activation, usually copper *(28)*. The enzymes involved are those identified as associated with tyrosine metabolism.

Hydralazine is rapidly absorbed and is 87-90% bound to plasma protein. It has a half-life in plasma of 2-3 h, and at equilibrium, concentrations of 0.1 to 0.8 mg/L were found to correlate with control of hypertension *(33,34)*. One of the principal metabolites is *N*-acetylhydralazine, and therefore one would expect a genetic dependence of drug disposition, and this indeed has been demonstrated *(34)*. As also identified in treatment with procainamide, a lupus-erythematosus-like syndrome develops in slow acetylators. This syndrome disappears when the drug is discontinued. Toxicity from hydralazine is dose- and blood-concentration related. Symptoms of toxicity include occipital headache, flushing, nausea, vomiting, tachycardia, palpitation, and angina in patients with coronary heart disease. Edema is common.

## Conclusion

The drugs reviewed here can be divided into five categories: 1) drugs for which therapeutic drug monitoring plays (or will play) a role in improved therapy; 2) drugs that theoretically should lend themselves well to therapeutic monitoring, but results do not correlate with the clinical situation as well as would be expected; 3) in-

active parent drugs that are metabolized to active intermediates, these lending themselves to therapeutic monitoring; 4) drugs that are safe and effective, and therefore require infrequent therapeutic monitoring; and 5) drugs for which there is no correlation between pharmacologic role and blood concentration.

*Category 1.* Prazosin, guanethidine, hydralazine, and clonidine have defined blood concentrations that correlate with their antihypertensive effect. Their concentrations in blood can be determined by currently available techniques, although these must be highly sensitive. These drugs display normal pharmacokinetic properties and their undesirable side effects can be expected when their concentrations in the blood exceed a defined limit. Interestingly two of the above four drugs have been available for years, but interest has developed only recently in measuring their concentrations routinely.

*Category 2.* Propranolol and metoprolol are drugs that have well-defined pharmacokinetic properties, yet the circulating concentrations of these drugs, even when combined with information on their metabolite concentrations, correlate poorly with the observed antihypertensive effect. This probably is attributable to interindividual variations in metabolism, protein binding, tissue distribution, and multiple mechanisms of action.

*Category 3.* $\alpha$-Methyldopa is a drug that is itself inactive. Current data suggest that the antihypertensive activity associated with $\alpha$-methyldopa is mediated by its metabolite, $\alpha$-methyldopamine, There appears to be a correlation between the concentration of $\alpha$-methyldopamine in blood and antihypertensive effect, but sensitive techniques are required to measure clinically significant concentrations of this analyte. These techniques are now available, and an increased interest in the ability to measure this analyte should be anticipated.

*Category 4.* Diuretics are drugs that are quite safe to use. The dosage of these drugs can easily be adjusted based upon the hypotensive response. The major problem associated with their use, hypokalemia, can easily be monitored by following serum potassium. The only use for therapeutic monitoring is to confirm patient compliance or abuse of the drug.

*Category 5.* Reserpine is the only drug reviewed here for which the role of therapeutic monitoring is negligible. The drug is highly membrane bound and is still active when so bound. Some attempts have been made to correlate dosage with decrease in tissue catecholamine content, but this practice is not common, nor are sufficient data available to document its general use.

My intent here has been to review briefly the application of therapeutic drug monitoring to the drugs most commonly used for control of essential hypertension. For more detailed pharmacokinetic data on each drug, readers are referred to the text by Gross (28) and the review by Israili (31). I have not dealt with the drugs used for control of hypertension resulting from renal failure, endocrine diseases, neoplasma, or other causes of secondary hypertension.

Recent knowledge of the biochemistry and physiology of the neuron, the baroreceptor system, and the impact of the central nervous system on the hypertension control factors has provided guidelines for design of new, more effective drugs specifically for control of hypertension that are safe and effective. With this increased knowledge has come the information needed to identify the critical analytes necessary to derive therapeutic drug monitoring information. More effective drugs, combined with the ability to monitor therapy when necessary, should result in better control of essential hypertension and improved health care in America.

## References

1. The Hypertension Detection and Follow-up Program Cooperative Group, Five-year findings of the hypertension detection and follow-up program. *J. Am. Med. Assoc.* **242,** 2562-2571 (1979).
2. Kannel, W.B., Sorlie, P., Castelli, W.P., and McGee, D., Blood pressure and survival after myocardial infarction: The Framingham study. *Am. J. Cardiol.* **45,** 326-330 (1980).
3. Cannon, M.L., Tannenbaum, R.P., and LaFranco, M., Diuretics in the treatment of hypertension. *Am. Pharm.* **18,** 34-40 (1978).
4. Laragh, J.H., A new and exciting look at hypertension. *Lab. Manage.* 31-39 (Nov. 1979).
5. Cooper, M.J., Sinaiko, A.R., Anders, M.W., and Mirkin, B.L., High pressure liquid chromatographic determination of hydrochlorothiazide in human serum and urine. *Anal. Chem.* **48,** 1110-1111 (1976).
6. Beerman, B., Groschinsky-Grind, M., and Lindstrom, B., Bioavailability of two hydrochlorothiazide preparations. *Eur. J. Clin. Pharmacol.* **11,** 203-205 (1977).
7. Shah, K.A., and Needham, T.E., Correlation of

urinary excretion with *in vitro* dissolution using several dissolution methods for hydrochlorothiazide formulations. *J. Pharmaceut. Sci.* **68,** 1486-1490 (1979).
8. Tisdall, P.A., Moyer, T.P., and Anhalt, J.P., Liquid-chromatographic detection of thiazide diuretics in urine. *Clin. Chem.* **26,** 702-706 (1980).
9. Moyer, T.P., Tisdall, P.A., and Anhalt, J.P., Simultaneous detection of thiazide diuretics, furosemide and ethacrynic acid in urine using liquid chromatography. In preparation.
10. Michelakis, A.M., and McAllister, R.G., The effect of chronic adrenergic receptor blockade on plasma renin activity in man. *J. Clin. Endocrinol. Metab.* **32,** 386-394 (1972).
11. Buhler, F.R., Laragh, J.H., Vaughan, E.D., et al. Antihypertensive action of propranolol. *Am. J. Cardiol.* **32,** 511-522 (1973).
12. Hollifield, J.W., Sherman, K., Vander Zwagg, R., and Shand, D.G., Proposed mechanisms of propranolol's antihypertensive effect in essential hypertension. *N. Engl. J. Med.* **295,** 68-73 (1976).
13. Nies, A.S., and Shand, D.G., Clinical pharmacology of propranolol. *Circulation* **52,** 6-15 (1976).
14. Walle, T., Conradi, E.C., Walle, U.K., et al., 4-Hydroxypropranolol and its glucuronide after single and long-term, doses of propranolol. *Clin. Pharmacol. Ther.* **27,** 22-31 (1980).
15. Koch-Weser, J., Drug therapy: Metoprolol. *N. Engl. J. Med.* **301,** 698-703 (1979).
16. Weinshilboum, R.M., Antihypertensive drugs that alter adrenergic function. *Mayo Clin. Proc.* **55,** 390-402 (1980).
17. Davies, D.S., Wing, L.M.H., Reid, J.L., et al., Pharmacokinetics and concentration-effect relationships of intravenous and oral clonidine. *Clin. Pharmacol. Ther.* **21,** 593-601 (1977).
18. Wing, L.H.M., Reid, J.L., Davies, D.S., et al., Pharmacokinetic and concentration-effect relationship of clonidine in essential hypertension. *Eur. J. Clin. Pharmacol.* **12,** 463-469 (1977).
19. Reid, I.A., MacDonald, D.M., Pachnis, B., and Ganong, W.F., Studies concerning the mechanism of suppression of renin secretion by clonidine. *J. Pharmacol. Exp. Ther.* **192,** 713-721 (1975).
20. Onesti, G., Schwartz, A.B., Kim, K.E., et al., Antihypertensive effect of clonidine. *Circ. Res.* **28,** Suppl. 2, 53-69 (1971).
21. Cho, A.K., and Curry, S.H., The physiological disposition of 2-(2,6-dichloroanilino)-2-imidazoline (St-155). *Biochem. Pharmacol.* **18,** 511-520 (1969).

22. Draffan, G.H., Clare, R.A., Murray, E., et al., The determination of clonidine in human plasma. *Proc. 3rd. Int. Symp. Mass Spectrom. Biochem. Med.,* Sardinia, Italy (1975).

23. Van Zweiten, P.A., The central action of antihypertensive drugs, mediated via central α-receptors. *J. Pharm. Pharmacol.* **25,** 89-95 (1973).

24. O'Dea, R.F., and Mirkin, B.L., Metabolic disposition of methyldopa in hypertensive and renal-insufficient children. *Clin. Pharmacol. Ther.* **27,** 37-43 (1980).

25. Freed, C.R., Quintero, E., and Murphy, R.C., Hypotension and hypothalamic amine metabolism after long-term α-methyldopa infusions. *Life Sci.* **23,** 313-322 (1978).

26. Saavedra, J.A., Reid, J.L., Jordan, W., et al., Plasma concentration of α-methyldopa and sulphate conjugate after oral administration of methyldopa and intravenous administration of methyldopa and methyldopa hydrochloride ethyl ester. *Eur. J. Clin. Pharmacol.* **8,** 381-386 (1975).

27. Walter, I.E., Khandelwal, J., Falkner, F., and Nies, A.S., The relationship of plasma guanethidine levels to adrenergic blockade. *Clin. Pharmacol. Ther.* **18,** 571-580 (1975).

28. *Antihypertensive Agents* (F. Gross, Ed.), *Handbook of Experimental Pharmacology,* **39,** Springer-Verlag, New York, NY, 1977.

29. Sen, G., and Bose, K.C., *Rawolfia serpentina,* a new Indian drug for insanity and high blood pressure. *Indian Med. World* **2,** 194-201 (1931).

30. Tripp, S.L., Williams, E., Wagner, W.E., and Lukas, G., A specific assay for subnanogram concentrations of reserpine in human plasma. *Life Sci.* **16,** 1167-1178 (1975).

31. Israili, Z.H., Correlation of pharmacological effects with plasma levels of antihypertensive drugs in man. *Ann. Rev. Pharmacol. Toxicol.* **19,** 25-52 (1979).

32. Verbesselt, R.M., Mullie, A., and Tjandramaga, T.G., The effect of food intake on the plasma kinetics and tolerance of prazosin. *Acta Ther.* **2,** 27-35 (1976).

33. Zacest, R., and Koch-Weser, J., Relationship of hydralazine plasma concentration to dosage and hypotension. *Clin. Pharmacol. Ther.* **13,** 420-425 (1972).

34. Zacest, R., and Stanley, R.E., The influence of acetylation phenotype on plasma hydralazine levels in man following oral and intravenous administration. In *Recent Advances in Hypertension.* R. Milliey and M. Safos, Eds., pp 343-350, Boehringer, New York, NY (1975).

# 52

# Hydrochlorothiazide: A Case Study

**Alexander G. Logan, M.D.**
**Steven J. Soldin, Ph.D.**

With current antihypertensive medication it is now possible to control hypertension in almost all instances. A failure to decrease blood pressure is most often due to poor compliance with drug therapy. In this regard, only about 65% of hypertensive patients consume enough of their prescribed medication to achieve adequate blood-pressure reduction (1,2).

Although there are now many strategies for improving patient compliance (3), quantitative measures of compliance are not available to most practicing physicians. Of the many methods to measure compliance, assessment of drug concentrations in body fluids is probably the most reliable and simplest. Asking patients about their compliance with therapy, although easy, will not detect the 50 to 60% of noncompliant individuals who do not admit to low compliance (4). Pill counts are not practical, because it is necessary to do a home visit to get the required information on compliance. Therapeutic response has not been found to be useful as a way to assess compliance (5).

Diuretics remain the cornerstone of antihypertensive drug therapy. In recent personal interviews with 75 Toronto general practitioners, 85% stated that they prescribed a diuretic as the drug of first choice in the treatment of hypertension. Furthermore, in a recently completed randomized controlled trial, 82% of hypertensive patients for whom drug therapy had been prescribed by their family doctor were taking hydrochlorothiazide, alone or in combination (2). Finally, the United States Joint National Committee on Antihypertensive Care advocates a thiazide diuretic as the first-line drug for antihypertensive therapy (6).

## Case Study

A 36-year-old man was referred to the Hypertension Clinic for evaluation of severe hypertension.

## Past History

This patient was first discovered to have hypertension 14 years ago. Although he was then started on antihypertensive drug therapy, he failed to renew his prescription or to return for follow-up assessment. Ten years

*Dr. Logan and Dr. Soldin are in the Departments of Medicine, Pharmacology and Clinical Biochemistry, University of Toronto, Hospital for Sick Children, and Mount Sinai Hospital, Toronto.*

later, at a pre-employment physical examination, his blood pressure again was noted to be above normal. He eventually saw his family physician, primarily because of an acute attack of gout. His blood pressure at that time was 190/140 mm Hg, and for this reason he was strongly advised to be admitted for investigation. For personal reasons he postponed his scheduled admission to the hospital for five months. When he was finally admitted, no secondary cause of hypertension was found and it was believed that his gross obesity was aggravating the hypertensive state.

After discharge from the hospital, his blood pressure remained poorly controlled despite antihypertensive drug therapy that included at different times hydrochlorothiazide, spironolactone, methyldopa, hydralazine, and propranolol. Furthermore, attempts at weight reduction were also unsuccessful. Although poor medication compliance was suspected, the patient maintained that he was following the prescribed drug regimen.

## Present Assessment

The patient was quite obese, weighed 116.5 kg and his blood pressure was 170/130 mm Hg in the sitting position. His pulse rate was 96 beats per minute and regular. Funduscopic examination revealed severe arteriolar narrowing but no exudates or hemorrhages. Although his heart was enlarged, there was no evidence of congestive heart failure. There was no abdominal bruit, and all peripheral pulses were palpable.

Laboratory examination revealed normal values for serum potassium and creatinine. Blood sugar, measured after a fast, was 1.82 g/L. The patient also had a secondary type IV hyperlipoproteinemia. The 24-h urine sodium excretion, a measure of salt intake, was high, 361 mmol/day.

This patient was initially treated with propranolol, 160 mg twice daily, and hydrochlorothiazide, 50 mg daily, to which apresoline, 100 mg twice daily, was later added. On this drug regimen his blood pressure declined to 130/100 mm Hg, but neither his weight nor the daily sodium excretion changed, despite repeated dietary instructions.

Shortly thereafter this patient's blood pressure increased to 200/160 mm Hg. For this reason, even though he was asymptomatic, he was admitted to the hospital for treatment. His blood pressure declined to 140/95 mm Hg on the same drug regimen prescribed to treat his hypertension as an outpatient. Figure 1 illustrates the results of the pharmacokinetic study of oral hydrochlorothiazide administration. Results of urinary catecholamine studies were normal.

In follow-up assessment, the patient's blood pressure, although initially normal, increased to 180/130 mm Hg. Blood was drawn and urine samples collected for hydrochlorothiazide assay; the analyses revealed no detectable hydrochlorothiazide in either serum or urine. When questioned again about his drug compliance, he admitted that he often had difficulty remembering to take his medication. By getting the patient to associate medication consumption with daily habits, compliance improved, as was evidenced by the then adequate concentrations of hydrochlorothiazide found in serum and urine specimens. His blood pressure remained under good control.

This case illustrates the importance of detecting poor compliance with prescribed drug therapy so that steps can be taken to overcome problems of noncompliance. Monitoring the therapeutic effect of a drug does not allow one to differentiate compliance problems from other factors that can influence clinical response.

Insufficient drug dosage, use of biologically ineffective agents, or poor drug bioavailability, or some combination of these may explain the lack of desired therapeutic effect. Moreover, there may be a good response to therapy despite poor compliance with a prescribed regimen that is greater than needed, or non-drug factors such as the placebo effect.

Although poor compliance should be strongly suspected in this case because of the patient's failure to keep appointments and to lose weight, the ability of physicians to predict future compliance with drug therapy has been shown to be poor (4). Thus, the development of simple and accurate measures of compliance by directly measuring serum and urinary drug concentrations should facilitate management of outpatients with chronic conditions.

### Characterization of Hydrochlorothiazide Mechanism of Drug Action

It is widely held that the antihypertensive effect of thiazide diuretics may be ascribed to two mechanisms. They lower blood pressure at first by depleting sodium, later by reducing the tone of precapillary arterioles,

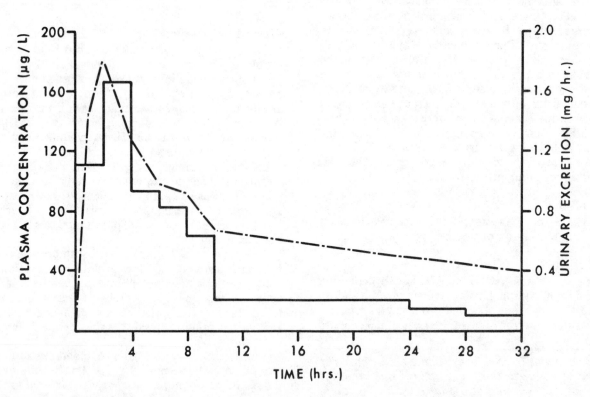

**Fig. 1.** Variation of drug concentrations in serum with time (— · —) and urinary drug excretion pattern (—) in a patient given a single 25 mg dose of hydrochlorothiazide, orally.

## HYDROCHLOROTHIAZIDE PROFILE

| | |
|---|---|
| **Generic name:** | Hydrochlorothiazide |
| **Chemical name:** | 6-chloro-7-sulfamyl-3, 4-dihydro-2H-1,2,4-benzothiadiazine-1, 1-dioxide |

**Chemical structure:**

| | |
|---|---|
| **Trade names:** | Hydrazide, Hydrid, Hydro-Aquil, Hydrodiuril, Novohydrazide, Hydrosaluret, Apo-Hydrochlorothiazide, Hydrodiuretex, Chemhydrazide, Esidrix Hydrozide, Urozide, Neocodema |
| **Relative molecular mass:** | 297.72 |
| **Melting point:** | 273-275° C |
| **Solubility in water:** | Practically insoluble. |
| **pK** | 7.0, 9.2 |
| **Dose absorption —** | |
| time to peak plasma concn, h: | 1.5 to 5.0 |
| percentage dose absorbed: | 65 to 72% |
| **Protein binding —** | |
| percentage bound: | About 93% |
| percentage free: | About 7% |
| **Tissue distribution Vd, L/kg:** | Not available |
| **Urinary excretion, % daily dose as unchanged drug:** | 65 to 72% |

### Clinical Pharmacology (9, 10, 11)

| | |
|---|---|
| **Recommended dose (mg/kg per d):** | Adults 12.5 to 100 mg |
| **Peak plasma level, h:** | 2 to 4 |
| **Biological half-life, h:** | 5 to 15 |
| **Time to steady-state, days:** | 1 to 3 |
| **Effective concentration — hypertension and diuresis:** | 10 to 300 $\mu g/L$ |
| **Monitoring Methods:** | TLC, GLC, HPLC, colorimetry |

and these actions appear to occur sequentially rather than simultaneously. Recent evidence has raised doubts that there is a direct action on arteriolar smooth muscle and suggests that the decrease in vascular tone may be a result of adaptation of reflex mechanisms to prolonged reduction in cardiac output (7).

## Drug Interactions

There is evidence that the natriuretic action of certain diuretics may be related to the intrarenal activation of the prostaglandin system (8). By the same token, their diuretic and antihypertensive effects may be reduced by the administration of an inhibitor of renal prostaglandin biosynthesis such as indomethacin. Thus, when the desired effect of diuretic therapy is not observed in hypertensive patients, concomitant administration of a prostaglandin inhibitor should be considered.

## Clinical Side Effects

The more common pharmacological effects of thiazide diuretics include hypokalemia, hyperuricemia, hyperglycemia, and increased serum urea nitrogen. These effects tend to be mild, usually do not produce symptoms, and only occasionally require specific therapy. Serious unpredictable adverse reactions to thiazide diuretics are rare, but include coma, pancreatitis, acute pulmonary edema, aplastic anemia, thrombocytopenia, and non-occlusive mesenteric infarction.

## References

1. Sackett, D.L., Haynes, R.B., Gibson, E.S., Hackett, B.C., Taylor, D.W., Roberts, R.S., and Johnson, A.L., Randomized clinical trial strategies for improving medication compliance in primary hypertension. *Lancet* **1**, 1205-1207 (1975).

2. Logan, A.G., Milne, B.J., Achber, C., Campbell, W.P., Haynes, R.B., Work-site treatment of hypertension by specially trained nurses. A controlled trial. *Lancet* **2**, 1175-1178 (1979).

3. Haynes, R.B., Sackett, D.L., Gibson, E.S., Taylor, D.W., Hackett, B.C., Roberts, R.S., and Johnson, A.L., Improvement of medication compliance in uncontrolled hypertension. *Lancet* **1**, 1265-1268 (1976).

4. Sackett, D.L., and Haynes, R.B. (Eds.), *Compliance with Therapeutic Regimens,* The Johns Hopkins University Press, Baltimore and London, 1976.

5. Haynes, R.B., Sackett, D.L., and Taylor, D.W., The practical management of low compliance with antihypertensive therapy. A guide for the busy practitioner. *Clinical Investigative Medicine* **1**, 175-180 (1979).

6. Report of the Joint National Committee on Detection, Evaluation, and Treatment of High Blood Pressure: A cooperative study. *JAMA* **237**, 255-261 (1977).

7. Shah, S., Khatri, I., and Freis, E.D., Mechanisms of antihypertensive effect of thiazide diuretics. *Am. Heart J.* **95**, 611-618 (1978).

8. Patak, R.V., Mookerjee, B.K., Bentzel, C.J., Hysert, P.E., Babej, M., and Lee, J.B., Antagonism of the effects of furosemide by indomethacin in normal and hypertensive man. *Prostaglandins* **10**, 649-653 (1975).

9. Beermann, B., and Groschinsky-Grind, M., Pharmacokinetics of hydrochlorothiazide in man. *Eur. J. Pharmacol.* **12**, 297-303 (1977).

10. Beerman, B., and Groschinsky-Grind, M., Antihypertensive effect of various doses of hydrochlorothiazide and its relation to the plasma level of the drug. *Ibid.* **13**, 195-201 (1978).

11. Soldin, S.J., Hach, E., Pollard, A., and Logan, A.G., High performance liquid chromatographic analysis of hydrochlorothiazide in serum and urine. *Therap. Drug Monitoring* **1**, 399-408 (1979).

# 53

# Nitroprusside

**Larry A. Broussard, Ph.D.**
**Christopher S. Frings, Ph.D.**

## Introduction

Sodium nitroprusside was shown to lower blood pressure in humans in 1929, but was not marketed for clinical use until 1974 (Nipride®, Roche Laboratories). Since then, nitroprusside has been shown to be an extremely effective and well-tolerated vasodilator drug and has been called the most effective vasodilator available for the management of acute hypertension, heart failure, and other vasoconstricted states, as well as for the induction of controlled hypotension during surgery (1).

## Chemistry

Nitroprusside is an iron coordination complex with a net negative charge of 2. The complex contains five cyanide (CN⁻) moieties and one nitroso (⁺NO) moiety complexed to a ferrous ion. Other chemical names include sodium nitroferricyanide, sodium nitrosylpentacyanoferrate (III), and sodium nitroprussiate. Nipride® is the dihydrate form $[Fe(CN)_5NO \cdot 2H_2O]$ and is a reddish brown, water soluble powder. In solution nitroprusside is photosensitive and should be protected from light.

## Clinical Uses

The primary use of nitroprusside is in the immediate treatment of hypertensive crisis. Nitroprusside has the following characteristics which make it the ideal drug for treating hypertensive emergencies: 1) rapid action, 2) relaxation of arterial and venous smooth muscle without affecting the central or autonomic nervous system, 3) no tachyphylaxis, and 4) high potency and low toxic:therapeutic ratio (3). Forms of acute hypertension that have been effectively treated with nitroprusside include the accelerated phase of essential or renovascular hypertension, pheochromocytoma, cerebral hemorrhage, toxemia of pregnancy, and postoperative hypertension (1).

---

*Dr. Broussard is Assistant Director of Clinical Chemistry and Dr. Frings is Director, Clinical Chemistry and Toxicology, Cunningham Pathology Associates (a.k.a. Medical Laboratory Associates), Birmingham, Alabama.*

---

Nitroprusside has been effectively used as hypotensive therapy in order to postpone surgery for patients with a dissecting aortic aneurysm until their condition stabilizes. Nitroprusside has also been used to reduce bleeding during many types of surgery, to treat patients with acute myocardial infarction, and to treat patients suffering from hypertension due to congestive heart failure. Ergot poisoning and lactic acidosis have also been successfully treated with nitroprusside.

## Metabolism and Toxicity

Nitroprusside should only be used as an infusion with sterile 5% dextrose in water and should not be given orally or by direct injection. The half-life of the drug is only a few minutes (2), and it is rapidly metabolized to cyanide, probably by direct combination of nitroprusside with sulfhydryl groups in red cells and tissue. The hepatic enzyme, rhodanase, converts cyanide to thiocyanate, with the rate of conversion apparently dependent on the availability of sulfur, usually thiosulfate (4). Thiocyanate is removed almost exclusively by the kidney, with a half-life of approximately 4 days in men with normal renal function (2). Due to hepatic conversion of cyanate to thiocyanate and subsequent renal excretion, nitroprusside must be used with extreme caution in patients with hepatic insufficiency or with diminished renal function.

Symptoms of toxicity are usually due to the accumulation of thiocyanate. Cyanide toxicity is extremely uncommon, although significantly elevated concentrations of cyanide in blood can be observed during prolonged therapy (2). Metabolic acidosis is the earliest sign of cyanide toxicity, and symptoms of thiocyanate toxicity include weakness, hypoxia, nausea, tinnitus, muscle spasms, disorientation and psychosis. Long-term treatment with nitroprusside may lead to hypothyroidism since thiocyanate displaces iodine from the thyroid gland. Blood thiocyanate levels can be used as a guide to impending toxicity (1).

Treatment of toxicity includes cessation of nitroprusside infusion and initiation of infusions of thiosulfate, sodium nitrite, and hydroxycobalamin, separately or together. Apparently, thiosulfate facilitates the conversion of cyanide to thiocyanate by furnishing sulfur. Sodium nitrite induces the formation of methemoglobin, which combines with the cyanide ion to form cyanomethemoglobin, and hydroxylcobalamin combines with cyanide to form cyanocobalamin. Hemodialysis may also be used to treat thiocyanate toxicity.

## Dosage and Therapeutic Monitoring

Nipride® is supplied in 50 mg vials which are diluted with 5% dextrose in water to achieve the desired concentration (usually 50, 100, or 200 mg/L). This solution should be protected from light and should not be kept or used longer than four hours. Freshly prepared solution has a faint brownish tint; if it becomes highly colored, it should be discarded.

The intravenous infusion of Nipride® should be administered by an infusion pump, micro-drip regulator, or any similar device that will allow precise measurement of the flow rate (4). The dosage range for nitroprusside infusion is broad with the average initial adult infusion rate between 0.5 and 1.5 $\mu g/kg/min$. The infusion rate can be adjusted to achieve the desired blood pressure because of the linear dose-response relation observed with nitroprusside.

Monitoring of the patient receiving nitroprusside infusion consists of observing for early signs of cyanide or thiocyanate toxicity and measuring blood levels of thiocyanate (1). Therapeutic levels of thiocyanate are considered to be 50-100 mg/L (5-10 mg/dl). Although there have been reports of patients tolerating levels to 200 mg/L, levels greater than 100 mg/L are generally associated with toxicity.

## Sodium Nitroprusside Profile

| | |
|---|---|
| Generic Name: | Sodium nitroprusside |
| Chemical names: | Sodium nitroferricyanide, sodium nitrosylpentacyanoferrate (III), sodium nitroprussiate |
| Chemical structure: |  |
| Molecular mass: | 261.91; 297.95 for the dihydrate |
| Recommended dosage: | Infusion rate regulated (usually initially between 0.5-1.5 $\mu g/kg/min$) to achieve the desired blood pressure |
| Metabolites: | Cyanide and thiocyanate |
| Thiocyanate: | Half-life:          approximately 4 days<br>Therapeutic range: 50-100 mg/L<br>Toxic range:       > 100 mg/L |

## References

1. Cohn, J.N., and Burke, L.P., Nitroprusside, *Ann. Int. Med.* **91**, 752-757 (1979).
2. *Goodman and Gilman's The Pharmacological Basis of Therapeutics,* Eds., Gilman, A.G., Goodman, L.S., and Gilman, A., Sixth Edition, Macmillan Publishing Co., Inc., New York, N.Y., 1980, pp 805-806.
3. Palmer, R.F., and Lasseter, K.C., Drug therapy-sodium nitroprusside, *N. Eng. J. Med.* **292**, 294-297 (1975).
4. *Physician's Desk Reference,* 35th edition, Medical Economics Company, Oradell, N.J., 1981, pp 1519-1521.

# 54

# Drug-Induced Cyanide Intoxication: Two Cases

**Thomas P. Moyer, Ph.D.**

## Introduction

Several commonly used therapeutic agents have the potential to undergo metabolic release (either systemic in vitro metabolism or microbial metabolism in the gut) of cyanide that may lead to subsequent cyanide intoxication. Two agents for which this may occur are nitroprusside (Nipride®) used for rapid blood pressure control in malignant hypertension, and amygdalin (laetrile) used in certain cancer chemotherapy programs.

## Case #1

In June of 1980 this healthy 10-year-old male developed bifrontal throbbing headaches which usually began upon his awakening in the morning and lasted from 1 h to all day long. The headaches were sometimes associated with nausea and vomiting. In August, weight loss became a problem. In October, he experienced episodes of blurred vision accompanying the symptoms listed above.

In late October of 1980 he sought medical assistance because of these problems. At the time of initial physical examination, the patient related no experience of diplopia, tinnitus, hearing or speech trouble, weakness, numbness, syncope or seizure activity. At the time, his blood pressure was 230/170 mmHg, experienced with tachycardia and flushing of the face. There was no family history of neurologic, thyroid, or adrenal disease, although both mother and father were hypertensive. The only other finding on routine physical examination was bilateral mild optic exudates and papiledema of 1 to 2 diopters elevation.

The patient was immediately admitted to the hospital with a tentative diagnosis of malignant hypertension and hypertensive retinopathy. All routine hematology and chemistry laboratory results were normal. The patient workup included tests to elucidate an intracranial mass, renal arterial stenosis,

*Dr. Moyer is associated with the Mayo Clinic, Rochester, Minnesota 55901.*

*This work was supported in part by grant No. CA 13650, Division of Cancer Treatment, National Cancer Institute.*

or a metabolic cause such as pheochromocytoma, neuroblastoma, or aldosteronoma.

Initial efforts to control his blood pressure included intravenous nitroprusside at 8 $\mu g/kg/min$ (patient weighed 35 kg). After 1 day of therapy on nitroprusside at 8 $\mu g/kg/min$, the blood pressure was reduced only to 200/120 mmHg. The dose was increased to 10 $\mu g/kg/min$. During physical examination that day a systolic bruit in the left upper quadrant was detected, directing attention to renal arterial stenosis as the cause for increased blood pressure.

On the afternoon of day 2, plasma sodium, potassium, chloride, bicarbonate and blood pH were noted to be "borderline low normal", with patient displaying symptoms of metabolic acidosis. Nitroprusside therapy was decreased to 3.3 $\mu g/kg/min$ after this observation.

On day 3 of hospitalization, the patient's blood pressure was still elevated, with laboratory reports coming back to rule out renal arterial stenosis, intracranial mass and metabolic disorders such as pheochromocytoma, neuroblastoma, or aldosteronoma. The only abnormal laboratory result was an elevated renin, at 36 mg/L/h (normal: 3-24 mg/L/h) which was cited to be consistent with the elevated blood pressure observed in this patient. Plasma thiocyanate concentration was 30 mg/L on this date.

Day 4 was taken up by a concerted effort to wean the patient off nitroprusside by adding prazocin and propranolol to the therapeutic regimen. Plasma thiocyanate on this day was observed to be 38 mg/L. Nitroprusside therapy was maintained at 3.3 $\mu g/kg/min$ with bolus of 10 $\mu g/kg/min$ given when blood pressure spikes were observed. During this time the blood pressure was holding at approximately 200/120 mmHg.

Day 6 of therapy continued in the attempt to wean the patient off nitroprusside. Thiocyanate concentration on this day was 60 $\mu g/mL$ and the patient continued in a state of worsening metabolic acidosis.

On day 7 of therapy, the blood pressure was greatly improved at 180/100, and the patient was off Nipride and taking propranolol, hydralazine, prazocin, and furosemide.

Day 7 was the first day that serum electrolytes returned to normal from the state of metabolic acidosis observed earlier.

Days 9 thru 15 involved continued investigation of the cause of hypertension and therapeutic manipulation to achieve best blood pressure control. At the time of dismissal, the patient had a blood pressure of 120/80 mmHg on therapy of furosemide, spironolactone, propranolol, captopril, α-methyldopa, and a sodium restricted diet.

Final diagnosis of malignant hypertension was assigned. One year later the patient returned with increased blood pressure. A 6 day hospitalization identified that the patient had been noncompliant. The drug regimen was reestablished and the patient returned home with blood pressure of 140/80 mmHg. Still no further etiology was identified, and a continued diagnosis of essential hypertension was assigned.

## Case #2

This 65-year-old female who experienced recurrent pancreatic adenocarcinoma with local and distant metastases had undergone previous resection of pancreas, spleen, and omentum. She was admitted to a National Cancer Institute sponsored oral laetrile clinical trial with informed consent. The clinical trial was carried out in the hospital Clinical Study Unit under constant nursing supervision directed by the physician trial coordinator.

Upon admission to the Clinical Study Unit, the patient was given a physical examination and was noted to be bright, cheerful, comfortable and in physical condition reasonable for her disease state. Amygdalin (laetrile) at a dose of 0.5 g was administered orally 3 times per day, 1/2 h before each meal. Two hours following the first administration of amygdalin, whole blood cyanide concentration peaked at 0.66 mg/L, with concurrent plasma thiocyanate concentration of 2.4 mg/L. A similar finding occurred on the second day of trial, with cyanide concentration peaking at 0.64 mg/L 2 h after the oral dose, with simultaneous thiocyanate at 6.7 mg/L. Two hours after the third morning dose, the whole blood cyanide concentration was 0.31 mg/L with concurrent thiocyanate 13.3 mg/L.

On day 4 of therapy, raw almonds were added to each meal according to diet plans of laetrile advocates. Two hours after the first morning dose of laetrile, cyanide concentration was 1.1 mg/L and thiocyanate was 14.4 mg/L. The patient maintained a bright, cheerful attitude, and neither displayed nor indicated any signs or symptoms of cyanide intoxication.

On the fifth day of therapy, 0.5 mg of amygdalin was administered at 7:45 A.M., followed by a breakfast at 8:15 A.M. including raw almonds. At 9:40 A.M. the patient vomited (unusual experience), and indicated

onset of severe headache, giddiness, and complained that her "arms felt like lead". Her physician was sitting at the bedside during this episode and indicated that she had a cyanotic appearance with greyish skin tone. At that time her respiration was 14/min, pulse was 92/min, blood pressure was 100/60 mmHg. A blood specimen was collected at 10:00 A.M. and the whole blood cyanide concentration at that time was 2.0 mg/L with plasma thiocyanate concentration of 11.5 mg/L. Electrolytes at 10:00 A.M. (all results in mmol/L) were sodium 128, potassium 4, ionized calcium 1.25, magnesium 2, bicarbonate 19, chloride 94, $pCO_2$ 1.2 (39.2 mmHg), protein 16 with an anion gap of 14, and blood pH 7.3, consistent with a mild episode of metabolic acidosis.

At 10:10 A.M. the headache was noted to be subsiding and dizziness was less apparent. At 10:35 A.M. headache and dizziness were no longer severe. At 10:55, the symptoms had totally cleared, and she was again bright and cheerful.

At 12 noon, her whole blood cyanide concentration was 1.74 mg/L with thiocyanate at 13.9 mg/L. All amygdalin therapy was stopped at this time and her condition was allowed to stabilize.

At 8:00 P.M. that evening her whole blood concentration of cyanide was 0.26 mg/L and thiocyanate was 15.6 mg/L. The following morning, without any additional amygdalin dose, her whole blood cyanide concentration was 0.13 mg/L and thiocyanate was 20.8 mg/L. At that time her electrolytes were as follows (all in mmol/L): sodium 136, potassium 4.1, ionized calcium 1.25, magnesium 2, bicarbonate 26, chloride 101, $pCO_2$ 1.30 (42.5 mmHg), protein 16 with an ion gap of 8, and blood pH 7.4.

On day 7 of the study, laetrile was again administered, and 2 hours after her morning dose her whole blood cyanide concentration was 0.91 mg/L and thiocyanate was 19.7 mg/L.

The study protocol then required that she be converted to intravenously administered amygdalin at a dose of 0.45 mg/kg/day over the next 15 days. During that study, her whole blood cyanide concentration dropped to not-detectable levels (less than 0.05 mg/L) and plasma thiocyanate concentration dropped back to 10 mg/L. This case has been reported in part elsewhere (1, 2).

## Method

The methods used here for analysis of whole blood cyanide and plasma thiocyanate are based on the methods of Feldstein and Klendshaj (3) and Bowler (4). Whole blood cyanide was determined by allowing hydrocyanic acid to diffuse across a permeable barrier (Conway diffusion cell) from strongly acidified whole blood. The diffusate was then quantitatively analyzed using the spectrophotometric properties of a condensation product of cyanopyridinium chloride and barbituric acid. Plasma thiocyanate was analyzed by complexing a protein-free filtrate of plasma with ferric ion which yields iron thiocyanate which can be analyzed spectrophotometrically. Details of these procedures have been described elsewhere (2).

## Discussion

Nitroprusside [sodium nitrosylpentacyanoferrate III, $Na_2Fe(CN)_5 NO \cdot H_2O$] is a potent vasodilator that is used to accomplish an immediate reduction in blood pressure in patients in hypertensive crisis. Its mechanisms of action is via peripheral neural ganglia blockade, and thus other agents that act by similar mechanisms (volatile anesthetics, circulatory depressants) will display an accumulated ganglionic blocking effect. It is never infused at a rate faster than 10 $\mu g/kg/min$, and the average dose is 3 $\mu g/kg/min$. At the normal infusion rate, 30-40% reduction in blood pressure would be expected within 10 min. For a more detailed review of the therapeutic use of the drug, readers are directed to the review by Tinker and Michenfelder (5).

Toxicity associated with nitroprusside use is directly related to release of cyanide during decomposition of nitroprusside. In the presence of hemoglobin, an electron transfer occurs such that heme iron ($Fe^{2+}$) is oxidized to $Fe^{3+}$ yielding methemoglobin, with simultaneous reduction of the nitroprusside iron complex to an unstable nitroprusside radical. This quickly breaks down to five molecules of cyanide, one of which reacts with methemoglobin to form cyanmethemoglobin (5). The remaining cyanide is free to circulate out of the red cell and is metabolized to thiocyanate by rhodanase (a sulfhydryl-dependent enzyme) in liver and kidney. Cyanide can also interact with the oxidative electron transport system in all tissues by inhibiting electron transfer from cytochrome $a$ to cytochrome $a^3$ which effectively blocks the final energy yielding step in the reduction of oxygen to water. To maintain physiologic activity tissues are thus forced to convert to glycolytic pathways for energy, the end result being accumulation of lactic acid and acetoacetic acid, which results in metabolic acidosis due to accumulation of organic anions.

Short term exposure to nitroprusside does not usually lead to any significant cyanide accumulation, as evidenced by the study of Bogusz et al. (6) which found whole blood cyanide concentrations in one patient peaking at 0.16 mg/L after dosage at 8 $\mu g/kg/min$ for 2 h. In a larger patient population exposed at 3 $\mu g/kg/min$ for periods of 2 h, whole blood cyanide concentrations were found to range from 0.01 to 1.8 mg/L. Plasma thiocyanate concentrations ranged from 0.3 to 18.0 mg/L in this same group of patients.

Toxicity due to cyanide accumulation in patients dosed with nitroprusside has been related to whole blood cyanide concentrations ranging from 2.9 to 28.7 mg/L (6). The fact that other studies suggest that whole blood concentrations of cyanide that are lethal range from 1.0 to 5.3 mg/L (summarized in references 5,6) points to a problem with the whole blood cyanide analysis as an index of systemic toxicity.

In nitroprusside therapy, cyanide release occurs in the red blood cell, and thus analysis of whole blood cyanide may yield an artificial elevation which may not directly relate to toxicity. Indeed, Vessey et al. (7) have suggested that the appropriate specimen for evaluation of systemic toxicity is a plasma sample. In cyanide intoxication unrelated to nitroprusside use, 90% of cyanide exists in the red blood cell. During nitroprusside therapy, the ratio of cyanide in red blood cells to plasma cyanide is as high as 200:1 (7). This presents an analytical problem in that the plasma concentration of cyanide during intoxication ranges from 0.1 to 0.5 mg/L (7), very near the limit of sensitivity for any clinically reasonable technique for analysis of cyanide.

To counter the discrepancy between whole blood cyanide and toxicity, monitoring plasma thiocyanate appears to offer a convenient index to follow using a test amenable to clinical laboratories. Early works suggested a reasonable limit associated with toxicity of 100 mg/L thiocyanate. Others (8) have identified patients without severe symptoms of intoxication with plasma thiocyanate concentrations as high as 230 mg/L. The rate of turnover of cyanide to thiocyanate will be dependent upon the pool of reducing substances to active sulfur donors in the conversion of cyanide to thiocyanate.

In our institution, we use the following thiocyanate concentration guidelines:

| | |
|---|---|
| 2-5 mg/L | normal |
| 5-20 mg/L | normal for nitroprusside therapy |
| 20-35 mg/L | borderline toxicity |
| 35-60 mg/L | increased potential for toxicity |
| > 60 mg/L | usually associated with metabolic acidosis |

At concentrations greater than 35 mg/L, concerted efforts are made to wean the patient off nitroprusside onto other hypertensive therapy. Obviously, these concentrations are only guidelines, and are used in light of the patient's status. It is important to remember it is easier to control a mild metabolic acidosis associated with cyanide intoxication with no long-term detrimental effects than it is to deal with the potential for cerebrovascular accident secondary to malignant hypertension.

Amygdalin is a cyanogenic glucoside (d-mandelo-nitrile-$\beta$-d-glucoside-6-$\beta$-d-glucoside, $C_6H_5CHCNOC_{12}H_{21}O_{10}$) found in certain plants. It is most commonly isolated from apricot seeds. It is reported to be effective in treatment of certain neoplastic diseases, although there appears to be no scientific basis for this claim [1,2]. When ingested orally, amygdalin undergoes metabolism in the gut (normal bacterial flora) to glucose and mandelonitrile [9]. The unstable mandelonitrile undergoes immediate decomposition to yield cyanide and benzaldehyde. This process can also be catalyzed by $\beta$-glucosidases and nitrile lyases, commonly found in nuts and seeds.

Our studies [1, 2] showed that when the drug is given orally, significant accumulation of cyanide and thiocyanate occurs. When the drug is given intravenously, there is no significant accumulation of cyanide, and thiocyanate increases to a small but significant degree. In a study of 250 patients treated with amygdalin on the protocol described in the case history, the highest whole blood cyanide experienced was 3.5 mg/L, and this patient did not display gross symptoms of cyanide intoxication (electrolyte analysis was not performed). Thus, there is some degree of variability from patient to patient in terms of their tolerance to blood cyanide concentration. A whole blood cyanide concentration greater than 2.0 mg/L should certainly be cause for concern.

Peak plasma thiocyanate was noted to lag behind peak cyanide concentrations by 24-48 h, and the highest thiocyanate observed in the study [1, 2] was 35 mg/L, and this was not associated with gross intoxication (electrolyte analysis was not performed).

## References

1. Moertel, C.G., Ames, M.W., Kovach, J.S., Moyer, T.P., Rubin, J.R., and Tinker, J.H., A pharmacologic toxicologicol study of amygdalin. *J. Am. Med. Assoc.* **245**, 591-594 (1981).

2. Ames, M.W., Moyer, T.P., Kovach, J.S., Moertel, C.G., and Rubin, J.R., Pharmacology of amygdalin (laetrile) in cancer patients. *Cancer Chemother. Pharmacol.* **6**, 51-57 (1981).

3. Feldstein, M., and Klendshaj, N., The determination of cyanide in biological fluids by micro diffusion analysis. *J. Lab. Clin. Med.* **44**, 166-170 (1954).

4. Bowler, R.G., The determination of thiocyanate in blood serum. *Biochem. J.* **38**, 385-388 (1944).

5. Tinker, J.H., and Michenfelder, J.D., Sodium nitroprusside: Pharmacology, toxicology and therapeutics. *Anesthesiology* **45**, 340-354 (1976).

6. Bogusz, M., Moroz, J., Karski, J., Giery, J., Regieli, A., Witkowski, R., and Golabek, A., Blood cyanide and thiocyanate concentrations after administration of sodium nitroprusside as hypotensive agent in neurosurgery. *Clin. Chem.* 60-63 (1979).

7. Vessey, C.J., Cole, P.V., and Simpson, P.J., Cyanide and thiocyanate concentrations following sodium nitroprusside infusion in man. *Br. J. Anesth.* **48**, 651-660 (1976).

8. Cohn, J.N., and Burke, L.P., Nitroprusside. *Ann. Int. Med.* **91**, 752-757 (1979).

9. Haisman, G.J., and Knight, D.J., The enzymatic hydrolysis of amygdalin. *Biochem. J.* **103**, 528-534 (1967).

# 55

# Heparin

**Gordon Ireland, Pharm.D.**

Episodes of thrombosis often complicate treatment of many different kinds of diseases. Medical practitioners must understand the medicinal approach to anticoagulation and how such therapy should be monitored by using appropriate laboratory tests.

I discuss here the use of heparin in treating thrombo-embolism, with specific emphasis on its mechanism of action, pharmacokinetics, laboratory monitoring, and activity inhibition.

## Mechanism of Action

Heparin was identified as an anticoagulant by McLean in 1916 but it was not until about 20 years later, when it became more available, that it was widely used clinically.

Heparin is generally considered the drug of choice in treatment of venous thrombo-embolism.

Heparin will not dissolve or remove the already-existing thrombus, but it can prevent the enlargement of thrombus and the formation of new thrombi.

Heparin, a naturally occurring mucopolysaccharide found in mast cells of many tissues such as liver, lung, and intestine, is derived from the intestine in the usual commercial preparation, the next most common source being lung tissue. Heparin derived from beef lung and pork intestinal mucosa are equivalent unit for unit in heparin activity.

Figure 1 shows the normal progression of the coagulation cascade. Once Factor XII and/or tissue factor are activated they activate the next factors in the cascade which then activate the next factors, etc. until fibrinogen is converted to fibrin and clotting ensues. Because it is a strong anion, heparin produces its effect by binding to positively charged coagulation factors. This enhancement of the effects of "heparin cofactor" (an $\alpha_2$-globulin that seems to be identical with antithrombin III) by heparin seems to be its primary action. The interaction of heparin and antithrombin III results in a conformational change in antithrombin III, which enhances its activity. "Heparin cofactor" neutralizes factor $X_a$, the catalyst for the conversion of prothrombin to thrombin. "Heparin cofactor" also inhibits the activity of thrombin and therefore blocks the conversion

---

*Dr. Ireland is Assistant Professor of Clinical Pharmacy at The Jewish Hospital of St. Louis, and the St. Louis College of Pharmacy.*

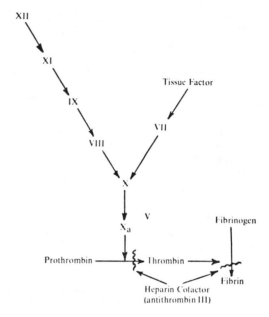

**Figure 1.** Coagulation Cascade.

of fibrinogen to fibrin "monomers," which lead to formation of the fibrin clot.

Because factor X occupies a central role in both the intrinsic and extrinsic thromboplastin pathways and because of the cascading of the coagulation sequence, inhibition of a relatively small amount of activated factor X blocks the formation of large quantities of the final coagulation products. Yin et al. showed that 1 $\mu$g of heparin cofactor neutralizes 32 USP units of factor $X_a$ but only 1.2 USP units of thrombin. Because each molecule of factor $X_a$ potentially can convert 50 molecules of prothrombin to thrombin, each microgram of cofactor may prevent the formation of 1500 units of thrombin.

The resolution of the thrombus that often occurs during therapy with heparin is primarily the result of endogenous mechanisms (e.g., thrombolysis, thrombus fragmentation, organization, recanalization, and development of collateral circulation) rather than the direct action of heparin.

## Pharmacokinetics

*Absorption:* Heparin is usually administered by the parenteral route, because on oral administration it loses its negative charges by the action of sulfatases in the

---

309

gastrointestinal tract. The preferable parenteral route is intravenous. Intramuscular injections are not used because there is a significant danger of bleeding into the muscle. Subcutaneous injection is also used, even though individual variation in heparin absorption by this route is well recognized.

Although there are few good studies addressing the absorption rate of subcutaneously injected heparin, some statements can be made. Heparin is absorbed slowly from the subcutaneous site. The anticoagulant effect of subcutaneous administration seems to support the fact that the heparin only gradually leaves the site of injection, because some studies have shown that subcutaneous administration of 15,000 to 20,000 units will prolong coagulation within the therapeutic range for as long as 10 to 24 hours.

*Distribution:* Recently, the apparent volume of distribution has been shown to correlate more closely to whole-blood volume (55—75 mL/kg) than to plasma volume (44 mL/kg), as previously thought. This volume of distribution of heparin varies with the dose of heparin, the age of the patient, the patient's body weight, and the disease state. Heparin does not cross the placenta, nor does it enter maternal milk.

*Metabolism:* The elimination and metabolic fate of heparin is very poorly understood, because a direct clinical assay for heparin is not readily available (an esterolytic method has been printed: *Clin. Chem.* 27: 526-529, 1981). Most studies examine the kinetics of its anticoagulant effect. The disappearance of heparin from plasma seems to follow a first-order rate process. The half-life (t½) of the anticoagulant effect of heparin increases from 0.5 to 2.5 h as the dose is increased. At normal doses the average t½ is 1.5 h. The t½ appears to decrease to about 45 min in patients with pulmonary embolism. Although only a small proportion of heparin is excreted unchanged in the urine, the anticoagulant activity of heparin has been shown to be prolonged in patients with impaired renal function (Table 1). The mechanism proposed to account for the major proportion of heparin elimination is its transfer to some extravascular compartment, probably the hepato-splenic reticuloendothelial system. Primarily, in this system, the heparin is metabolized by *N*-and *O*-desulfation to inactive metabolites. There may be a secondary site of metabolism in the kidneys.

## Administration

Currently, heparin is administered by intermittent intravenous injection or constant intravenous infusion. If hemostasis processes are normal, the incidence of bleeding after full therapeutic doses of heparin is about 10-15%. It is considerably greater in elderly women and in patients with impaired hemostasis. The

**Table 1.** Anticoagulant Half-Life of Heparin (from Perry et al.)

| Heparin concn. USP units/mL | Normal | Renal failure |
|---|---|---|
| | Time, min | |
| 0.6 | 36.8 | 47.5 |
| 0.3 | 22.7 | 37.6 |

initial dose is 75 units/kg of total body weight for diagnoses other than pulmonary embolism, for which the dose is 100 units/kg followed by intermittent bolus doses or continuous infusion dosing.

*Intermittent bolus dosing:* Traditionally, heparin maintenance doses by intermittent bolus intravenous injection have been between 5000 and 15,000 units every 4 to 6 h. This method provides infinitely prolonged clotting times immediately after the injection, declining to subtherapeutic values just before the next dose.

*Constant infusion dosing:* Constant infusion offers several advantages over intermittent bolus dosing: flexibility in dosage adjustment; less total heparin required; clotting times can be measured at any time; risk of hemorrhage appears less; and the clotting time can be maintained continuously within the therapeutic range.

Continuous intravenous infusion also prevents large variations between peak and trough effects of heparin. Following a loading dose of 5000-15,000 units, a dose of 35-50 units/kg is required to anticoagulate blood to a clinically desirable level. Therefore, in a 70-kg adult it will be necessary to maintain a level of 2500 to 3500 units in the body at all times which can be achieved by an infusion rate of 900-1200 units/hour. The heparin infusion should be administered with a constant-infusion pump.

*Low-dose subcutaneous dosing:* Clinical evidence indicates that patients are at a higher risk for deep venous thrombosis for about seven days postoperatively. Studies with use of [125]I-labeled fibrinogen show that about 20-30% of all surgical patients, 40-50% of elderly surgical patients, and half the patients who undergo hip procedures develop postoperative venous thrombosis, which may or may not be clinically evident.

At least seven recently published clinical trials with use of [125]I-labeled fibrinogen have demonstrated that low-dose heparin prophylaxis, initiated 2 to 12 h before surgery and continued through the first seven to 10 postoperative days, significantly decreased the incidence of deep-vein thrombosis. The effect of low-dose heparin prophylaxis in the prevention of postoperative pulmonary emboli remains to be established.

The protocols for low-dose heparin usually suggest 5000 units of heparin be administered subcutaneously (usually in the fat of the abdomen) 2 to 12 h before surgery. Postoperatively, heparin dosage is 5000 units administered subcutaneously every 8 to 12 h for seven to 10 days, or until the patient is fully mobile.

Following the effects of therapy with heparin by laboratory coagulation tests may not be of great value, because with low-dose subcutaneous heparin the activated partial thromboplastin time may be only moderately prolonged for a few hours after the administration of heparin. There are no established therapeutic values for coagulation studies to follow in low-dose therapy with heparin.

## Laboratory Monitoring

Historically, the method most used for measuring the effects of heparin has been the whole blood clotting time, or Lee-White clotting time. Although the Lee-White clotting time has been abandoned as too cumbersome, time consuming, insensitive, and crude, the test does detect the effects of heparin activity. The prolongation of the Lee-White time essentially parallels the amount of heparin present. Most of its variability can be attributed not to properties of the test itself, but to the lack of care with which it is performed. Properly done, it is usually quite a satisfactory test.

Prolongation of whole-blood clotting times from 1½ to 3 times that of normal controls is necessary to prevent thrombus formation and enlargement. The increased incidence of hemorrhagic complications makes the increase of clotting times by greater than 3 undesirable. Generally the more recently introduced tests are preferred over the Lee-White clotting time. These tests, which are more rapid and more reproducible, include the whole blood activated partial thromboplastin time (WBAPTT), the activated partial thromboplastin time (APTT), and partial thromboplastin time (PTT). All these tests provide similar estimates of the half-life of the anticoagulant effect of heparin. The APTT seems to provide the greatest precision (Table 2); this test is done in most clinical laboratories, but the specimen must be processed quickly, to avoid any effect from platelet factor 4, which may be released while the specimen is being held in the collection container and decrease the effect of the heparin.

Basu et al., in studying 234 patients, showed that the risk of recurrent thrombosis was 7% if the patient had an APTT of less than 1½ times control for two consecutive days and a risk of 21% if the APTT was less than 1½ times control for three consecutive days. There was no recurrence of venous thromboembolism in any pa-

tient when the APTT was prolonged to at least 1½ times the control value.

It seems very important, therefore, that patients with venous thromboembolism should be given enough heparin to prolong the APTT to within the therapeutic range, no matter how much heparin is required to obtain this result.

Samples for the measurement of clotting times may be collected at any time while the patient is receiving a constant infusion of heparin but should be collected just prior to administration of the dose in intermittent bolus dosing.

**Table 2.** Comparison of Four Coagulation Tests

|  | Relative precision | Relative economy |
|---|---|---|
| Whole-blood partial thromboplastin time (WBPTT) | 1.00 | 1.00 |
| Whole-blood clotting time (WBCT) | 0.61 | 0.16 |
| Activated partial thromboplastin time (APTT) | 1.57 | 0.42 |
| Partial thromboplastin time (PTT) | 0.58 | 0.15 |

## Duration of Heparin Therapy

As mentioned above, the objectives of therapy with heparin are to arrest the thrombotic process and prevent the propagation of existing thrombi. The risk of continued thrombosis remains until there has been endothelialization of the thrombus and, probably, until collateralization and recanalization restore adequate blood flow. The interval required for this varies from patient to patient. Generally seven to 10 days is thought, on the basis of experiments in animals, to be the time required for endothelialization of the thrombus. Some current studies are trying to determine if such data can appropriately be extrapolated to humans.

When oral anticoagulants are used for prophylaxis, their administration should overlap full-dose heparin therapy for three to five days, at which time the heparin can be rapidly discontinued. This interval is required for the full antithrombin effect of orally administered anticoagulants which inhibit the synthesis of vitamin K dependent factors II, VII, IX, and X. It takes three to five days for the activity of existing factors to end. It must be remembered that heparin may prolong the prothrombin time (PT), the test used to follow oral anticoagulant activity, because of its antithrombin effect. When patients are taking both heparin and oral anticoagulants, the PT should be measured at a time when heparin activity is at its lowest point, i.e. just before the next heparin dose. A PT should be measured on the day heparin is discontinued, to ensure that the value on oral anticoagulant alone is within therapeutic range.

## Complications of Therapy with Heparin

*Hemorrhage.* The most important factor predisposing a patient to hemorrhage during therapy with heparin is an anatomical or functional defect. The actual amount of heparin seems to be less significant. These factors include recent surgical incision, thrombocytopenia, uremia, deep intramuscular injections, prior history of bleeding, or concurrent administration of drugs known to alter platelet function, such as aspirin, dipyridamole, anturane, and phenylbutazone.

There is still some controversy regarding the decreased incidence of bleeding with continuous intravenous infusion as compared to intermittent bolus heparin administration. Salzman et al. and Glazier et al., in their respective studies, showed a significant difference in favor of continuous infusion therapy, whereas Wilson and Lampman could show no statistical difference in the occurrence of bleeding between continuous infusion and intermittent bolus administration.

*Thrombocytopenia.* The onset of thrombocytopenia may occur within three to five days of initiating heparin therapy. The clinical picture may resemble disseminated intravascular coagulopathy with reduction in fibrinogen and an increase in fibrin degradation products. The platelet count usually returns to normal within three to five days of discontinuing the heparin. The mechanism of this reaction is thought to be immunological.

*Osteoporosis.* Osteoporosis usually occurs only after chronic heparin therapy of greater than 10,000 units per day for six months.

## Inhibition of Heparin Activity

Discontinuing the administration of heparin usually suffices when there is minor bleeding secondary to the anticoagulation therapy. The effects will usually vanish within a few hours.

In the case of a more severe complication, such as extremely prolonged APTT or major bleeding, or both, the effect of heparin can be rapidly neutralized by administering protamine sulfate, a basic molecule that combines with heparin to form a stable complex with no anticoagulant activity. It is injected intravenously at a rate of 1 mg of protamine per 100 units of total heparin thought to be present in the blood at the time of protamine administration. For example, given the half-life of intravenously administered heparin (about 0.5-1.5 h), the dose of protamine would be half the amount required to neutralize the heparin dose, if the protamine is given 30 min after the heparin was administered.

Excess protamine sulfate should be avoided because it also inhibits the thrombin/fibrinogen reaction and thus can have a further anticoagulant activity in the patient.

## References

1. Rosenberg, R.D., Actions and interactions of antithrombin and heparin. *N. Engl. J. Med.* **292**, 146 (1975).

2. Coon, W., Some recent developments in the pharmacology of heparin. *J. Clin. Pharmacol.* **337** (July 1979).

3. Salzman, E.W., Deykin, D., Shapiro, R.M., and Rosenberg, R., Management of heparin therapy: Controlled prospective trial. *N. Engl. J. Med.* **292**, 1046 (1975).

4. Glazier, R.L., and Crowell, E.B., Randomized prospective trial of continuous vs intermittent heparin therapy. *J. Am. Med. Assoc.* **236**, 1365 (1976).

5. Wilson, J.R., and Lampman, J., Heparin therapy: A randomized prospective study. *Am. Heart J.* **97**, 155 (1979).

6. Basu, D., Gallus, A., Hirsch, J., and Cade, J., A prospective study of the value of monitoring heparin treatment with activated partial thromboplastin time. *N. Engl. J. Med.* **287**, 324 (1972).

7. Genton, E., Guidelines for heparin therapy. *Ann. Intern. Med.* **80**, 77 (1974).

# 56

# Heparin Monitoring during Cardiopulmonary Bypass

**Paul Didisheim, M.D.**

## Case Report

A 59-year-old woman was admitted to St. Mary's Hospital in Rochester because of a prolonged episode of intractable chest pain. She had had an inferior myocardial infarction six years earlier and had had moderate angina pectoris since that time. Her symptoms had usually been relieved with nitroglycerin and Inderal. Cardiac catheterization on this admission demonstrated total occlusion of the left anterior descending and right coronary arteries. Because of persistent angina, coronary artery bypass surgery was performed. The saphenous vein was harvested from the left thigh. After heparinization, adequate hypothermia, and infusion of cardioplegic solution, two bypass grafts were implanted with reversed segments of saphenous vein from the aorta to the two occluded coronary arteries distal to their occluded segments. The patient was rewarmed and weaned from bypass, heparin was neutralized with protamine, and incisions were closed. Heparin levels in plasma after heparinization, hypothermia, rewarming, and protamine neutralization were 6.6, 7.3, and .04 units/mL, respectively. Hemostasis was satisfactory throughout, and the postoperative course was uneventful.

## Discussion

Heparin (*1,2*) is a heterogeneous group of straight-chain anionic mucopolysaccharides called glycosaminoglycans (GAGs) of variable molecular weight averaging 15,000 but extending from 4,000 to 40,000 daltons. There is a general tendency for their anticoagulant activity to increase with molecular weight. They have certain essential structural features which distinguish them from related GAGs that have little or no *in vitro* anticoagulant activity: The GAG chains consist of alternating uronic acids and glycosamines, both in the pyranose form; heparin also differs from other GAGs by its greater extent of sulfation, about 2 to 2.5 sulfate ions per disaccharide unit compared with one or more. First isolated from liver (hence its name), heparin is

*Dr. Didisheim is Professor of Laboratory Medicine (Hematology), Mayo Medical School; and Director, Coagulation Area, Hemotology Laboratory, Mayo Clinic, Rochester, MN 55905.*

found in many tissues and is particularly abundant in mast cells.

Heparin requires a plasma cofactor for its anticoagulant activity, and it is now generally accepted that this heparin cofactor is antithrombin III (AT III), an $\alpha_2$ globulin and protease inhibitor present in normal plasma. It has been suggested that heparin binds to lysine residues on the AT III molecule forming a 1:1 complex inducing a conformational change and rendering its active site more accessible to thrombin and other serine proteases. Heparin markedly accelerates the velocity at which AT III complexes with and inactivates thrombin. About two thirds by weight of commercial heparin does not bind to AT III and has little anticoagulant activity.

Heparin also inhibits serine proteases which act earlier than thrombin in the blood coagulation cascade, in particular factor Xa. This action appears to be concentrated in the low-molecular-weight fractions. There is some evidence that this may be the most important mechanism *in vivo* for heparin's antithrombotic action, especially when administered in low dose. Another mechanism whereby heparin exerts its anticoagulant action is in preventing the formation of a stable fibrin clot: Heparin inhibits the activation of fibrin-stabilizing factor (factor XIII) by thrombin. Heparin administration also causes release of lipoprotein lipase from tissues into the blood.

Heparin is used clinically in three main ways: (1) in low dose, by subcutaneous injection, for the prophylaxis of venous thrombosis; (2) in standard dose, intravenously for the treatment of venous or arterial thrombosis or embolism; and (3) in high dose, for maintaining the fluidity of blood in extracorporeal circulatory devices such as cardiopulmonary bypass for open heart surgery or the artificial kidney for hemodialysis. When given intravenously the inhibitory effect on blood coagulation is noted almost immediately, as soon as it is distributed throughout the circulation. When added *in vitro*, heparin acts immediately. Commercial heparins are from two sources. Most are prepared from porcine intestinal mucosa while some are from bovine lung. There is no convincing evidence of difference in their efficacy or incidence of side-effects.

The principal risk associated with heparin administration is hemorrhage. This is not a problem with low

313

dosage but may occur in standard and high dosage, particularly if treatment is prolonged. The antidote is protamine which is administered intravenously and almost immediately forms an inactive complex with heparin. Rarely thrombocytopenia severe enough to contribute to hemorrhage may follow heparin therapy. Paradoxically, thrombosis has been associated with heparin treatment but this complication is very unusual. Alopecia occurs rarely, and osteoporosis and spontaneous fractures have occurred in patients who have received large amounts of heparin daily for six months or more.

Heparin is poorly absorbed sublingually or gastrointestinally because of its polarity and molecular size. Its entry into the placental circulation or maternal milk is also minimal. Deep subcutaneous (intrafat) administration is used with low-dose therapy and for treatment of ambulatory patients. Intramuscular injection is not recommended because this can cause large hematomas at the injection site. High-dose administration is accomplished by continuous or intermittent intravenous injection. The disappearance rate of intravenously injected heparin is proportional to the dose administered. This is assumed to be due to uptake by the reticuloendothelial system and possibly other extravascular sites from which it is slowly released. The approximate biological half-life in the circulation after 100, 200, and 400 units/kg of heparin is 1.0, 1.6, and 2.5 h, respectively. Heparin is metabolized in the liver by an enzyme named heparinase. The inactive metabolic products are then excreted in the urine. Heparin itself may appear in the urine after large intravenous doses. In patients with hepatic or renal failure, the half-life of heparin is significantly prolonged. Patients with pulmonary embolism may require increased doses to achieve anticoagulation because of accelerated clearance of heparin from the circulation. At sites of active thrombosis, the increased concentrations of both thrombin and platelet-derived platelet factor 4, a cationic, low-molecular-weight protein which binds heparin, may explain the accelerated removal of heparin from circulating blood.

The U.S.P. unit of heparin is the quantity that will prevent 1.0 mL of citrated sheep plasma from clotting for 1 h after the addition of 0.2 mL 1% $CaCl_2$. Heparin sodium U.S.P. must contain at least 120 U.S.P. units/mg. Because different heparin preparations vary in their purity and potency, heparin should always be prescribed and described on a unit basis. Monitoring of heparin therapy was first done by determining the coagulation time of whole blood (Lee-White test). The variability of this procedure has led to substitution of the activated partial thromboplastin time (APTT) in most centers. Recently specific assays for heparin have been developed in which a chromogenic or fluorogenic

## Heparin Profile

### Chemical Information

Trade names: Hepthrom, Lipo-hepin, Liquaemin, Panheparin, Calciparine

Chemical name: Heparin sodium, heparin calcium

pKa: Not applicable

Mol. mass: 4,000-40,000

Melting point, °C: Not applicable

Water solubility: 1 g in 20 mL

### Absorption and Distribution

Dose absorbed: None orally, sublingually, or rectally

Peak plasma level, time: Intravenous, immediate; subcutaneous, 4-8 h

Protein bound: Not applicable

$V_d$: Not applicable

Form in urine:
Unchanged drug: % dependent on dose
Unchanged drug is detectable in blood
Half-life is dependent on dose (see text)

### Dosage and Blood Levels

| Recommended dose[1] | Adults | Children |
|---|---|---|
| Deep subcutaneous intrafat (low dose) | 5,000-10,000 units q 8-12 h | 50-100 units/Kg/8-12 h |
| Intravenous (standard dose) | 5,000-10,000 units q 4-6 h | 50-100 units/Kg/4-6 h |
| Intravenous (high dose) for hemodialysis | 2,000-3,000 units prime; 1,000-2,000 units/h | variable |
| For cardiopulmonary bypass | 8,000-10,000 units/m² | variable |

### Effective levels[2]

| | | |
|---|---|---|
| Low dose | 0.1-0.3 units/mL plasma | same |
| Standard dose | 0.3-2.0 units/mL plasma | same |
| High dose | 3.0-7.0 units/mL plasma | same |

### Monitoring Methods

Lee-White coagulation time (whole blood)

Activated clotting time (whole blood)

Activated partial thromboplastin time (APTT) (plasma)

Specific assay for heparin (plasma)
Chromogenic
Fluorogenic

[1] Typical examples. Many variants have been proposed.
[2] Estimates. Limited data are avilable.

peptide is used (3). In our experience the fluorometric assay for heparin (4) is a sensitive, specific method which has the advantage over the Lee-White or APTT test of being unaffected by variability of levels of coagulation and fibrinolytic factors of the blood or by other drugs such as oral anticoagulants of the coumarin family which may be concurrently given. The fluorometric assay is useful in monitoring heparin and protamine therapy during cardiopulmonary bypass (5).

Heparin is stable in citrated blood at room temperature for 2 h (4) and at 4° C for 24 h. Monitoring heparin therapy by determining heparin levels in plasma with a specific assay is too recent a practice for much experience to have been accumulated; approximate effective levels are indicated in the following table.

## References

1. O'Reilly, R.A., Anticoagulant, antithrombotic, and thrombolytic drugs. In *The Pharmacologic Basis for Therapeutics*, A.G. Gilman, L.S. Goodman, and A. Gilman, Eds., Sixth Edition, Macmillan, New York, NY, 1980, pp 1347-1366.

2. Barrowcliffe, T.W., and Thomas, D.P., Antithrombin III and heparin. In *Haemostasis and Thrombosis*, A.L. Bloom, and D.P. Thomas, Eds.,Churchill Livingstone, New York, NY, 1981, pp 712-724.

3. Mitchell, G.A., Gargiulo, R.J., Huseby, R.M., Lawson, D.E., Pochron, S.P., and Sehuanes, J.A., Assay for plasma heparin using a snythetic peptide substrate for thrombin: Introduction of the fluorophore aminoisophthalic acid, dimethyl ester. *Thromb. Res.* **13**, 47-52 (1978).

4. Choo, I.H.F., Didisheim, P., Doerge, M.D., Johnson, M.L., Bach, M.L., Melchart, L.M., Johnson, W.J., and Taylor, W.F., Evaluation of a heparin assay method using a fluorogenic synthetic peptide substrate for thrombin. *Thromb. Res.* **25**, 115-123 (1982).

5. Hughes, D.R., Faust, R.J., Didisheim, P., and Tinker, J.H. Heparin monitoring during cardiopulmonary bypass in man: Use of fluorogenic heparin assay to validate activated clotting time. *Anesth. Analg.* **61**, Supp. 2, 189-190 (1982).

# 57

# Warfarin: A Case Report

**Alexander Duncan, M.D.**

A 30-year-old white woman presented with several complaints including chest pain, recurrent blackouts, and a tender right calf, all of which had been present for several months. She had also experienced an episode of hemoptysis about five days previously. She gave an interesting history of 17 previous hospitalizations in the past four and one-half years for recurrent thrombophlebitis, usually involving the right lower limb, and three episodes of pulmonary embolism, presumably secondary to her thrombophlebitis. No records of these hospitalizations were available at this presentation.

Because of her recurrent thrombotic episodes, she had been taking 25 mg of warfarin daily for four and one-half years, and 5000 int. units of subcutaneous heparin twice daily for three months.

The patient was noted to be grossly obese, weighing 113 kg (249 lb.) with a regular pulse of 100, and a normal blood pressure of 130/85 mmHg. The only significant examination findings were tenderness in the ribs beneath her left breast and some diffuse tenderness of the right lower limb with a negative Holmes sign. All her peripheral pulses were palpable, and both lower limbs were considered normal with no clinical evidence of phlebitis. Chest examination revealed normal lung fields with no evidence of pulmonary embolism.

Results of initial lab studies revealed she had normal complete blood count and chemistries and a prothrombin time of 10.8 s (normal: 9.5-11.3 s). An electrocardiogram indicated normal sinus rhythm, arterial blood gases were $p_{O_2}$ 95 mmHg (normal: 80-90 mmHg) and $p_{CO_2}$ 39 mmHg (normal: 35-45 mmHg), and pH was 7.41 (normal: 7.32-7.42).

Despite no clinical evidence of thrombosis, on the basis of her previous history it was decided to continue both warfarin and heparin treatment as before while investigating her presenting complaints.

One immediate concern was the apparent lack of therapeutic anticoagulation indicated by her normal prothrombin time, despite long-term therapy with a high dose of warfarin. Patients on warfarin therapy rarely require a daily dose of more than 15 mg to provide stable therapeutic anticoagulation, and despite this patient's weight, 25 mg should have been sufficient to treat her successfully. This raised the questions of was

*Dr. Duncan is in the Departments of Clinical Pathology and Hematology Research, Mayo Clinic, Rochester, MN 55901.*

the patient resistant to warfarin, and was she taking her medication as prescribed.

For the next two days, the patient continued to experience chest pain and dyspnea, but all electrocardiograms were normal except for intermittent sinus tachycardia (SVT) in the range of 110-150/min. One arterial blood gas sample was taken, and results had not changed since admission.

At this juncture a cardiologist assessed the patient and suggested that her recurrent chest pains were from her ribs and not cardiac in origin. He considered it very unlikely that the pains were caused by recurrent small pulmonary emboli.

Because of the continuing lack of evidence of thrombosis, her anticoagulant therapy was discontinued. Her prothrombin time was 10.3 s, and a test for warfarin concentration in serum detected no drug.

During the next two days the patient's lower limbs were examined with Doppler ultrasound and venous plethysmography, but neither test indicated a venous obstruction in either leg. Because of continuing complaints of chest pain and dyspnea the patient was put on a Holter monitor for 24 h. This indicated episodes of SVT, but no other significant arrhythmia. By now, her previous records had become available, revealing no concrete evidence of thrombophlebitis despite repeated Doppler ultrasounds and phlebogram studies. There was even less evidence to support a diagnosis of pulmonary embolism: numerous previous perfusion lung scans were all normal, as was a pulmonary angiogram done during an episode of "pulmonary embolism." Moreover, in the previous four and one-half years none of her prothrombin times had been in the therapeutic range, despite the patient's insistence that she was taking 25 mg of warfarin every day during that time.

It was now felt necessary to establish whether the patient was indeed refractory to warfarin or if patient compliance was the problem. On the third day after her anticoagulants were stopped, a hemostatic survey was done to make sure there were no more effects from the warfarin and the heparin on the results of the coagulation test. The screen revealed a prothrombin time of 11 s, an activated partial thromboplastin time of 30 s (normal: 25-35 s), platelets $335 \times 10^3$ (normal: $130\text{-}370 \times 10^3$), fibrinogen 4.56 g/L (normal: 1.90-3.60 g/L), thrombin time 22 s (normal: 20-25 s), and a functional antithrombin III value 75% of normal. All these results were close to the normal values for that laboratory.

The patient was then started on 25 mg of warfarin daily. After 24 h her prothrombin time was 13.8 s, and serum warfarin concentration was 1.3 mg/L (normal therapeutic: 2-5 mg/L). After 48 h her prothrombin time had increased to 16.7 s and the serum warfarin to 1.7 mg/L. After 72 h her prothrombin time was 22.8 s and serum warfarin was 3.2 mg/L. These results — the expected prolongation of her prothrombin time and the increased drug concentrations in the therapeutic range — indicated that the patient was not refractory to oral warfarin, but that she had not been taking her medication as she claimed. A psychiatric assessment of the patient was consistent with a functional rather than organic origin for her presenting symptoms.

This woman exemplifies a case where the normal method for assessing the efficacy of anticoagulant therapy, i.e., a prolongation of her prothrombin time, could not provide information on the supposed failure of a high dose of warfarin to anticoagulate this patient. Instead, the measurement of serum warfarin concentrations was the answer to this dilemma.

## Pharmacology of Warfarin

Warfarin is the most widely prescribed oral anticoagulant in the United States. It owes its origin to a report in 1924 *(1)* of a hemorrhagic disorder in cattle after the ingestion of spoiled sweet clover. This disorder was later shown to be due to a decrease in plasma prothrombin, and in 1949 the causative agent was identified as 3-($\alpha$-acetonylbenzyl)-4-hydroxycoumarin, the chemical name for warfarin *(2)*.

At first it was used as a rodent poison, being thought too toxic for humans, but a suicide attempt involving repeated large doses of a warfarin-containing rodenticide led to clinical trials that eventually established the safe use of warfarin in human therapeutics. Long known to be a vitamin K antagonist, its exact mode of action has become apparent only in the past few years.

The vitamin K-dependent clotting factors II, VII, IX, and X are synthesized in the liver in an inactive zymogen form *(3-7)*. The main difference between the zymogenic and active form of these coagulation factors is the inability of the zymogens to bind divalent cations, especially calcium, and still be able to bind to phospholipid-containing membranes as part of the normal blood-clotting mechanism.

In 1974 the discovery of $\gamma$-carboxyglutamic acid *(8)* led to the finding that the difference in the active factors was the conversion of certain glutamic acid residues in the zymogens to $\gamma$-carboxyglutamic acid residues. Binding of calcium to these specific residues initiates binding of the clotting factor to membrane phospholipid *(13)*.

The enzymic carboxylation of these glutamic acid residues requires vitamin $K_1$ as a cofactor. In hepatic microsomes, vitamin $K_1$ is reduced to a hydroquinone form, vitamin $KH_2$. The carboxylation reaction involving the clotting factor zymogens is coupled with a reaction in which an enzyme, vitamin $KH_2$, epoxidase, converts vitamin $KH_2$ to the biochemically inert vitamin K epoxide or vitamin KO. This is enzymically reduced back to vitamin $KH_2$ by epoxide reductase. This sequence of reactions constitute the vitamin $K_1$ epoxide cycle. Warfarin has been shown to inhibit the action of epoxide reductase *(14,15)* and thus leads to a buildup of the inert vitamin KO and a decrease in the urinary excretion of $\gamma$-carboxyglutamic acid, secondary to a decrease in the synthesis of the clotting factors II, VII, IX, and X *(16)*.

The onset of warfarin's anticoagulant effect is influenced both by its inhibition of clotting factor syntheses and the unchanged degradation rates for each coagulation factor. The half-lives of these factors in circulation are quite different (6, 24, 40, and 60 h for factors VII, IX, X, and II), so that warfarin affects factor VII concentrations much more quickly than concentrations of prothrombin (Factor II). This is why the maximum efficacy of anticoagulant therapy, as assessed by the prolongation of the prothrombin time, appears three days after therapy begins. Because larger doses have no effect on these factor degradation rates, only enough warfarin to inhibit the synthesis is required to produce the maximum rate of anticoagulation, and the practice of giving patients large loading doses of warfarin at the beginning of therapy has been discontinued.

Warfarin is rapidly absorbed after an oral dose and a peak plasma concentration is reached 1 h after ingestion. It is 99% bound to albumin and has a half-life of 35 h. The drug is a racemic mixture of D and L enantiomorphs, which are metabolized differently, but are both excreted as glucuronide esters in urine and feces. Alterations in the metabolism that influence the action of warfarin include various forms of liver disease that lead to a decrease in protein synthesis *(17)* and any gastrointestinal disease that leads to vitamin K deficiency. Both of these enhance the response to warfarin. During pregnancy there is an increase in the synthesis of the clotting factors, which results in a decreased response to warfarin. Because warfarin crosses the placenta and may cause hypoprothrombinemia in the fetus, it should not be used in pregnant patients.

Phenylbutazone displaces warfarin from albumin, thus increasing the active free warfarin and increasing the effect of a given dose of warfarin. Phenylbutazone also inhibits the metabolism of the more potent enantiomorph, L-warfarin *(18)*. Metranidazole and cotrimoxazole both prolong the half-life of L-warfarin and thus potentiate its effect.

Drugs that decrease the response to oral warfarin include barbiturates and glutethimide, which cause induction of hepatic microsomes and thus increase the metabolism of warfarin.

The main toxic effect of warfarin is hemorrhage occurring as hematuria, melena uterine bleeding, epistaxis, or hemoptysis. The hemorrhage usually occurs because of inadequate control, caused by failure to determine prothrombin time frequently enough. To maintain the patient in the therapeutic range, a hemorrhage is treated by withdrawing the drug and giving the patient 10-20 mg of oral vitamin $K_1$ which converts prothrombin times to normal within 24 h. If the hemorrhage is severe or critical, the clotting factor defect can be reversed in a few hours by giving 20-50 mg of vitamin $K_1$ intravenously.

The prolongation of the prothrombin time remains the primary way to measure the anticoagulant effect of warfarin, but measuring concentrations in serum, as described here or in someone with a possible inability to absorb the drug, can provide useful information.

## References

1. Schofield, F.W., Damaged sweetclover: The cause of a new disease in cattle simulating hemorrhagic septicemia and blackleg. *J. Am. Vet. Med. Assoc.* **64**, 553-575 (1924).

2. Ikawa, M., Stahmann, M.A., and Link, K.P., Studies on 4-hydroxycoumarins. V. Condensation of $\alpha$, $\beta$-unsaturated ketones with 4-hydroxycoumarins. *J. Am. Chem. Soc.* **66**, 902-906 (1944).

3. Hemker, H.C., Veltkamp, J.J., Hensen, A., and Loeliger, E.A., Nature of prothrombin biosynthesis: Preprothrombinaemia in vitamin K deficiency. *Nature* **200**, 589-590 (1963).

4. Ganrot, P.O., and Nilehn, J.E., Plasma prothrombin during treatment with dicumarol. II. Demonstration of an abnormal prothrombin fraction. *Scand. J. Clin. Lab. Invest.* **22**, 23-28 (1968).

5. Denson, K.W.E., The levels of factors II, VII, IX and X by antibody neutralization techniques in the plasma of patients receiving phenindione therapy. *Br. J. Haematol* **20**, 643-648 (1971).

6. Larrieu, M.J., and Meyer, D., Abnormal factor IX during anticoagulant treatment. *Lancet ii*, 1085 (1970).

7. Pryoz, H., Immunological techniques and coagulation factors. In *Immunological Mechanisms in Blood Coagulation. Thrombosis and Hemostasis.*, F. Duckert, Ed., Schattauer Press, Stuttgart, 1971, pp 296-299.

8. Stenflo, J., Fernlund, P., Egan, W., and Roepstorff, P., Vitamin K dependent modifications of glutamic acid residues in prothrombin. *Proc. Natl. Acad. Sci. USA* **71**, 2730-2733 (1974).

9. Nelsestuen, G.L., Zytkovicz, T.H., and Howard, J.B., The mode of action of vitamin K. Identification of $\gamma$-carboxyglutamic acid as a component of prothrombin. *J. Biol. Chem.* **249**, 6347-6350 (1974).

10. Kisiel, W., and Davie, E.W., Isolation and characterization of bovine factor VII. *Biochemistry* **14**, 4928-4934 (1975).

11. DiScipio, R.G., Hermodson, M.A., Yates, S.G., and Davie, E.W., A comparison of human prothrombin, factor IX (Christmas factor), factor X (Stuart factor) and protein S. *Biochemistry* **16**, 698 (1977).

12. Fujikawa, K., Legaz, M.E., and Davie, E.W., Bovine factors $X_1$ and $X_2$ (Stuart factor). Isolation and characterization. *Biochemistry* **11**, 4882 (1972).

13. Olson, R.E., and Sottie, J.W., Vitamin K and $\gamma$-carboxyglutamate biosynthesis. *Vitam. Horm.* **35**, 59-108 (1977).

14. Willingham, A., and Matschiner, J.T., Changes in phylloquinone epoxidase activity related to prothrombin synthesis and microsomal clotting activity in the rat. *Biochem. J.* **140**, 435-441 (1974).

15. Whitlon, D.S., Sadowski, J.A., and Suttie, J.W., Mechanism of coumarin action: Significance of vitamin K epoxide reductase inhibition. *Biochemistry* **17**, 1371-1377 (1978).

16. Levy, R.J., Lian, J.B., Gundberg, C., and Gallop, P.M., $\gamma$-Carboxyglutamate excretion and vitamin K metabolism. In *Vitamin K Metabolism and Vitamin K Dependent Protein*, J.W. Suttie, Ed., University Park Press, College Park, MD, 1980 pp 375-379.

17. Williams, R.L., Schary, W.L., Blaschke, T.F., et al., Influence of acute viral hepatitis on disposition and pharmacologic effect of warfarin. *Clin. Pharmacol. Ther.* **20**, 90-97 (1976).

18. Lewis, R.J., Trager, W.F., Chan, K.K., et al., Warfarin: Stereochemical aspects of its metabolism and the interaction with phenylbutazone. *J. Clin. Invest.* **53**, 1607-1617 (1974).

# Pharmacokinetics of Morphine: A Review

**H.M. Vandenberghe, Ph.D.**
**S.J. Soldin, Ph.D.**
**S.M. MacLeod, Ph.D.**

Morphine (Figure 1), the oldest analgesic drug, is still widely administered for relief of chronic and acute pain in adults and children. Although this drug is extensively used, it is only in recent years that the development of sensitive and specific assays for determination of morphine concentrations in serum has allowed study of the drug's disposition in more depth. More pharmacokinetic data are becoming available but a clear dose-response relationship with respect to analgesic effect remains undefined. Clinical quantitation of the analgesic effect is complicated as the intensity of pain is highly variable depending on the type of pain, while the individual reaction to pain is subject to even greater variation. Better understanding of the pharmacokinetics of morphine and of changes in this drug's disposition in disease should aid in the improvement of pain relief when morphine is administered.

Morphine is a naturally occurring alkaloid, prepared by extraction from opium, the dried juice of unripe seed pods of *Papaver somniferum*. It is available in two salt forms: morphine sulfate pentahydrate and morphine hydrochloride trihydrate.

The following topics will be discussed: absorption, distribution, biotransformation, first-pass effect, excretion, clearance, and relation of concentrations in plasma and pharmacological activity.

## Absorption

Morphine is readily absorbed through all mucous membranes, but not through the intact skin. After intramuscular (IM) injection in healthy volunteers and surgical patients, morphine is rapidly absorbed and reaches peak concentrations within 20 min (*1,2*). The absorption half-life averages 8 min and the systemic availability is 100% (*2*). Absorption and elimination patterns following subcutaneous administration of morphine are similar to those after IM injections.

After oral administration of morphine, the fraction absorbed is difficult to assess because of a major first-pass effect. Morphine is mainly absorbed from the small intestine. It has a pKa of 7.95 and is highly

*The authors are affiliated with the Departments of Clinical Biochemistry and Pharmacology, University of Toronto, and the Research Institute, Hospital for Sick Children, Toronto, Canada.*

ionized in the stomach. The peak concentration after an oral dose was obtained after 15 min in healthy volunteers and the concentration was 5 to 7 times lower than after the same parenteral dose (*1*). In six cancer patients the peak serum concentrations were reached between 10 and 120 min after dosing and the absorption half-life ranged from 4 to 57 min (*3*).

The oral bioavailability in healthy volunteers was estimated to be 30% when the areas under the serum-concentration time curves after oral and intravenous administration of morphine were compared (*1*). In six cancer patients the bioavailability ranged between 15 and 64% with a mean value of 38% (*3*). This low bioavailability can be explained by the first-pass effect; oral morphine is lost during passage through the intestinal mucosa and the liver, where extensive metabolism takes place. Controlled studies have shown that oral administration of morphine is only one-sixth as effective as parenteral administration of the same dose when peak analgesia is measured (*4*). Thus, the oral-to-parenteral dose ratio for morphine is 6 to 1 compared with 4 to 1 for hydromorphone and meperidine, and 2 to 1 for methadone and codeine (*5*). In cancer patients an oral dose 5.5 to 7 times greater

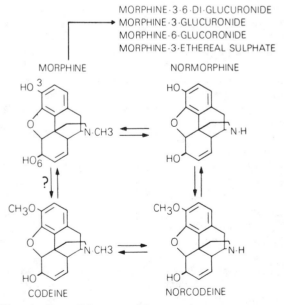

**Fig. 1. Possible morphine pathway**
Adapted from Boerner et al. (*14*)

than the parenteral dose appeared adequate for effective therapy (*3*). Because of its high first-pass effect morphine is designated a *flow-limited hepatic clearance* drug. Drugs which alter hepatic blood flow such as cimetidine may be able to affect morphine clearance by the liver.

In man, the contributions of intestinal and hepatic metabolism to first-pass elimination have not been studied. In the rat, however, the oral bioavailability following first-pass elimination of morphine by both gut mucosa and liver was 15% (*6*). This indicates that 85% of the administered oral dose is metabolized or sequestered before reaching the systemic circulation. Intraportal administration of morphine bypasses the gut mucosa and results in a first-pass elimination by the liver of 72% when compared to the same intravenous dose. Subsequent calculation of the amount of morphine sequestered in the gut mucosa and contributing to the first-pass elimination yields a value of 46%. Thus 54% of the original dose passes through the gut into the portal blood and only 28% of this reaches the systemic circulation, i.e., a net systemic bioavailability of 15%.

## Distribution

Morphine leaves the blood very rapidly after intravenous (IV) injection in both anesthetized and healthy individuals, and within 5 min 93% of the dose has disappeared from the extracellular compartment (*1*, *2*). Organ sampling in animals has shown that the drug is readily distributed into highly perfused tissues such as the kidney, lungs, liver, and spleen. Skeletal muscle may contain low absolute concentrations of morphine, but this reservoir generally accounts for the major fraction of morphine not distributed to kidney, lungs, liver, or spleen. Only small amounts of morphine cross the blood-brain barrier and are detectable in the central nervous system; however, even small amounts are capable of producing significant analgesia after reacting with specific opiate receptors. Newborn infants are more susceptible to morphine-induced respiratory depression, and it has been postulated that the increased sensitivity is related to the ease with which morphine gains access to the central nervous system receptor sites (i.e., permeates the blood-brain barrier).

In older patients, serum concentrations at 2 to 5 min after an IV injection of morphine were significantly higher and more variable in patients over 50 than in patients under 50 years of age (*7*). The 2-min serum concentration of morphine correlated directly with age. This can be explained by the fact that the distribution of morphine is influenced by the cardiac output, which decreases with increasing age, while certain tissues where morphine is concentrated may be less well perfused. Older patients are more sensitive to morphine and the higher and more variable concentrations may contribute to this phenomenon.

Morphine freely passes the placental barrier as indicated by the fact that babies born to addicted mothers present withdrawal symptoms. Neonatal sedation also occurs when morphine is given close to delivery. The drug also appears in breast milk.

In plasma, morphine is bound 35% to albumin and 6% to the $\gamma$-globulins (*8*). The binding to both proteins is independent of the morphine concentration and dependent upon the concentration of proteins. In uremic patients without hepatic failure, in patients with hepatic failure, and in hepatorenal disease, the percentage binding of morphine to protein has been shown to decrease depending on the decrease in albumin. An increased sensitivity to morphine in uremic patients and in patients with hepatic cirrhosis may, at least in part, be due to decreased morphine protein binding with resulting higher concentration in the central nervous system (*9*).

Different studies (*2*, *3*, *10-13*) have reported an apparent volume of distribution ($V_d$) falling in a range from 1.0 to 6.3 L/kg.

## Biotransformation

A possible morphine metabolic pathway in man suggested by Boerner et al. (*14*) is shown in Figure 1 and the percentages of metabolites identified in urine are presented in Table 1. The major metabolite of morphine is morphine-3-glucuronide, which is an analgetically inactive product formed by glucuronidation of the phenol ring. In vivo, glucuronidation takes place mainly in the liver microsomes and to a limited extent in the intestine, the kidney, and probably the placenta. Morphine-3-glucuronide appears in serum 1 min after IV injection of morphine, and within 90 min the metabolite represents more than

## Table 1. Morphine Metabolites Identified in Urine (*14, 15, 18, 19*)

| | |
|---|---|
| Morphine-3-glucuronide | 54-74% |
| Normorphine | |
|   Free | 0.5-1.5% |
|   Conjugates | 3-5% |
| Morphine-6-glucuronide | <1% |
| Morphine-3-ethereal sulfate | 0.5-4% |
| Morphine-3,6-diglucuronide | <1% |
| Codeine | |
|   Free | 1-6% |
|   Conjugates | |

90% of the total morphine serum concentration (*11*).

Small amounts of morphine-6-glucuronide have been recovered from urine, and although a minor metabolite, it was shown to be 45 times more potent than morphine after intracerebral injection in mice (*14*).

A third metabolite obtained by synthetic reaction is morphine-3-ethereal sulfate. In urine 0.5 to 4% of an administered dose of morphine is recovered as morphine-3-ethereal sulfate. The formation of codeine from morphine by *O*-methylation and excretion of codeine and presumably glucuronidated metabolites are controversial (*15, 16*).

Oxidative biotransformation of morphine to normorphine takes place in the liver catalyzed by the microsomal oxidative system. A parallel biotransformation may also occur in the brain. Formation of normorphine appears to be greater after an oral dose than after parenternal administration of the drug. The amount of normorphine conjugates in the urine represents 0.5 to 1.5% and 3 to 5% of the administered dose, respectively (*14*). This metabolite has analgesic potency similar to morphine (*17*).

The metabolite morphine-*N*-oxide has been demonstrated only in urine of cancer patients also receiving amiphenizole. Other minor metabolites of morphine have been isolated from urine in different animal species but at present have not been found in man.

## Excretion

The elimination half-life of morphine in healthy volunteers and in surgical patients has been found to average about 2 h following any mode of administration (*1, 2, 10-13*). A significant correlation between age and elimination half-life in patients between 23 and 75 years could not be demonstrated (*7*). Interindividual half-lives vary greatly and cover, for example, a range from 1 to 7.8 h in cancer patients (*3*) and 1 to 5 h in surgical patients (*13*). The preoperative and postoperative elimination half-lives in 10 patients indicated great intraindividual variation (*13*).

After an oral dose only 3% of morphine is excreted unchanged by the kidneys, primarily through glomerular filtration and to a lesser extent by tubular secretion, while after parenteral dosage about 8 to 10% is excreted unchanged during the first 48 h (*1*).

The elimination half-life of the metabolite morphine-3-glucuronide averaged 3 h (*11*) and 71% was found in the urine in the first 48 h after an oral dose, while 67% was found in this form after a parenteral morphine dose (*1*).

The major route of elimination is the kidney, but to a small extent morphine and morphine-3-glucuronide are excreted into bile. Bile is gradually released into the duodenum where morphine-3-glucuronide is hydrolyzed by enzymes in the gut, primarily in the cecum by bacteria. The liberated morphine can be reabsorbed in the cecum and this establishes enterohepatic recirculation. This has been demonstrated in rats and some data suggest a similar phenomenon in man. In man, data on biliary excretion are sparse. In feces of normal volunteers 6.7 to 10.4% of an intramuscularly administered dose of morphine-*N*-methyl-$^{14}$C was recovered within 72 h. Morphine is also secreted into saliva and analysis of saliva by spin immunoassay (FRAT, Syva Co.) has been suggested as a suitable indicator of nonprotein-bound morphine.

## Clearance

The reported clearance values for morphine vary widely. Several reported studies are presented in Table 2. A possible explanation for the clearance differences may be found in the major variations in study design. Where morphine serum concentrations were measured by radioimmunoassay, a 27% overestimation of concentration values has been indicated (*21*). However, this method was used by Stanski et al. (*2, 10*) who reported a clearance of 5.6 mL/kg/min in one study and 12.4 and 14.7 mL/kg/min in another. Other similar differences in clearances cannot be explained on this basis.

### Table 2. Clearance of Morphine

| Mode of Administration | Clearance mg/kg/min | Age, years | Ref. |
|---|---|---|---|
| Single IV bolus before surgery | 6.2 | 1-7 | |
| | 6.7 | 7-15 | *12* |
| Multiple IV bolus during surgery | 13.8 | 7-15 | *12* |
| Single IV dose in cancer patients | 9.2 | 49-76 | *3* |
| Single IV bolus in healthy volunteers | 14.7 | 26-32 | *2* |
| IV infusion over 15 min before surgery | 12.4 | 61-80 | *2* |
| Single IV bolus during anesthesia | 23.1 | 18-39 | *11* |
| Single IV high dose (1 mg/kg) before surgery | 5.6 | 37-66 | *10* |
| Single IV dose during anesthesia + postoperative programmable IV injections | 21.0 | 22-58 | *13* |
| Single IV dose 3 to 7 days after surgery | 21.0 | 22-58 | *13* |
| Single IV bolus + continuous IV infusion during anesthesia | 21.1 | 0-5 | *20* |

Assuming a hepatic blood flow of 21 mL/kg/min, a clearance of 21 to 23 mL/kg/min suggests that the hepatic blood flow is the limiting step in elimination of morphine. Because morphine elimination is primarily via metabolism in the liver and hepatic blood flow may be a rate-limiting step, liver disease may therefore change the disposition of morphine. A comparison of morphine pharmacokinetics in healthy individuals and patients with cirrhotic disease did not reveal any difference in clearance (22). Intra- and extra-hepatic shunting was present in cirrhotic patients. It was postulated that a significant amount of morphine conjugation occurs at extrahepatic sites in the gut and kidney. Similarly, in a rat model with passive hepatic venous congestion, the expected detrimental effects on biotransformation and disposition of morphine could not be demonstrated (23).

## Relationship of Concentrations in Plasma and and Pharmacological Activity

The relationship between pharmacokinetics and pharmacodynamics of morphine remains difficult to assess, although we have overcome the lack of sensitive techniques to determine morphine serum concentrations. The analgesic response to pain is highly variable among individuals, because the perception of pain and particularly the reaction to pain are very diverse. In addition, the pain intensifies following trauma and surgery may vary.

Berkowitz et al. (7) indicated that the decline in morphine concentration in serum after intramuscular injection in anesthetized patients roughly correlated with the decline in analgesia obtained in cancer patients receiving an intramuscular dose of morphine. They suggested that a serum morphine concentration of 0.050 mg/L (175 x $10^{-6}$ mol/L) provided moderate analgesia; however, analgesic effect and drug concentrations were not determined in the same patients.

Using continuous intravenous morphine, the measurement of pain relief after upper abdominal operations has been evaluated by means of a linear color-coded light analog, and on this basis it was concluded that a morphine concentration in serum of 0.023 to 0.025 mg/L (80.6 x $10^{-6}$ to 87.6 x $10^{-6}$ mol/L) would give adequate analgesia (24). The relief of pain in patients who have had abdominal surgery has been studied during patient-controlled administration of intravenous doses of morphine by a programmable drug injector. The mean morphine consumption was 2.6 ± 1.2 mg/h, which produced a mean concentration in serum ± SD of 0.021 ± 0.012 mg/L (73.6 x $10^{-6}$ ± 42.1 x $10^{-6}$ mol/L) with a calculated mean

minimum effective concentration ± SD of 0.016 ± 0.009 mg/L (56.1 x $10^{-6}$ ± 31.5 x $10^{-6}$ mol/L). This procedure achieved satisfactory analgesia in all patients. The mean morphine consumption of 2.6 ± 1.2 mg/h proved equivalent to the traditional dosage of 10 to 15 mg IM administered at 4 h intervals. The latter regimen yields high peaks and low troughs associated with drowsiness and pain, respectively. More frequent smaller doses as in patient-controlled administration of IV doses of morphine or administration of a bolus followed by a continuous IV infusion provides more continuous relief of pain and correspondingly greater comfort (24).

In most cancer patients receiving oral morphine in doses of 20 to 30 mg, serum concentrations above 0.020 mg/L (70.1 x $10^{-6}$ mol/L) could be achieved after a single dose. Oral morphine can be used effectively but great variability in bioavailability and half-life must be taken into account for adjustment of oral doses.

In children undergoing surgery and receiving 70% nitrous oxide in addition to intravenous doses of morphine, effective pain relief was tested by monitoring increase in blood pressure, pulse frequency, and sweating. Adequate analgesia during surgery corresponded with a mean morphine concentration in serum of 0.0650 mg/L (228 x $10^{-6}$ mol/L). The range was between 0.0463 and 0.0827 mg/L (162 x $10^{-6}$ to 290 x $10^{-6}$ mol/L) (95% confidence limits) and evaluations did not differ among several anesthesiologists (12).

## Summary

Morphine is the most important analgesic drug in clinical practice and is widely used. It has an elimination half-life of approximately 2 h and is extensively metabolized mainly to morphine-3-glucuronide, which is excreted via the kidneys. The drug is well absorbed after intramuscular injection and possibly after oral administration. The oral bioavailability varies widely (15% in rats; 15-64% in cancer patients; 30% in healthy volunteers: see above), due to the first-pass effect with extensive metabolism of morphine in the gut mucosa and the liver. Morphine is widely distributed in the body and only 35% is bound to albumin and 6% to the γ-globulins. The therapeutic range for morphine has not been defined clearly, although recent studies have suggested a morphine concentration in serum of 0.020 to 0.025 mg/L (70.1 x $10^{-6}$ to 87.6 x $10^{-6}$ mol/L) as adequate for analgesia in postoperative adult patients. During surgery, a concentration of 0.065 mg/L (228 x $10^{-6}$ mol/L) has been suggested in children between seven and 15 years of age to provide analgesia in balanced anesthesia.

# References

1. Brunk, S.F., and Delle, M., Morphine metabolism in man. *Clin. Pharmacol. Ther.* **16**, 51-57 (1974).

2. Stanski, D.R., Greenblatt, D.J., and Lowenstein, E., Kinetics of intravenous and intramuscular morphine. *Clin. Pharmacol. Ther.* **24**, 52-59 (1978).

3. Sawe, J., Dahlstrom, B., Paalzow, L., and Rane, A., Morphine kinetics in cancer patients. *Clin. Pharmacol. Ther.* **30**, 629-635 (1981).

4. Jaffe, J.H., and Martin, W.R., Opioid analgesics and antagonists. In *The Pharmacologic Basis of Therapeutics*, A.G. Gilman, L.S. Goodman, and A. Gilman, Eds., Macmillan Publishing Co., Inc., New York. N.Y., 1980, pp 494-534.

5. Houde, R.W., Analgesic effectiveness of the narcotic agonist-antagonists. *Brit. J. Clin. Pharmacol.* **8** (Suppl. 3), 279S-308S (1979).

6. Dahlstrom, B.E., and Paalzow, L.K., Pharmacokinetic interpretation of the enterohepatic recirculation and first-pass elimination of morphine in the rat. *J. Pharmacokin. Biopharm.* **6**, 505-519 (1978).

7. Berkowitz, B.A., Ngai, S.H., Yang, J.C., Hempstead, J., and Spector, S., The disposition of morphine in surgical patients. *Clin. Pharmacol. Ther.* **17**, 629-635 (1975).

8. Olsen, G.D., Morphine binding to human plasma proteins. *Clin. Pharmacol. Ther.* **17**, 31-35 (1975).

9. Olsen, G.D., Bennett, W.M., and Porter, G.A., Morphine and phenytoin binding to proteins in renal and hepatic failure. *Clin. Pharmacol. Ther.* **17**, 677-684 (1975).

10. Stanski, D.R., Greenblatt, D.J., Lappas, D.G., Koch-Weser, J., and Lowenstein, E., Kinetics of high-dose intravenous morphine in cardiac surgery patients. *Clin. Pharmacol. Ther.* **19**, 752-756 (1976).

11. Murphy, M.R., and Hug, C.C., Pharmacokinetics of intravenous morphine in patients anesthetized with enflurane-nitrous oxide. *Anesthesiology* **54**, 187-192 (1981).

12. Dahlstrom, B., Bolme, P., Feychting, M., Noack, G., and Paalzow, L., Morphine kinetics in children. *Clin. Pharmacol. Ther.* **26**, 354-365 (1979).

13. Dahlstrom, B., Tamsen, A., Paalzow, L., and Hartvig, P., Patient-controlled analgesic therapy, Part IV: Pharmacokinetics and analgesic plasma concentrations of morphine. *Clin. Pharmacokin.* **7**, 266-279 (1982).

14. Boerner, U., Abbott, S., and Roe, R.L., The metabolism of morphine and heroin in man. Review. *Drug Metab. Rev.* **4**, 39-73 (1975).

15. Boerner, U., and Abbott, S., New observations in the metabolism of morphine, The formation of codeine from morphine in man. *Experientia* **29**, 180-181 (1973).

16. Yeh, S.Y., Absence of evidence of biotransformation of morphine to codeine in man. *Experientia* **30**, 264-266 (1974).

17. Johannesson, T., and Milthers, K., Morphine and normorphine in the brain of rats. A comparison of subcutaneous, intraperitoneal, and intravenous administration. *Acta Pharmacol. Toxicol.* **19**, 241-246 (1962).

18. Yeh, S.Y., Krebs, H.A., and Gorodetzky, C.S., Isolation and identification of morphine $N$-oxide $\alpha$-and $\beta$-dihydromorphines, $\beta$- or $\gamma$-isomorphine, and hydroxylated morphine as morphine metabolites in several mammalian species. *J. Pharm. Sci.* **68**, 133-140 (1979).

19. Yeh, S.Y., Gorodetzky, C.W., Krebs, H.A., Isolation and identification of morphine 3- and 6-glucuronides, morphine 3,6-diglucuronide, morphine-3-ethereal sulphate, normorphine and normorphine 6-glucuronide as morphine metabolites in humans. *J. Pharm. Sci.* **66**, 1288-1293 (1977).

20. Vandenberghe, H.M., Chinyanga, H., Edrenyi, L., MacLeod, S.M., and Soldin, S.J., IV morphine for young children based on total body clearance. *Pediatr. Res.* **16**, 132A (1982).

21. Stanski, D., Paalzow, L., and Edlund, P.O., Morphine pharmacokinetics. Gas-liquid chromatographic assay vs. radioimmunoassay. *J. Pharmacokin. Biopharm.*, in press, 1982.

22. Patwardhan, R.V., Johnson, R.F., Hoyumpa, A., Sheehan, J.J., Desmond, P.V., Wilkinson, G.R., Branch, R.A., and Schenker, S., Normal metabolism of morphine in cirrhosis. *Gastroenterology* **81**, 1006-1011 (1981).

23. Knodell, R.G., Farleigh, R.M., Steele, H.M., and Bond, J.H., Effects of liver congestion on hepatic drug metabolism in the rat. *J. Pharmacol. Exp. Ther.* **221**, 52-57 (1982).

24. Nayman, J., Measurement and control of postoperative pain. *Ann. R. Coll. Surg. Engl.* **61**, 419-426 (1979).

# 59

# Acetaminophen: Clinico–Pathologic Correlations and Case History

Daniel T. Teitelbaum, M.D.

## Case History

In February 1978, a 19-year-old woman was transferred to St. Anthony Hospital Poisoning Treatment Center, 24 h after admission to a local community hospital because she had ingested an overdose of acetaminophen. The patient's family physician indicated that 6 h before her admission to the community hospital, the patient had ingested 75 0.5-g tablets of a proprietary medication subsequently identified as acetaminophen.

The patient had been in good health before admission to the hospital but had recently been in psychiatric crisis because of difficulties with her boyfriend. She stated that she took the acetaminophen tablets in an attempt at suicide.

The patient's past medical history was not remarkable. She denied any hospitalizations for serious illness. She specifically denied any neurological problems. She had never had any liver dysfunction. There was no history of hepatitis in any close family member, either in the recent or distant past. The patient had never been noted to be anemic and was not known to have any aberration in hemoglobin or abnormality of the erythrocytes that might lead to hemolysis. She had had no previous surgery. She had never been pregnant and had no gynecologic problem. She had been taking a "minidose" estrogen/progesterone combination birth-control pill for 2.5 years. She took no other medication, except acetaminophen occasionally for headache or other minor pains and discomforts.

She was a moderate user of coffee and tea, and drank alcohol on social occasions in moderation. She occasionally used marijuana.

The patient was employed as a dry cleaner in a small dry-cleaning establishment. She worked extensively with chlorinated hydrocarbon solvents and had done

*Dr. Teitelbaum is President of the Center for Toxicology, Man and Environment, Inc. at 6858 East Tennessee Avenue, Suite 365 in Denver, Colorado, 80224.*

so for about three years before this admission to the hospital (1).

On the day before admission, the patient became despondent about her personal problems, which had intensified to a degree that she believed unmanageable. At about 10:00 p.m. she took 75 0.5-g tablets of acetaminophen. Within 2 h she became moderately nauseated, without much vomiting. She became dizzy at approximately 3:00 a.m. and became quite frightened as the night progressed. At 6:00 a.m. she presented herself in the emergency room of her local community hospital. Thirty milliliters of ipecac was administered, followed by an oral fluid load. Copious vomiting resulted about 20 min later. No tablets were recovered in the vomitus.

At this time the patients blood pressure was 110/80 mm Hg, her pulse rate 120 per minute, and she was alert and oriented. There was no evidence of scleral icterus, abnormal extraocular movements, or increased intercranial pressure.

Results of examination of the head, neck, chest, and heart were within normal limits. There was a slight tenderness over the liver, which was of normal size. No abdominal masses were noted. The rest of the physical examination, including a neurologic examination, revealed no abnormalities.

Laboratory data at the time of admission revealed an erythrocyte count of 4.6 million/mm³, a hemoglobin concentration of 145 g/L, a hematocrit of 40%, and a leukocyte count of 10,600 cells/mm³, with a normal differential count. Platelets were considered to be adequate in number. Serum electrolytes were: sodium, 142 mmol/L; potassium, 4.8 mmol/L; chloride, 101 mmol/L; and total $CO_2$, 30 mmol/L. Other laboratory values were: calcium, 96 mg/L; phosphorus, 45 mg/L; alkaline phosphatase, 250 U/L; aspartate aminotransferase, 850 U/L; alanine aminotransferase, 2050 U/L; and bilirubin, 23 mg L. The blood glucose concentration was 1.05 g/L.

The patient was admitted to the Intensive Care Unit. A sample of blood was submitted to the toxicology reference laboratory for emergency determination of serum acetaminophen concentration (2). The acetaminophen concentration at the time of admission to community hospital was found to be 400 mg/L.

About 6 h after the initial determination of acetaminophen concentration and biochemical profile at this hospital, the patient was noted to be confused and to have developed scleral icterus. No asterixis was noted and no bleeding developed. A repeat determination of acetaminophen revealed that the acetaminophen concentration was now 370 mg/L. This persistently high acetaminophen concentration, combined with neurological and hepatic deterioration, suggested severe acetaminophen poisoning(3). The aspartate aminotransferase concentration was now 4000 U/L, the alanine aminotransferase 7200 U/L, and the bilirubin 30 mg/L. The prothrombin time was normal, as was the blood ammonia concentration.

Consultation was requested from the St. Anthony Poisoning Treatment Center. They recommended that the patient be begun on acetylcysteine (Mucomyst, TM Mead Johnson) and that the protocol recommended by the Rocky Mountain Poison Center(4) be followed to prevent further hepatic damage.

The patient was transferred to the Center for further therapy, and was given 140 mg of acetylcysteine per kilogram body weight by mouth, plus a maintenance dose of 70 mg/kg orally administered, shortly after her arrival at the Center. A standing dose of 70 mg/kg was given every 4 h for the next 3 days, for a total of 17 such maintenance doses. During this time, the patient was carefully evaluated for change in neurological status, bleeding, respiratory complications, fluid and electrolyte imbalance, and other problems. Her hepatic status was followed very closely.

Twelve hours after she was admitted to St. Anthony Hospital, her neurological status had deteriorated significantly, and she had asterixis and evidence of hepatic coma. She was moderately jaundiced and the liver was enlarged and tender. The AST value exceeded 10 000 U/L. The serum alkaline phosphatase activity was 5500 U/L, 857 of which appeared to be liver-derived. The leukocyte count was 17,500 cells/mm$^3$, and the serum acetaminophen concentration was 85 mg/L.

The patient began to improve clinically 24 h after admission to St. Anthony Hospital. The AST was noted to be 3000 U/L and the ALT 2500 U/L. The bilirubin was 26 mg/L. By this time the patient's neurological status was significantly improved. Her asterixis and confusion had disappeared, and the acetaminophen value was 20 mg/L.

On the third day after this admission, the patient's acetaminophen concentration could no longer be measured. The AST value was 1200 U/L, the ALT 2000 U/L, the liver was enlarged and tender, the bilirubin was now 26 mg/L. The patient was alert and oriented.

She continued to improve, and was discharged from the hospital on the 10th day after this admission, at which time results of liver function tests were normal.

About six months later her liver was biopsied, and no significant abnormalities were seen (5). She was considered to be well.

### Mechanism of Action

The mechanism of action of acetaminophen is much like that of salicylate. It is the common metabolite of both acetanilide and phenacetin, both of which have been used for many years. Analgesic and antipyretic effects are quite similar to those of aspirin. However, acetaminophen does not have potent anti-inflammatory effects, and cannot be used as an anti-rheumatic agent. It is useful for relieving pain of moderate intensity. Acetaminophen has a direct effect on the heat-regulating mechanisms of the body. The analgesic effect on peripheral pain is moderate, it is insignificant when pain comes from a hollow viscus. Because the mechanism of action of acetaminophen is quite similar to that of aspirin and its biological half-life not very different from that of aspirin, its analgesic and antipyretic effects approximate those of aspirin.

### Site of Action

Antipyretic action is central, controlled by the hypothalamus. Although there are few data on the penetration of the blood-brain barrier by acetaminophen, its ability to affect the heat-regulating mechanism implies such access. The site of the analgesic effect has not been precisely located. From various studies central, peripheral, and combined mechanisms have been proposed.

### Drug–Drug Interactions

The only clearly demonstrated drug - drug interaction is in the ability of acetaminophen to inhibit prothrombin formation. Ascorbic acid or salicylamide, if administered at the same time as acetaminophen, may inhibit the metabolism of acetaminophen to acetaminophen sulfate, its most important nontoxic metabolite. The resulting limitations on its production by depletion of glutathione is accompanied by an increase in the more toxic metabolites. Interference with the normal formation and excretion of acetaminophen sulfate by any competitive compound will result in an increase in the toxic metabolites. Thus symptoms of toxicity may appear at lower doses of acetaminophen than generally expected.

Enzyme inducers such as phenobarbital, chlorinated hydrocarbon, birth-control pills, alcohol, and some other commonly used medications will produce an increased potential for hepatic damage, owing to formation of the epoxide and other oxymetabolites. Patients who are occupationally exposed to these substances and take unusually large doses of acetaminophen will be more likely to develop liver failure than those not so exposed.

## Side Effects

Side effects of treatment with acetaminophen are negligible in ordinary therapeutic dosage. The drug is well tolerated, does not cause gastrointestinal bleeding, and is not believed to affect platelet function. Hepatic disease as a result of normal doses is almost unknown. Some dizziness, nausea, and mild psychic effects have been described.

The principal problem with acetaminophen is the severe liver disorder caused by massive overdoses, a problem first described about 10 years ago, in Britain. At first, it was believed to be a phenomenon confined to a relatively limited genetic population in the British Isles, but more recently it has been reported in almost every country wheren the drug is used. Clearly, the problem arises from a rate-limited shift from the usual metabolism of acetaminophen.

In the presence of massive overdoses of the drug, the liver's ability to provide sulfhydryl groups for the formation of its sulfate metabolite is overwhelmed, and a disproportionate amount of the hepatotoxic oxymetabolites, cysteinate, and mercaptate are produced. The production of these more toxic metabolites increases with the dose, and this may totally destroy the liver. If the disorder is recognized, a large excess of sulfhydryl groups can be provided by administering a sulfhydryl donor such as acetylcysteine. This apparently helps protect the liver. Other sulfhydryl donors such as glutathione and D-penicillamine have been utilized successfully, but are much more difficult to give.

## Specimen Collection, Storage, Transport, and Stability

The specimen used in the analysis for acetaminophen may be either serum or plasma. Methods are now available for every type of analysis, ranging from thin-layer chromatography to gas chromatography/mass spectroscopy, any of which will give reliable results if well controlled. Proper set-up requires standards and blanks. Perhaps the most convenient current method is "high-performance" liquid chromatography, which is reasonably fast, quite specific, and requires only a small specimen.

Specimens need not be refrigerated and are reasonably stable for at least 5 days. They may be transported by mail or by air. It should be recognized that if the patient is admitted into the hospital with a history of significant overdose, it is essential quickly to obtain a 4-h and a repeat 8-h determination, which must be analyzed on an emergency basis. This is a classic example of the need for emergency toxicology services, either in the hospital or in a nearby specialty laboratory. Therapy should not be delayed if the history strongly suggests massive acetaminophen overdosage. Results of the laboratory determinations can be used as indications for termination of therapy, rather than initiation of therapy.

## When Should One Obtain Specimens?

Specimens should be obtained on admission to hospital if at least 4 h have passed since the overdose of acetaminophen was taken. A second specimen should be obtained 4 h after that and the half-life determined; if it exceeds 4 h and the total concentration exceeds 150 g/L, there is a very high probability that liver disorder will be detected.

## Clinical Pharmacology

Acetaminophen is rarely used in ongoing therapy. Because it is not effective as an antirheumatic, and is only a mild analgesic, patients rarely take the medication for more than a few days. Its toxicity in normal therapeutic doses is very low. Only in situations of significant overdose do problems appear. Accordingly, therapeutic monitoring is probably indicated only in cases of acute overdosage. Then it is clearly indicated. Recent statistics from the Poison Information Centers demonstrate that acetaminophen is now the second or third most common drug involved in accidental overdosage by children. As it is also commonly used by adolescents and adults, all hospitals must be able, either in house or on an emergency referral basis, to analyze biological materials for acetaminophen.

The usual dose range is 8 - 10 mg/kg for children, 10 - 20 mg/kg for adults. As long as adults take no more than 2 g per day, there is no problem of liver damage. After a 10 - g dose clinical evidence of liver damage is seen.

The metabolic dispositon of acetaminophen is interesting. The excretion of the drug varies with the dose ingested. In ordinary therapeutic doses, about 4.2% is exreted as acetaminophen, unchanged. Two primary metabolites are noted, the glucuronide and the sulfate, and in addition a small percentage of the ingested dose may be excreted as the mercaptate and the cysteinate, both of which are the result of oxidative

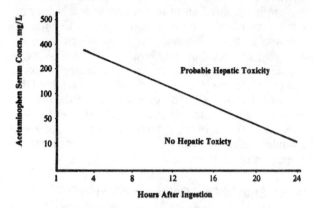

**Fig. 1.** Semilogarithmic plot of plasma acetaminophen concentration vs. time (From Rumack and Matthew, *Pediatrics* 55: 871, 1975.)

metabolism of acetaminophen. An intermediate oxymetabolite, which has not been identified, is believed to be the toxic material associated with liver necrosis. It has been demonstrated that this oxymetabolite can bind covalently to liver macromolecules and cause destruction of the hepatocyte function. Fortunately, the oxymetabolite is a very minor product in acetaminophen metabolism under ordinary circumstances. The liver can readily provide glutathione for the formation of the sulfate metabolite, but if the ingested dose exceeds 2 g, the oxymetabolite may increase in concentration, with a relative decrease in the proportion excreted as sulfates and an increase in the excretion of the cysteinate and mercaptate conjugates of acetaminophen. After a single dose of 30 g, one that is almost always associated with severe liver disorder, the percentages of the excreted drug may appear as follows: acetaminophen, 13.8%, acetaminophen glucuronide, 32.7%, acetaminophen sulfate, 8.66%, and acetaminophen cysteinate and mercaptate, 44.8%.

When a patient is admitted who has ingested more than one or two tablets (if a small child) or more than five or 10 tablets (if an adult), acetaminophen should be measured within 4 h of the ingestion, and if the results exceed 150 mg/L there is a significant probability of acute hepatic disorder. If the initially determined value is less than this 4 h after ingestion, the probability of hepatic necrosis is extremely small. If the patient is hospitalized and therapy with acetylcysteine begun for acetaminophen intoxication, the laboratory should be prepared to repeat the acetaminophen determination approximately 4 h after the initial determination. A demonstrated half-life of longer than 4 h would be consistent with a very high probability of acetaminophen-induced liver toxicity. All patients should have emergency baseline studies of hepatic function on admission, including AST, ALT, and γ-glutamyltransferase. These should be repeated daily until all evidence of liver disorder has passed.

The now recommended protocol for management calls for the administration of a loading dose of acetylcysteine of 140 mg/kg, and a maintenance dose of 70 mg of acetylcysteine per kilogram body weight every 4 h for 3 days. Throughout this period and for about three to four days afterwards, or until the results of liver-function tests return to normal, AST, ALT, and γ-glutamyltransferase should be measured.

It may not be safe to biopsy the liver in this acute phase, because there may be significant disturbance of coagulation. However, if the patient's prothrombin time is normal, and a liver biopsy is done, evidence of

## ACETAMINOPHEN PROFILE

| | |
|---|---|
| Generic name: | Acetaminophen |
| Chemical name: | N–(4–hydroxyphenyl) acetamide |
| Chemical structure: | |

$$CH_3CONH-\!\!\langle\ \rangle\!\!-OH$$

| | |
|---|---|
| Trade name: | Tylenol, Valadol, Datril, Tempra |
| Molecular weight: | 151.16 |
| Melting point, °C: | 169–170.5 |
| Solubility in water, mg/mL: | very slightly in cold water, ater, much more so in hot water |
| pK$_a$: | not available |
| Partition coefficient: | not available |
| Dose absorption – | |
|   time to peak plasma conc., h: | ½–1 |
|   percentage dose absorbed: | virtually complete |
| Protein binding – | |
|   percentage bound: | 20–50% in acute overdosage |
|   percentage free: | 50–80% |
| Tissue distribution, V$_d$, L/kg: | .85 |
|   CSF/plasma: | not available |
|   Brain/plasma: | not available |

| Urinary excretion, % daily dose – | 10–g dose | 30–g dose |
|---|---|---|
|   as unchanged drug: | 4.27 | 13.8 |
|   as acetaminophen glucuronide: | 59.4 | 32.7 |
|   as acetaminophen sulfate: | 22.5 | 8.66 |
|   as acetaminophen cysteinate or mercaptate: | 13.9 | 44.8 |

| | Adults | Children |
|---|---|---|
| Recommended dose, mg/kg/d: | 10–20 | 8–15 |
| | 1-g dose - 3 h | 1-g dose - 3 h |
| Half-life, h: | 1-g dose - 3 h | |
| | 10-g dose - 6.5 h | |
| Time to steady state, h: | not relevant | not relevant |
| Effective levels, µg/mL: | 10, in 4 h after dose | |
| Toxic levels, µg/mL: | 150, in 4 h after dose | |
| Steady-state level expected from 1 mg/kg/d, µg/mL: | not relevant | |
| Methodologies available for analysis: | HPLC, UV, Colorimetric | |

acute centrilobular necrosis with hepatocyte death may be expected.

Acetaminophen should be monitored at eight-hour intervals until concentrations reach 50 mg/ L or less. In patients with severe hepatic necrosis this may take several days. If adequate glutathione is provided through the administration of acetylcysteine, one may expect to see a reasonably good disposition of the overdose of acetaminophen.

In summary, acetaminophen is not typical of drugs monitored in therapeutic situations. In ordinary doses, its toxicity is negligible; one would not expect to see severe disorders of any sort. However, in the event of overdosage significant hepatic necrosis may well develop. Overdosage demands direct monitoring of liver-function, and determination *on an emergency basis* of the acetaminophen concentration. There are many methods for assaying for acetaminophen; which is used by an individual hospital or laboratory need be determined only by the available resources. If the hospital has a heavy pediatric load, "high-performance" liquid chromatography has a great advantage over all other methods, because as little as 300 $\mu$L of serum is adequate for a duplicate determination. If, however, the principal patient load of a hospital is adolescent or adult, then a spectrophotometric method or a gas chromatography method would be quite acceptable since these can be carried out effectively on samples in the range of 2 to 5 mL.

## References

1. Goldfinger, *et.al.,* Concomitant alcohol and drug abuse enchancing acetaminophen toxicity. *Am. J. Gastroenterology.* 70 385-388 (1978).
2. Hackett, L.P., and Dusci, L.J., Determination of paracetamol in human serum. *Clin. Chem. Acta* 74 187-190 (1977).
3. Gazzard, B.G., *et.al.,* Early prediction of the outcome of a paracetamol overdose based on an analysis of 163 patients. *Postgrad Med. J.* 53 243-247.
4. Rumack, B.H., and Peterson, R.G., Acetaminophen overdose: incidence, diagnosis and management in 416 patients. *Pediatrics* 62: 989-903 (1978).
5. Hamlyn, A.N., *et.al.,* Liver function and structure in survivors of acetaminophen poisoning. *Am. J. Dig. Dis.* 22 605-10 (1977).

# Appendixes

# Appendix I.

# Self-Assessment Questions

## Chapter 1

1. Which of the following seizure types is a grand mal convulsion?

a. absence
b. generalized tonic-clonic
c. partial complex
d. atonic
e. partial simple

2. Seizures are a common manifestation of poisoning with all of the following drugs except:

a. tricyclic antidepressants
b. acetaminophen
c. theophylline
d. penicillin
e. local anesthetics

3. Epilepsy caused by brain tumor is most common in which decade of life?

a. first
b. third
c. fifth
d. seventh
e. eighth

4. The most common CT brain scan finding in patients with epilepsy is:

a. normal
b. brain atrophy
c. brain tumor
d. brain infarction (stroke)
e. hydrocephalus

5. All of the following statements about the EEG are true except:

a. in epilepsy the EEG may be normal
b. the EEG indicates the electrical activity of the underlying brain surface
c. scalp electrical potentials must be amplified greatly to produce the EEG
d. an abnormal EEG proves a diagnosis of epilepsy
e. the EEG is usually abnormal during a seizure

6. The most common seizure type in patients with epilepsy is:

a. generalized tonic-clonic
b. generalized absence
c. partial complex
d. simple partial
e. myoclonic

7. Frequently repeated or continuous seizures lasting more than 30 min are called:

a. Lennox-Gestaut syndrome
b. status epilepticus
c. infantile spasms
d. partial complex seizures
e. reflex epilepsy

8. The most common cause of epilepsy is:

a. birth asphyxia
b. trauma
c. brain tumor
d. drug ingestion
e. infection

## Chapters 2-5

9. Which of the following statements describes the absorption of phenytoin?

a. oral Dilantin is absorbed slowly
b. generic phenytoin is absorbed slowly
c. intramuscular phenytoin is well absorbed
d. oral Dilantin is rapidly absorbed
e. none of the above

10. The therapeutic range of phenytoin is 10-20 mg/L. A patient whose seizure disorder is uncontrolled with a serum concentration of 12 mg/L:

a. will require another anticonvulsant in addition to phenytoin as the serum level is therapeutic
b. may not require an additional anticonvulsant if serum concentrations are increased to between 15 and 20 mg/L
c. should have the phenytoin dosage increased by 50% to produce a concentration of 18 mg/L
d. should continue therapy and be monitored as control may suddenly develop
e. none of the above

11. Renal-failure patients treated with phenytoin:

a. require lower daily dosages than patients with normal renal function
b. have higher free phenytoin fractions
c. have lower free phenytoin fractions
d. will have artificially reduced serum concentrations measured by EMIT
e. none of the above

12. Each of the following drugs will interact with phenytoin. Which one may increase the free phenytoin fraction while reducing the total serum concentration?

a. phenobarbital
b. carbamazepine
c. ethosuximide
d. valproic acid
e. all of the above

13. During pregnancy, pregnant epileptics treated with phenytoin will require:

a. additional anticonvulsants
b. smaller dosages of phenytoin
c. higher dosages of phenytoin
d. no anticonvulsant therapy
e. more frequent doses

14. An adult receiving Dilantin® for seizure control should have his phenytoin serum sample collected:

a. 4-10 h after the dose
b. just prior to a dose
c. 30 min after a dose
d. anytime within the dosing interval
e. at peak and trough times determined for the individual

15. An 8-year-old epileptic receiving phenytoin for seizure control should be expected to:

a. respond at serum concentrations below the therapeutic range
b. require at least two daily doses
c. have a longer half-life than an adult
d. require multiple anticonvulsants for seizure control
e. be poorly responsive to phenytoin until age 12

16. An epileptic adult is admitted to the hospital in status epilepticus. She responds to intravenous diazepam and receives a loading dose of phenytoin. Serum phenytoin concentration 6 h after the loading dose is 18 mg/L. Oral or intravenous maintenance dosages of 400 mg per day are administered; however, 4 days later the patient begins to have seizures again and the serum phenytoin concentration is 9 mg/L. Why has the serum phenytoin concentration declined?

a. inadequate maintenance therapy
b. poor oral absorption
c. poor bioavailability
d. increased metabolic rate due to diazepam
e. increased renal elimination due to changes in acid-base status

17. Which of the following adverse effects is *not* a dose-related side effect of phenytoin?

a. osteomalacia
b. drowsiness
c. blurred vision
d. ataxia
e. dysarthria

18. Which of the following drugs may reduce the phenytoin serum concentration as a result of increased hepatic metabolism?

a. salicylates
b. chloramphenicol
c. phenothiazines
d. carbamazepine
e. diazepam

19. In epilepsy:

a. patient compliance is a major factor in the success or failure of drug therapy
b. seizures may occur with variable frequency
c. 30-40% of the plasma phenytoin values <10 mg/L are the failure of the patients to receive their prescribed medication
d. all of the above
e. none of the above

20. The rate of metabolism of many drugs is:

a. lower in infancy and childhood than later in life
b. higher in infancy and childhood than later in life
c. lower when the patient is about to enter puberty
d. both a and c
e. both b and c

21. In adjusting the dosage of phenytoin, it is essential to realize:

a. that the relationship between the change in dose of drug and the change in plasma concentration is not always linear
b. that at relatively low plasma phenytoin levels, the rate of metabolism of the drug is proportional to drug concentration
c. that at some point within the therapeutic range, the metabolizing system may become saturated and the rate of metabolism will be unable to increase, regardless of drug concentration
d. all of the above
e. none of the above

22. The amount of phenytoin that is bound to plasma proteins is usually approximately:

a. 30%
b. 60%
c. 90%
d. 100%
e. none of the above

23. In a patient who is taking phenytoin on a regular basis, it takes about how many days before a plasma steady-state concentration of phenytoin occurs?

a. 1-2
b. 3-4
c. 5-7
d. 9-10
e. none of the above

24. The phenotype of isoniazid inactivator is determined by:

a. genetic counseling
b. chromosome analysis
c. amino acid analysis
d. giving a test dose of isoniazid
e. family history

25. Four hours after a test dose, a fast isoniazid inactivator is likely to have:

a. high concentration of isoniazid
b. low concentration of isoniazid
c. drowsiness and vomiting
d. tingling of fingers

26. The major pathway in phenytoin biotransformation is:

a. dealkylation
b. aromatic hydroxylation
c. direct conjugation of parent compound
d. acetylation

27. Phenytoin intoxication is manifested in most patients by:

a. extreme drowsiness
b. nausea and vomiting
c. poor coordination
d. low blood sugar
e. stomach cramps

28. Phenytoin is usually not used to treat the following seizure types:

a. generalized tonic-clonic (grand mal)
b. absence (petit mal)
c. partial complex (psychomotor)
d. partial simple (jacksonian)

29. Phenytoin-isoniazid interaction occurs as a result of:

a. altered nerve cell sensitivity
b. altered intestinal absorption
c. altered biotransformation
d. altered plasma protein binding
e. interference with laboratory assay

30. Phenytoin biotransformation is carried out by enzymes in:

a. kidney tubules
b. liver microsomes
c. liver mitochondria
d. liver cell cytoplasm

31. The chemical name for phenytoin is:

a. 3-ethyl-5-phenylhydantoin
b. 5-ethyl-3-methyl-5-phenylhydantoin
c. 1-(2-phenylacetyl)-urea
d. 5,5-diphenylhydantoin
e. 5-ethyl-5-phenylbarbituric acid

32. Although phenytoin was introduced in 1938, it is still most commonly used for treating all types of epilepsy except:

a. psychomotor
b. petit mal
c. grand mal
d. myoclonic seizures
e. all of the above

33. The relationship between seizure control and plasma level of phenytoin was first demonstrated in:

a. 1957
b. 1947
c. 1951
d. 1960
e. 1912

34. The methods for phenytoin analysis that are now mostly of historical interest are:

a. ultraviolet spectrophotometry
b. colorimetry
c. benzophenone-extraction
d. thin-layer chromatography
e. all of the above

35. The most commonly used current methods are:

a. radioimmunoassay
b. fluorescent immunoassay
c. homogeneous enzyme immunoassay
d. gas-liquid chromatography
e. "high-performance" liquid chromatography

36. The most accurate and sensitive method, which can be used to validate all other methods, is:

a. homogeneous enzyme immunoassay
b. gas-liquid chromatography
c. "high-performance" liquid chromatography
d. thin-layer chromatography
e. gas chromatography-mass spectrometry

37. The method that can be used for "stat" analyses but is inappropriate for uremic patients is:

a. EMIT
b. RIA
c. GLC
d. HPLC
e. TLC

38. An advantage in using a gas-liquid chromatographic method specific for phenytoin is that simultaneously one can determine:

a. 5-(4-hydroxphenyl)-5-phenylhydantoin
b. 5-(3,4-dihydroxyphenyl)-5-phenylhydantoin
c. 5-(3-O-methyl-4-hydroxyphenyl)-5-phenylhydantoin
d. HPLC

39. Disadvantages in use of GLC methods are:

a. difficulty in maintaining reproducible GLC as well as extraction parameters
b. a need for highly trained and dedicated analysts
c. that only thermally stable and volatile analytes can be used
d. that derivitization is usually necessary for better volatility, sensitivity, and reduction in peak tailing
e. all of the above

40. HPLC columns of significantly less cost and increased column life are:

a. 3%-OV17
b. SP-1000
c. GP 2% SP-25.O-DA on 100/120 Supelcoport
d. radial compression
e. GP 2% SP-2110/1% SP-2510DA on 100/120 Supelcoport

## Chapters 6-10

41. Phenobarbital (intramuscular) is not effective as an immediate drug in status epilepticus because of:

a. slow absorption from injectton site
b. high percentage of protein binding
c. slow distribution into all tissues
d. insolubility at injection site
e. slower distribution into brain tissue

42. After an initial oral dose of 125 mg of primidone one could expect to detect the drug in serum within:

a. 1 min
b. 30 min
c. 12 h
d. 24 h
e. not at all

43. The primary active metabolite(s) of primidone is:

a. phenobarbital and p-hydroxyphenobarbital
b. phenylethylmalonamide
c. p-hydroxyphenobarbital
d. phenylethylmalonamide and phenobarbital
e. phenylethylmalonamide and p-hydroxyphenobarbital

44. The dose of phenobarbital was altered in a patient's regimen from 30 mg twice a day to 60 mg twice a day. A sample should be obtained for analysis in:

a. 24 h
b. 14-21 days
c. 3 days
d. 7 days
e. any of the above

45. Phenytoin (400 mg per day) was added to a patient's regimen that had been 250 mg primidone four times a day. Approximately two weeks later the patient presented with nystagmus and ataxia. Which of the following is most likely to be responsible for these toxic signs?

a. phenytoin
b. primidone
c. phenobarbital
d. phenylethylmalonamide
e. p-hydroxyphenobarbital

46. The therapeutic range of primidone is (mg/L):

a. 15-30
b. 10-20
c. 6-15
d. 50-100
e. 4-8

47. Clinical signs of phenobarbital intoxication usually occur at concentrations in plasma (mg/L) in excess of:

a. 18
b. 50
c. 10
d. 30
e. 80

48. Steady-state concentrations of primidone will usually be present in what length of time after a constant dose?

a. 24 h
b. 30 min
c. 2-3 days
d. 4-5 h
e. 7-14 days

49. Which factor below is most likely to affect the rate at which primidone is absorbed?

a. pK
b. solubility and tablet disintegration
c. gastric acidity
d. relative molecular mass
e. presence of other medications

50. Combination phenobarbital/phenytoin therapy is commonly used in treatment of:

a. generalized motor seizures
b. petit mal seizures
c. focal motor seizures
d. all of the above
e. a and c

51. New onset of a generalized motor seizure disorder in adults is initially treated with:

a. combination phenobarbital/phenytoin
b. combination phenobarbital/phenytoin if the patient has had more than three seizures in the past week
c. phenobarbital
d. phenytoin
e. c or d

52. Phenobarbital is frequently prescribed in split daily dose:

a. because the half-life may be less than 24 h
b. to minimize sedative effects
c. to minimize interaction with serum phenytoin binding
d. all of the above
e. two of the above

53. In vitro studies have shown that phenobarbital and phenytoin behave similarly in:

a. limiting calcium influx in nerve terminal preparations
b. facilitating sodium-potassium-ATPase (sodium pump)
c. enhancing a slow potassium-dependent outward membrane current
d. all of the above
e. two of the above

54. Metabolism of phenobarbital and phenytoin are similar in that:

a. the major metabolite of each is formed via $p$-hydroxylation
b. water solubility is enhanced by glucuronide conjugation
c. less than 10% of each is excreted unmetabolized in the urine
d. all of the above
e. a and b

55. Phenobarbital pretreatment:

a. tends to increase the half-life of phenytoin
b. tends to decrease the half-life of phenytoin
c. consistently lowers the phenytoin concentrations in blood
d. may increase the serum concentration of phenytoin
e. b and d

56. Adding phenytoin if a patient is already taking phenobarbital:

a. tends to raise the concentration of phenobarbital
b. requires reduction of the phenobarbital dose when phenytoin is first begun
c. tends to inhibit hepatic enzyme metabolism of phenobarbital
d. all of the above
e. a and c

57. Serum protein binding of phenytoin:

a. is about 90%
b. drops with the addition of phenobarbital
c. rises with the addition of phenobarbital
d. is mainly to alpha$_1$-globulins
e. two of the above

58. Low serum concentrations of phenytoin may be due to:

a. erratic drug taking
b. changes in serum binding secondary to phenobarbital
c. enhanced metabolism by phenobarbital
d. all of the above
e. a and c

59. Plasma unbound ("free") phenytoin concentration is:

a. closely correlated with total plasma phenytoin concentration
b. greater than 95% of the plasma total phenytoin concentration
c. less than 5% of the plasma total phenytoin concentration
d. so low that it cannot be measured by current techniques
e. more clinically relevant than the plasma total phenytoin concentration

60. After changing a patient's phenobarbital dose given once per day, how long may it take for the plasma concentrations to reach 95% of steady state?

a. 2 days
b. 4 days
c. 8 days
d. 12 days
e. approximately 3 weeks

61. After starting a patient on a high dose of phenytoin, approximately how long may it take to reach 95% of steady state?

a. 2 days
b. 4 days
c. 8 days
d. 14 days
e. approximately 3 or more weeks

62. When are samples usually drawn for routine monitoring of phenytoin?

a. 1 h after the last dose
b. 4 h after the last dose
c. 8 h after the last dose
d. just before the next dose is to be taken

63. Usually a newly diagnosed grand mal epileptic is initially treated wtih:

a. one antiepileptic drug
b. two antiepileptic drugs
c. two antiepileptic drugs, then changed to only one drug
d. three antiepileptic drugs
e. no drugs unless the seizures are very severe and frequent

64. Effective concentrations (mg/L) of phenobarbital in adults are usually:

a. 10-20
b. 8-12
c. 15-30
d. 50-100
e. 6-15

65. Steady-state concentrations of primidone will be reached in how many days after a constant dose?

a. 7-14
b. 21
c. 6
d. 2-3
e. 14-21

66. The presence of ataxia, nystagmus, and confusion indicate intoxication with which of the following drugs?

a. phenobarbital
b. phenytoin
c. primidone
d. carbamazepine
e. all of the above

67. Steady-state concentrations of phenobarbital (as derived from primidone) should be reached how soon after a change in primidone dose?

a. 14-30 h
b. 2-3 days
c. 14-30 days
d. 8-10 days
e. several months

68. Addition of 400 mg per day of phenytoin to a daily regimen of 1000 mg of primidone and 15 mg of phenobarbital:
a. is a useful approach to control of tonic-clonic seizures
b. is likely to result in phenytoin intoxication
c. is likely to result in primidone intoxication
d. is likely to result in phenobarbital intoxication
e. is likely to have no effect on the phenobarbital serum concentration

69. Which of the following methods will give results for phenobarbital in the shortest time?

a. gas-liquid chromatography
b. "high-performance" liquid chromatography
c. enzyme-mediated immunoassay
d. spectrophotometry
e. radioimmunoassay

70. Which of the following procedures requires no prior preparation of the plasma before analysis of phenobarbital or primidone?

a. enzyme-mediated immunoassay
b. "high-performance" liquid chromatography
c. gas-liquid chromatography
d. spectrophotometric assay

71. If a patient is on a therapeutic regimen of primidone, plasma samples should be assayed for:

a. primidone only
b. phenobarbital only
c. primidone and phenobarbital
d. primidone, phenobarbital, and phenylethylmalon-amide

72. More accurate and reproducible results for the assay of phenobarbital and primidone will be obtained with which of the following combinations?

a. comparison of peak-height ratio of unknown to peak-height ratio of standards
b. on-column derivatization with internal standards added to the plasma and peak-height ratios of standards to internal standard used to prepare calibration curve
c. plasma extract directly injected with no internal standards
d. utilization of specific internal standards for each drug, calibration curve not necessary

73. How often should calibration curves be determined when enzyme-mediated immunoassay is used as method of analysis?

a. daily
b. weekly
c. with a new lot of reagents
d. with a new lot of calibrators
e. monthly

74. Which of the following procedures will permit duplicate determinations of either phenobarbital or primidone with a single 200-$\mu$L tube of blood?

a. "high-performance" liquid chromatography
b. gas-liquid chromatography
c. enzyme-mediated immunoassay
d. none of the above

## Chapters 11 and 12

75. Peak concentrations of ethosuximide in plasma after oral administration occur after how many hours?

a. 0.25-0.50
b. 0.50-1.0
c. 1-2
d. 3-7
e. 10-12

76. The apparent volume of distribution is a pharmacokinetic parameter that:

a. relates the amount of drug in the body to the dose administered
b. relates the amount of drug in the body to the concentration in plasma
c. represents the physiologic space into which a drug distributes
d. relates drug clearance to concentration in plasma
e. relates the half-life of a drug to the time it takes to attain steady state

77. The magnitude of the apparent volume of distribution of ethosuximide (0.62 L/kg in adults and 0.69 L/kg in children) suggests uniform distribution of ethosuximide into:

a. lean tissue
b. skeletal muscle
c. body water
d. fat tissue
e. adipose tissue

78. Ethosuximide concentrations in saliva cannot be used to reflect ethosuximide concentrations in plasma because:

a. ethosuximide does not distribute into saliva
b. ethosuximide saliva concentrations bear no relationship to concentrations in plasma
c. correlations between ethosuximide concentrations in saliva and plasma are variable
d. ethosuximide is unstable in saliva
e. concentrations of ethosuximide in saliva are much greater than those in plasma

79. Ethosuximide elimination is characterized by:

a. complete renal elimination of unchanged drug
b. predominant renal elimination of unchanged drug with some hepatic metabolism
c. hepatic metabolism with no renal elimination of unchanged drug
d. predominant hepatic metabolism with a minor degree of renal excretion of unchanged drug
e. hepatic blood flow limited metabolism

80. The clearance of ethosuximide from the body:

a. decreases with increasing age
b. increases with increasing age
c. is unaltered by coadministration of carbamazepine
d. has no effect on the ultimate mean steady-state concentration of ethosuximide in plasma
e. is independent of dose

81. On a body weight basis, children require larger maintenance doses of ethosuximide than an adult does because of their:

a. reduced metabolic clearance of ethosuximide
b. enhanced volume of distribution for ethosuximide
c. greater metabolic clearance of ethosuximide
d. lesser volume of distribution for ethosuximide
e. need for higher concentrations in plasma for seizure control

82. In steady-state, the most appropriate time within a dosing interval to obtain a blood sample for monitoring ethosuximide concentration in plasma is:

a. 1 h after the dose
b. 5 h after the dose
c. 12 h after the dose
d. 15 h after the dose
e. anytime within the dosing interval

83. Steady-state concentrations of ethosuximide in plasma:

a. occur within a day after drug administration
b. occur when the dosing rate of ethosuximide matches its elimination rate from the body
c. occur in a shorter time for adults than children
d. are unimportant for assessing the adequacy of a given dosage regimen for seizure control
e. bear no relationship to the size of the dose

84. Assessment of a particular dosing rate of ethosuximide in providing adequate seizure control can only be made:

a. at steady state
b. after a single dose of a drug
c. once the bioavailability is known
d. after intravenous infusion of ethosuximide
e. none of these

85. The minimum ethosuximide concentration (mg/L) in plasma needed for adequate seizure control in most patients is:

a. 10
b. 40
c. 60
d. 100
e. 285

86. The disproportionate change in ethosuximide concentrations in plasma with changes in dose is presumably due to:

a. saturable hepatic metabolism of ethosuximide
b. enhanced bioavailability of ethosuximide
c. reduced volume of distribution of ethosuximide
d. enhanced clearance of ethosuximide
e. lesser renal elimination of ethosuximide

87. Which of the following toxicities from ethosuximide therapy is not related to dose?

a. nausea
b. pancytopenia

c. vomiting
d. lethargy
e. headaches

88. To achieve a steady-state ethosuximide concentration in plasma of 70 mg/L in a patient who is not controlled at a steady-state concentration in plasma of 35 mg/L, one should administer:

a. twice the dose
b. less than twice the dose
c. three times the dose
d. half of the present dose
e. none of these

## Chapters 13-15

89. The effects and (or) toxicity of carbamazepine are best related to:

a. administered carbamazepine dosage
b. total plasma carbamazepine concentration
c. Total plasma carbamazepine 10,11-epoxide concentration
d. free plasma carbamazepine 10,11-epoxide concentration
e. urinary carbamazepine concentration

90. The dose-rate of carbamazepine in a patient previously unexposed to this drug must be increased gradually because:

a. the apparent clearance of carbamazepine is initially high and then decreases
b. the apparent volume of distribution of carbamazepine increases with continued therapy
c. the half-life of carbamazepine increases with continued therapy
d. the apparent clearance of carbamazepine increases with continued therapy
e. the patient develops a tolerance to the side effects of carbamazepine

91. The dose-rate of carbamazepine is necessarily higher in children than in adults because:

a. the half-life of carbamazepine is longer in children
b. the apparent volume of distribution is larger in children
c. the apparent clearance of carbamazepine is higher in children
d. children require higher plasma carbamazepine concentrations to attain the same effect as adults
e. children can tolerate higher plasma carbamazepine concentrations than adults can

92. Carbamazepine may need to be given in higher doses and more frequently in patients who are concurrently receiving other anticonvulsants because:

a. other anticonvulsants may induce enzymes responsible for the metabolism of carbamazepine, causing a higher clearance and shorter half-life
b. autoinduction may be accelerated in these patients
c. apparent volumes of distribution tend to be higher in these patients
d. other anticonvulsants tend to inhibit the effects of carbamazepine
e. the seizure threshold is decreased in patients taking other anticonvulsants

93. A plasma carbamazepine concentration measured at the end of a dosage interval may not necessarily be the lowest concentration during the interval because:

a. the rate of carbamazepine absorption varies from patient to patient
b. the apparent clearance of carbamazepine increases with prolonged treatment
c. the half-life of carbamazepine decreases with continued therapy
d. the apparent volume of distribution changes during a dosage interval
e. the extent of carbamazepine absorption may change from dose to dose

94. Plasma carbamazepine concentrations should be carefully monitored during pregnancy because:

a. carbamazepine is toxic to the fetus
b. the apparent clearance of carbamazepine decreases during pregnancy, causing toxicity
c. the protein binding of carbamazepine increases during pregnancy
d. the apparent clearance of carbamazepine increases during pregnancy, necessitating an increase in the dose-rate
e. the apparent volume of distribution of carbamazepine decreases as the pregnancy progresses

95. The dose-rate of carbamazepine should be adjusted in all of the following cases except:

a. when a patient is uncontrolled with a steady-state plasma carbamazepine concentration of 4 mg/L
b. when a patient is completely controlled, demonstrates no toxicity, and has a steady-state plasma carbamazepine concentration of 10 mg/L

c. when a patient is controlled, but exhibits toxicity to carbamazepine with a steady-state plasma carbamazepine concentration of 13 mg/L
d. when a patient is uncontrolled with a steady-state salivary carbamazepine concentration of 1 mg/L

96. An adult epileptic has been taking carbamazepine and phenobarbital for two years, during which no seizures were reported. The physician discontinues the phenobarbital in an attempt to control this patient with carbamazepine alone. Which of the following situations do you anticipate?

a. plasma carbamazepine concentrations probably increasing over the next 2 to 3 weeks, then reaching a new steady-state
b. phenobarbital plasma concentrations increasing over the next week
c. salivary carbamazepine concentrations decreasing
d. carbamazepine 10, 11-epoxide concentrations gradually increasing over 2 to 3 weeks
e. the half-life of carbamazepine decreasing

97. Carbamazepine may:

a. never be administered in combination with other drugs
b. cause a decrease in warfarin concentrations in blood
c. increase the blood concentrations of phenytoin and warfarin
d. shorten the plasma half-life of phenytoin
e. b and d

98. Sudden cessation of carbamazepine medication may produce:

a. cardiac and renal dysfunction
b. marrow depression
c. status epilepticus
d. skin and hematologic manifestations
e. all of the above

99. Which of the following are common signs of intoxication in patients taking antiepileptic drugs?

a. psychomotor seizures
b. drowsiness and ataxia
c. fever
d. anxiety
e. a and d

100. Other disorders where treatment with carbamazepine is beneficial are:

a. hepatic and renal disease
b. rheumatoid arthritis
c. trigeminal neuralgia and multiple sclerosis
d. severe depression in combination with imipramine
e. none of the above

101. The most common carbamazepine-associated side effects are:

a. bone marrow depression
b. hyperactivity
c. skin and hematologic manifestations
d. arrhythmia
e. a and c

102. Which of the following would *not* explain why an adult patient demonstrates typical signs of carbamazepine toxicity at a plasma concentration of 6.8 mg/L?

a. the patient is also taking phenytoin and primidone
b. the salivary carbamazepine concentration is 3.5 mg/L
c. the patient is taking 600 mg of carbamazepine per day in three divided doses
d. the extent of plasma protein binding of carbamazepine and its epoxide metabolite is very low in this patient, as compared with the average patient
e. the assay was in error and provided an underestimate of the true carbamazepine plasma concentration

103. In a patient who is taking both carbamazepine and phenytoin, the occurrence of side effects is probably most related to:

a. the sum of carbamazepine and phenytoin plasma concentration
b. only the plasma carbamazepine concentration
c. only the salivary carbamazepine concentration
d. only the phenytoin plasma concentration
e. the sum of urinary carbamazepine and phenytoin concentrations

104. Saliva should not be collected from a patient less than 2 h after drug administration, particularly if carbamazepine was given as a crushed tablet or suspension, because:

a. the half-life of carbamazepine is longer than 2 h
b. protein is saliva can bind to the drug, thus yielding an overestimate of the true salivary concentration
c. carbamazepine 10,11-epoxide concentrations in saliva will be overestimated
d. carbamazepine can remain in the mouth for up to 2 h, thus yielding artifactually high salivary concentrations
e. carbamazepine inhibits salivary secretion for approximately 2 h after intake

105. The percentage of carbamazepine bound to plasma protein:

a. is relatively constant from patient to patient, averaging 75%
b. is variable from patient to patient and probably related to interindividual differences in plasma protein concentration
c. cannot be estimated by measuring carbamazepine in saliva and plasma
d. varies from 10 to 20% in most patients
e. varies from 13 to 33% in most patients

106. Poor precision may result with some GLC assays for CBZ and CBZ-EP because:

a. these compounds are unstable under alkaline conditions
b. these compounds are not stable at ambient temperature
c. these compounds are unstable at the high temperatures necessary for GLC
d. appropriate internal standards cannot be found for these compounds
e. the sensitivity of these methods is poor

107. Simultaneous analyses of CBZ, CBZ-EP, and other anticonvulsants are not possible with which method?

a. HPLC
b. GLC
c. EMIT
d. TLC

108. The response parameter of the EMIT assay that is related to known drug concentration in the standard curve is:

a. peak height
b. peak-height ratio
c. enzyme reaction rate
d. peak area
e. relative fluorescence

109. Spectrophotometric procedures for analysis of CBZ are considered inferior to chromatographic methods for all the following reasons except:

a. nonspecificity
b. insensitivity
c. inability to allow simultaneous analysis of other anticonvulsants
d. inability to quantify CBZ at ambient temperatures
e. inability to quantify CBZ metabolite

110. The protein-precipitation method used for sample preparation in some HPLC methods may suffer from which of the following disadvantages?

a. it is time consuming
b. it requires derivitization
c. there may be progressive loss in HPLC column efficiency
d. the epoxide metabolite decomposes
e. an internal standard cannot be used

111. The EMIT® system for determining CBZ is more cost-effective than chromatographic methods in:

a. a clinical laboratory well equipped with GLC and HPLC instruments
b. a laboratory that performs assays for various convulsants but only about 10 per week
c. a laboratory that performs 50 CBZ assays per week

112. Simultaneous analysis of CBZ-EP and CBZ might be desirable because:

a. CBZ is degraded to CBZ-EP
b. CBZ-EP is degraded to CBZ
c. CBZ-EP may be pharmacologically active
d. CBZ-EP is carcinogenic
e. CBZ and CBZ-EP cannot be separated on chromatographic systems

## Chapter 16

113. Valproic acid is thought to exert its anticonvulsant activity by:

a. promoting sodium efflux from neurons
b. inhibiting the mechanism for re-uptake of norepinephrine into adrenergic neurons
c. increasing brain levels of $\gamma$-aminobutyric acid
d. inhibiting glial cell carbonic anhydrase
e. decreasing the release of acetylcholine from central cholinergic neurons

114. The therapeutic concentration of valproic acid is thought to be:

a. 55 - 100 $\mu g/mL$
b. 15 - 40 $\mu g/mL$
c. 2 - 5 $mg/dL$
d. 100 - 200 $\mu g/mL$
e. 1 - 10 $mg/L$

115. Chemically, valproic acid is:

a. related to the barbiturates
b. one of the benzodiazepines
c. a carboxylic acid

d. similar to phenytoin
e. a succinimide

116. At present, the best analytical approach for determining serum concentrations of valproate is:

a. "high-pressure" liquid chromatography
b. spectrophotometry
c. gas-liquid chromatography
d. radioimmunoassay
e. EMIT

117. Valproic acid reaches steady-state concentrations in:

a. 5 days
b. 10 days
c. 2.5 days
d. 1 day
e. 8 days

118. Which of the following statements about the interaction of drugs with physiological systems is true?

a. drugs alter only the physiological system responsible for eliciting a therapeutic effect
b. a drug may alter the activity of more than one physiological system
c. because drugs can alter more than one physiological system, it is possible to elicit therapeutic and undesirable side effects at the same serum concentration
d. b and c

119. Drug action to produce a therapeutic effect can be attributed to an alteration of the cell's normal activity related to:

a. cell growth
b. cell repair
c. cell reproduction
d. biochemical activity within the cell
e. all of the above

120. Unexpected analyte concentrations observed in routine diagnostic procedures after chronic drug therapy can be attributed to:

a. a direct pharmacological effect of the drug on a physiological or biochemical system to decrease the concentration of an analyte
b. a direct pharmacological effect of the drug on a physiological or biochemical system to increase the concentration of analyte
c. a direct interference with a chemical or biochemical analytical technique
d. all of the above
e. none of the above

121. Factors that may affect therapeutic drug monitoring and interpretations are:

a. age
b. sex
c. renal function
d. liver function
e. all of the above

122. To properly interpret a patient's serum drug concentration, one must know:

a. the usual therapeutic range
b. concomitant drug therapy
c. the time relationship between dose and specimen collection
d. the specificity of the assay
e. all of the above

123. The fluctuation of a drug concentration in serum during a dosing interval may be due to:

a. length of the dosing interval
b. rate of elimination from the body
c. volume of distribution of the drug in the body
d. fluid intake
e. all of the above

124. Steady-state serum concentrations are those values that recur with each dose once an equilibrium is reached between the dose of the drug and the amount being eliminated during the dosing interval. How much time must lapse before steady-state is reached if the dosing interval is equivalent to the half-life of the drug?

a. after 50% of the original dose has been metabolized or excreted
b. after 3 doses have been administered
c. after 5 half-lives of the drug
d. just before the dose
e. none of the above

125. The most common cause of suboptimal drug concentrations, and consequent failure to achieve the desired therapeutic response, is:

a. malabsorption
b. excess stomach acid
c. depressed stomach acid
d. patient noncompliance
e. none of the above

126. As a rule of thumb, to maintain a constant, steady-state plasma drug concentration without excessive fluctuations, a drug dosage interval should be _____ that drug's half-life.

a. equal to
b. one-fourth of
c. one-eighth of
d. one-half of
e. twice

127. The intensity of the pharmacological effect of a drug is most nearly proportional to:

a. the amount of drug taken
b. the dosage from the drug
c. the concentration of drug at the receptor site
d. the concentration of drug at the absorption site
e. none of the above

## Chapters 17-19

*For questions 128-137, use the following key:*

a— if 1, 2, and 3 are correct
b— if 1 and 3 are correct
c— if 2 and 4 are correct
d— if 4 only is correct
e— if all are correct

128. Quinidine and procainamide have similar electrophysiologic actions in that they:

1. decrease automaticity
2. increase excitability
3. increase effective refractory period duration relative to action potential duration
4. decrease action potential duration

129. *N*-Acetylprocainamide:

1. is an active procainamide metabolite, equipotent to the parent drug
2. is mostly eliminated by renal excretion
3. concentrations usually exceed those of procainamide in rapid acetylators
4. has a half-life in normal individuals of about 6 h

130. The pharmacokinetic properties of lidocaine would lead you to think that it would:

1. be a good drug to give orally
2. have a longer half-life when severe liver disease is present
3. be present in high concentrations in the urine
4. take some hours for a continuous infusion to produce concentrations in blood greater than 90% of steady-state values

131. Which of the following drugs are beta blockers?

1. propranolol
2. verapamil
3. metoprolol
4. quinidine

132. For which of the following antiarrhythmics have active metabolites been discovered?

1. disopyramide
2. procainamide
3. propranolol
4. lidocaine

133. High doses of digitalis affect the transmembrane action potential of Purkinje fibers in which of the following ways?

1. decreased resting potential
2. decreased slope of phase 4
3. decreased slope of phase 0
4. decreased duration of phase 3

134. The bioavailability of tablet digoxin:

1. is normally around 70%
2. is increased by anticholinergics
3. is decreased by cholestyramine and antacids
4. is decreased if taken with meals, because the total amount of digoxin absorbed is decreased

135. Which of the following pharmacokinetic statements apply to digoxin?

1. it is eliminated from the body mostly by liver metabolism
2. the "apparent volume of distribution" is about 0.5 L/kg
3. the "apparent volume of distribution" is increased in severe renal failure
4. the half-life of digoxin in the body is approximately 1.5 days for subjects with normal renal function

136. "Sensitivity" to digitalis is increased in:

1. hypokalemia
2. hypomagnesemia
3. hypercalcemia
4. hypothyroidism

137. Digoxin toxicity:

1. occurs in about 1% of hospitalized patients treated with digoxin
2. in most, but not all, patients is accompanied by digoxin in blood exceeding 2 ng/mL

3. means that quinidine and procainamide are especially suitable for patients developing prolonged atrioventricular conduction
4. is frequently accompanied by gastrointestinal and neurologic symptoms

138. The most clinically important alteration in digoxin pharmacokinetics is:

a. decreased bioavailability as a result of slow tablet dissolution
b. decreased bioavailability because it is bound in the gut by antacids and kaolin-pectin antidiarrheal compounds
c. decreased bioavailability because of intestinal disease states characterized by diarrhea
d. produced by renal impairment
e. produced by liver failure

139. The bioavailability of oral digoxin tablets is approximately:

a. 50%
b. 60%
c. 70%
d. 80%
e. 90%

140. Digoxin concentrations are of value to the physician:

a. in helping diagnose digitalis toxicity
b. in guiding dosage adjustments in patients with altered digoxin pharmacokinetics
c. in assessing patient compliance
d. all of the above
e. none of the above

141. All of the following statements are true *except:*

a. quinidine results in decreased serum digoxin levels
b. digoxin values are of no clinical value when obtained within several hours of a given dose
c. renal failure greatly prolongs the serum half-life of digoxin
d. there is good correlation between serum and myocardial concentrations of digoxin
e. there is good correlation between the serum concentrations of digoxin and its pharmacological effects

142. The usual "therapeutic" range (ng/mL) for serum digoxin is:

a. 0.5-1.0
b. 1.0-2.0
c. 1.5-2.5
d. 2.0-3.0
e. 2.5-3.5

143. Digitalis toxicity:

a. can be accurately diagnosed by measuring the concentrations of digoxin in serum
b. frequently is caused by a change in digoxin pharmacokinetics that increases the body stores of digoxin
c. does not occur with digoxin concentrations in the accepted "therapeutic" range
d. has not been associated with concomitant use of quinidine
e. all of the above

144. The large volume of distribution of digoxin is due to:

a. serum protein binding
b. tissue sequestration
c. active renal reabsorption
d. all of the above
e. none of the above

145. The clearance of a drug is defined as:

a. the product of the half-life and the serum concentration
b. the product of the half-life and the volume of distribution
c. the product of the elimination rate constant and the volume of distribution
d. the urine concentration divided by the serum concentration
e. the product of the dose and the volume of distribution

146. The two pharmacological factors observed in the digoxin-quinidine interaction are:

a. an increase in the volume of distribution of digoxin
b. a decrease in the volume of distribution of digoxin
c. a decrease in the volume of distribution of quinidine
d. an increased clearance of quinidine
e. a decreased clearance of digoxin

147. The time course of the change in digoxin concentration when quinidine is added is:

a. a few minutes
b. a few hours
c. a few days
d. a few weeks
e. a month or more

148. Digoxin is used in atrial flutter and fibrillation to:

a. increase cardiac contractility
b. block A-V node transmission
c. suppress spontaneous atrial depolarization
d. all of the above
e. a and b

## Chapters 20-28

149. Lidocaine's effects are short-lived after a single intravenous bolus because it is:

a. rapidly metabolized in the liver
b. highly protein bound
c. rapidly metabolized by plasma esterases
d. rapidly distributed
e. taken up by the heart

150. Procainamide is usually given every 3-4 h. Giving larger doses less often might:

a. produce a decreased antiarrhythmic effect just before a dose
b. produce side effects just after a dose
c. lead to excessive accumulation of N-acetylprocainamide
d. all of the above
e. a and b

151. Monitoring N-acetylprocainamide as well as procainamide plasma concentrations during procainamide therapy is:

a. useful because the total effect is equal to the sum of the two
b. useful if one remembers that the total effect is equal to the procainamide concentration plus half the N-acetylprocainamide concentration
c. useful because N-acetylprocainamide accumulation can explain some clinical effects during procainamide therapy
d. useless because there is no predictable concentration-response relationship
e. useless because N-acetylprocainamide is only weakly active

152. After an appropriate loading dose of lidocaine, a patient with severe heart failure is treated with a maintenance lidocaine infusion. When will steady state be achieved?

a. immediately, because loading was appropriate
b. very quickly, because lidocaine's t½ α is 8 min
c. After 4-5 elimination half-lives, i.e., 8-10 h
d. answer c is correct in normals; for the patient described, 4-5 elimination half-lives is 16-20 h
e. answer c is correct in normals; for the patient described, 4-5 elimination half-lives is 24-30 h

153. Higher than usual quinidine dosages are required in:

a. the elderly
b. patients receiving phenytoin
c. patients with heart failure
d. patients with cirrhosis
e. patients receiving digoxin

154. A patient with a plasma concentration of phenytoin 15 $\mu$g/mL develops renal failure and the plasma concentration drops to 6 $\mu$g/mL. Which is the most likely explanation?

a. malabsorption due to uremic gastritis
b. decreased binding to plasma proteins
c. enhanced hepatic metabolism compensating for decreased renal function
d. increased volume of distribution
e. none of the above; non-compliance is the only reasonable explanation

155. Which loading dose would be appropriate for an adult with normal cardiac and liver function?

a. 50-75 mg
b. 500-700 mg
c. 200-300 mg
d. 900-1000 mg
e. 2 mg/min continuous infusion

156. An adverse effect that may occur from lidocaine is:

a. drowsiness
b. paresthesia
c. dizziness
d. dysarthria
e. all of the above

157. Which of the following factor(s) may increase plasma lidocaine concentrations?

a. congestive heart failure
b. hepatocellular liver disease
c. propranolol
d. norepinephrine
e. all of the above

158. Which statement is true regarding the pharmacokinetics of lidocaine?

a. half-life is two days
b. volume of distribution is 5 L
c. it is excreted unchanged by the kidneys
d. binding occurs predominantly to albumin
e. none of the above

159. The plasma half-life of lidocaine in normals is approximately:

a. 24 h
b. 30 h
c. 1.5 h
d. 1.5 days
e. 10 h

160. Which of the following factors may decrease plasma lidocaine concentrations?

a. liver disease
b. rubber-stoppered collection tubes
c. congestive heart failure
d. propranolol
e. norepinephrine

161. The metabolism and elimination of lidocaine is best described as:

a. excreted unchanged by the kidneys
b. primarily metabolized by the liver
c. 50% excreted unchanged by the kidney and 50% metabolized by the liver
d. primarily eliminated by the lungs
e. 50% eliminated by the lungs and 50% excreted unchanged by the kidney

162. Procainamide:

a. can always be used safely with concomitant quinidine administration
b. is a good drug for the treatment of digitalis-induced arrhythmias
c. may have additive effects to those of quinidine and lidocaine
d. has a higher central nervous system/myocardial ratio of activity than procaine
e. was introduced for clinical use in 1965

163. The most reliable time for collection of plasma specimens for procainamide/NAPA determination is:

a. just before the next dose
b. just after the last dose
c. midway between specified times of administration
d. as soon as arrhythmias have decreased by 10% per hour
e. none of the above

164. Which of the following is the recommended method for therapeutic drug monitoring of procainamide/NAPA?

a. chromatographic
b. TLC
c. EMIT
d. HPLC
e. c and d

165. The appearance of a lupus erythematosus-like syndrome after the use of procainamide:

a. usually becomes manifest shortly after initiation of treatment
b. is seen in "fast acetylators"
c. is seen in "slow acetylators"
d. is extremely rare, such that long-term therapy with procainamide is safe and recommended
e. is never seen in oriental patients

166. Which of the following can be linked either causally or as a consequence of high initial procainamide/NAPA concentrations?

a. decreased renal perfusion
b. low left ventricular output
c. continued ventricular dysrhythmias
d. collection of samples too close to intravenous lines of drug infusion
e. all of the above

167. The actions of procainamide on the myocardium include:

a. decreased effective refractory period
b. increased AV node conduction
c. blockage of intracellular calcium transport
d. all of the above

168. If quinidine is given to a patient who is receiving a constant dose of digoxin, you should expect to find:

a. a decreased half-life of quinidine
b. an increase in plasma digoxin
c. no change in plasma digoxin
d. an increased renal clearance of digoxin

169. The mechanisms by which quinidine affects plasma concentrations of digoxin probably include:

a. a reduced renal clearance of digoxin
b. a decreased absorption of digoxin
c. a direct interference to diminish digoxin's effect
d. induction of liver microsomes

170. The major route of elimination of quinidine is by:

a. excretion of unchanged drug in urine
b. methylation during hepatic first-pass
c. hydroxylation by liver oxidases
d. excretion of glucuronide conjugate

171. Older people have a higher intrinsic clearance of quinidine than would a younger control group.

a. true
b. false

172. Quinidine and dihydroquinidine have essentially identical pharmacologic and pharmacokinetic properties.

a. true
b. false

173. The main use of quinidine is in he therapy of:

a. congestive heart failure
b. relapsing vivax malaria
c. atrial fibrillation
d. hypertension
e. angina pectoris

174. Quinidine acts by:

a. altering myocardial membrane conductance to specific cations
b. smooth muscle relaxation
c. stimulation of $\alpha$-adrenergic receptors
d. increasing the discharge potential of ectopic pacemakers
e. all of the above

175. The effective concentration of quinidine in serum is:

a. 2-5 mg/L
b. 2-5 $\mu$g/L
c. 1-2 $\mu$g/L
d. 10-20 mg/L
e. 15-40 mg/L

176. Phenobarbital may interfere with quinidine therapy:

a. by prolonging the half-life of quinidine
b. by increasing the rate of quinidine metabolism
c. by counteracting the vagal effects of quinidine
d. by increasing the rate at which dihydroquinidine is formed
e. not at all

177. Quinidine toxicity can be manifest by:

a. ventricular tachycardia
b. hypertension
c. hypotension
d. edema
e. seizures

178. Disopyramide is excreted mainly as:

a. N-desisopropyl disopyramide in urine
b. unchanged in urine
c. N-desisopropyl disopyramide in feces
d. unchanged in feces
e. none of the above

179. Effective plasma concentrations (mg/L) of dis-opyramide are:

a. 1-2
b. 5-7
c. 2-5
d. 0.1-0.2
e. 0.2-0.5

180. A very effective antidote for disopyramide over-dosage is:

a. atropine
b. digitalis
c. epinephrine
d. all of the above
e. not yet known

181. Most of disopyramide's adverse reactions are due to:

a. allergic reactions
b. anticholinergic properties of the drug
c. arrhythmias
d. central nervous system depression
e. adrenergic $\beta$-blocker activity

182. Disopyramide's mean elimination half-life, in hours, in adults is about:

a. 2
b. 5

c. 9
d. 18
e. 24

183. A serum disopyramide concentration of 8.5 mg/L should be considered:

a. insufficient for a good response
b. below the therapeutic range
c. within the therapeutic range
d. toxic
e. none of the above

184. Propranolol:

a. is rapidly absorbed from the gastrointestinal tract
b. is rapidly cleared by the renal tubules
c. is excreted via the lungs
d. is not metabolized by the hepatic drug metabolizing systems
e. none of the above

185. Which of the following statements about first-pass effects are true?

a. less drug per dose will reach the systemic circulation after an oral dose than after an intravenous dose of the same magnitude
b. first-pass effects are more commonly observed for those drugs with very short half-lives
c. first-pass effects are associated with hepatic drug-metabolizing enzymes
d. these effects occur because drugs, after absorption, are transported via the hepatic portal system to the liver
e. all of the above

186. The toxic range, above which propranolol's side effects are commonly observed, is:

a. 80 $\mu$g/L
b. 150 $\mu$g/L
c. 350 $\mu$g/L
d. 1000 $\mu$g/L
e. not clearly established

187. Protein-binding of propranolol is:

a. 70-75%
b. 90-96%
c. 0%
d. 50-60%
e. none of the above

188. The mechanism by which propranolol exerts its pharmacological effects in various disease states is attributable to the fact that propranolol:

a. blocks beta receptors
b. blocks alpha receptors
c. blocks gamma receptors
d. a and b
e. b and c

189. The effects of propranolol on receptors can be reversed by the administration of:

a. strychnine
b. procainamide
c. a beta agonist
d. a and b
e. b and c

## Chapters 29-32

190. Persons interested in antibiotic choice include:

a. the patient and physician
b. the nurse and pharmacist
c. the clinical laboratory
d. the drug representative
e. all of the above

191. Which of the following is true?

a. fever is treated with antibiotics
b. a viral infection with cough and runny nose will respond to antibiotics
c. antibiotics are not innocuous drugs
d. failure to produce a cure is often due to administration of insufficient antibiotic
e. newer antibiotics are always more efficacious

192. Which of the following is true?

a. some antibiotics have no adverse effects
b. the administration of an antibiotic involves a risk-benefit analysis
c. chloramphenicol is an innocuous drug
d. gentamicin is an innocuous drug
e. clindamycin is an innocuous drug

193. Therapeutic drug monitoring is currently recommended for the following:

a. phenobarbital and phenytoin
b. theophylline
c. gentamicin
d. chloramphenicol
e. all of the above

194. Appropriate therapeutic drug monitoring for antibiotics is dependent upon obtaining:

a. peak and trough concentrations
b. drawing the peak and trough samples at the correct times
c. knowing the therapeutic range
d. administering the antibiotic at the appropriate dose and interval
e. all of the above

195. Sodium dodecyl sulfate can be added to serum to retard degradation of which of the following drugs?

a. carbenicillin
b. cephalothin
c. gentamicin
d. chloramphenicol
e. vancomycin

196. For practical purposes and allowing for distribution, serum for measuring a "peak" concentration of an aminoglycoside should be obtained:

a. 1 h after an intramuscular or intravenous dose
b. 1 h after an intramuscular dose and immediately after an intravenous dose
c. 1 h after an intramuscular dose and 30 min after an intravenous dose
d. immediately after an intramuscular or intravenous dose
e. just before a subsequent dose

197. Which of the following drugs is most active against *Pseudomonas aeruginosa?*

a. tobramycin
b. kanamycin
c. streptomycin
d. vancomycin
e. chloramphenicol

198. Based on the usual apparent volume of distribution, a single 100-mg dose of gentamicin to a 70-kg person will give a peak concentration (mg/L) of:

a. 1 to 2
b. 2 to 4
c. 4 to 6
d. 6 to 8
e. 8 to 10

199. A child who weighs 15 kg has a trough concentration of chloramphenicol of 10 mg/L. How much chloramphenicol (mg) should be given to attain a peak concentration of 20 mg/L?

a. 5
b. 10
c. 15
d. 20
e. none of the above

200. For which of the following drugs does impaired renal function *least* affect elimination?

a. amikacin
b. gentamicin
c. streptomycin
d. chloramphenicol
e. vancomycin

201. Nephrotoxicity occurs in what percentage of patients receiving aminoglycoside therapy?

a. 5-40%
b. over 50%
c. less than 5%
d. over 70%
e. 0%

202. Aminoglycosides are used in the treatment of:

a. fungal infections
b. Gram-negative infections
c. Gram-positive infections
d. viral infections
e. all of the above

203. Which of the following is not an aminoglycoside?

a. tobramycin
b. gentamicin
c. streptomycin
d. amikacin
e. vancomycin

204. Which of the following factors affects the clinical efficacy of aminoglycoside therapy?

a. microbiological susceptibility
b. drug concentration at the site of infection
c. host defense factors
d. all of the above
e. none of the above

205. Peak serum concentrations of amikacin (mg/L) should be:

a. 5-10
b. 20-30
c. 10-20
d. less than 10
e. less than 2

206. Microorganisms:

a. do not usually develop resistance to aminoglycosides
b. are more likely to be resistant to amikacin than to gentamicin
c. resistant to gentamicin are often sensitive to tobramycin
d. develop resistance to gentamicin by plasmid-mediated transfer of inactivating enzyme activity
e. c and d

207. Which of the following factors could affect a patient's immune function?

a. neutropenia
b. steroid administration
c. radiation therapy
d. severe systemic illness
e. all of the above

208. Which of the following is observed in cases of aminoglycoside-related nephrotoxicity?

a. impaired urine-concentrating ability
b. proximal tubular dysfunction
c. proteinuria
d. increased excretion of $\beta_2$-microglobulin
e. all of the above

209. A major risk associated with gentamicin therapy is:

a. ototoxicity
b. hepatotoxicity
c. neutropenia
d. respiratory depression
e. blindness

210. Older patients are at greater risk for the development of aminoglycoside-related nephrotoxicity than younger patients.

a. true
b. false

211.   How many serum samples are required after the first dose of aminoglycoside to improve our kinetic estimates without adding unnecessary costs?

a. two
b. three
c. four
d. five
e. six

212.   Rapid, sensitive, and precise assay methodologies for aminoglycoside antibiotics are:

a. radioimmunoassays
b. radioenzymic assays
c. "high-performance" liquid chromatography
d. gas-liquid chromatography
e. all of the above

213.   Differences between fitting serum concentrations vs time data by linear regression analysis or by nonlinear regression analysis are that:

a. the data may be weighted with linear regression analysis
b. peak concentration is obtained with nonlinear regression analysis
c. nonlinear regression provides a practical clinical approach
d. nonlinear regression analysis is complex and requires a sophisticated computer base
e. all of the above

214.   After the serum specimens have been analyzed, the next step in analyzing the data is:

a. determining peak concentrations
b. determining the elimination rate constant
c. determining the drug's half-life
d. plotting for serum concentration vs time data on semi-log paper
e. determining the drug's distribution volume

215.   Infusion of the aminoglycoside antibiotics should be:

a. over 30-60 min
b. by a rapid bolus
c. over 2 h
d. intramuscular in patients who are hypotensive
e. by intramuscular injection for all patients

216.   The drug's distribution volume:

a. describes a pharmacologic space within which a particular drug is distributed
b. approximates the extracellular fluid compartment for the aminoglycosides
c. may vary from patient to patient
d. depends on the patient's rate of elimination
e. all of the above

## Chapters 33 and 34

217.   Vancomycin is effective in the treatment of:

a. Gram-negative infections
b. fungal infections
c. staphylococcal infections
d. meningococcal infections
e. all of the above

218.   Vancomycin functions by:

a. inhibiting bacterial cell-wall synthesis
b. inhibiting bacterial protein synthesis
c. acting as an antimetabolite
d. affecting cell-membrane permeability
e. affecting nucleic acid metabolism

219.   The half-life of vancomycin in adults is:

a. 2-3 h
b. 5-11 h
c. 10-30 h
d. 20-44 h
e. more than 5 days

220.   The major toxic effects of vancomycin administration are:

a. ototoxicity
b. nephrotoxicity
c. hypersensitivity reactions
d. diarrhea
e. none of the above

221.   Vancomycin concentrations in serum can be determined by:

a. HPLC
b. spectrophotometry
c. enzyme immunoassay
d. fluorescence immunoassay
e. gas-liquid chromatography

222. Radioenzymic assays for chloramphenicol:

a. are based on the ability of chloramphenicol to specifically inhibit certain enzyme-catalyzed reactions
b. are actually assays for the acetylated derivatives of chloramphenicol
c. make use of specific chloramphenicol acetylating enzymes isolated from chloramphenicol-resistant variants of *Escherichia coli*
d. are competitive binding assays involving radio-labeled chloramphenicol and specific chloramphen-icol-binding proteins found in some bacteria
e. suffer from interference by non-active chloram-phenicol metabolites

223. The recommended therapeutic concentrations for chloramphenicol are:

a. 10-20 mg/dL
b. less than 25 $\mu$g/mL
c. 100-200 $\mu$g/mL
d. 10-20 $\mu$g/mL
e. less than 50 $\mu$g/mL

224. Chloramphenicol acts by:

a. inhibiting protein synthesis by binding to 30$S$ ribosomes, therby preventing access of aminoacyl tRNA to the mRNA-ribosome complex
b. inhibiting the final cross-linking reaction involved in the synthesis of peptidoglycan, a bacterial cell-wall component
c. suppressing the activity of peptidyl transferase, therby preventing peptide bond formation
d. binding to the cell membrane, thereby disorienting the lipoprotein structure sufficiently to allow for loss of intracellular contents
e. inhibiting RNA polymerase activity by virtue of its ability to bind to DNA

225. "Gray-baby" syndrome is:

a. a common, benign side effect of chloramphenicol administration
b. a teratogenic effect due to the administration of chloramphenicol during the last trimester of preg-nancy
c. a serious, dose-independent hypersensitivity to chloram-phenicol seen in newborns
d. a severe, often fatal consequence of excessively high-dose chloramphenicol therapy in infants
e. a consequence of simultaneous therapy with chlor-amphenicol and phenytoin in newborns

226. A severe blood dyscrasia:

a. occurs in about 1 in 24 000 to 200 000 patients receiving chloramphenicol
b. can be a dose-independent consequence of chlor-amphenicol therapy
c. sometimes, with complete bone marrow aplasia, can occur during chloramphenicol therapy
d. that is often fatal appears to be a hypersensitivity to chloramphenicol
e. all of the above

227. Chloramphenicol is an effective antibiotic in the treatment of infections from:

a. *Schistosoma,* yeast, and fungi
b. *Pseudomonas*
c. *Hemophilus influenzae*
d. *Plasmodium falciparum*
e. all of the above

## Chapter 35

228. The presence of a second compound with anti-microbial activity will most often produce erroneous results with which assay methodology?

a. radioimmunoassay
b. bioassay
c. EMIT
d. HPLC

229. Advantages of the radioimmunoassay techni-ques over bioassay techniques generally include:

a. more rapid turnaround time
b. higher specificity
c. higher sensitivity
d. all of the above

230. Advantages of HPLC techniques over other methods for antimicrobial assays include:

a. ability to distinguish between parent compound and biologically active metabolites
b. less cost by reagents and instrumentation
c. less personnel training required
d. all of the above

231. Which of the following techniques is most limited to the variety of antimicrobial assays available?

a. bioassay
b. RIA
c. EMIT
d. HPLC

232. Monitoring aminoglycoside concentrations and adjusting dosage regimens have been demonstrated to:

a. improve safety
b. improve efficacy
c. be cost-effective in burn patients
d. all of the above

233. To optimally utilize antibiotic assay results, one must interpret the data by incorporating which of the following?

a. other antibiotics the patient is receiving
b. timing of the specimen in relation to the dose administered
c. clinical status of the patient
d. all of the above

234. The specificity of bioassay can be enhanced by:

a. inactivating other antimicrobials in the specimen
b. using the pathogen responsible for the patient's infection as the test organism
c. using a strain of test organism that is selectively sensitive to one of the antibiotics
d. a and c
e. a and b

235. Potential advantages of using EMIT® procedures for aminoglycoside assays include:

a. rapid turnaround time
b. availability of other quantitative drug assays
c. minimal personnel training required
d. all of the above

## Chapters 36-38

236. Which of the following statements about the pathology of asthma are true?

a. mucus plugs may be present in the trachea and bronchial tubes
b. the lungs are overdistended
c. there is bacterial infection in the lungs and pus is present
d. an increased number of eosinophils may be found on microscopic section of the lung
e. there is edema in the lining of the conducting airways (the tracheae and the bronchial tubes)

237. Which of the following laboratory tests are useful for a patient with acute asthma?

a. arterial blood gases
b. serum creatinine
c. serum bilirubin

d. total leukocyte count and differential from which total eosinophil count is derived
e. "acute" serum for viral studies

238. In young patients with asthma which of the following disorders are often present concurrently?

a. eczema
b. bacterial pneumonia
c. allergic rhinitis
d. allergy to drugs
e. headaches

239. Theophylline is a safe, effective bronchodilator that can be best used when serum concentrations are monitored. Which of the following illnesses or situations decrease theophylline clearance in the liver and make a patient vulnerable to theophylline toxicity?

a. erythromycin treatment
b. congestive heart failure
c. cirrhosis of the liver
d. pulmonary edema
e. smoking

240. Treatment of severe acute asthma in the hospitalized patient should always include the following:

a. intravenous fluids
b. oxygen
c. bronchodilators such as theophylline and $\beta$-adrenergic agonists
d. corticosteroids
e. antibiotics

241. Which of the following statements about asthma are true?

a. asthma attacks are always caused by exposure to allergens
b. young patients with asthma often have family members who also have asthma
c. asthma is a common disease
d. asthma is never fatal
e. most patients with asthma should be able to lead normal lives if they receive appropriate treatment

242. Asthma, especially in young patients with allergies, is often associated with an elevated eosinophil count. Which other disorders are commonly associated with an elevated eosinophil count?

a. parasitic diseases
b. immunodeficiency diseases
c. adverse reactions to drugs
d. emphysema
e. heart disease

243. The major metabolic pathway for theophylline in neonates is:

a. demethylation
b. oxidation
c. decarboxylation
d. *N*-methylation

244. After theophylline therapy in neonates, the serum caffeine concentration relative to that of theophylline:

a. is always lower
b. is about equal
c. may vary with dose
d. is always higher

245. The serum half-life of theophylline relative to that of caffeine in neonates is:

a. longer
b. shorter
c. about equal
d. not known

246. In the treatment of neonatal apnea, caffeine as the sole therapeutic agent:

a. is ineffective, except when combined with theophylline
b. effectively reduces apneic episodes
c. may be used without therapeutic monitoring
d. has a well-established therapeutic range

247. The toxicity of caffeine relative to theophylline is:

a. greater
b. less
c. about equal
d. not well defined in infants

## Chapters 39-42

248. Tricyclic antidepressants are used to treat:

a. depressive disorders in adults
b. depressive disorders in children
c. childhood enuresis
d. chronic pain
e. all of the above

249. The relationship between plasma concentrations of tricyclic antidepressants and clinical efficacy is reasonably well established for:

a. depressive disorders in adults
b. childhood enuresis

c. childhood depression
d. anorexia nervosa
e. all of the above

250. The principal action of tricyclic antidepressant drugs is thought to result from these compounds' ability to:

a. block biogenic amine re-uptake
b. enhance biogenic amine re-uptake
c. produce anticholinergic effects
d. produce antihistaminic effects
e. cause sedation

251. The tricyclic antidepressant most likely to block the re-uptake of the neurotransmitter serotonin is:

a. amitriptyline
b. nortriptyline
c. imipramine
d. desipramine
e. doxepin

252. The major routes of metabolism of the tricyclic antidepressants are:

a. *N*-demethylation of the side chains
b. hydroxylation of the ring nucleus
c. dealkylation (removal of the side chain)
d. a and b
e. a and c

253. Which of the following tricyclic antidepressants are metabolized by aromatic ring hydroxylation to form 2-hydroxy derivatives?

a. amitriptyline and nortriptyline
b. imipramine and desipramine
c. doxepin
d. protriptyline
e. all of the above

254. Which tricyclic antidepressant or metabolite is not thought to be pharmacologically active?

a. imipramine
b. desipramine
c. 2-hydroxyimipramine
d. 2-hydroxydesipramine
e. iminodibenzyl

255. Plasma concentrations of tricyclic antidepressants are usually increased by:

a. barbiturates
b. chloral hydrate
c. neuroleptics
d. glutethimide
e. benzodiazepines

256. When tricyclic antidepressants and sedatives are administered together, the effect of the sedative is usually:

a. unchanged
b. increased
c. diminished
d. unchanged, because tricyclics and sedatives are not given together
e. not predictable

257. The principal side effects of the tricyclic antidepressants are caused by their:

a. ability to block norepinephrine re-uptake
b. anticholinergic activity
c. antihistaminic activity
d. ability to block serotonin re-uptake
e. sedative activity

258. Among the most serious adverse effects of tricyclic antidepressants are their:

a. anticholinergic effects
b. sedative effects
c. antihistaminic effects
d. cardiotoxic effects
e. sleep disturbance

259. The principal pharmacological action of a tricyclic antidepressant drug like imipramine is thought to be:

a. inhibition of re-uptake of biogenic amines
b. inhibition of acetylcholine re-uptake
c. sedative activity
d. cardiovascular activity
e. all of the above

260. Which of the following antidepressant drugs or metabolites can inhibit the uptake of biogenic amines?

a. imipramine
b. desipramine
c. imipramine and desipramine
d. imipramine, desipramine, and their 2-hydroxy metabolites
e. only the 2-hydroxy metabolites of imipramine and desipramine

261. Which of the following actions are responsible for many of the untoward side effects of tricyclic antidepressant drugs?

a. inhibition of neurotransmitter re-uptake
b. anticholinergic action
c. sedative action
d. drug interactions
e. none of the above

262. Monitoring tricyclic antidepressant drugs in plasma can be most useful when:

a. drug toxicity is suspected
b. the patient is elderly
c. the patient is taking more than one drug
d. compliance with prescribed dose schedules is poor
e. all of the above

263. The maximum recommended dose of imipramine (mg/day) in elderly patients is:

a. 20
b. 100
c. 150
d. 250
e. 300

264. The antidepressant response rate to imipramine therapy generally:

a. is low when concentrations in plasma are <150 $\mu$g/L
b. is proportional to dose between 150 and 250 $\mu$g/L
c. reaches a plateau at 250 $\mu$g/L
d. does not increase further with increasing concentrations in blood >250 $\mu$g/L
e. all of the above

265. The maximum recommended dose of imipramine (mg/day) in middle-aged, physically healthy patients is:

a. 20
b. 100
c. 150
d. 250
e. 300

266. Monitoring tricyclic antidepressants in plasma is particularly useful in elderly patients because they:

a. have a decreased tolerance for tricyclic antidepressants
b. attain lower concentrations in blood from given doses
c. require much higher doses of medication
d. metabolize tricyclic antidepressant drugs rapidly
e. all of the above

267. The relationship between plasma concentrations and clinical response in patients treated with amitriptyline is:

a. curvilinear
b. always therapeutic between 120 and 250 ng/mL
c. nonexistent
d. dependent on amitriptyline concentration
e. not well established

268. Which of following actions is thought to be responsible for the principal pharmacological actions of tricyclic antidepressant drugs?

a. inhibition of neurotransmitter re-uptake
b. anticholinergic action
c. sedative action
d. drug interactions
e. cardiovascular action

269. In physically healthy, middle-aged patients of average weight, the usual therapeutic dose of amitriptyline (mg/day) is between:

a. 50 and 100
b. 50 and 200
c. 100 and 200
d. 150 and 300
e. 200 and 300

270. Plasma concentrations of amitriptyline at 120 $\mu g/L$ and nortriptyline at 80 $\mu g/L$ would generally be:

a. too low
b. within the acceptable range
c. too high, but not toxic
d. mildly toxic
e. highly toxic

271. Amtriptyline is the most potent tricyclic antidepressant with respect to:

a. antidepressant activity
b. anticholinergic activity
c. cardiovascular activity
d. inhibition of biogenic amines
e. all of the above

## Chapters 43-45

272. The principal action of the "traditional" tricyclic antidepressants is thought to result from the compounds' ability to:

a. block biogenic amine re-uptake
b. enhance biogenic amine re-uptake
c. produce anticholinergic effects
d. produce antihistamine effects
e. cause sedation

273. Traditional tricyclic antidepressants must be used with extreme caution in patients who:

a. are young
b. are elderly
c. have a history of heart disease
d. have a history of drug allergy
e. have been treated previously for depression

274. The tricyclic antidepressant most likely to block re-uptake of the neurotransmitter serotonin is:

a. amitriptyline
b. imipramine
c. doxepin
d. desipramine
e. trimipramine

275. Long-term studies indicate that the antidepressant that may be safe for extended treatment is:

a. trimipramine
b. trazodone
c. alprazolam
d. maprotiline
e. zimelidine

276. Tricyclic antidepressants can be lethal when exceeding the usual dose by:

a. 2 times
b. 5 times
c. 10-20 times
d. 20-50 times
e. 50-100 times

277. The following antidepressant is a tetracyclic antidepressant:

a. trimipramine
b. maprotiline
c. trazodone
d. alprazolam
e. all of the above

278. Overdosage of amoxapine is characterized primarily by:

a. severe anticholinergic reactions
b. oversedation
c. arrhythmias, tachycardia
d. severe antihistaminic effects
e. central nervous system overactivity, convulsions

279. The principal pharmacologic effects (i.e., antidepressant effects) of amoxapine are due to:

a. amoxapine alone
b. 7-hydroxy and 8-hydroxy amoxapine
c. amoxapine and 7-hydroxy amoxapine
d. amoxapine and 8-hydroxy amoxapine
e. other metabolites

280. The therapeutic concentration of amoxapine in plasma is thought to be ($\mu$g/L):

a. 100-250
b. 100-300
c. 200-400
d. 200-500
e. 200-600

281. The antidepressant that has no effect on re-uptake of either serotonin or norepinephrine is:

a. trimipramine
b. maprotiline
c. alprazolam
d. trazodone
e. amoxapine

282. Maprotiline most nearly resembles which tricyclic antidepressant with respect to its pharmacological action?

a. imipramine
b. amitriptyline
c. desipramine
d. nortriptyline
e. trimipramine

283. Studies conducted to date indicate that the therapeutic range for maprotiline ($\mu$g/L) is:

a. 80-200
b. 180-400
c. 200-500
d. 180-600
e. 300-600

284. In middle-aged, physically healthy adults of average weight, the usual average dose of maprotiline (mg/day) is:

a. 50-100
b. 75-100
c. 150-250
d. 300-400
e. >400

285. The usual upper limit for dosage of maprotiline (mg/day) is:

a. 100
b. 150
c. 200
d. 300
e. 400

286. The relationship between plasma concentration and clinical response in patients treated with maprotiline:

a. is curvilinear
b. is always therapeutic between 180 and 400 $\mu$g/L
c. does not exist
d. is age dependent
e. is not well established

287. The principal metabolite of norepinephrine originating in the brain appears to be:

a. normetanephrine
b. metanephrine
c. 3-methoxy-4-hydroxyphenylglycol
d. 3-methoxy-4-hydroxyphenylacetic acid
e. 3-methoxy-4-hydroxyvanillylmandelic acid

288. Some studies suggest that depressed patients with "high" pretreatment concentrations of MHPG may respond more favorably to:

a. maprotiline
b. trimipramine
c. nortriptyline
d. amitriptyline
e. desipramine

289. Research indicates that certain depressed patients with low pretreatment urinary concentrations of MHPG respond favorably to all but which antidepressant?

a. amitriptyline
b. imipramine
c. desipramine
d. maprotiline
e. nortriptyline

290. Based on an arterial-venous study published recently, the percentage of urinary MHPG that originates in the brain is:

a. 20%
b. 30%
c. 40%
d. 60%
e. 100%

# Chapter 46

291. Lithium carbonate is indicated for:

a. treatment of acute mania
b. prophylaxis of bipolar depression
c. prophylaxis of unipolar depression
d. all of the above
e. none of the above

292.   The therapeutic range of lithium (mmol/L) is:

a. between 0.2 and 0.8
b. between 0.4 and 1
c. between 0.6 and 1.2
d. between 1 and 1.6
e. not supported by actual data

293.   All of the following statements are true except:

a. plasma lithium concentration may not necessarily reflect the severity of an overdose
b. lithium concentrations can be quite high, while symptoms of intoxication might be only mild
c. lithium concentrations may be relatively low, while toxic symptoms might be severe
d. lithium toxicity will always appear at concentrations of 1.5 mmol/L
e. chronic toxicity of lithium may occur at lower concentrations than acute toxicity

294.   All of the following are common early signs of lithium toxicity except:

a. nausea
b. vomiting
c. diarrhea
d. somnolence
e. seizures

295.   The concomitant use of lithium and diuretics:

a. will always cause lithium intoxication
b. should follow an appropriate upward adjustment of lithium dose
c. should have no effect on lithium plasma concentrations
d. should follow an appropriate downward adjustment of lithium dose
e. will in itself lead to a decrease in lithium plasma concentration

296.   Which of the following is not true about lithium pharmacokinetics?

a. it has no active metabolites
b. it is not protein bound
c. it is rapidly absorbed after an oral dose
d. steady-state is reached in 24 h
e. it is mainly excreted through the kidneys

## Chapters 47-50

297.   The most appropriate time to collect a blood sample for methotrexate TDM after a high-dose treatment is:

a. immediately before and at 96 h after the dose
b. at 8 and 12 h after the dose
c. at 24 and 48 h after the dose
d. at 72 h after the dose

298.   The methotrexate concentration at which toxicity does *not* usually occur is:

a. 1 mmol/L at 24 h
b. 0.5 mmol/L at 24 h
c. 0.5 mmol/L at 48 h
d. 5 $\mu$mol/L at 48 h

299.   Citrovorum factor (CF) is provided after high-dose methotrexate therapy to rescue the patient from the cytotoxic effects of methotrexate by:

a. binding directly to methotrexate before cytotoxic effects occur
b. supplying tetrahydrofolate, which is necessary for DNA synthesis
c. competing with methotrexate at the binding site on the cell surface
d. limiting absorption of oral doses of methotrexate

300.   Excretion of methotrexate is directly related to:

a. adequate renal function
b. enterohepatic circulation
c. the pH of the urine
d. all of the above

301.   Methotrexate is an effective antitumor agent because it:

a. competes with folate for binding sites on the nuclear membrane
b. disrupts hydrogen bonding in DNA
c. prevents formation of reduced folates required for purine synthesis
d. is converted to leucovorin, a cytotoxic drug

302.   Toxicity from high-dose methotrexate infusion is likely if the serum concentration of methotrexate at 48 h after the dose is:

a. greater than 5 $\mu$mol/L
b. less than 0.1 $\mu$mol/L
c. equal to 0.05 $\mu$mol/L
d. equal to or less than 1 $\mu$mol/L

303.   The major metabolite of methotrexate, 7-hydroxymethotrexate, is:

a. less soluble in water than methotrexate
b. more soluble in alkaline urine
c. appears in serum during high-dose therapy
d. may be primarily responsible for renal failure associated with methotrexate therapy
e. all of the above

304. After high-dose infusion, methotrexate is excreted primarily:

a. as the unchanged drug
b. as a 7-hydroxymethotrexate metabolite
c. in urine with an acid pH
d. in the feces as a result of enterohepatic circulation
e. all of the above

305. The primary purpose of giving the patient vincristine during high-dose methotrexate influsion is to:

a. partially block the action of methotrexate in healthy cells
b. promote cellular uptake of methotrexate
c. provide a synergistic antitumor agent
d. promote tubular reabsorption of methotrexate
e. all of the above

306. By definition, a cytotoxic drug:

a. is cell specific
b. enhances the body's immune response
c. kills all cells
d. is generally not life threatening
e. all of the above

307. Antimetabolite drugs act by:

a. intercalating into DNA
b. mimicking naturally occurring compounds important in nucleoside synthesis
c. alkylation of guanine
d. promoting accumulation of chemotherapeutic agents in certain cells

308. At which phase of replication are antimetabolite cytotoxic agents most effective?

a. $G_1$
b. S
c. $G_2$
d. M
e. none of the above

309. Methotrexate is:

a. a phase-specific antimetabolite
b. a vinca alkaloid
c. an alkylating agent
d. an activator of tetrahydrofolate dehydrogenase
e. none of the above

310. Therapeutic monitoring of alkylating agents has realized limited success because most of them:

a. are active via one or more metabolites
b. do not follow normal pharmacokinetic principles
c. are consumed during the process of alkylation
d. have short half-lives
e. all of the above

311. A sensitive laboratory index of cytotoxicity is:

a. serum creatinine
b. leukocyte count
c. hematocrit
d. serum thyroxin
e. all of the above

312. The concentration of methotrexate ($\mu$mol/L) after 72 h of therapy consistent with no renal damage is:

a. 30
b. 3.2
c. 1.0
d. 0.2
e. 2.5

313. External symptoms of toxicity due to vinblastine are:

a. nausea and vomiting
b. alopecia
c. tremors
d. hyperpigmentation
e. all of the above

314. Serum creatinine concentration is a good index of nephrotoxicity due to cytotoxic agents.

a. true
b. false

315. At which phase of replication is adriamycin most effective?

a. $G_1$
b. S
c. $G_2$
d. M
e. a and b

316. MTX does not inhibit the synthesis of:

a. DNA
b. reduced folates
c. folic acid
d. RNA
e. protein

317. The 24-h and 48-h 7OH-MTX/MTX ratios generally vary between:

a. 10-100
b. 0-50
c. 20-40
d. 30-70
e. 10-60

318. Nephrotoxicity after high-dose MTX is mainly averted by:

a. monitoring serum creatinine
b. alkalinization of the urine
c. maintenance of a high urine output
d. b and c
e. a, b, and c

319. In the osteogenic sarcoma chemotherapy protocol, doxorubicin is administered:

a. concurrently with MTX
b. once a month
c. for two days in a row
d. every third week
e. up to a toal dose of 550 mg/m$^2$

320. Which is the least important parameter to monitor during high-dose MTX?

a. creatinine
b. AST
c. urine pH
d. urine output
e. plasma MTX concentration

321. The total body clearance of MTX is:

a. independent of urine flow
b. independent of urine pH
c. similar to that of 7-OH-MTX
d. faster than that of 7-OH-MTX
e. slower than that of 7-OH-MTX

322. Which statement is false?

a. leucovorin is administered for 72 h after high-dose MTX
b. leucovorin is a competitive inhibitor of dihydrofolate reductase
c. leucovorin is not necessary after low-dose MTX therapy
d. leucovorin is necessary for high-dose MTX therapy
e. leucovorin is a reduced folate derivative

323. Which is least likely to occur after high-dose MTX therapy?

a. vomiting, nausea
b. alopecia, skin rashes
c. nephrotoxicity
d. renal toxicty
e. cardiotoxicity

## Chapters 51 and 52

324. The principal hormone that controls re-absorption of sodium in the distal tubule of the kidney is:

a. cortisol
b. aldosterone
c. ACTH
d. α-methylnorepinephrine

325. The diuretic that competes with the mineralocorticoid binding site in the distal tubule is:

a. hydrochlorothiazide
b. triamterene
c. chlorthalidone
d. spironolactone

326. The baroreceptor mechanism consists of a group of cells that control the release of:

a. renin
b. cortisol
c. hydrochlorothiazide
d. norepinephrine

327. The important factor in thiazide therapy to ensure that natriuresis occurs is:

a. blood concentration
b. duration of drug in blood
c. low bioavailability
d. blood pH

328. α-Methyldopa is not active until it is metabolized to:

a. norepinephrine
b. homovanillic acid
c. serotonin
d. α-methyldopamine

329. The active metabolite of hydralazine is

a. hydralazine-O-glucuronide
b. 1-phthalazinone
c. triazolo phthalazine
d. N-acetyl hydralazine

330. The best method of monitoring therapy of hypertension with thiazide diuretics combines measurement of plasma potassium concentration with:

a. use of a sphygmomanometer
b. plasma sodium concentration
c. plasma renin concentration
d. plasma aldosterone concentration

331. Monitoring hydrochlorothiazide concentrations in serum or plasma allows the clinician to:

a. correlate clinical response with serum concentration
b. determine patient compliance
c. assess whether the drug regimen should be altered
d. all of the above
e. none of the above

332. Patients receiving thiazide diuretics should be carefully monitored for:

a. hyperkalemia, hypernatremia, hyperglycemia, and hyperuricemia
b. hypokalemia, hyponatremia, hypoglycemia, and hypouricemia
c. hypokalemia, hyperuricemia, and hyperglycemia
d. all of the above
e. none of the above

333. In the case history in Chapter 52, failure to achieve adequate blood pressure control initially was due to:

a. use of an inappropriate drug
b. patient noncompliance
c. inadequate drug dosage
d. failure to use multiple drug regimens
e. none of the above

334. Hydrochlorothiazide has the following properties:

a. it is strongly protein bound
b. it is eliminated renally, predominantly as the unchanged drug
c. it has a half-life of 5-15 h
d. peak plasma concentrations are achieved 2-4 h after the dose
e. all of the above

## Chapters 53 and 54

335. The primary use of nitroprusside is:

a. treatment of toxemia of pregnancy
b. immediate treatment of hypertensive crisis

c. treatment of pheochromocytoma
d. treatment of acute myocardial infarction
e. none of the above

336. The half-life of nitroprusside is about:

a. 5 min
b. 1 h
c. 6 h
d. 48 h
e. 72 h

337. A guide to nitroprusside toxicity is monitored by measuring blood concentrations of:

a. cyanide
b. nitroprusside
c. thiocyanate
d. nitrite
e. sulfur

338. Therapeutic concentrations of thiocyanate are approximately:

a. 5-10 mg/L
b. 50-100 mg/L
c. 0.5-2 mg/mL
d. 10-20 mg/L
e. 100-200 mg/L

339. The dose range for nitroprusside infusion ($\mu$g/kg of body weight per minute) is approximately:

a. 0.2-0.5
b. 50-60
c. 1.5-3
d. 0.5-1.5
e. 100-200

340. Nipride® (nitroprusside) is a coordination complex of cyanide with which transition metal?

a. copper
b. cobalt
c. iron
d. manganese
e. nickel

341. The mechanism of action of nitroprusside is similar to that of:

a. propranolol
b. hydralazine
c. ether
d. phenobarbital
e. lidocaine

342. Cyanide is released from nitroprusside during the oxidation/reduction reaction with:

a. cytochrome $P_{450}$
b. monoamine oxidase
c. hemoglobin
d. $Na^+K^+$-ATPase

343. The normal concentration of thiocyanate (mg/L) in patients treated with nitroprusside is:

a. 2-5
b. 5-20
c. 30-50
d. 60-100
e. 100-500

344. Amygdalin is converted to cyanide by enzymes commonly found in the following:

a. normal intestinal flora
b. bitter almonds
c. apricot pits
d. all of the above

345. The concentration (mg/L) of whole-blood cyanide commonly associated with severe intoxication by cyanide is usually:

a. much greater than 60
b. less than 0.5
c. greater than 5
d. always greater than 30

## Chapters 55-57

346. Heparin is a mucopolysaccharide that has an anticoagulant effect by virtue of:

a. blocking the synthesis of vitamin K
b. inhibiting the conversion of prothrombin to thrombin
c. binding calcium ion, necessary cofactors in clotting
d. inhibiting the activity of thrombin in formation of fibrin
e. lysing the polymerized fibrin of the clot

347. Administration of heparin is most often by:

a. the oral route
b. intramuscular injection
c. subcutaneous injection
d. intermittent intravenous injection
d. constant intravenous infusion

348. Laboratory monitoring of anticoagulant therapy is most reliably done by:

a. Lee-White clotting time
b. whole-blood activated partial thromboplastin time (WBAPTT)
c. activated partial thromboplastin time (APTT)
d. partial thromboplastin time (PTT)
e. prothrombin time (PT)

349. In changing from heparin to dicumarol therapy it is necessary to:

a. delay dicumarol administration until heparin concentrations are insignificant
b. measure the APTT (in the period when both are being administered) immediately after an intravenous injection of heparin
c. start dicumarol administration 3 to 5 days before discontinuing heparin
d. measure the prothrombin time before beginning the dicumarol
e. administer heparin only before surgery and dicumarol only after surgery

350. The metabolism of heparin produces a half-life of:

a. 30 min
b. 1.5 h for normal doses, but increasing with larger doses
c. 4.5 h or longer with patients with pulmonary embolism
d. less than normal half-life in patients with impaired renal function
e. 1.5 h for normal subcutaneous administration

351. APTT measurements:

a. are reliable up to 12 h after collection
b. are expected to be about 1.5 times that for the controls for patients in the therapeutic range for anticoagulant therapy
c. should be less than 50 s for post-operative patients on anticoagulant therapy
d. are invalid for patients also receiving aspirin
e. should be compared with PT measurements

352. For patients on heparin therapy who suffer hemorrhagic complications:

a. there is no remedy except to surgically repair the anatomical or functional defect
b. the best procedure is to give transfusions
c. in case of severe bleeding, discontinuation of heparin will usually clear the problem in a few hours
d. the APTT time can be returned to normal by administration of protamine sulfate
e. secure alteration of platelet function by aspirin dose

353.   Heparin is ineffective if given:

a. orally
b. subcutaneously
c. intramuscularly
d. intravenously
e. rectally

354.   The biological half-life of heparin in the circulation after intravenous administration is:

a. 30-60 min
b. 60-90 min
c. 90-120 min
d. 120-180 min
e. dependent on the dose administered

355. The half-life of heparin is affected by:

a. thrombocytopenia
b. hepatic failure
c. pulmonary insufficiency
d. pulmonary embolism
e. renal failure

356.   Heparin interacts with all but one of the following:

a. antithrombin III
b. thrombin
c. dicumarol
d. platelet factor 4
e. protamine

357.   Monitoring of heparin therapy is done with:

a. the Lee-White test
b. the APTT test
c. the ACT test
d. the chromogenic assay for heparin
e. all of the above

358.   Heparin is stable in blood for:

a. 30 min at 4 °C
b. 2 h at room temperature
c. 24 h at 4 °C
d. 48 h at room temperature
e. 72 h at room temperature

359.   Patients taking warfarin are usually monitored by which of the following tests?

a. bleeding time
b. serum warfarin concentration
c. partial thromboplastin time
d. prothrombin time
e. fibrinogen concentration

360.   Vitamin K is involved in the synthesis of the clotting factors II, VII, IX, and X. By which of the following mechanisms does it act?

a. by introducing $\gamma$-carboxyglutamic acid residues into the zymogen form of the clotting factors
b. by preventing the binding of calcium
c. by inhibiting the enzyme phospholipase
d. by inhibiting the enzyme vitamin KO epoxide reductase
e. by increasing the urinary excretion of $\gamma$-carboxyglutamic acid

361.   Warfarin takes three days to exert its maximum effect because:

a. all the clotting factors have the same half-life
b. the normal degradation rates of the clotting factors are unaffected by warfarin
c. only a small dose of the drug is used in the first 24 h
d. warfarin is poorly absorbed orally
e. warfarin has a short half-life, 35 min

362.   In the body, warfarin:

a. is 99% bound to fibrinogen
b. is metabolized in the liver to a glucuronide and excreted in urine and feces
c. reaches a peak plasma concentration in 24 h
d. does not interact with drugs such as barbiturates or glutethimide
e. is safe to use in pregnancy because it does not cross the placenta

363.   The most important toxic effect of warfarin is:

a. thrombocytopenia
b. jaundice
c. thrombophlebitis
d. pulmonary embolism
e. hemorrhage such as epistaxis, hematuria, or gastrointestinal bleeding

364.   In a warfarin-treated patient with a life-threatening hemorrhage, which is the most appropriate treatment?

a. warfarin therapy should be continued at a reduced dosage and 20 mg of vitamin $K_1$ given orally
b. warfarin therapy should be continued at a reduced dosage and 50 mg of vitamin $K_1$ given intravenously
c. warfarin therapy should be discontinued and 50 mg of vitamin $K_1$ given intravenously
d. warfarin therapy should be discontinued and 50 mg of vitamin $K_1$ given orally
e. warfarin therapy should be discontinued and no vitamin $K_1$ given

## Chapter 58

365.   Morphine can be metabolized in the:

a. brain
b. gut
c. kidney
d. liver
e. all of the above

366.   The low bioavailability of orally administered morphine is the result of the following factors:

a. sequestration in the gut mucosa
b. metabolism in the liver
c. acidity of the stomach, preventing absorption of ionized morphine
d. metabolism in the intestinal mucosa
e. all of the above

367.   The oral/intravenous dose ratio for effective treatment when morphine is given orally is:

a. 4 to 1
b. 2 to 1
c. 6 to 1
d. 10 to 1
e. 7 to 1

368.   The reported oral bioavailability of morphine in humans is:

a. 5-10%
b. 10-20%
c. 15-60%
d. 30-75%
e. 100%

369.   The percentage of morphine bound to albumin is:

a. 90%
b. 35%
c. 41%
d. 6%
e. 15%

370.   The major metabolite of morphine is:

a. morphine-3-ethereal sulfate
b. morphine-6-glucuronide
c. normorphine
d. morphine-3-glucuronide
e. codeine

371.   Morphine is excreted in the urine mainly:

a. unchanged

b. as morphine-3-glucuronide
c. as normorphine
d. as morphine-3-ethereal sulfate
e. as codeine

372.   Morphine is detectable in which of the following during treatment?

a. urine
b. saliva
c. bile
d. breast milk
e. all of the above

## Chapter 59

373.   Acetaminophen is primarily a problem when it is taken

a. in 8 - 10 mg/kg doses by children
b. in 10 - 20 mg/kg doses by adults
c. in doses of 2 g per day or less
d. in doses of 2 g at a time
e. in doses of 10 g at a time

374.   Some degree of acetaminophen toxicity is inevitable when doses exceed the maximum therapeutic dose because:

a. bleeding from the gastrointestinal tract occurs
b. depression of prothrombin time leads to purpura
c. there is a decrease in the percentage of unmetabolized acetaminophen excreted
d. acetaminophen cysteinate excretion increases
e. the body has a limited capacity to form the nontoxic sulfate metabolite of acetaminophen

375.   When a patient is admitted with an acute overdosage of acetaminophen, acetaminophen should be measured:

a. 4 h after admission
b. 8 h after admission
c. every 12 h until it is $< 50 \ \mu g/L$
d. all of the above
e. none of the above

376.   Measurement of acetaminophen concentrations should be accompanied by emergency determination of:

a. AST
b. ALT
c. prothrombin time
d. all of the above
e. none of the above

377.   Acetaminophen may be measured successfully by:

a. HPLC
b. GLC
c. spectrophotometry
d. all of the above
e. none of the above

378.   The antidepressant response rate to imipramine therapy is low when plasma concentrations (ng/mL) are:

a. up to 250
b. greater than 250
c. below 150
d. below 100
e. none of the above

# Appendix II.

# Answers to Self-Assessment Questions

**Chapter 1**

1-b, 2-b, 3-c, 4-a, 5-a, 6-a, 7-b, 8-a.

**Chapters 2-5**

9-a, 10-b, 11-b, 12-d, 13-c, 14-d, 15-b, 16-a, 17-a, 18-d, 19-d, 20-e, 21-d, 22-c, 23-c, 24-d, 25-b, 26-b, 27-c, 28-b, 29-c, 30-b, 31-d, 32-b and d, 33-d, 34-e, 35-c, d, and e, 36-e, 37-a, 38-a, 39-e, 40-d.

**Chapters 6-10**

41-c, 42-b, 43-d, 44-b, 45-c, 46-c, 47-b, 48-c, 49-b, 50-c, 51-c, 52-b, 53-a, 54-c, 55-c, 56-c, 57-a, 58-c, 59-a, 60-e, 61-b, 62-d, 63-a, 64-c, 65-d, 66-e, 67-c, 68-d, 69-c, 70-a, 71-c, 72-b, 73-a, 74-b and c.

**Chapters 11 and 12**

75-d, 76-b, 77-c, 78-c, 79-d, 80-a, 81-c, 82-e, 83-b, 84-a, 85-b, 86-a, 87-b, 88-b.

**Chapters 13-15**

89-b, 90-d, 91-c, 92-a, 93-a, 94-d, 95-b, 96-a, 97-e, 98-c, 99-b, 100-c, 101-e, 102-e, 103-a, 104-d, 105-b, 106-c, 107-c, 108-c, 109-d, 110-c, 111-b, 112-c.

**Chapter 16**

113-c, 114-a, 115-c, 116-c, 117-c, 118-d, 119-e, 120-d, 121-e, 122-e, 123-e, 124-c, 125-d, 126-a, 127-c.

**Chapters 17-19**

128-b, 129-e, 130-c, 131-c, 132-e, 133-b, 134-a, 135-d, 136-e, 137-c, 138-d, 139-c, 140-d, 141-a, 142-b, 143-b, 144-b, 145-c, 146-b, 147-c, 148-b.

**Chapters 20-28**

149-d, 150-e, 151-c, 152-c, 153-b, 154-b, 155-c, 156-e, 157-e, 158-e, 159-c, 160-b, 161-b, 162-c, 163-a, 164-e, 165-b, 166-e, 167-a, 168-b, 169-a, 170-c, 171-b, 172-a, 173-c, 174-a, 175-a, 176-b, 177-c, 178-b, 179-c, 180-e, 181-b, 182-c, 183-d, 184-e, 185-e, 186-e, 187-d, 188-a, 189-c.

**Chapters 29-32**

190-e, 191-c, 192-b, 193-e, 194-e, 195-b, 196-c, 197-a, 198-c, 199-c, 200-d, 201-a, 202-b, 203-e, 204-d, 205-b, 206-d, 207-e, 208-e, 209-a, 210-a, 211-b, 212-e, 213-e, 214-d, 215-a, 216-e.

**Chapters 33 and 34**

217-c, 218-a, d, and e, 219-b, 220-e, 221-a, 222-c, 223-d, 224-c, 225-d, 226-e, 227-c.

**Chapter 35**

228-b, 229-d, 230-a, 231-c, 232-d, 233-d, 234-d, 235-d.

**Chapters 36-38**

236-a, b, d, and e, 237-a, d, and e, 238-a and c, 239-a, b, c, and d, 240-a, b, c, and d, 241-b, c, and e, 242-a, b, and c, 243-d, 244-c, 245-b, 246-b, 247-d.

**Chapters 39-42**

248-e, 249-a, 250-a, 251-a, 252-d, 253-b, 254-e, 255-c, 256-b, 257-b, 258-d, 259-a, 260-d, 261-b, 262-e, 263-b, 264-e, 265-e, 266-a, 267-e, 268-a, 269-d, 270-b, 271-b.

**Chapters 43-45**

272-a, 273-c, 274-a, 275-b, 276-d, 277-b, 278-e, 279-d, 280-d, 281-c, 282-c, 283-b, 284-c, 285-d, 286-e, 287-c, 288-d, 289-a, 290-d.

**Chapter 46**

291-d, 292-a, 293-b, 294-b, 295-e, 296-c.

**Chapters 47-50**

297-c, 298-d, 299-b, 300-d, 301-c, 302-a, 303-e, 304-a, 305-b, 306-c, 307-b, 308-b, 309-a, 310-e, 311-b, 312-d, 313-d, 314-b, 315-b, 316-c, 317-e, 318-d, 319-e, 320-b, 321-d, 322-b, 323-e.

**Chapters 51 and 52**

324-b, 325-d, 326-a, 327-b, 328-d, 329-d, 330-a, 331-d, 332-e, 333-b, 334-e.

**Chapters 53 and 54**

335-b, 336-a, 337-c, 338-b, 339-d, 340-c, 341-c, 342-c, 343-b, 344-d, 345-c.

**Chapters 55-57**

346-b, 347-d, 348-c, 349-c, 350-b, 351-b, 352-d, 353-a, and e, 354-e, 355-b, d, and e, 356-a, b, d, and e, 357-e, 358-b, and c, 359-d, 360-a, 361-b, 362-b, 363-e, 364-c.

**Chapter 58**

365-e, 366-e, 367-c, 368-c, 369-b, 370-d, 371-b, 372-e.

**Chapter 59**

373-e, 374-e, 375-d, 376-e, 377-d, 378-d.

# Index to Volumes I and II